IMMUNOLOGY

A slide atlas of Immunology, based on the contents of this book, is available. In the slide atlas format, the material is split into volumes, each of which is presented in a binder together with numbered 35mm slides of each illustration. Each slide atlas volume also contains a list of abbreviated slide captions for easy reference when using the slides. Further information can be obtained from:

Gower Medical Publishing, Middlesex House
34–42 Cleveland Street, London W1P 5FB

Gower Medical Publishing
101 5th Avenue, New York, NY 10003, USA

Cover picture shows a diagrammatic representation of the pentameric polypeptide structure of human IgM (see page 5.5).

IMMUNOLOGY

IVAN M. ROITT
MA DSc(Oxon) Hon MRCP (Lond)
FRCPath FRS
Professor and Head of Department of Immunology
University College and Middlesex School of Medicine
London, UK

JONATHAN BROSTOFF
MA DM(Oxon) DSc
FRCP FRCPath
Reader in Clinical Immunology
Department of Immunology
University College and Middlesex School of Medicine
London, UK

DAVID K. MALE
MA PhD
Lecturer in Neuroimmunology
Department of Neuropathology
Institute of Psychiatry
London, UK

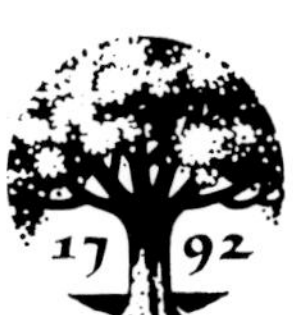

J.B. Lippincott Company PHILADELPHIA

Gower Medical Publishing · London · New York

PROJECT TEAM

Publisher	Fiona Foley
Project Editor	Lindy van den Berghe
Design & Illustration	Celia Welcomme
Linework	Karen Cochrane Marion Tasker
Paste-up	Pete Wilder
Index	Anita Reid
Production	Seamus Murphy

Gower Medical Publishing

DISTRIBUTORS

USA and Canada
J.B. Lippincott Company
East Washington Square
Philadelphia, PA 19105, USA

Japan
Igaku Shoin Ltd
Tokyo International
P.O. Box 5063
Tokyo, Japan

UK and rest of world
Churchill Livingstone
Medical Division of Longman Group UK Limited
Robert Stevenson House
1/3 Baxter's Place
Leith Walk, Edinburgh EH1 3AF, UK

British Library Cataloguing in Publication Data
Roitt, Ivan M. (Ivan Maurice) *1927–*
Immunology – 2nd ed.
I. Immunology
I. Title II. Brostoff, Jonathan
III. Male, David K.
574.2'9 QR181

ISBN 0-443-04204-7 (Churchill Livingstone)
0-397-44696-9 (J.B. Lippincott) (cased)
0-397-44573-3 (Gower/Lippincott) (limp)

Typeset by Dawkins Typesetting Limited
Typeset in Antikva Margaret Light and Univers
Originated in Hong Kong by Mandarin Offset
Printed in Hong Kong by Mandarin Offset
Reprinted in Hong Kong in 1990 by Mandarin Offset

Preface to 1st edition

We believe this to be a remarkably unusual book. We have attempted to present the subject primarily with appealing visual images, many of which are the distillation of much complicated scientific research. These illustrations are complemented specifically by individual captions, and more generally by a concise narrative text which links these images into an evolving conceptual thread. The book covers basic immunology and the fundamental principles relating to clinical immunology. The subject is covered in some depth and much attention is given to the underlying experimental studies. We hope that anyone interested in immunology, be they undergraduate, postgraduate or clinician, will find this an attractive but nonetheless thorough account, which they will find difficult to put down once they have opened it.

We would like to acknowledge the many immunologists and molecular biologists whose research findings have been included to explain particular immunological reactions, and to develop ideas on the function of the immune system. We greatly admire their work, and hope we will be forgiven for not mentioning all these scientists individually. In some cases, we have selected particular items, or simplified experiments to make points more readily understood. Readers who wish to grapple with the fine details of the experiments and hypotheses may locate the original papers by reference to review articles included as further reading at the end of each chapter.

IMR
JB
DKM

Preface to 2nd edition

With the rapid advances in immunology and the increase in our understanding of basic processes, substantial revisions have been made to both the text and diagrams in this edition and new sections have been added to many chapters to bring the book completely up to date. The revisions are too numerous to detail but include new data on the T cell antigen receptor, the genes and proteins of the major histocompatibility complex, and the ways in which T cells recognize antigen. The elucidation of many leucocyte surface molecules and the use of the CD nomenclature throughout serves to clarify cell functions, their differentiation pathways and activation steps. The explosion of detailed information on cytokines has necessitated a complete rewriting of the central chapters on the development of the immune response. Finally, in order to improve the conceptual flow of the book the order of the chapters has been changed and some have been retitled to encompass the new data and understanding of the subject.

IMR
JB
DKM

Acknowledgements

P. M. Lydyard and C. E. Grossi would like to thank Prof. M. W. Fanger, Dr D. Katz, Dr P. Crocker and Dr N. Hogg for helpful discussions (Chapter 2) and Dr K. McLennan for providing photographs for Chapter 3.

The editors would like to thank Lindy van den Berghe and Celia Welcomme for their sterling work in bringing this edition to fruition. They would also like to thank Pete Wilder, Marian Tasker, Mark Willey, Sue Tyler, Linda Payne, Michael Rabess and Nicola Bowen for their contributions. The slide atlas would not have appeared without the help of Lazlo Purdy and Shahla Nouri. Michele Campbell stepped into the breach on many occasions. Ensuring that the production went smoothly and to time we thank Seamus Murphy. Lastly we thank Fiona Foley who gave us unfailing help and advice.

Contents

6 THE GENERATION OF DIVERSITY

Dr Frank Hay

7 ANTIGEN RECOGNITION

Professor Michael Steward

8 CELL COOPERATION IN THE IMMUNE RESPONSE

Professor Marc Feldmann and Dr David Male

9 CELL-MEDIATED IMMUNE RESPONSES

Dr Graham Rook

Contents

14 DEVELOPMENT OF THE IMMUNE SYSTEM

Dr Peter Lydyard and Professor Carlo Grossi

15 EVOLUTION OF IMMUNITY

Dr John Horton and Dr Ann Lackie

16 IMMUNITY TO VIRUSES, BACTERIA AND FUNGI

Dr Graham Rook

17 IMMUNITY TO PROTOZOA AND WORMS

Dr Janice Taverne

Contents

22 HYPERSENSITIVITY – TYPE IV

Professor Ross St.C. Barnetson and Dr David Gawkrodger

23 AUTOIMMUNITY AND AUTOIMMUNE DISEASE

Professor Ivan Roitt

24 TRANSPLANTATION AND REJECTION

Dr Ken Welsh and Dr David Male

25 IMMUNOLOGICAL TECHNIQUES

Professor Michael Steward and Dr David Male

Contributors

Professor Ross St. C. Barnetson
Department of Dermatology
University of Sydney, NSW 2006, Australia

Dr Anne Cooke
Wellcome Trust Senior Lecturer, Department of Immunology
University College and Middlesex School of Medicine
40–50 Tottenham Street, London W1N 8AA, UK

Dr Jonathan Brostoff
Reader in Clinical Immunology, Department of Immunology
University College and Middlesex School of Medicine
40–50 Tottenham Street, London W1N 8AA, UK

Dr Maureen Dawson
Research Fellow, Paterson Institute for Cancer Research
Christie Hospital & Holt Radium Institute
Wilmslow Road, Manchester M20 9BX, UK

Professor Marc Feldmann
Charing Cross Sunley Research Centre
Lurgan Avenue, Hammersmith, London W6 8LW, UK

Dr David J. Gawkrodger
Consultant Dermatologist
University Department of Dermatology
Royal Hallamshire Hospital, Sheffield S10 2JF

Professor Carlo E. Grossi
Professor of Anatomy and Director of Division of Clinical Pathology
National Cancer Institute, Genova, Italy

Dr Tony J. Hall
Merrell Dow Research Institute
67084 Strasbourg, France

Dr Frank C. Hay
Reader in Immunology
Departments of Immunology and Rheumatology Research
University College and Middlesex School of Medicine
40–50 Tottenham Street, London W1N 8AA, UK

Dr John Horton
Reader in Immunology, Department of Biological Sciences
University of Durham, Durham DH1 3LE, UK

Dr James G. Howard
Assistant Director, The Wellcome Trust
1 Park Square West, London NW1 4LJ, UK

Dr Ann M. Lackie
Lecturer in Zoology, Department of Zoology
The University, Glasgow G12 8QQ, UK

Dr Peter M. Lydyard
Senior Lecturer
Departments of Immunology and Rheumatology Research
University College and Middlesex School of Medicine
40–50 Tottenham Street, London W1N 8AA, UK

Dr Michael Moore
Head, Department of Immunology
Paterson Institute for Cancer Research
Christie Hospital & Holt Radium Institute
Wilmslow Road, Manchester M20 9BX, UK

Dr David K. Male
Lecturer in Neuroimmunology, Institute of Psychiatry
Department of Neuroimmunology
Denmark Hill, London SE5 8AF, UK

Dr Michael J. Owen
Senior Research Scientist
Imperial Cancer Research Fund Laboratories
St Bartholomew's Hospital
Dominion House, London EC1A 7BE, UK

Professor Ivan M. Roitt
Professor and Head of Department of Immunology
University College and Middlesex School of Medicine
40–50 Tottenham Street, London W1N 8AA, UK

Dr Graham Rook
School of Pathology
University College and Middlesex School of Medicine
Ridinghouse Street, London W1P 7PN, UK

Professor Michael Steward
Professor of Immunology
London School of Hygiene and Tropical Medicine
Keppel Street, London WC1E 7HT, UK

Dr Janice Taverne
Research Associate, Department of Immunology
University College and Middlesex School of Medicine
40–50 Tottenham Street, London W1N 8AA, UK

Dr Roger Taylor
Reader in Immunology, Department of Pathology
University of Bristol, Bristol BS8 1TH, UK

Dr Malcolm W. Turner
Reader in Immunochemistry, University of London
30 Guildford Street, London WC1N 1EH, UK

Dr Mark Walport
Senior Lecturer in Medicine
Royal Postgraduate Medical School
Hammersmith Hospital
DuCane Road, London W12 0HS, UK

Dr Ken Welsh
Head, SE Thames Regional Tissue Typing Laboratory
Guy's Hospital, St Thomas Street, London SE1 9RT, UK

1 Adaptive and Innate Immunity

Our environment contains a large variety of infectious microbial agents – viruses, bacteria, fungi and parasites. These can cause pathological damage and if they multiply unchecked will eventually kill their host. Most infections in normal individuals are of limited duration and leave little permanent damage due to the individual's immune system, which combats infectious agents.

The immune system has two functional divisions: the innate immune system and the adaptive immune system. Innate immunity acts as a first line of defence against infectious agents and most potential pathogens are checked before they establish an overt infection. If these first defences are breached, the adaptive immune system is activated and produces a specific reaction to each infectious agent which normally eradicates that agent. The adaptive immune system also remembers the infectious agent and can prevent it causing disease later (Fig. 1.1). For example, diseases such as measles and diphtheria produce lifelong immunity following an infection. The two key features of the adaptive immune system are thus specificity and memory.

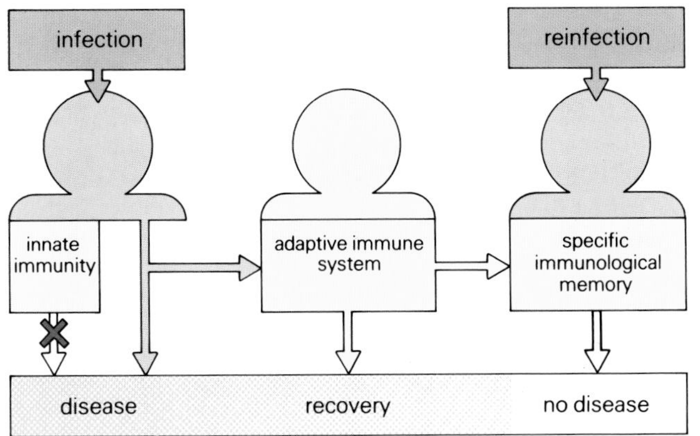

Fig. 1.1 Adaptive and innate immunity. When an infectious agent enters the body it first encounters elements of the innate immune system. These may be sufficient to prevent disease but if not, a disease will result and the adaptive immune system is activated. The adaptive immune system produces recovery from the disease and a specific immunological memory is established so that following reinfection with the same agent no disease results; the individual has acquired immunity to the infectious agent.

The innate and adaptive immune systems consist of a variety of molecules and cells, distributed throughout the body, whose functions are described in Fig. 1.2. The most important cells are the leucocytes or white blood cells which are described fully in Chapter 2. The leucocytes fall into two broad categories: phagocytes, including neutrophil polymorphs, monocytes and macrophages, which form part of the innate immune system, and lymphocytes, which mediate adaptive immunity. Cells of the immune system (lymphoid cells) are organized into lymphoid organs (see Chapter 3).

	innate immune system	adaptive immune system
	resistance not improved by repeated infection	resistance improved by repeated infection
soluble factors	lysozyme, complement, acute phase proteins e.g. CRP, interferon	antibody
cells	phagocytes natural killer (NK) cells	T lymphocytes

Fig. 1.2 The major elements of the innate and adaptive immune systems. There is considerable interaction between the two systems. Immunity due to soluble factors is sometimes referred to as humoral immunity.

THE INNATE IMMUNE SYSTEM

The exterior of the body presents an effective barrier to most organisms; in particular, most infectious agents cannot penetrate intact skin (Fig. 1.3).

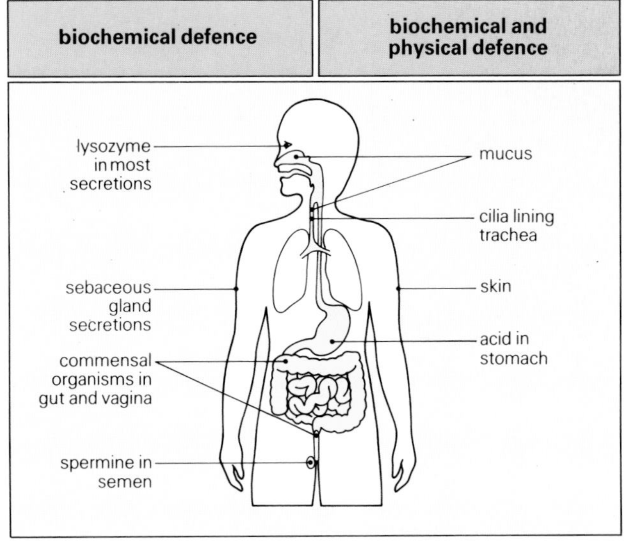

Fig. 1.3 Exterior defences. Most of the infectious agents which an individual encounters do not penetrate the body surface, but are prevented from entering by a variety of biochemical and physical barriers. The body tolerates a number of commensal organisms which compete effectively with many potential pathogens.

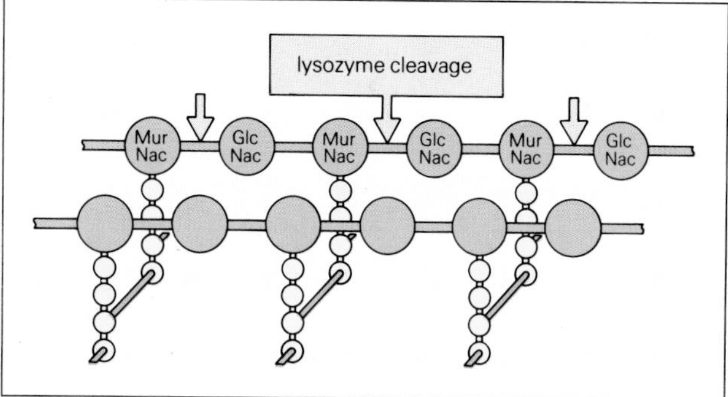

Fig. 1.4 Action of lysozyme on the cell wall of *Staphylococcus aureus*. In the structure of *S. aureus* cell wall proteoglycan, the backbone of *N*-acetylglucosamine (GlcNac) alternates with *N*-acetylmuramic acid (MurNac), cross-linked by amino acid side chains (yellow) and bridges of 5-glycine residues (orange). Lysozyme splits the molecule at the places indicated.

The importance of this barrier is made abundantly clear when an individual suffers serious burns. In this case prevention of infection via the damaged skin is a major concern. Most infections enter the body via the epithelial surface of the nasopharynx, gut, lungs and genitourinary tract. A variety of physical and biochemical defences protects these areas from most infections. For example, lysozyme is an enzyme distributed widely in different secretions and is capable of splitting a bond found in the cell walls of many bacteria (Fig. 1.4).

PHAGOCYTES AND NK CELLS

If an organism penetrates an epithelial surface it encounters phagocytic cells of the monocyte/macrophage lineage. These cells are of several different types but are all derived from bone marrow stem cells and their function is to engulf particles, including infectious agents, internalize them and destroy them. For this purpose they are strategically placed where they will encounter such particles; for example, the Kupffer cells of the liver line the sinusoids along which blood flows, while the synovial A cells line the synovial cavity (Fig. 1.5). The blood phagocytes include the neutrophil polymorph and the blood monocyte (Fig. 1.6). Both these cells can migrate out of the blood vessels into the tissues in response to a suitable stimulus but they differ in that the polymorph is a short-lived cell while the monocyte develops into a tissue macrophage.

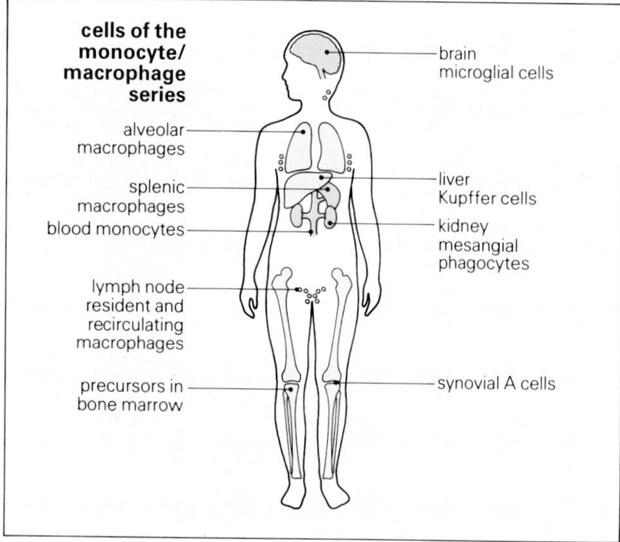

Fig. 1.5 Phagocytes of the monocyte/macrophage series. Many organs contain phagocytic cells derived from blood monocytes which are manufactured in the bone marrow. Monocytes pass out of the blood vessel and become macrophages in the tissues. Resident phagocytic cells of different tissues (listed right) were previously referred to as the reticuloendothelial system, but they too appear to belong to the monocyte lineage.

Natural killer (NK) cells are leucocytes which can recognize cell surface changes that occur on some virally infected cells and some tumour cells. They bind to these target cells and kill them. This kind of reaction, in which a lymphocyte kills a target cell, is called cytotoxicity. The cells responsible for natural killer activity are primarily large granular lymphocytes, and the target cells may be rendered more susceptible by soluble factors such as interferons.

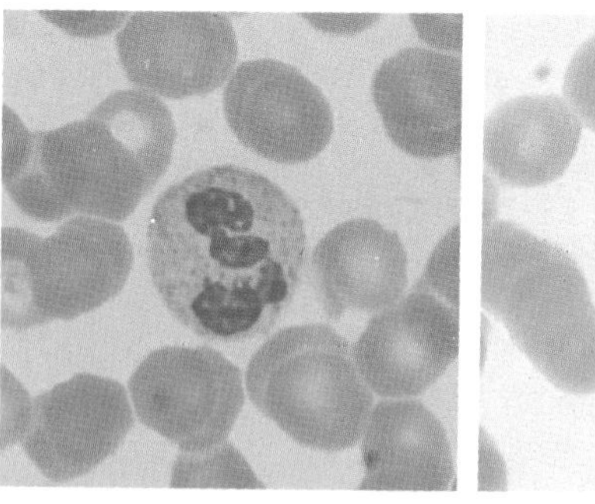
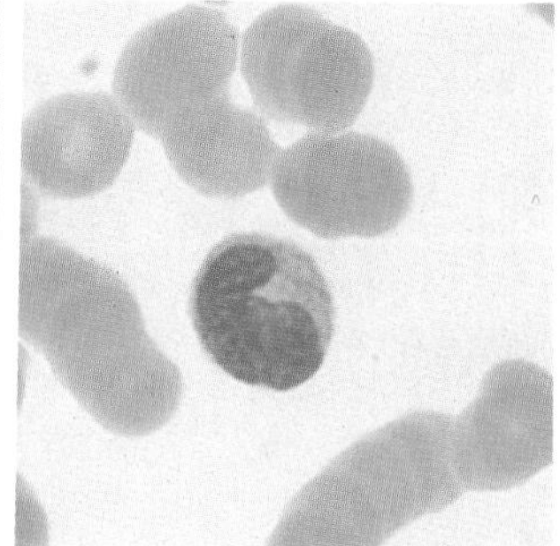

Fig. 1.6 Phagocytes. Apart from the fixed cells, there are polymorphonuclear neutrophils (left) and blood monocytes (right), both derived from bone marrow stem cells. (Courtesy of Dr P. M. Lydyard.)

ACUTE PHASE PROTEINS: COMPLEMENT; INTERFERONS

The serum concentration of a number of proteins, referred to as acute phase proteins, increases rapidly during infection. Concentrations can increase 2- to 100-fold and remain elevated throughout infection. One example is C-reactive protein, so-called because of its ability to bind the C protein of pneumococci. C-reactive protein bound to bacteria promotes the binding of complement, which facilitates their uptake by phagocytes; this process of protein coating to enhance phagocytosis is known as opsonization (Fig. 1.7).

The complement system is a group of about twenty serum proteins whose overall function is the control of inflammation. Several of the components are acute phase proteins, as they increase during infection. The components interact with each other and with other elements of the innate and adaptive immune systems. For example, a number of microorganisms spontaneously activate the complement system via the so-called 'alternative pathway'; the system can also interact with antibodies of the adaptive immune system by activation of the 'classical pathway'.

Complement activation occurs with each component sequentially acting on others in a similar way to the operation of the blood clotting system. Activation by either the classical or alternative pathway generates various peptides which have the following effects.

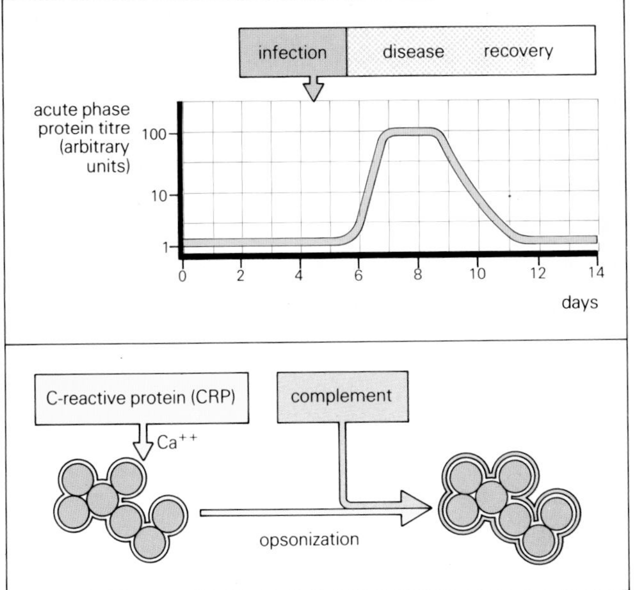

Fig. 1.7 Acute phase proteins. Acute phase proteins (here exemplified by C-reactive protein) are serum proteins which increase rapidly in concentration (up to 100-fold) following infection (graph). They are important in the innate immunity to infection. C-reactive protein (CRP) recognizes and binds, in a Ca^{2+}-dependent fashion, to molecular groups found on a wide variety of bacteria and fungi. In particular it binds the phosphorylcholine moiety of pneumococci. CRP acts as an opsonin and also activates complement with all the associated sequelae.

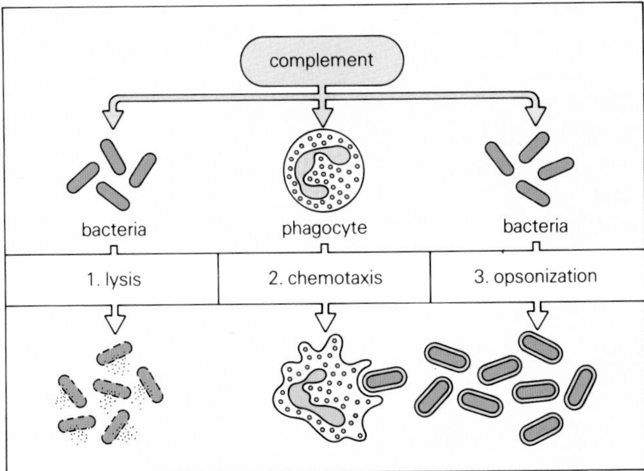

Fig. 1.8 Complement functions. The complement system has an intrinsic ability to lyse the cell membranes of many bacterial species (1). Complement products released in this reaction attract phagocytes to the site of the reaction – chemotaxis (2). Once they arrive at the site of reaction other complement components coating the bacterial surface allow the phagocyte to recognize the bacteria and facilitate bacterial phagocytosis – opsonization (3). These are all functions of the innate immune system, although the reactions can also be triggered by the adaptive immune system.

1. Opsonization of microorganisms for uptake by phagocytes.
2. Attraction of phagocytes to sites of infection (chemotaxis).
3. Increased blood flow to the site of activation and increased permeability of capillaries to plasma molecules.
4. Damage to plasma membranes of cells, viruses or organisms which have induced the activation. This in turn can produce lysis of the cell (Fig. 1.8).

The complement system acts in concert with other components of the innate and adaptive immune systems. For example, the destruction of bacterial cell walls by lysozyme facilitates an attack on the cell membrane by the complement system. The functions of the complement system are discussed in full in Chapter 13.

Interferons (IFNs) comprise a group of proteins that are important in viral infections. One group of interferons is produced by cells which have become virally infected; another type is released by certain activated T lymphocytes. Interferons induce a state of antiviral resistance in uninfected tissue cells. They also have several other effects on protein metabolism in these cells and affect how they respond to lymphocytes and NK cells (Fig. 1.9). IFNs are produced very early in infection and are the first line of resistance against many viruses.

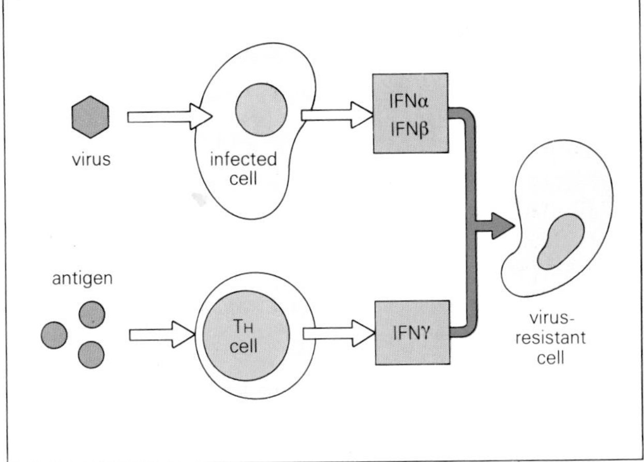

Fig. 1.9 Interferons. When cells become infected by virus, they may produce interferon. Different cell types produce interferon α (IFNα) or interferon β (IFNβ); interferon γ (IFNγ) is also produced by some types of lymphocyte (TH) after activation by antigen. Interferons act on other cells to induce a state of resistance to viral infection. IFNγ has many other effects as well.

INFLAMMATION

Inflammation is the body's reaction to an injury such as an invasion by an infectious agent. In just the same way as it is necessary to increase the blood supply to active muscles during exercise to provide glucose and oxygen so it is also necessary to direct elements of the immune system into sites of infection. Three major events occur during this response.

1. An increased blood supply to the infected area.
2. Increased capillary permeability caused by retraction of the endothelial cells. This permits larger molecules to traverse the endothelium than would ordinarily be

capable of doing so and thus allows the soluble mediators of immunity to reach the site of infection.
3. Leucocytes, particularly neutrophil polymorphs and to a lesser extent macrophages, migrate out of the capillaries and into the surrounding tissue. Once in the tissue they migrate towards the site of infection by a process known as chemotaxis.

These events manifest themselves as inflammation.

CHEMOTAXIS

Chemotaxis is the process by which phagocytes are attracted to sites of inflammation (Fig. 1.10). *In vitro* phagocytes will actively migrate up a concentration gradient of certain (chemotactic) molecules. Particularly active is C5a, a fragment of one of the complement components. When purified C5a is applied to the base of an ulcer *in vivo*, neutrophil polymorphs can be seen sticking to the endothelium of the nearby capillaries shortly afterwards. Initially this occurs on the side of the capillary nearest the point of application but as the C5a diffuses further the neutrophils stick to all sides of the endothelium before traversing the endothelium, crossing the basement membrane and migrating up the gradient of the chemotactic molecule. Adherence and diapedesis of leucocytes is shown in Figs 1.11 and 1.12. Both neutrophil polymorphs and macrophages are attracted by C5a, but neutrophils are the predominant cell in sites of acute inflammation, reflecting their numerical preponderance in the blood.

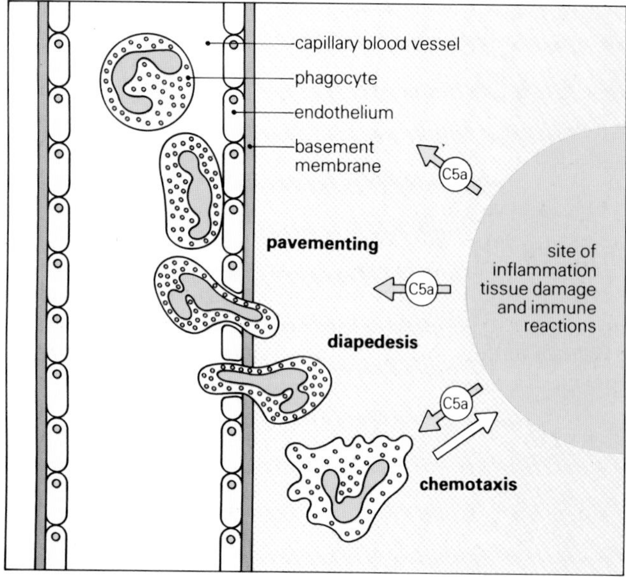

Fig. 1.10 Chemotaxis. At a site of inflammation, tissue damage and complement activation by the infectious agent cause the release of chemotactic peptides (e.g. C5a, a fragment of one of the complement components, which is one of the most important chemotactic peptides). These peptides diffuse to the adjoining capillaries, causing passing phagocytes to adhere to the endothelium (pavementing). The phagocytes insert pseudopodia between the endothelial cells and dissolve the basement membrane (diapedesis). They then pass out of the blood vessel and move up the concentration gradient of the chemotactic peptides towards the site of inflammation.

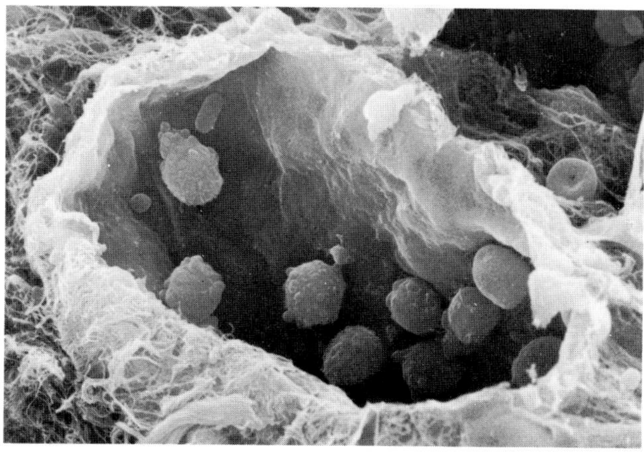

Fig. 1.12 Scanning electronmicrograph showing leucocytes adhering to the wall of a venule in inflamed tissue. x16,000. (Courtesy of Professor M. J. Karnovsky.)

PHAGOCYTOSIS

Once they have arrived at a site of inflammation the phagocytes have to recognize the infectious agent. They have receptors on their surface which allow them to attach non-specifically to a variety of microorganisms, but the attachment is greatly enhanced if the microorganism has been opsonized by the C3b component of complement. Complement activation at the site of infection causes C3b to be deposited on the infectious agent; since both neutrophils and macrophages have receptors which specifically bind to C3b, this allows the

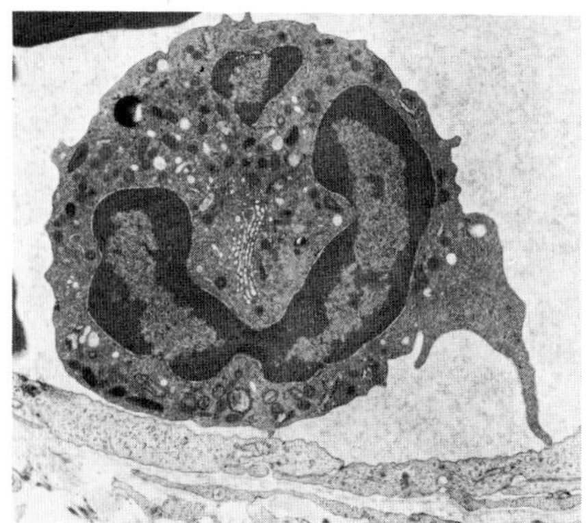

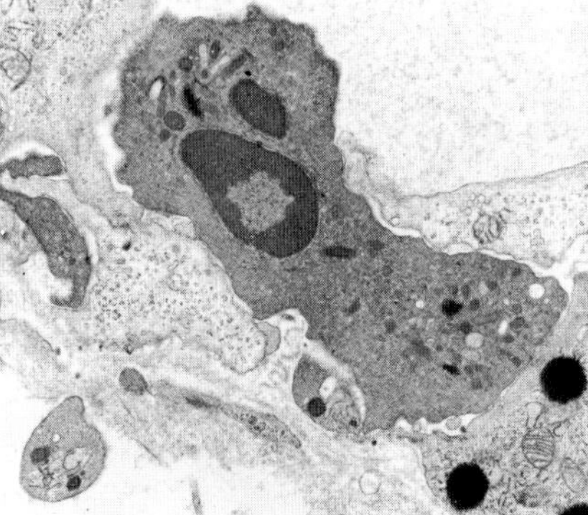

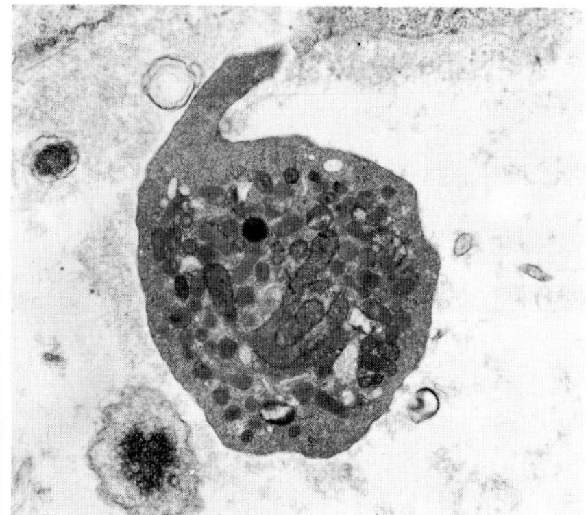

Fig. 1.11 Electronmicrographs showing the three phases of diapedesis. A leucocyte adheres to the capillary endothelium (left) before it penetrates the endothelium (middle). The third micrograph illustrates a leucocyte which has traversed the endothelium. x4000. (Courtesy of Dr I. Jovis.)

phagocytes to recognize their targets (Fig. 1.13). The importance of complement opsonization can be seen in those very rare patients who are genetically deficient in complement component C3. These patients suffer from recurrent bacterial infections and septicaemia.

complement (opsonization)
attachment by non-specific receptors
attachment by C3b receptors
phagosome forming
lysosome
damage and digestion
phagocytosis
lysosome fusion
release of microbial products

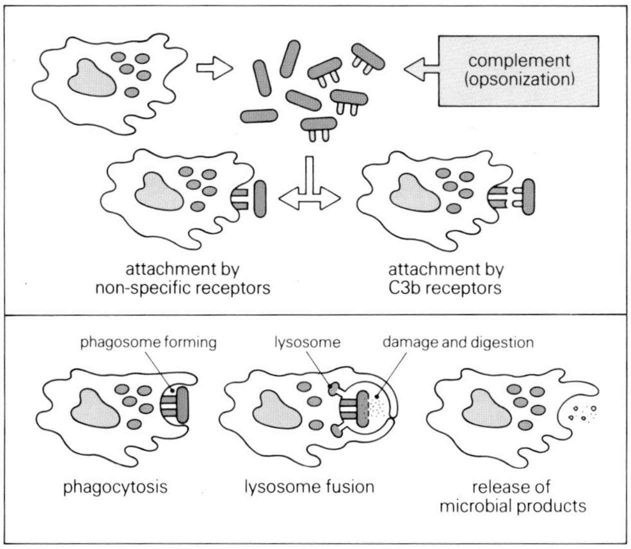

Fig. 1.13 Phagocytosis. Phagocytes arrive at a site of inflammation by chemotaxis. They may then attach to microorganisms via their non-specific cell surface receptors or, if the organism is opsonized with a fragment of the third complement component (C3b) through activation of the complement system, attachment will be through the cell surface receptors for C3b. If the membrane now becomes activated by the attached infectious agent, it is taken into a phagosome by pseudopodia which extend around it. Once inside, lysosomes fuse with the phagosome to form a phagolysosome and the infectious agent is killed by a battery of microbicidal mechanisms. Undigested microbial products may be released to the outside.

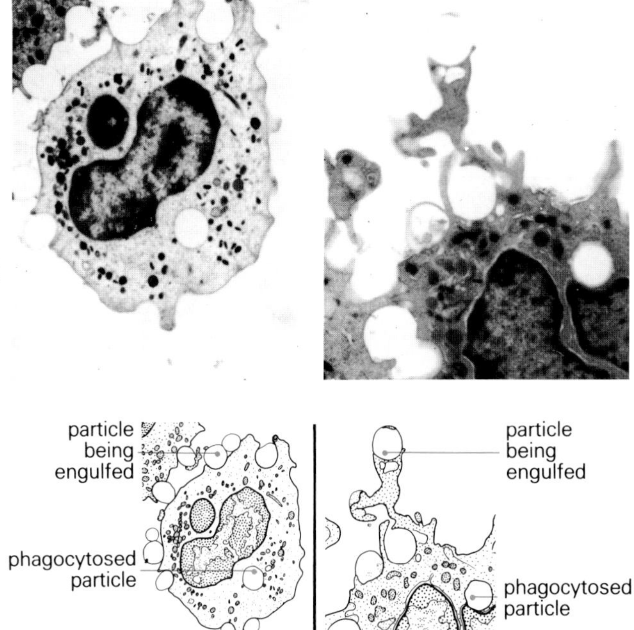

Fig. 1.14 Electronmicrographic study of phagocytosis. These two micrographs show human phagocytes engulfing latex particles. x3000 (left); x4500 (right). (Courtesy of Professor C. H. W. Horne.)

After attachment the phagocytes proceed to engulf the microorganism by extending pseudopodia around it. These fuse and the microorganism is internalized in a phagosome (Fig. 1.14). Lysosomes fuse with the phagosome and destroy the trapped microorganism. The mechanisms involved are described more fully in Chapters 16 and 17.

ANTIBODY – A FLEXIBLE ADAPTOR

Problems arise when the phagocytes are unable to recognize the infectious agent, either because they lack a suitable receptor for it or because the microorganism does not activate complement and so cannot become attached to the phagocyte via the C3b receptor. Ideally, what is needed is a flexible adaptor that can attach at one end to the microorganism and at the other to the phagocyte. In answer to this requirement, molecules known as antibodies have evolved and these are fully described in Chapter 5. Antibodies are a class of molecules produced by B lymphocytes of the adaptive immune system. They have several functions, including acting as flexible adaptors which bring about adherence of infectious agents to phagocytes (Fig. 1.15).

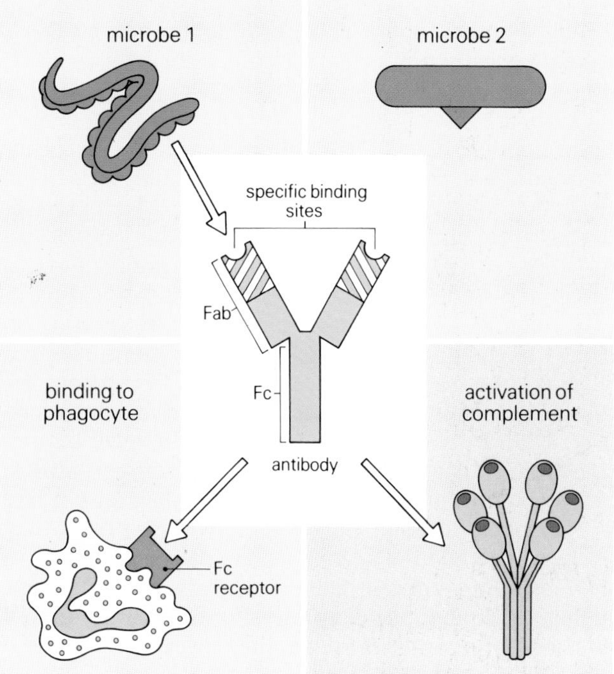

Fig. 1.15 Antibody – a flexible adaptor. When a microorganism lacks the inherent ability to activate complement or bind to phagocytes, the body provides a class of flexible adaptor molecules with a series of different shapes which can attach to the surface of different microbes. These flexible adaptor molecules are antibodies and the body can make several million different antibodies able to recognize a wide variety of infectious agents. Thus the antibody illustrated binds microbe 1, but not microbe 2, by its 'antigen-binding portion' (Fab) while the 'Fc portion' (which may activate complement) binds to Fc receptors on host tissue cells, particularly phagocytes.

phagocyte	opsonin	binding
1	–	±
2 C3b, C3b receptor	complement C3b	+ +
3 Ab, Fc receptor	antibody	+
4	antibody and complement C3b	+ + + +

Fig. 1.16 Opsonization. Phagocytes have some intrinsic ability to bind directly to bacteria and other microorganisms (1), but this is much enhanced if the bacteria have activated complement (C3b) so that the cells can bind the bacteria via C3b receptors (2). Opsonization of organisms which do not activate complement well, if at all, is performed by antibody (Ab) which acts as a bridge to attach the microbe to the Fc receptor on the phagocyte (3). Antibody can also activate complement and if both antibody *and* C3b opsonize, binding is greatly enhanced (4).

An antibody molecule can only bind to one type of infectious agent; the other end of the molecule binds to the phagocyte via a receptor, the Fc receptor. Macrophages, neutrophils and all other cells of the monocyte/macrophage series have Fc receptors. As antibodies also cause activation of complement by the classical pathway, infectious agents often have both antibody and C3b bound to their surface. The phagocyte recognizes the agent via both its Fc receptors and its C3b receptors; thus attachment and phagocytosis are greatly enhanced (Fig. 1.16). Antibodies are therefore effectively bifunctional molecules. One part, which is extremely variable between different antibodies, is responsible for binding to the many different infectious agents the body may encounter, while the second, constant portion binds to the Fc receptors of cells and also activates complement. In fact, antibodies act as adaptors for other cells, as well as phagocytes, and different antibodies can act as adaptors for different cell types.

ANTIGEN

Antibody molecules do not bind to the whole of an infectious agent. Each antibody molecule binds to one of many molecules on the microorganism's surface. Molecules to which antibodies bind are called antigens (*anti*body *gen*erators). Different antibodies will bind to different antigens since each antibody is specific for a particular antigen. Indeed, a particular antigen specifically induces the production of the antibodies which can bind to it. The way in which a sufficient diversity of antibody molecules is generated to recognize different antigens is explained in Chapter 7. Each antibody binds to a particular part of the antigen called an antigenic determinant, or epitope (the terms antigenic determinant and epitope are synonymous). A particular antigen can have several different epitopes or several identical epitopes (Fig. 1.17). Antibodies are specific for the epitopes rather than for the whole antigen molecule but since each antigen has its own particular set of epitopes, which are not usually shared with other antigens, the collection of antibodies in an antiserum is effectively specific for the antigen. The characteristics of antigen–antibody combination are discussed in Chapter 6.

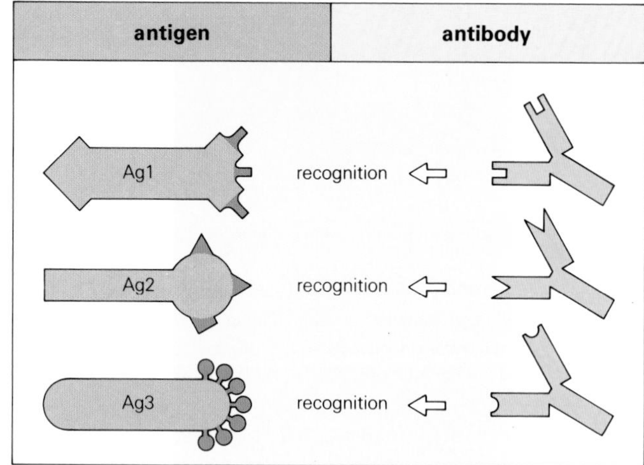

Fig. 1.17 Antigens. Foreign molecules which generate antibodies are called antigens. Antigen molecules each have a set of antigenic determinants also called epitopes. The epitopes on one antigen (Ag1) are usually different from those on another (Ag2). Some antigens (Ag3) have repeated epitopes. Epitopes are molecular shapes recognized by the antibodies and cells of the adaptive immune system. Each cell recognizes one epitope rather than the whole antigen. Even simple microorganisms have many different antigens.

ADAPTIVE IMMUNITY AND CLONAL SELECTION

The specificity of the adaptive immune system is based on the specificity of the antibodies and lymphocytes. Each lymphocyte is only capable of recognizing one particular antigen. As the immune system as a whole can specifically recognize many thousands of antigens, the lymphocytes recognizing any particular antigen are a very small proportion of the total. How then is an adequate response to an infectious agent generated? The answer is by clonal selection. Antigen binds to the small number of cells which can recognize it and induces them to proliferate so that they constitute sufficient cells to mount an adequate immune response; that is, the antigen selects the specific clones of antigen-binding cells (Fig. 1.18). This occurs both for the B lymphocytes, which proliferate and mature into antibody-producing cells, and for the T lymphocytes, which are involved in the recognition and destruction of virally infected cells.

The immune system generates antibodies which can recognize all of the different antigens, even before it encounters them. So many different antibodies are

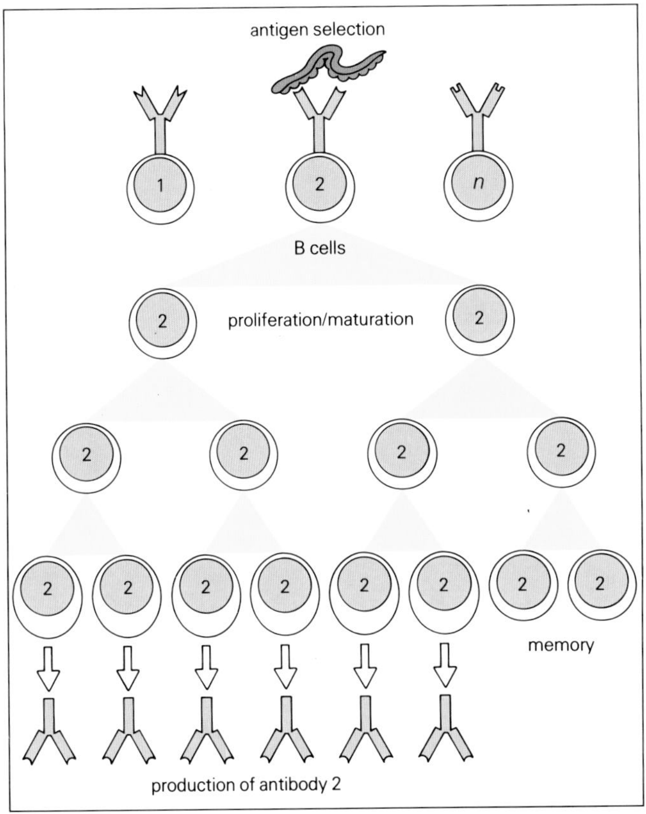

Fig. 1.18 Clonal selection. Each antibody-producing cell (B cell) is programmed to make just one antibody, which is placed on its surface as an antigen receptor. Each B cell has a different antigen-binding specificity (1–*n*). Antigen binds to only those B cells with the appropriate surface receptor. These cells are stimulated to proliferate and mature into antibody-producing cells and the longer-lived memory cells, all with the same antigen-binding specificity (2).

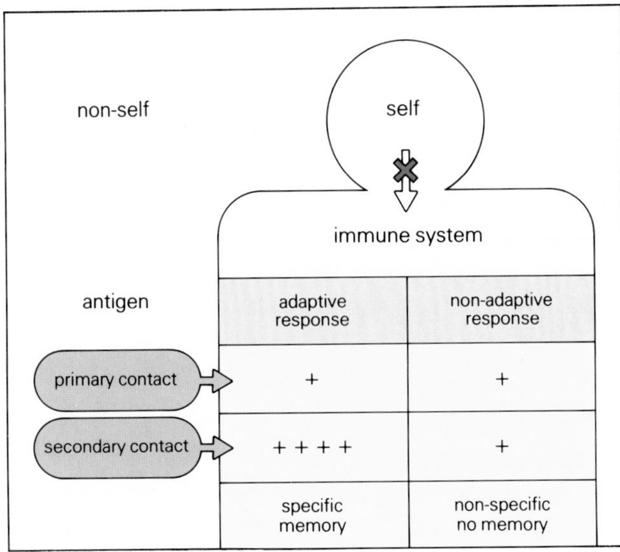

Fig. 1.19 Summary of self/non-self discrimination. The immune system discriminates self from non-self, and reacts against non-self molecules (antigens). Following a primary contact with antigen, there are weak adaptive, and non-adaptive responses, but if the same antigen persists or is encountered a second time there is a much enhanced specific response to that antigen. The characteristics of the adaptive immune response are specificity and memory.

produced that most of them will never be called upon to protect the individual against infection. However the tremendous number of infectious organisms and their further diversification through continual mutation makes it necessary for all these antibodies to be available.

This raises the question of exactly what the immune system is capable of recognizing. Broadly speaking, the immune system regards all molecules not belonging to the individual as 'non-self' and reacts against them, and it recognizes many of the individual's own molecules as 'self' and does not react against them. Failure to react to a potentially antigenic molecule is referred to as tolerance (see Chapter 12). The critical importance of self/non-self discrimination is outlined in Fig. 1.19 in the context of the adaptive and non-adaptive immune response. The body must both tolerate its own tissues and react effectively against all infective agents if disease is to be avoided.

INTEGRATED DEFENCE MECHANISMS

It will be appreciated that the innate and adaptive immune systems do not act in isolation. Antibodies produced by lymphocytes help phagocytes to recognize their targets. Following clonal activation by antigen, T lymphocytes produce lymphokines which stimulate phagocytes to destroy infectious agents more effectively. The macrophages in turn help the lymphocytes by transporting antigen from the periphery to lymph nodes and other lymphoid organs, where it is presented to lymphocytes in a form they can recognize (Fig. 1.20).

The immune system is not the only system which protects the body from injury; the clotting, fibrinolytic and kinin systems are also involved in mediating inflammation and in the resolution of tissue damage. These systems interact to maintain the integrity of the vascular system and to limit the spread of tissue damage whether it is caused by physical injury or infectious agents.

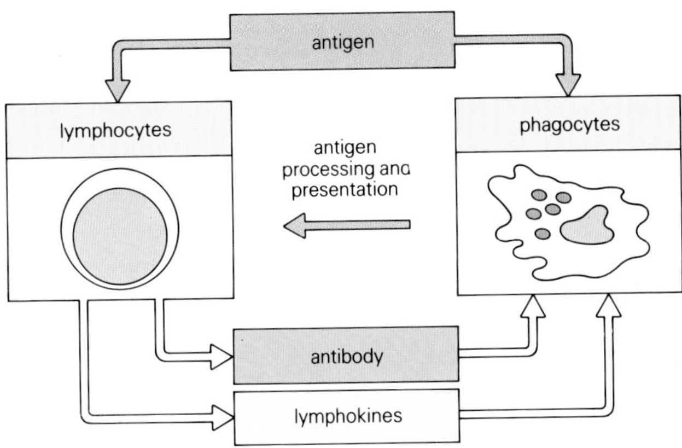

Fig. 1.20 Interaction between lymphocytes and phagocytes. The adaptive and non-adaptive areas of the immune system interact at all levels. Lymphocytes are responsible for specific recognition: they produce antibody and lymphokines, soluble molecules which help the phagocytes combat the infection. Antigens are processed by phagocytes and other cells which cannot themselves specifically recognize antigens, and are presented to lymphocytes which can recognize them.

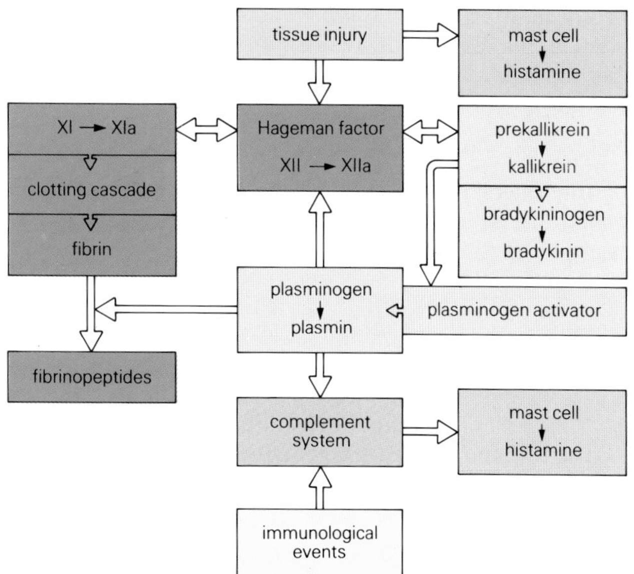

Fig. 1.21 The plasma enzyme systems in inflammation. The four plasma enzyme systems which interact in the control of inflammation are the clotting system (turquoise), the kinin system (light blue), the fibrinolytic system (pink) and the complement system (green). When tissue injury occurs, enzymes are released and surfaces are exposed which activate Hageman factor XII and trigger mast cells to release histamine. Activated Hageman factor (XIIa) activates, and is reciprocally activated by, factor XIa and kallikrein. The kinin system produces bradykinin which induces pain, increased vascular permeability and vasodilation. Kallikrein activates the fibrinolytic system to produce plasmin which can activate Hageman factor and complement components and splits fibrin to produce chemotactic fibrinopeptides. Immunological events, for example, the combination of antibody with antigen, interact with these systems and modulate inflammation via the complement system. Different components (for example, C3a and C5a) trigger mast cells to release histamine producing vasodilation, increased capillary permeability and chemokinesis. (Other factors act as spasmogens, cause endothelial cell retraction, and are chemotactic for phagocytes.)

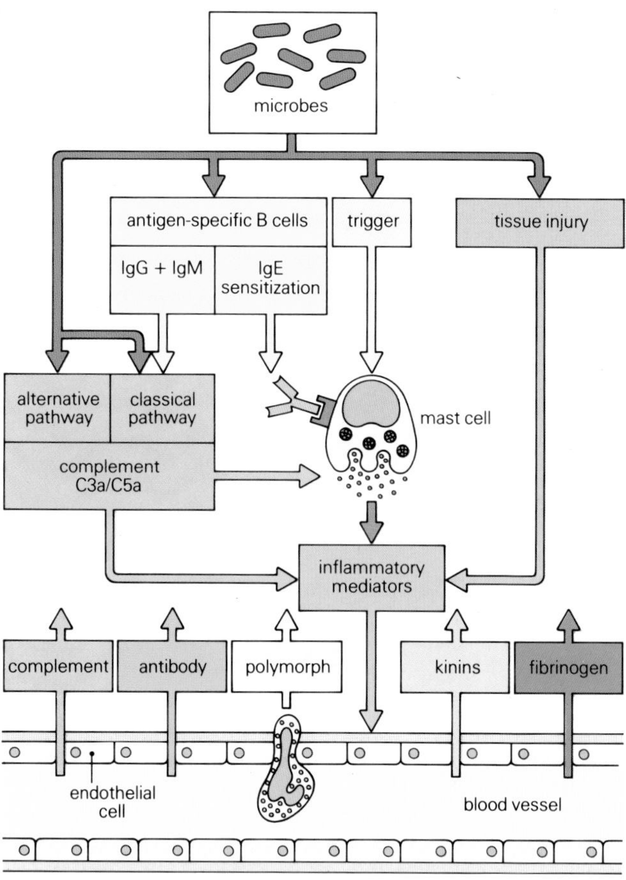

Fig. 1.22 Immune system in acute inflammation. The adaptive immune system modulates inflammatory processes via the complement system. Antigen from microbes stimulates antigen-specific B cells to produce antibodies; some (IgE) bind to mast cells while others (IgG and IgM) activate complement. Complement can also be activated directly by microbes via the alternative pathway. When triggered by microbial antigens, the sensitized mast cell releases mediators. In association with complement (which also activates mast cells via C3a and C5a) the mediators induce local inflammation, facilitating the arrival of phagocytes and more plasma enzyme system molecules.

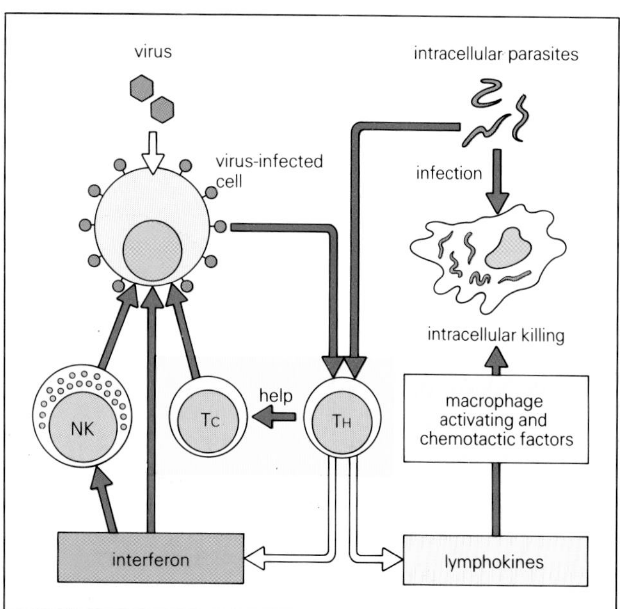

Fig. 1.23 Innate and acquired mechanisms of killing intracellular organisms. Viruses and intracellular parasites stimulate T cells of the adaptive immune system (yellow). T helper cells (TH) cooperate in the maturation of T cytotoxic cells (Tc) and release lymphokines, including interferon. Tc cells and NK cells can kill virally infected cells. Interferons (also produced by the infected cell) stimulate NK cells and inhibit viral replication directly. Other lymphokines attract macrophages to the site of infection and enable them to kill intracellular organisms which would otherwise persist.

Immunological events can interact with this integrated system of damage control via the complement system (Fig. 1.21). Complement components released from sites of inflammation act directly on the local vasculature, and fragments C3a and C5a can also activate mast cells. These cells are widely distributed throughout the body and contain mediators which cause vasodilation and increased vascular permeability. The immune system can also interact directly with mast cells via a type of antibody (IgE) which binds to Fc receptors on the mast cell (Fig. 1.22). The inflammatory reaction effects the arrival of molecules and cells to the site of infection where they activate the macrophages to destroy their intracellular parasites (Fig. 1.23).

VACCINATION

Specificity and memory, the two key elements of the adaptive immune response, are exploited in vaccination, since the adaptive immune system mounts a much stronger response on second encounter with antigen. This secondary immune response is both faster to appear and more effective than the primary response. The principle is to alter a microorganism or its toxins in such a way that they become innocuous without losing antigenicity. Take, for example, vaccination against diphtheria. The diphtheria bacterium produces a toxin which is cytotoxic for muscle cells. The toxin can be chemically modified by formalin treatment so that it retains its antigenic epitopes but loses its toxicity; the resulting toxoid is used as a vaccine (Fig. 1.24). Other infectious agents, such as the polio virus, can be attenuated so that they retain their antigenicity but lose their pathogenicity.

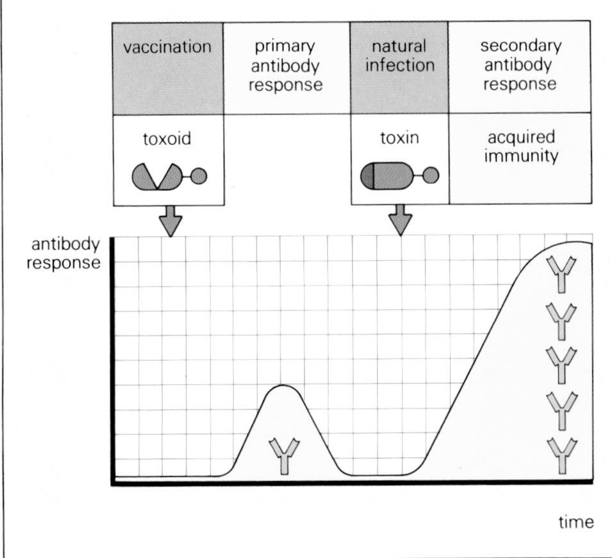

Fig. 1.24 Principle of vaccination. The principle of vaccination is illustrated by immunization with diphtheria toxoid. Diphtheria toxoid retains some of the epitopes of the diphtheria bacillus toxin so that a primary antibody response to these epitopes is produced following vaccination with toxoid. In a natural infection the toxin restimulates B memory cells which produce the faster and more intense secondary antibody response to the epitope, so neutralizing the toxin.

IMMUNOPATHOLOGY

Up to this point the immune system has been presented as an unimpeachable asset. It is certainly true that deficiencies in any part of the immune system leave the individual exposed to a greater risk of infection, although other parts of the system often partly compensate for such deficiencies. Clearly, strong evolutionary pressures from infectious agents have led to the development of the system in its present form, but there are occasions when the immune system is itself a cause of disease or other undesirable consequences (Fig. 1.25).

It has been stated that the immune system is established on a principle of self/non-self recognition. In some cases tolerance of self antigens breaks down and autoimmune disease may develop (see Chapter 23). In other cases innocuous antigens such as pollen are recognized and the immune system mounts an inappropriate response to them, giving rise to symptoms of hypersensitivity discussed in Chapters 19–22. Hypersensitivity reactions can also occur during infections. In some infections the amount of tissue damage produced by the immune reactions to a resistant microorganism may be comparable to that produced by the infection itself. In spite of these drawbacks it must always be remembered that overwhelming selective pressures have led to the development of the immune system as we see it today.

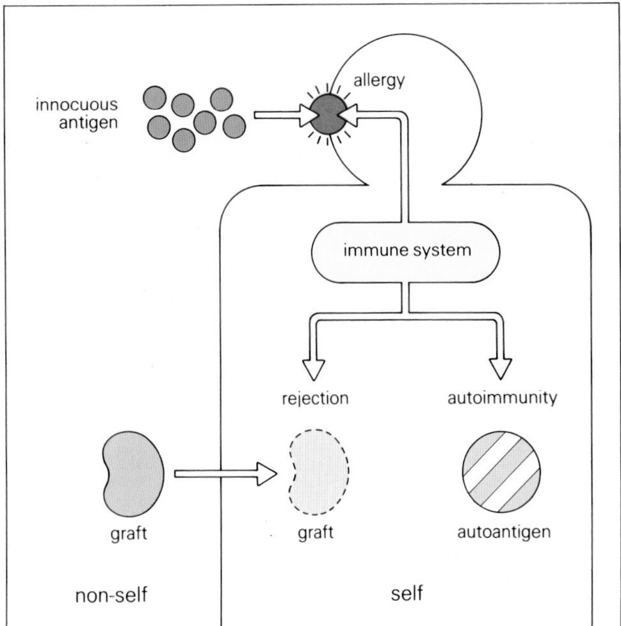

Fig. 1.25 Undesirable consequences of immunity. Tissue damage may occur through the operation of immune mechanisms, either because the immune response is excessive or if the antigen is persistent. Thus, in allergic patients, some innocuous antigen such as pollen provokes an immune reaction out of proportion to any damage it might do; we speak of hypersensitivity reactions. The immune system recognizes foreign tissue grafts like any other antigen and rejects them. Sometimes the self/non-self recognition system breaks down and the body's own components are recognized as non-self (autoantigens) in which case autoimmune disease can ensue.

FURTHER READING

Law, S. K. A. & Reid, K. B. M. (1988) *Complement*. Oxford: IRL Press.

Roitt, I. M. (1987) *Essential Immunology*. 6th edition. Oxford: Blackwell Scientific Publications.

Ryan, G. B. & Mayno, G. (1977) *Inflammation*. Michigan: The Upjohn Company.

Stites, D. P., Stobo, J. D., Fudenberg, H. H. & Wells, J. V. (1987) *Basic and Clinical Immunology*. 6th edition. California: Lange Medical Publications.

Taussig, M. J. (1984) Inflammation: Section 1, *Processes in Pathology and Microbiology*. 2nd edition. Oxford: Blackwell Scientific Publications.

2 Cells Involved in the Immune Response

The immune system of vertebrates consists of a number of organs and several different cell types which have evolved to accurately and specifically recognize non-self antigens on microorganisms and to eliminate those organisms. By contrast, lower animals have more primitive defence mechanisms to protect themselves. These include proteins (with low specificity) which can recognize and agglutinate a wide variety of microorganisms, and cells which are capable of engulfing and digesting the microbes – phagocytes.

Phagocytes are an important defence in all animals, including the vertebrates. The key development which has occurred in vertebrate immune systems is the evolution of lymphoid cells and lymphoid organs. The lymphoid cells function to produce the high degree of specificity involved in the recognition of non-self antigens by vertebrate immune systems.

All the cells of the immune system arise from pluripotent stem cells through two main lines of differentiation (Fig. 2.1):

1. the lymphoid lineage – producing lymphocytes
2. the myeloid lineage – producing phagocytes (monocytes and neutrophils) and other cells.

There are two different kinds of lymphocytes which subserve different functions; these are T cells and B cells, which are both equipped with surface receptors for antigen. There is also a 'third population' of cells which does not possess these conventional receptors. T cells develop in the thymus whilst B cells differentiate in fetal liver and, in mammals, in the adult bone marrow. In birds, B cells differentiate in an organ found only in avian species, the bursa of Fabricius. These are the central or primary lymphoid organs where the mature lymphocyte precursors acquire the ability to recognize antigens through the development of surface receptors. The 'third population' of lymphocytes (TPCs), also called non-T, non-B cells or 'null cells', probably develop in the bone-marrow but their differentiation sequence is still uncertain. This population contains cytotoxic lymphocytes.

The phagocytes are also of two basic kinds – monocytes and polymorphonuclear granulocytes. The latter are more usually referred to as polymorphs and may be neutrophils, basophils, or eosinophils depending on the differential staining of their granules. In addition, there are a number of auxiliary cells which include:

1. a variety of cells specialized to present antigen to T and B cells, referred to as antigen-presenting cells (APCs)
2. platelets, which are involved in blood clotting and inflammation

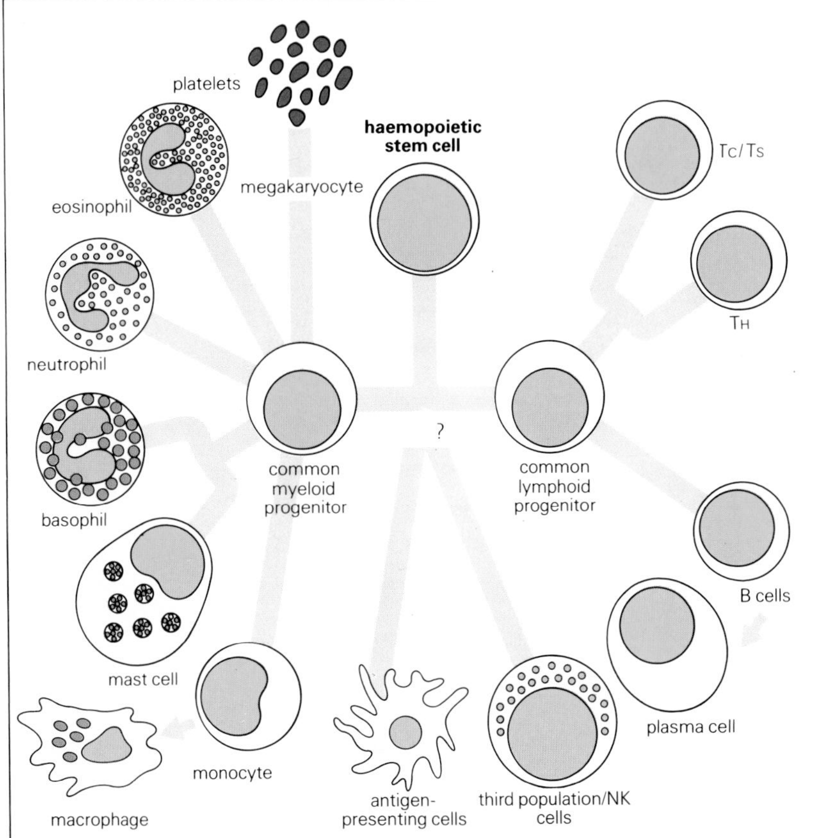

Fig. 2.1 Origin of cells involved in the immune response. All these cells are derived from pluripotent stem cells which give rise to two main lineages; one for lymphoid cells and the other for myeloid cells. The common lymphoid progenitor has the capacity to differentiate into either T cells or B cells depending on the microenvironment to which it homes. T cells develop in the thymus while B cells develop in the fetal liver or bone marrow. The precise origin of the antigen-presenting cells and the third population of lymphoid cells is not certain, although they do develop ultimately from the haemopoietic stem cell. The myeloid cells differentiate into the committed cells shown on the left.

3. mast cells, which have structural and functional similarities to basophil polymorphs.

The important features of these cell types will now be described in greater detail.

LYMPHOID CELLS

Lymphocytes are produced in the primary or central lymphoid organs (thymus and adult bone marrow) at a high rate (10^9/day). Some of these cells migrate via the circulation into the secondary lymphoid tissues namely, the spleen, lymph nodes, tonsils, and unencapsulated lymphoid tissue. The average human adult has about 10^{12} lymphoid cells and the lymphoid tissue as a whole represents about 2% of total body weight. Lymphoid cells represent about 20% of the total white blood cells (leucocytes) present in the adult circulation – the majority of white cells being polymorphonuclear (PMNs). Many mature lymphoid cells are long-lived and may persist as memory cells for several years.

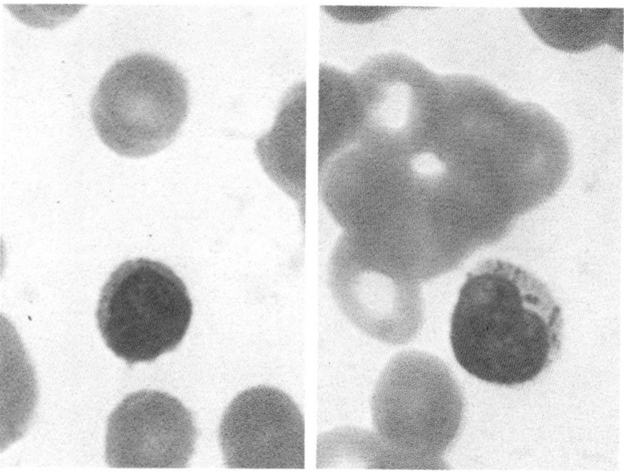

Fig. 2.2 Morphological heterogeneity of lymphocytes. The small lymphocyte (left) is agranular with a high N/C ratio. The large granular lymphocyte (right) has a lower N/C ratio and azurophilic granules in the cytoplasm. Condensed chromatin produces dark nuclear staining. Giemsa stain, × 1000.

MORPHOLOGICAL HETEROGENEITY OF LYMPHOCYTES

Lymphocytes in a conventional blood smear are heterogeneous in both size (6–10 μm in diameter) and morphology. Differences are seen in the nuclear (N) to cytoplasmic (C) ratio, the degree of cytoplasmic staining with histological dyes and the presence or absence of azurophilic granules.

Two distinct types of resting lymphoid cells can be distinguished in the circulation by light microscopy using a haematological stain such as Giemsa. The typical small lymphocyte is agranular and possesses a high N/C ratio. Others, with a lower N/C ratio and containing intracytoplasmic azurophilic granules are currently referred to as large granular lymphocytes (LGLs), not to be confused with granulocytes or monocytes which also have granules. (Fig. 2.2). Resting blood T cells show two distinct morphological patterns. The majority of both functional T cell populations – T-helper (TH) cells and suppressor or cytotoxic T (Tc/s) cells – carry a cytoplasmic structure termed the 'Gall body', which consists of a cluster of primary lysosomes associated with a lipid droplet. The Gall body is easily identified by lysosomal enzyme cytochemistry and electron microscopy (Fig. 2.3). Up to 20% of TH cells and 35% of Tc/s cells display granular lymphocyte morphology with primary lysosomes dispersed in the cytoplasm and a well-developed Golgi-apparatus (Fig 2.4).

Resting blood B cells do not display Gall bodies or granular lymphocyte morphology and their cytoplasm is predominantly occupied by single ribosomes (Fig. 2.5). Occasionally activated B cells are found with developing rough endoplasmic reticulum (Fig. 2.6).

Third population cells are all characterized by granular lymphocyte morphology. In comparison with granular T cells they display a larger number of azurophilic/electron dense granules.

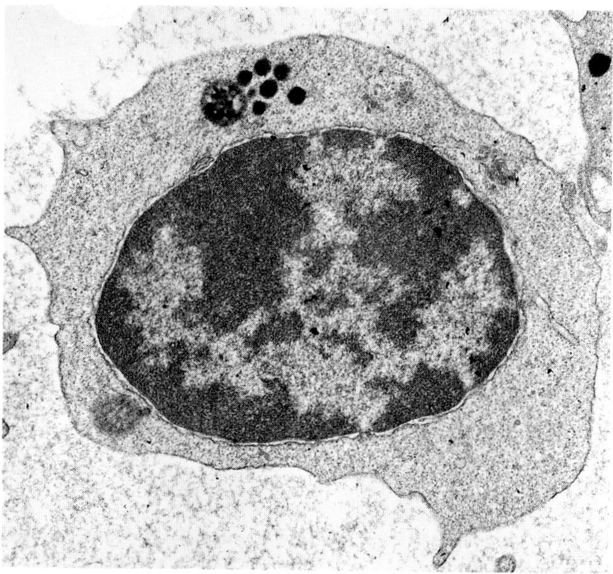

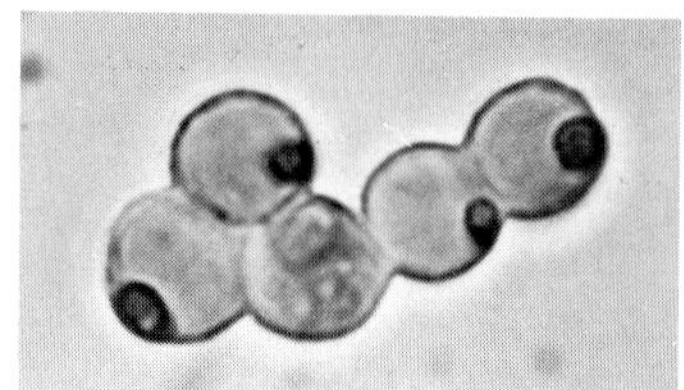

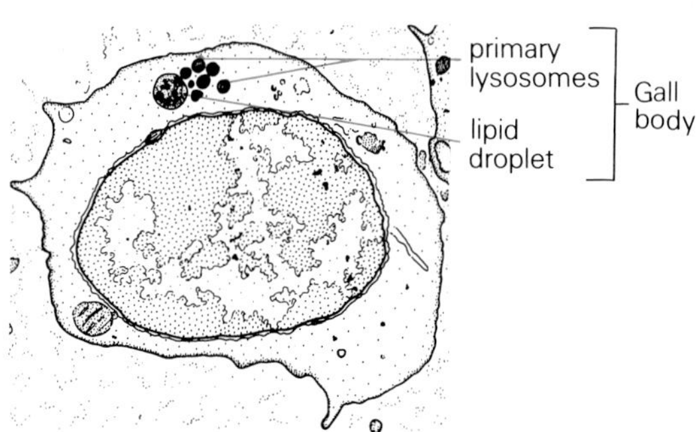

Fig. 2.3 Ultrastructure of a non-granular T cell. This electronmicrograph shows the Gall body which is characteristic of the majority of resting T cells (× 10,500). This structure is also seen as a single 'spot' following staining for non-specific esterase in light microscopy (insert, × 400).

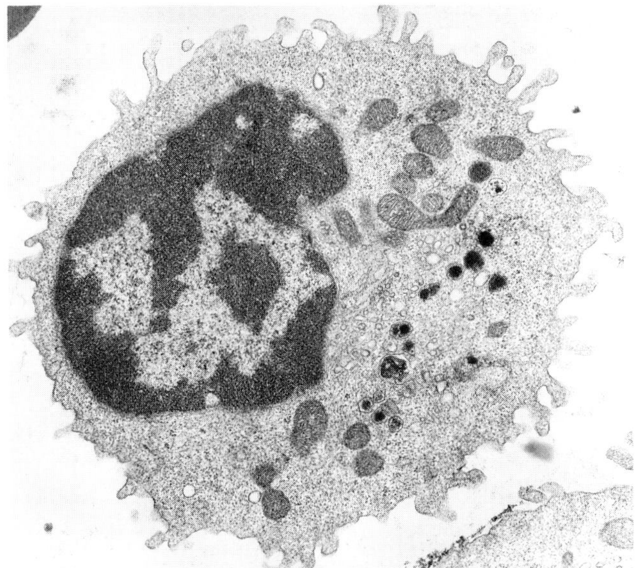

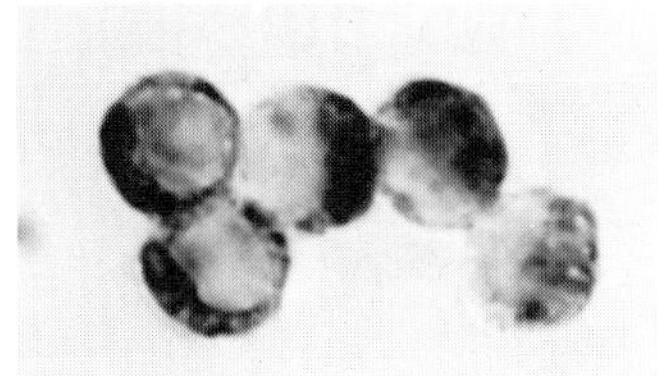

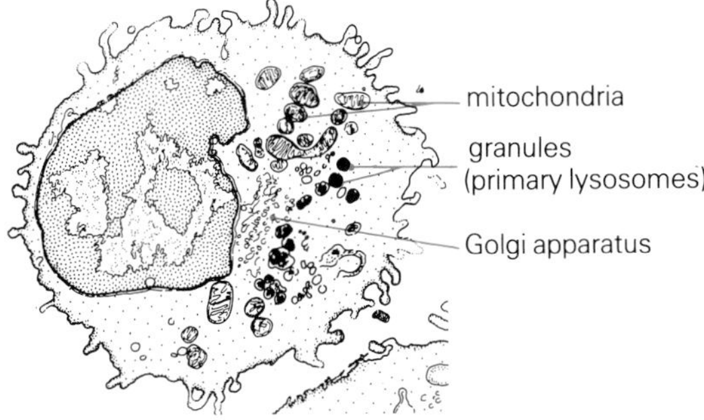

Fig. 2.4 Ultrastructure of T cells with granular morphology. These cells characteristically have electron-dense peroxidase-negative granules (primary lysosomes). These granules are dispersed in the cytoplasm with some close to the well-developed Golgi apparatus. There are many mitochondria present (× 10,000). Cytochemical staining for acid phosphatase shows a granular pattern of staining under light microscopy (insert, × 400).

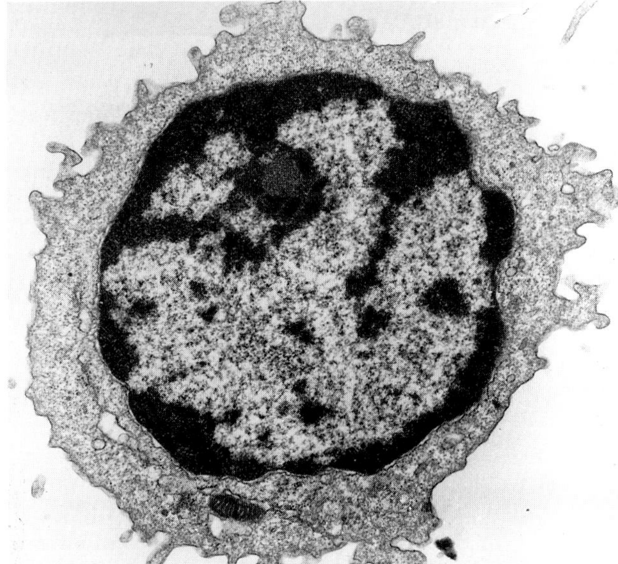

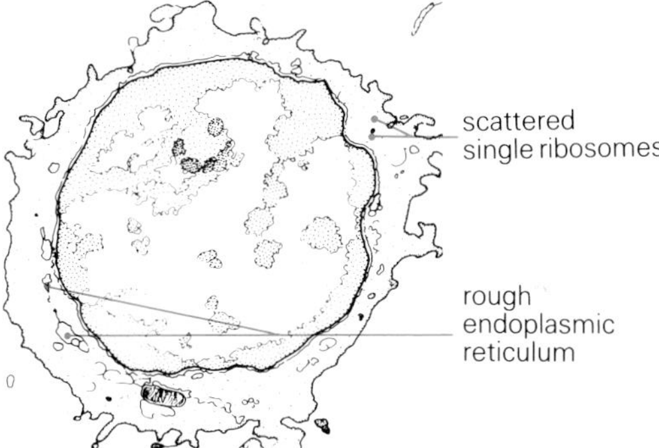

Fig. 2.5 Ultrastructure of a resting B cell. These cells have no Gall body or granules. Scattered ribosomes and isolated profiles of rough endoplasmic reticulum (RER) are seen in the cytoplasm (× 11,500).

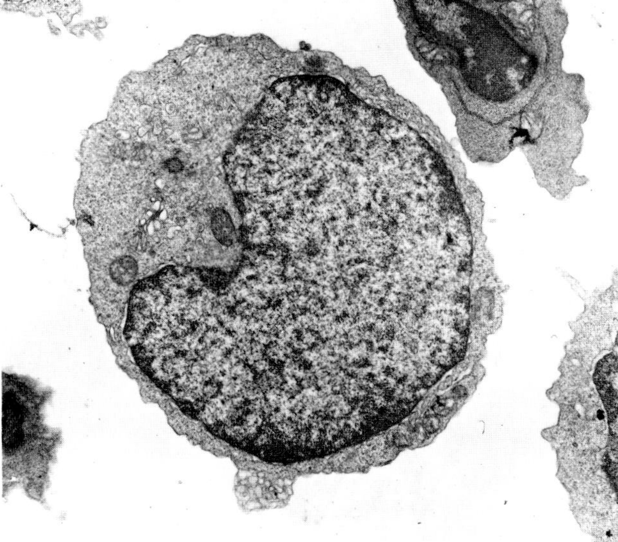

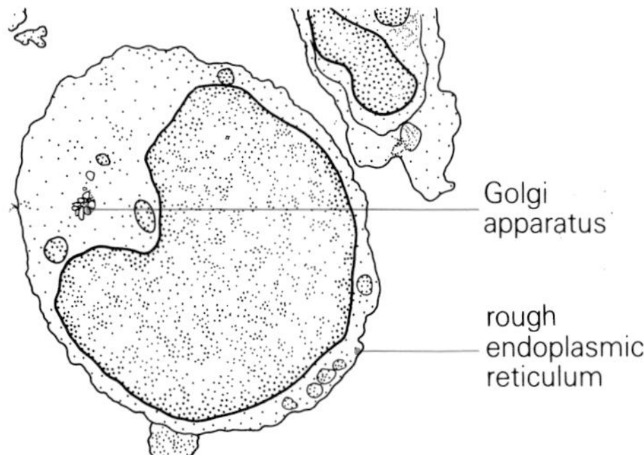

Fig. 2.6 Electronmicrograph showing the ultrastructure of a B cell blast. The main feature of activated B cells is the development of the machinery for immunoglobulin synthesis. This includes rough endoplasmic reticulum, free polyribosomes and the Golgi apparatus, which is involved in glycosylation of the immunoglobulins. × 7500.

MARKERS

Lymphocytes and other leucocytes express a large number of different molecules on their surfaces. Some of these appear at particular stages of cell differentiation or activation for short periods, while others are characteristic of different cell lineages. Such molecules which can be used to distinguish cell populations are called markers, and many of them can be identified by specific monoclonal antibodies. Recently a systematic nomenclature has been developed for these cell surface molecules – the CD system, in which the markers are numbered CD1, CD2, etc. The term CD (cluster designation) was derived by computer analysis of monoclonal antibodies raised in different laboratories worldwide against human leucocyte antigens. An international workshop determined their patterns of staining on leucocytes and the weights of the molecules precipitated by the antibodies. Monoclonal antibodies with similar specificity characteristics were grouped together and given a CD number. This number is now also used to indicate the specific molecule recognized by a group of monoclonal antibodies (see Fig. 2.11). In many cases the functions of the molecules are known, for example the marker CD35 is a complement C3b receptor (CR1).

Markers may be demonstrated using fluorescent antibodies as probes. In this case the surface markers act as antigens (Fig. 2.7). Hybridoma technology for making these antibodies, together with flow cytometry techniques, which allows enumeration and the separation of cells on the basis of their size and fluorescence intensity (see Chapter 25) has revolutionized studies on the functional activities of lymphoid cell populations.

T CELLS

One of the first ways of distinguishing human T cells from B cells was by their ability to bind to sheep erythrocytes which is through the CD2 molecule (Fig. 2.8). However the definitive T cell marker is the T cell antigen receptor (TCR). There are presently two defined types of TCR; TCR-2 is a heterodimer of 2 disulphide-linked polypeptides (α and β), TCR-1 is structurally similar but consists of γ and δ polypeptides. Both receptors are associated with a complex of polypeptides making up the CD3 complex (see Chapter 5). Thus a T cell is defined either by TCR-1 or TCR-2 which is associated with CD3.

Approximately 95% of blood T cells express TCR-2 and up to 5% have TCR-1. The TCR-2 bearing cells can be subdivided further into two distinct non-overlapping populations; the TH subset which is $CD4^+$ and the Tc/s subset which is $CD8^+$. $CD4^+$ T cells recognize antigens in association with major histocompatibility complex (MHC) class II molecules (see Chapter 4), while $CD8^+$ T cells recognize antigens in association with MHC class I molecules.

The $CD4^+$ set can be further divided functionally into:

1. those cells which positively influence the immune response of T cells and B cells – the helper cell function, which are $CDw29^+$
2. cells inducing suppressor/cytotoxic functions in $CD8^+$ cells – the suppressor inducer function, which are themselves $CD45R^+$.

Other monoclonal antibodies and criteria have been used to subdivide the $CD4^+$ set. For example, all $CD4^+$

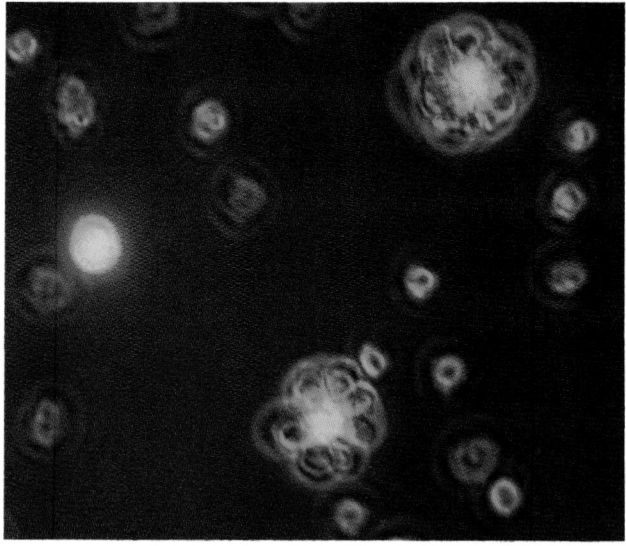

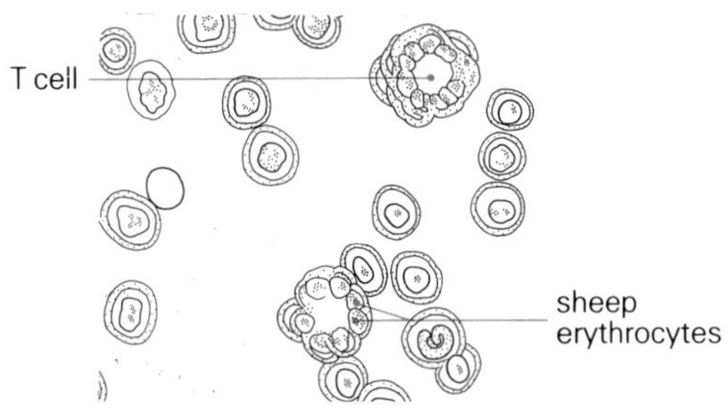

Fig. 2.8 Typical marker of human T cells. Human T cells from blood and tissues have the fortuitous property of binding to sheep erythrocytes (SE). Following their centrifugation together, T cells are distinguishable by their ability to form rosettes with SE. The nucleated cells are distinguished from the SE by green fluorescent staining of the nuclei and cytoplasm with acridine orange. The formation of rosettes with SE by T cells also provides a means for the physical separation of T from non-T cells (see Chapter 25).

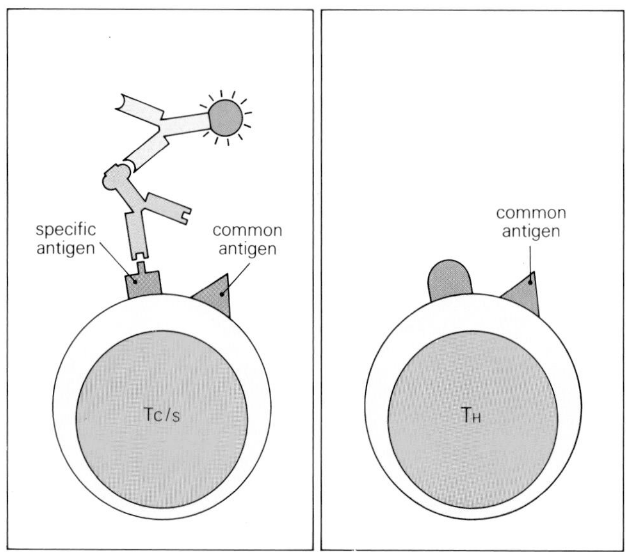

Fig. 2.7 Immunofluorescent method for the demonstration of T cell markers. Mouse antibodies directed towards T cell subset-specific antigen on a cytotoxic or suppressor T cell (Tc/s) will bind to this antigen but not to the T cell-specific antigen common to the T-helper (TH) subset. The bound antibody is detected using antibodies to mouse immunoglobulin coupled to a fluorescent molecule.

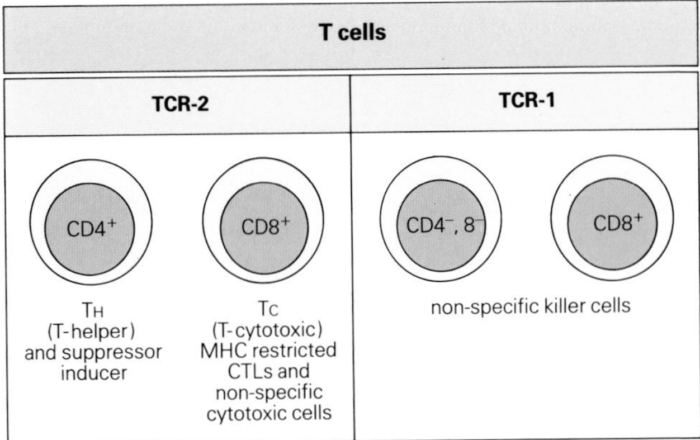

Fig. 2.9 T cell lineages. T cells may be differentiated according to their expression of the antigen receptors TCR-1 or TCR-2 and expression of surface molecules CD4 or CD8. These correspond with the functional categories of cells.

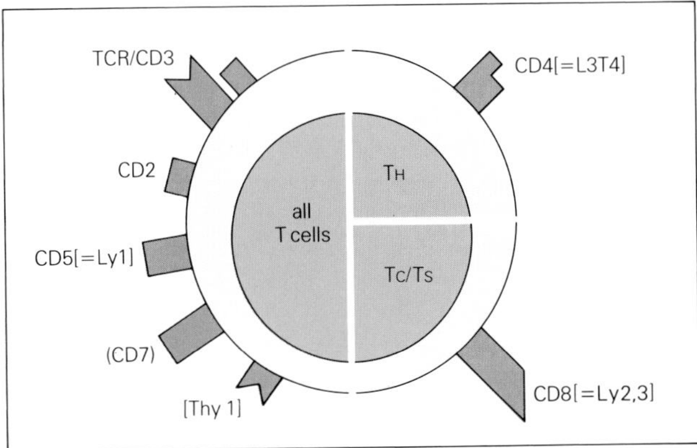

Fig. 2.10 Major T cell markers in man and mouse. The molecule CD7 is bracketed to indicate that it is only detected thus far in man. Markers in square brackets are specific for mouse (Thy-1) or mouse equivalents.

Fig. 2.11 Summary of the main CD molecules. This table shows some of the CD molecules characterized so far. The majority do not show absolute lineage specificity, but some are more lineage related than others.

antigen	mol.wt (kD)	distribution	identity/function
CD1a	49	thymocytes, Langerhans' cells	
CD1b	45	thymocytes	
CD1c	43	thymocytes	
CD2	50	T cells	sheep erythrocyte receptor
CD3	20–26	T cells	part of T cell antigen receptor complex
CD4	60	T cell subset TH	MHC class II restricted immune recognition
CD5	67	T cells, B cell subset	
CD6	120	T cells	
CD7	40	T cells	? IgM Fc receptor
CD8	32	T cell subset (Tc/s)	MHC class I restricted immune recognition
CD10	100	pre B cells	
CD11a	180	leucocytes	α chain of LFA-1 (adhesion molecule)
CD11b	160	monocytes, granulocytes	α chain of complement receptor CR3 (MAC-1)
CD11c	150	monocytes, granulocytes	α chain of p150, 95 (complement receptor/adhesion molecule)
CD13	150	granulocytes, monocytes	
CD14	55	monocytes, (granulocytes)	
CD15	50–180	granulocytes, monocytes	carbohydrate hapten
CD16	50–60	granulocytes (macrophages)	Fc receptor (Fc_{γ}R III) low affinity
CD17		granulocytes, monocytes, platelets	
CD18	95	leucocytes	β chain of LFA-1, CR3 and p150, 95
CD19	95	B cells	
CD20	35	B cells, dendritic cells	
CD21	140	B cells, dendritic cells	complement receptor CR2
CD22	135	B cells	
CD23	45	activated B cells	IgE receptor (low affinity)
CD25	55	activated T cells, B cells and macrophages	IL-2 receptor (low affinity polypeptide); α chain
CD28	44	T cell subset	
CDw29	135	T cell subset and many non-leucocytes	
CDw32	40	monocytes, granulocytes, platelets, B cells	Fc receptor (Fc_{γ}R II)
CD33	67	granulocyte/monocyte precursors, monocytes	
CD34	115	granulocyte/monocyte precursors	
CD35	220	B cells, erythrocytes, granulocytes, dendritic cells, T cells, plasma cells	complement receptor CR1
CD38	45	plasma cells, T cells	
CDw41	140 + 95	megakaryocyte , platelets	Gp11b/111a
CDw42	150	megakaryocytes, platelets	Gp1b
CD45	180–220	leucocytes	leucocyte common antigen
CD45R	220, 205	B cells, T cell subsets, granulocytes, monocytes	restricted leucocyte common antigen

cells expressing natural killer (NK) cell markers produce the lymphokine interleukin-2 (IL-2), and do not proliferate in response to antigens and mitogens. In fact, recent *in vitro* studies on $CD4^+$ clones in mouse and man have defined two separate populations (TH1 and TH2) based on the production of different lymphokines.

$CD8^+$ T cells can also be subdivided by a number of criteria and a variety of monoclonal antibodies into specific functional subsets. For example cells which recognize antigen in association with MHC molecules and produce IL-2 ($CD28^+$) and cells which do not recognize antigen in association with MHC molecules or produce IL-2 ($CD11b^+$).

$CD3^+$/TCR-1^+ cells represent a minority of circulating T cells which are also $CD4^-$, $CD8^-$. These cells home in to surface epithelia such as the epidermis and mucosal epithelia and are termed intra-epithelial lymphocytes (IEL). In interstitial mucosal epithelium TCR-1^+ cells also express CD8. It is probable that these cells represent a primitive cytotoxic population operating at the sites of entry of pathogens. Division of the TCR, CD4 and CD8 bearing cells into different functional subsets is illustrated in Figs 2.9 and 2.10.

Thus far we have described the antigen-specific receptors and markers allowing definition of T cell subsets. There are also a number of other surface molecules, expressed on all T cells (pan T cell markers) which are also found on cells of other lineages. For example, as shown above, all T cells express receptors for sheep erythrocytes (CD2). This molecule together with the TCR/CD3 complex and other membrane bound glycoproteins is involved in activating T cells when recognized by the appropriate ligand. CD2 is also found on about 50% of $CD3^-$ NK cells. CD5 molecules are expressed on all T cells, and also on a subpopulation of B cells which are involved in autoantibody production. CD7 is seen on all third population cells, and this molecule may be the receptor for the Fc portion of IgM. A summary of the more important CD markers is given in Fig. 2.11, which includes those seen on T cells and those present on other haemopoietic cells.

Murine T cells express markers similar to those detected on human T cells (see Fig. 2.10). In addition, all murine T cells carry a molecule, Thy-1 or θ, with a molecular weight of 19–35 kD. With regard to suppressor cells in the mouse, a small proportion of T cells carry I–J molecules, the expression of which is controlled by genes in the MHC (see Chapter 10). The binding of the lectin *Vicia villosa* might also mark a population in man and mouse which is involved in 'contrasuppression'.

B CELLS

B lymphocytes represent about 5–15% of the circulating lymphoid pool and are classically defined by the presence of endogenously produced immunoglobulins (antibody). These molecules are inserted into the surface membrane where they act as specific antigen receptors. They are detected on the surface of mature cells by staining cell suspensions with fluorochrome-labelled specific antibodies to the appropriate immunoglobulin of the species under investigation. Staining of cells in the cold results in the detection of the fluorescence with a 'ring-like' (or patchy) appearance over the cell (Fig. 2.12).

The majority of human peripheral blood B lymphocytes express both surface IgM and IgD molecules, which share the same specificity on the same cell. Very few

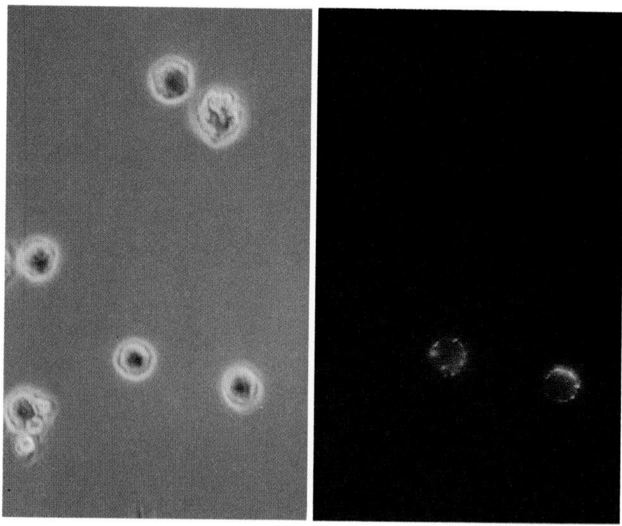

Fig. 2.12 B cells stained for surface immunoglobulin. Human blood B cells stained in the cold with fluoresceinated anti-human immunoglobulin show a patchy surface fluorescence viewed under ultraviolet light (right). Under phase contrast light microscopy (left) it can be seen that only 2 out of the 6 cells in this field are B lymphocytes. The lower cell shows 'capping' of the fluorescent antibody.

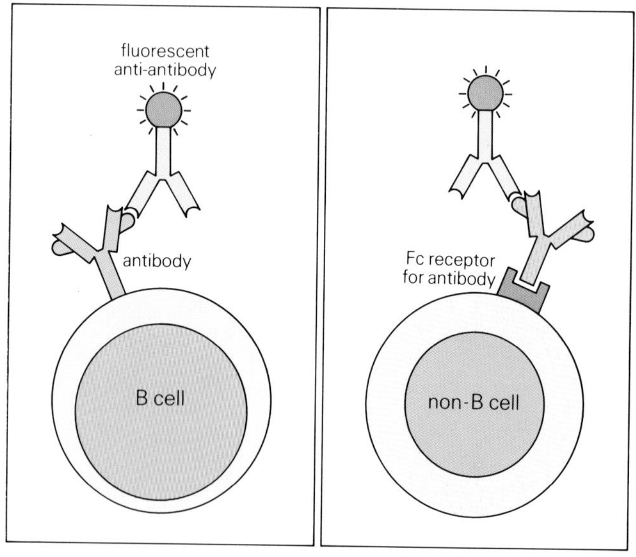

Fig. 2.13 Visualization of antibody bound to B cells and non-B cells by immunofluorescence. The surface antibody on the B cell is detected using a fluorescein anti-antibody conjugate (left). This conjugate will also 'detect' non-B cells carrying receptors for the Fc part of the antibody and which have antibody on their surface (right).

cells express surface IgG, IgA or IgE in the circulation although these are present in larger numbers in specific locations in the body, for example, IgA-bearing cells in the intestinal mucosa. Since other cells, in addition to B cells also carry surface receptors which non-specifically bind to antibodies, care should be taken in evaluating the number of B cells when using anti-immunoglobulin reagents. Antibodies bound to these receptors (Fc receptors) can also stain with fluoresceinated anti-human immunoglobulin (Fig. 2.13).

Divalent antibodies will cross-link antigens on surface

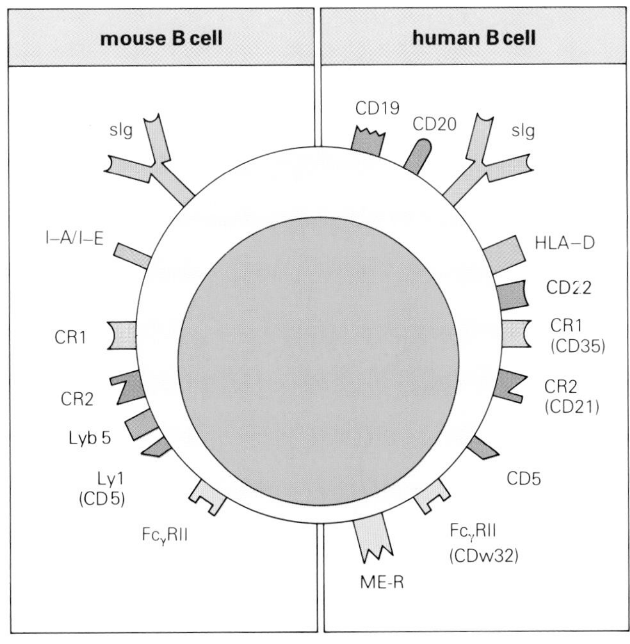

Fig. 2.14 Summary of the surface markers on mouse and human peripheral B cells. Equivalent molecules are in the same colour.

surface markers of human TPCs	
marker	**shared specificities**
CD16	minority of T cells, granulocytes, some macrophages
CD11b	granulocytes, monocytes, some T cells
CD38*	activated T cells, plasma cells, haemopoietic precursors
CD2*	all T cells
CD7	all T cells
CD8*	some T cells
Leu19,NHK-1 (270 kD)	some T cells
Leu7* (110 kD)	some T cells
IL-2R (β chain, p70)	activated T cells

*Expressed on 10–80% of TPCs only.

Fig. 2.15 Surface markers of human TPCs.

surface markers of murine TPCs	
marker	**shared specificities**
Thy 1*	T cells
Lyb5 (T200)	B cells
NK1	–
NK2	–
FcγR*	some T cells, granulocytes some monocytes/macrophages
Asialo GM1	–
CR3 (CD11b, MAC-1)	granulocytes, monocytes

*Expressed on some but not all murine TPCs.

Fig. 2.16 Surface markers of mouse TPCs.

membrane glycoproteins and be seen as 'patches' of cross-linked antigen–antibody complexes on the cell surface. Most of these complexes are actively swept along the cell surface and are seen as a 'cap' over one pole of the cell (see Fig. 2.12, right). This phenomenon is not peculiar to immunoglobulin on B cells but may also be seen with surface glycoproteins on other cell types when multivalent antibodies are attached to them.

A number of other markers are carried by both mouse and human B cells but not by resting T cells (Fig. 2.14). B cells are defined as those cells carrying endogenously produced immunoglobulins. The majority of B cells carry MHC class II antigens which are important in cooperation with T cells. These are I–A/I–E in the mouse and HLA–DP, DQ and DR antigens in man. Complement receptors for C3b (CR1, CD35) and C3d (CR2, CD21) are commonly found on B cells and are associated with activation and possibly homing of the cells. In this regard, the CR2 molecule is also the receptor for the Epstein-Barr virus (EBV) which on entry leads to the activation of the B cell. Fc receptors for IgG (FcRII, CDw32) are also present. CD19, CD20 and CD22 are the main markers currently used to identify human B cells. A marker originally found only on T cells (Ly1, CD5) has now been shown to be present on some B cells and identify a subset which is predisposed to autoantibody production. Some human B cells bind to mouse erythrocytes. The mouse erythrocyte rosette (ME-R), together with CD5, probably identifies an immature B cell population and both markers have been useful in the diagnosis of human lymphoproliferative disorders. Lyb5(T200) is a mouse alloantigen found on all B cells.

THIRD POPULATION CELLS

Third population cells (TPCs) have already been defined by morphology as large granular lymphocytes (see Fig. 2.2). TPCs possess larger numbers of electron-dense granules than granular T cells. They account for up to 20% of blood lymphocytes and can be negatively defined as cells lacking conventional surface antigen receptors, that is, TCR or immunoglobulin. Most surface antigens detectable on TPCs by monoclonal antibodies are shared with T cells or cells of the myelomonocytic series. The major markers of human TPCs and their shared specificities are shown in Fig. 2.15. A reagent commonly used to identify TPCs in purified lymphocyte populations is the monoclonal antibody to CD16 (Fc_γR III, Fc_γRlo). This is also expressed by a small proportion of T cells, by granulocytes and by some macrophages. Resting TPCs also express the α chain of the IL-2 receptor, an intermediate affinity receptor of 70 kD. Therefore, direct stimulation with IL-2 results in activation of TPCs. The phenotypic features of murine TPCs have been defined primarily by using allo- or heteroantisera. A distinctive morphologic difference between human and murine TPCs is the presence in the latter of fewer, but much larger, azurophilic granules. A summary of phenotypic markers of murine TPCs is shown in Fig. 2.16.

TPCs can also be functionally identified through their ability to kill certain tumour cells, virus infected cells, and targets coated with IgG antibodies. These lytic activities are referred to as natural killer (NK) activity and antibody-dependent cellular cytotoxicity (ADCC) respectively (Fig. 2.17). TPCs may also release interferon-γ (IFNγ) and other cytokines which may be important in the regulation of haemopoiesis and the immune response.

B cells, T cells and 'third population' cells have other important surface molecules which are common to all leucocytes. For example, the leucocyte function antigen (LFA-1) is also found on granulocytes and macrophages and is important in cell adhesion and intercellular communication. CD2 on T cells is also an LFA molecule (LFA-2).

LYMPHOCYTE ACTIVATION

Both T and B cells are activated when they bind their specific antigen in the presence of accessory cells; the resting 'virgin' lymphocytes then proliferate and mature into effector cells. This clonal selection through antigen

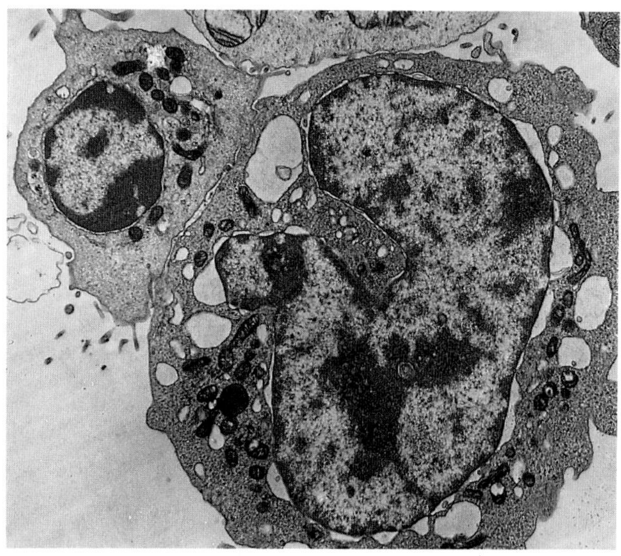

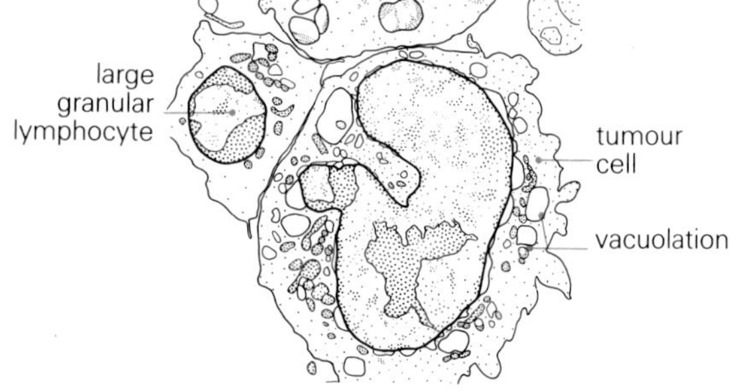

Fig. 2.17 Electronmicrograph of a large granular lymphocyte (LGL) killing a tumour cell. LGLs bind to and kill IgG antibody-coated, and even non-coated, tumour cells. It is essential for the membranes of the two cells to be closely apposed in order for the LGL to deliver its cytotoxic factors. Note the vacuolation of the tumour cell cytoplasm, characteristic of a dying cell. × 4500.

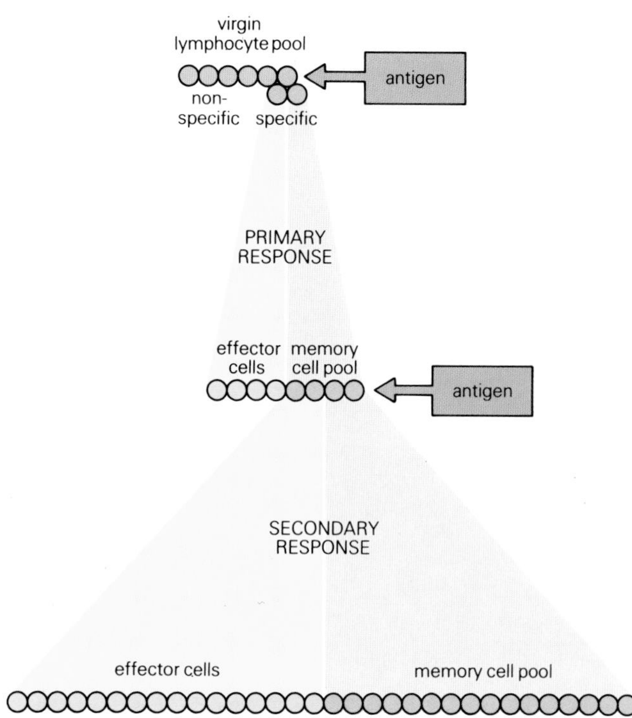

Fig. 2.18 Primary and secondary clonal expansion of lymphocytes in response to specific antigenic stimulation. T and B lymphocytes carrying specific antigen receptors are produced in the primary lymphoid organs and form the 'virgin' lymphoid pool. Following stimulation by specific antigen these cells proliferate and differentiate as clones into either effector cells (e.g. T cells with cytotoxic or other functions, or antibody-secreting plasma cells from mature B cells), or memory cells constituting the memory cell pool. This cellular proliferation is the primary response. When the memory cells are again stimulated by antigen they also proliferate (the secondary response) and some cells of the clone mature into effector cells whilst other cells remain as memory cells, thus increasing the size of both effector and memory cell pools.

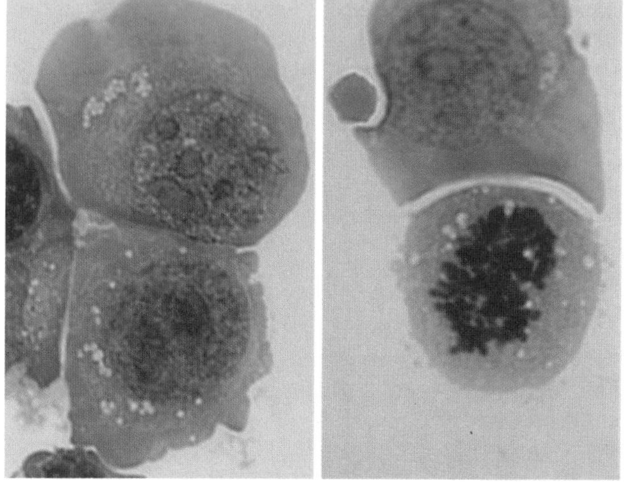

Fig. 2.19 Mitogen/antigen-induced lymphocyte blastogenesis. The human T cells and B cells shown here have been stimulated by the pokeweed mitogen. There is increased basophilia in the cytoplasm and an increase in the cell volume (left). The chromosomes condense and can be clearly seen during metaphase (right). Giemsa stain, × 2000.

recognition results in expansion of specific clones which either terminally differentiate into effectors or give rise to memory cells (Fig. 2.18). The memory cells recirculate through the body tissues and lymphoid organs via the blood and the thoracic duct thus allowing surveillance of the body tissues for invading microorganisms.

Antigen-induced lymphocyte proliferation normally occurs outside the blood and thoracic duct and can be visualized *in vitro* by cultivating lymphoid cells with specific antigens. Using the same experimental system, it can be demonstrated that mitogenic lectins (a lectin is a protein which binds and cross-links specific cell surface carbohydrate residues), will polyclonally stimulate lymphoid cells. These mitogenic lectins (mitogens) are derived from various plants and bacteria. Monoclonal antibody to the surface molecules CD3, TCR and one epitope of CD2, are also mitogenic. Their use *in vitro* has shown that activation of T and B cells results in the production of cytokines, for example, interleukins, and of receptors for those cytokines which together drive the cells through cell cycle (proliferation) and ultimately to effector function (maturation). Lymphocyte activation by either antigens or mitogens results in intracellular changes and subsequent development into a lymphoblast. Mitogen stimulation of lymphocytes *in vitro* is believed to mimic the series of events which occur *in vivo* following their stimulation by specific antigens.

T and B cells are activated by different mitogens. Phytohaemagglutinin (PHA) and Concanavalin A (Con A) stimulate human and mouse T cells. Lipopolysaccharide (LPS) stimulates mouse B cells. Pokeweed mitogen (PWM) stimulates both human T and B cells (Fig. 2.19).

Following T and B cell activation by mitogen or antigen, distinctive differentiation features are observed at the ultrastructural level (Figs 2.6 and 2.20). Ultimately, many B cell blasts mature into terminally differentiated plasma cells. Some B blasts do not develop rough endoplasmic reticulum cisternae. These cells are found in germinal centres and named follicle centre cells or centroblasts and centrocytes – they are the putative B memory cells (Fig. 2.21).

Under light microscopy, the cytoplasm of the plasma cell is basophilic; this is due to the large amount of RNA being utilized for antibody synthesis in the rough endoplasmic reticulum (Fig. 2.22). At the ultrastructural level, the rough endoplasmic reticulum can often be seen in parallel arrays (Fig. 2.23). Plasma cells are seldom seen in the circulation (less than 0.1% of lymphocytes) and are normally restricted to the secondary lymphoid organs and tissues. Antibodies produced by a single plasma cell are of one specificity and immunoglobulin class. Immunoglobulins are visualized in the plasma cell cytoplasm by staining with fluorochrome-labelled specific antibodies (Fig. 2.24).

nucleolus
mitochondria
lipid
granules

Fig. 2.20 Electronmicrographs showing the ultrastructure of T cell blasts. T cell blasts developing after antigen or mitogen stimulation are large cells with extended cytoplasm containing a variety of organelles, including mitochondria and free polyribosomes. The blasts may be 'agranular' (left) or granular (right) depending on the presence or absence of electron-dense granules. Note also the lipid droplets in the granular blast. Studies on T cell clones (i.e. populations derived from a single cell) have shown that in humans all cytotoxic clones are granular. Studies on the mouse have shown that both cytotoxic and suppressor clones are granular, whilst those clones without these functions are agranular. × 3200.

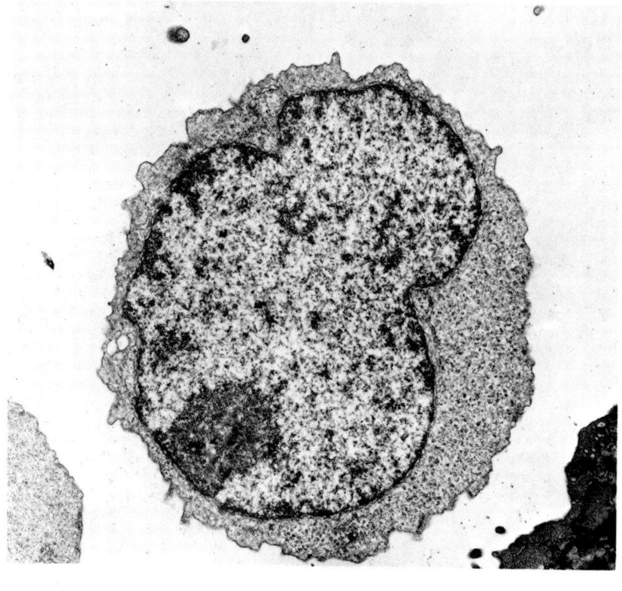

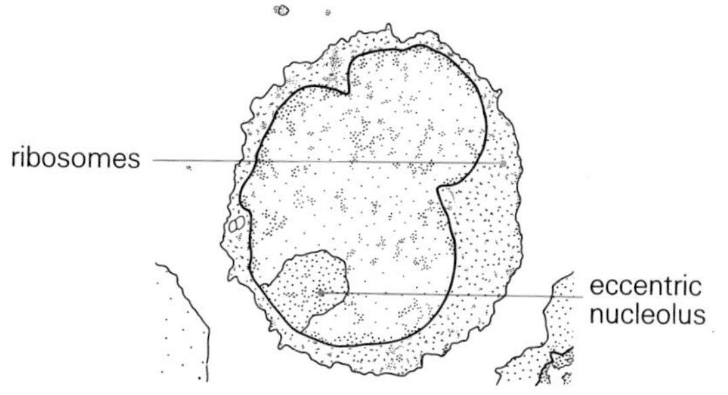

Fig. 2.21 Electronmicrograph showing a small follicle centre cell. This shows extended cytoplasm largely occupied by polyribosomes and a few strands of rough endoplasmic reticulum. The large eccentric nucleolus adjacent to the nuclear envelope is of note. This cell is frequently seen as a tumour cell in lymphomas. × 8500.

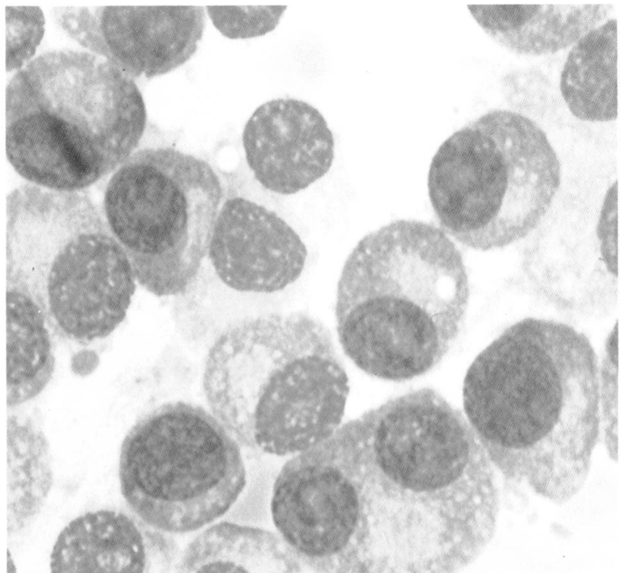

Fig. 2.22 Morphology of the plasma cell. The mature plasma cell has an eccentric nucleus and a large amount of basophilic cytoplasm, which is due to the abundant RNA required for protein synthesis. May-Grünwald-Giemsa stain, × 1500.

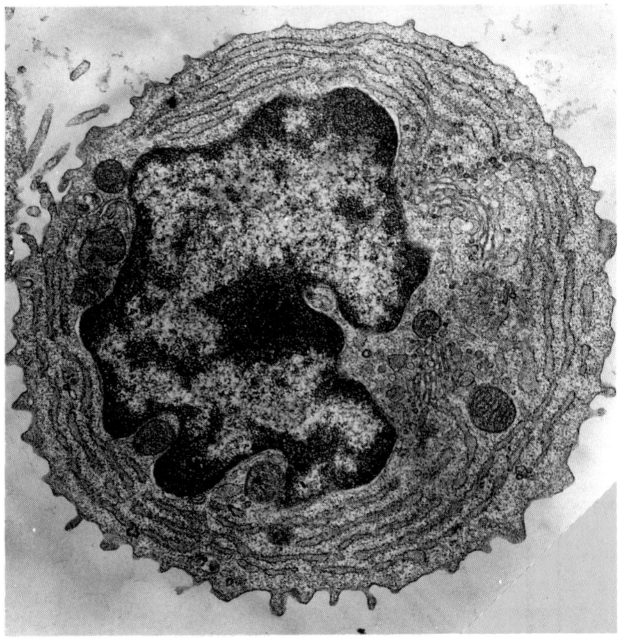

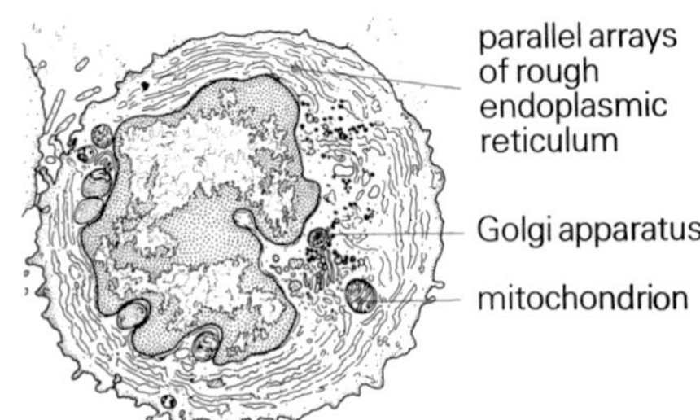

Fig. 2.23 Electronmicrograph showing the ultrastructure of the plasma cell. The plasma cell is characterized by parallel arrays of rough endoplasmic reticulum. In mature cells these cisternae become dilated with immunoglobulins. Mitochondria and a well-developed Golgi apparatus are also seen. x 9500.

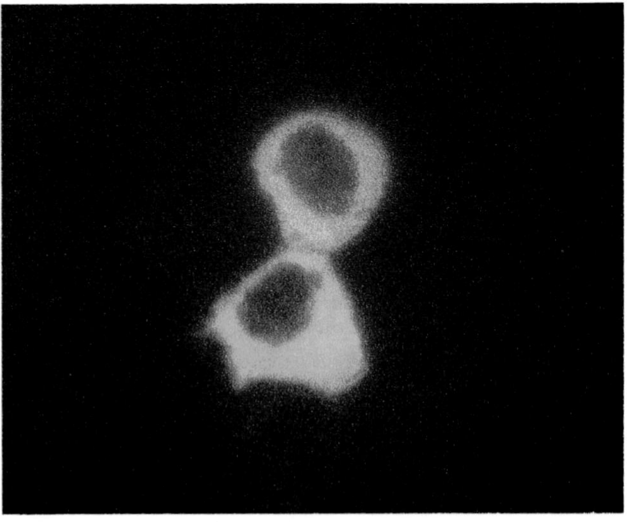

Fig. 2.24 The immunofluorescent staining of intracytoplasmic immunoglobulin in plasma cells. Fixed human plasma cells treated with fluoresceinated anti-human IgM (green) and rhodaminated anti-IgG (red) show extensive intracytoplasmic staining. The distinct staining (red or green) of the two plasma cells indicates that plasma cells normally only manufacture one class of antibody. × 3000.

ACTIVATION ANTIGENS

Activation of T or B cells increases the expression of several surface molecules and induces the *de novo* appearance of additional markers (of activation). This allows a more efficient interaction of the activated cells with other cells.

The IL-2 receptor (IL-2R) is expressed following T cell activation. This is made up of a low affinity receptor (CD25) and a larger medium affinity molecule of 70 kD. Together they make up a dimer – the high affinity IL-2R. Class II MHC molecules, transferrin receptors (important for proliferation) and CD38 are also generated on activated T cells. The latter two markers are expressed in the early phases of T cell ontogeny but disappear during intrathymic development (see Chapter 14).

Molecules which are found on activated B cells include high affinity IL-2R, but also less well defined receptors for growth and different ation factors such as IL-3, IL-4, IL-5 and IL-6 (see Chapter 8). Transferrin receptors and elevated levels of membrane class II MHC molecules are also detected. CD23 (low affinity IgE receptor) is present on murine and human activated B cells and involved in driving B cells into proliferation. Markers of terminally differentiated plasma cells not found on earlier stages of activation are the CD38 and PCA-1 molecules.

TPCs are activated by interaction with the appropriate target and T cell derived lymphokines such as IL-2 and IFNγ. This results in an increase in their cytolytic ability and the expression of additional markers, notably HLA–DR, class II MHC molecules.

MONONUCLEAR PHAGOCYTIC SYSTEM (MONOCYTES)

Bone marrow derived stem cells give rise to the cells of the mononuclear phagocyte system which has two main

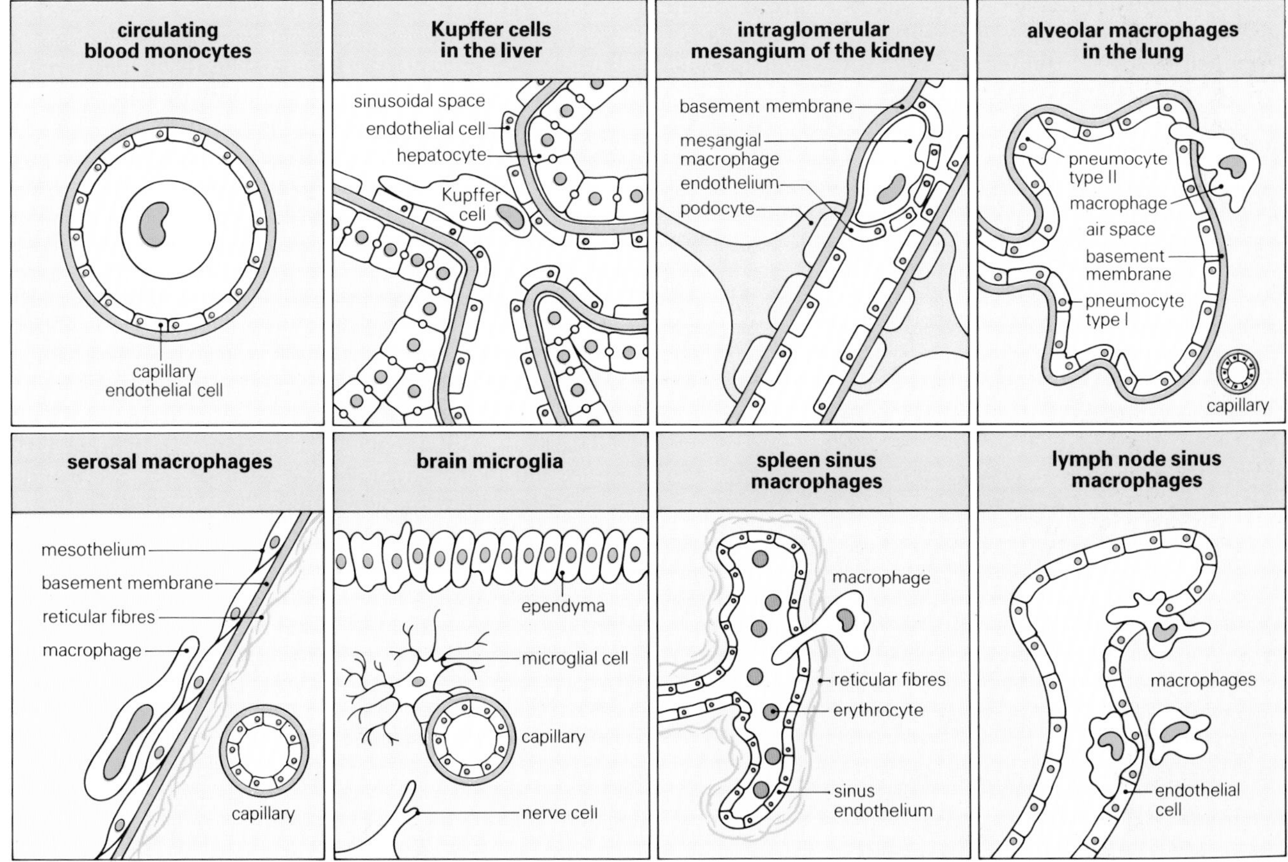

Fig. 2.25 The mononuclear phagocyte system. The cells of this system include circulating blood monocytes, and dispersed phagocytes in connective tissue or fixed to the endothelial layer of the blood capillaries which in the liver are known as Kupffer cells. Endothelium-fixed phagocytes include the intraglomerular mesangial cells in the kidney. Alveolar and serosal macrophages are examples of 'wandering' macrophages, while brain microglia are cells which enter the brain around the time of birth and differentiate into fixed tissue cells.

functions, performed by the following two different types of cells:

1. the 'professional' phagocytic macrophages whose predominant role is to remove particulate antigens
2. antigen-presenting cells (APCs) whose role is to present antigen to specific lymphocytes.

THE RETICULOENDOTHELIAL SYSTEM

The phagocytic tissue macrophages form a network – the reticuloendothelial system (RES) which is found in many organs (Fig. 2.25). Intravenously injected carbon particles become localized in these tissues (Fig. 2.26).

Progenitors common to the granulocytic and monocytic series give rise to promonocytes in the bone marrow (see Chapter 14). These differentiate into blood monocytes which represent a circulating pool and migrate into the various organs and tissue systems to become macrophages. Since the blood monocyte is the most easily obtainable phagocytic cell of this class it has been studied in greatest detail. The human blood monocyte is large (10–18 μm diameter) relative to the lymphocyte; it usually has a horseshoe-shaped nucleus and often contains faint azurophilic granules (Fig. 2.27). Ultrastructurally, the monocyte possesses ruffled membranes, a well-developed Golgi complex and many intracytoplasmic lysosomes (Fig. 2.28). These lysosomes contain several acid hydrolases and peroxidase which is important in intracellular killing of microorganisms.

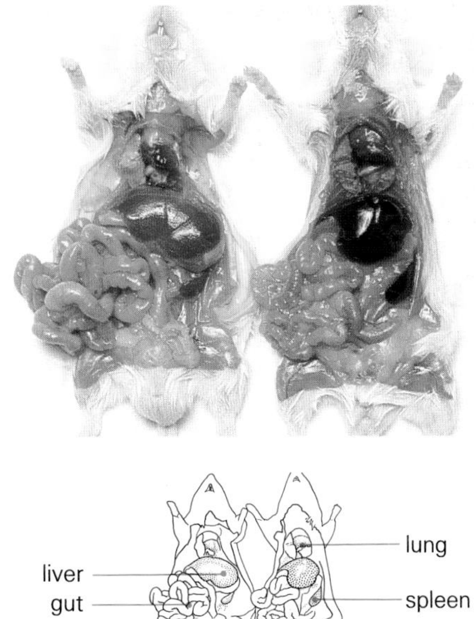

Fig. 2.26 Localization of intravenously injected particles in the reticuloendothelial system. A mouse was injected intravenously with fine carbon particles and killed 5 minutes later. Carbon accumulates in organs rich in mononuclear phagocytes – lungs, liver, spleen and areas of the gut wall. The normal organ colour is shown in the control mouse on the left.

Monocytes/macrophages will adhere strongly to glass and plastic surfaces and will actively phagocytose organisms or even tumour cells *in vitro*. Ingestion and adherence by monocytes is promoted when the cells bind the microorganisms through specialized receptors for certain carbohydrates, IgG and complement, with which the microorganism is coated.

Mannosyl-fucosyl receptors (MFR) on human and murine monocyte/macrophages can bind to non-encapsulated microorganisms carrying these surface sugars. There are three distinct Fc receptors for IgG on human and murine macrophages. $Fc_{\gamma}RI$ on human cells has a high affinity for IgG. This is homologous to the $Fc_{\gamma}R2a$ receptor in the mouse. $Fc_{\gamma}RII$ (CDw32) is of medium affinity and is equivalent to the $Fc_{\gamma}R2b/1$ receptor in the mouse and $Fc_{\gamma}RIII$ or FcR1o (CD16), has low affinity. These receptors probably have different functions which include triggering extracellular killing, opsonization and phagocytosis. This function is also performed by other molecules including the CR1 (C3b receptor, CD35). Other molecules, probably involved mainly in adhesion include CR3 (C3bi receptor, CD11b, MAC-1), present especially on activated macrophages together with the 'leucocyte function antigens' LFA-1 (CD11a) and p150/95 kD (CD11c). Both CD11b and CD11c are found in intracytoplasmic vesicles and are rapidly expressed following activation. Class II MHC antigens are present on some of the monocytes/macrophages and are important in presentation of antigens to T cells. A low affinity receptor for the Fc of IgE (CD23) is also present on some macrophages. Other molecules found primarily on human macrophages include CD13, CD14 and CD15. It should be stressed that none of these markers discussed are lineage specific. Lineage specific markers in the mouse include F4.80(160 kD), sheep erythrocyte receptor (SER, not to be confused with CD2) and erythroblast receptor (EbR). The latter two are also site specific . The main markers on human and mouse monocytes are summarized in Fig. 2.29. In addition to all of these molecules, monocytes and macrophages must also have receptors for lymphokines such as IFNY and migration inhibition factor.

Like neutrophils, monocytes and macrophages contain peroxidase, which inactivates peroxide ions generated during killing of ingested microorganisms.

The functions of monocytes and macrophages can be enhanced by factors released from T cells. Monocyte/macrophages also produce complement components,

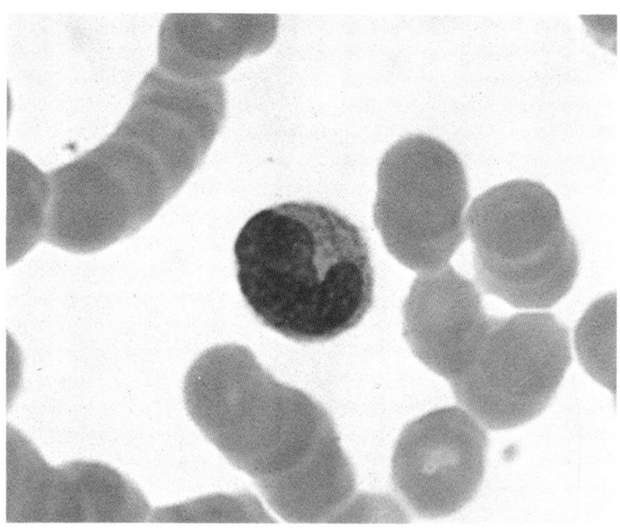

Fig. 2.27 Morphology of the monocyte. Blood monocytes have a characteristic horseshoe-shaped nucleus and are larger than most circulating lymphocytes. Giemsa stain, × 1200.

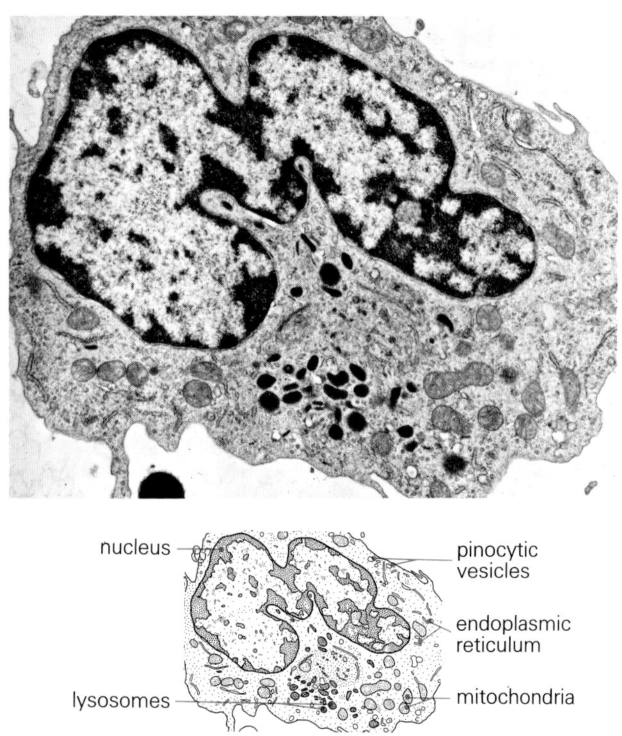

Fig. 2.28 Electronmicrograph showing the ultrastructure of the monocyte. This shows the horseshoe-shaped nucleus, pinocytic vesicles, lysosomal granules, mitochondria and isolated rough endoplasmic reticulum cisternae. × 8000. (Courtesy of Dr B.Nichols; from the *Journal of Cell Biology* 1971, **50,** 498, by copyright permission Rockefeller University Press.)

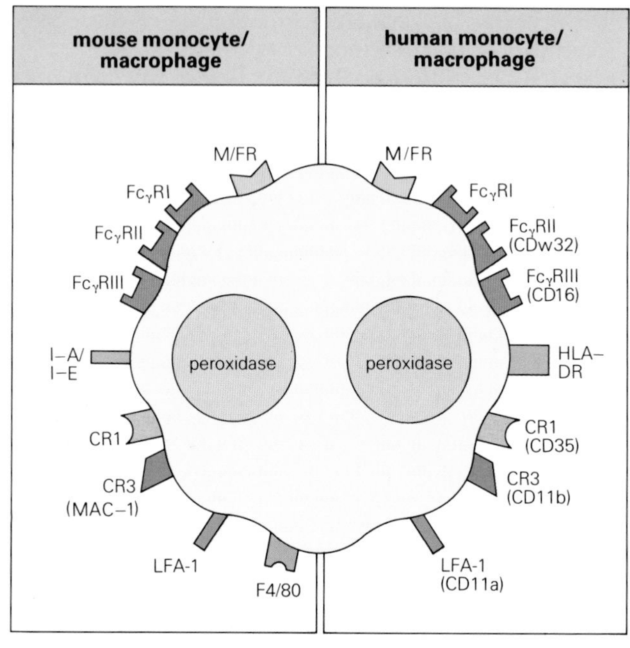

Fig. 2.29 Summary of the main surface markers on mouse and human monocytes/macrophages. Equivalent molecules are shown in the same colour.

prostaglandins, interferons and monokines such as interleukin-1 and tumour necrosis factor (TNF) (see Chapter 9).

ANTIGEN-PRESENTING CELLS

APCs are a heterogeneous population of leucocytes with exquisite immunostimulatory capacity. Some have a pivotal role in the induction of funtional activity of T- helper cells; some communicate with other leucocytes. Cells other than leucocytes can acquire the ability to 'present' antigens under the influence of cytokines. This usually corresponds to the induction of class II MHC molecules by cells which do not normally express them, for example, endothelial cells.

APCs are found primarily in the skin, lymph nodes, spleen and thymus (Fig. 2.30). The archetypal APC is the Langerhans' cell in the skin. These cells with characteristic 'tennis-racket' granules termed Birbeck granules migrate via the afferent lymphatics as 'veiled cells' into the paracortex of the draining lymph nodes. Within the paracortex the cells 'interdigitate' with many T cells (Fig. 2.31) providing an efficient mechanism to present antigen carried from the skin to T cells in the draining lymph nodes. These APCs are rich in class II MHC molecules which are important for presenting antigen to the $CD4^+$ T cells.

Other specialized APCs, the follicular dendritic cells, are found in the secondary follicles of the B cell areas of the lymph nodes and spleen and communicate with B cells; these APCs lack class II MHC molecules, and possess CR1 (CD35). Some markers on different kinds of APCs are shown in Fig. 2.32.

Recently APCs have been found in the thymus. These interdigitating cells which are especially abundant in the thymic medulla are rich in self antigens (including class II MHC molecules). The thymus is of crucial importance in the development and maturation of T cells. It appears that the immature T cells learn to discriminate self antigens from non-self antigens during this maturation step. The interdigitating cells carry self antigen and are therefore thought to play a role in selecting out T cells that react against self antigen.

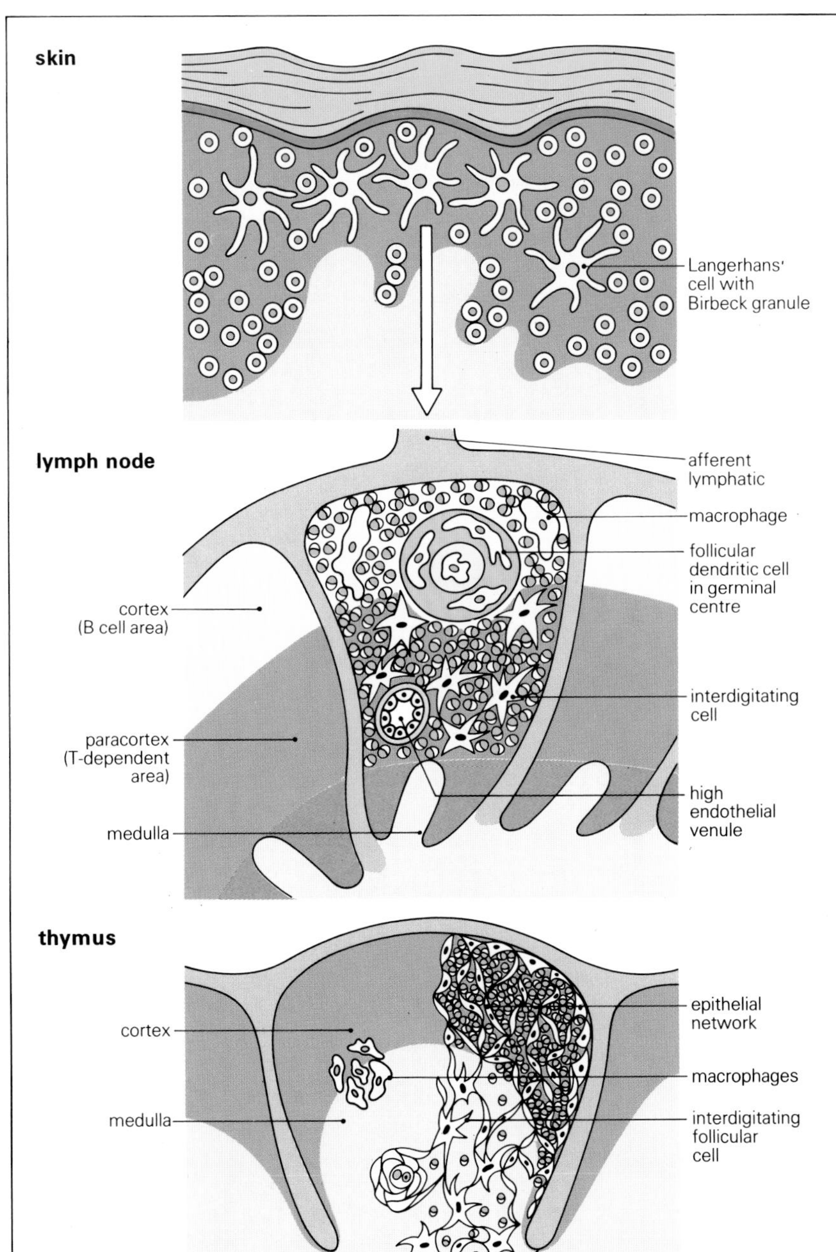

Fig. 2.30 Antigen-presenting cells. Bone-marrow derived antigen-presenting cells (APCs) are found especially in lymphoid tissues and in the skin. APCs are represented in the skin by Langerhans' cells, present in the epidermis and characterized by specialized granules (the tennis racket-shaped Birbeck granules). These cells, rich in Ia (mouse) or HLA–DR (human) determinants, are believed to carry antigens and migrate via the afferent lymphatics (where they appear as 'veiled' cells) into the paracortex of the draining lymph nodes where they interdigitate with T cells. These 'interdigitating cells' localized in the T cell-dependent areas of the lymph node present antigen to the antigen-sensitive lymphocytes. Follicular dendritic cells are found in the B cell areas of the lymph nodes and in particular in the germinal centres. Some macrophages located in the outer cortex and marginal sinus may also act as APCs. In the thymus, APCs occur as interdigitating follicular cells.

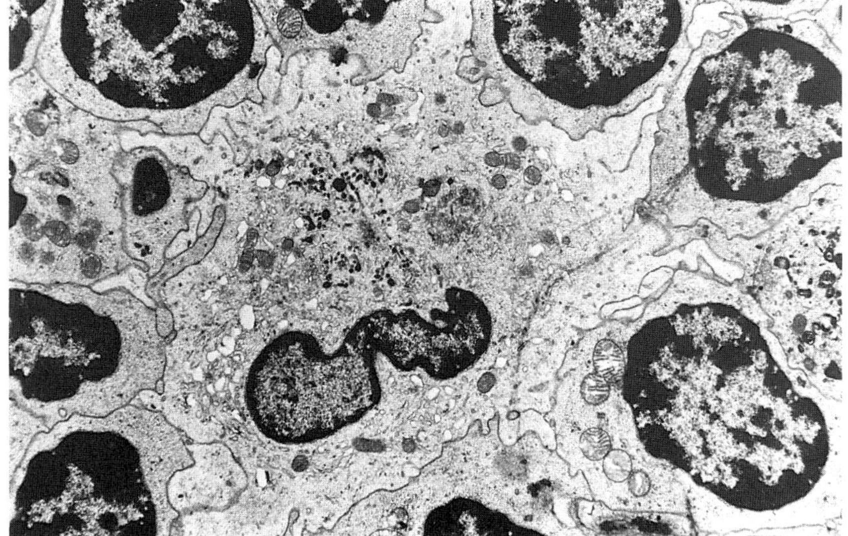

Fig. 2.31 Electronmicrograph showing the ultrastructure of an interdigitating cell (IDC) in the T cell area of the rat lymph node. Intimate contacts are made with the membranes of the surrounding T cells. The cytoplasm contains relatively few organelles and does not show the Birbeck granules characteristic of the skin Langerhans' cell, but these appear after antigenic stimulation. × 2000. (Courtesy of Dr B. H. Balfour.)

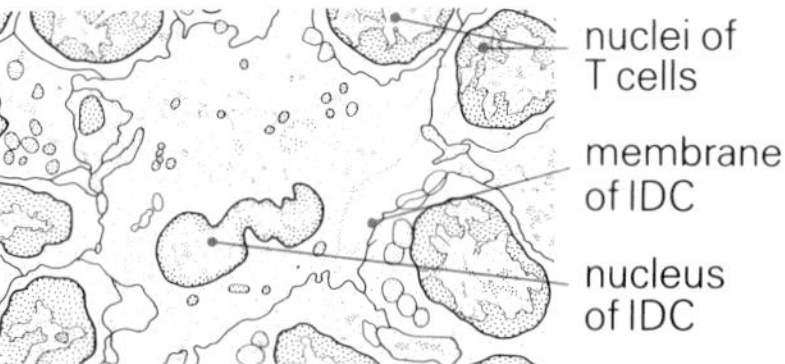

markers	Langerhans' cells	interdigitating cells	follicular dendritic cells	B cells	macrophages
MHC class II	+	+	−	+	(+)
$Fc_{\gamma}R$	+	−	+	+	+
CR1 (CD35)	+	−	+	+	+
phagocyte function	−	−	−	−	+

Fig. 2.32 Markers on different antigen-presenting cells. The Langerhans' cells (LCs) and interdigitating cells derived from them are rich in class II MHC for communicating with $CD4^+$ T cells. LCs also possess receptors for IgG and C3b (CR1). Follicular dendritic cells located within the secondary follicles do not express class II MHC but have high levels of $Fc\gamma R$ and the type I complement receptor (CR 1) to enable them to trap immune complexes and interact with B cells. B cells and macrophages are also efficient as antigen-presenting cells and have been included for completeness.

B cells which are rich in class II MHC molecules (especially after 'activation') have also been shown to be efficient in processing and presenting antigen particularly when the B cell is specific for the antigen being presented (see Chapter 8).

It is now clear that many somatic cells of the body normally do not express class II MHC molecules. However, cytokines such as IFNγ and TNF can induce these molecules and thus potentiate antigen presentation. It has been suggested that such induction of expression of 'inappropriate' class II MHC molecules might contribute to the pathogenesis of a variety of autoimmune diseases.

THE POLYMORPHONUCLEAR GRANULOCYTES (POLYMORPHS) AND PLATELETS

Granulocytes are produced in the bone marrow at a rate of 80 million/minute and are short-lived (2/3 days) relative to monocyte/macrophages which may live for months or years. Granulocytes represent about 60–70% of the total normal blood leucocytes but are also found in extravascular sites. Polymorphs are able to adhere to and penetrate the endothelial cells lining the blood vessels. As the name suggests, the mature forms usually contain a multilobed nucleus and many granules. They are classified into neutrophils, eosinophils and basophils on the basis of the staining reaction of their granules by histological dyes.

Although polymorphs do not show any specificity for antigens they play an important role in acute inflammation and, together with antibodies and complement, in protection against microorganisms. Their predominant role is phagocytosis and their importance in protection is emphasized by the great increase in susceptibility to infections found in individuals with low numbers of circulating polymorphs.

NEUTROPHILS

Neutrophils represent over 90% of the circulating granulocytes and are 10–20 μm in diameter (Fig. 2.33).

A variety of chemotactic agents for neutrophils are activated complement components, for example C5a, or are derived from the fibrinolytic and kinin generating systems, or are products derived from other leucocytes, platelets and certain bacteria. Margination (adhesion to endothelial cells) and diapedesis (movement through the capillary wall) occurs when a chemoattractant is produced in intravascular sites.

Neutrophils possess two main types of granules. The primary (azurophilic) granules (lysosomes) contain acid hydrolases, myeloperoxidase and muramidase (lysozyme) whilst the secondary or specific granules contain

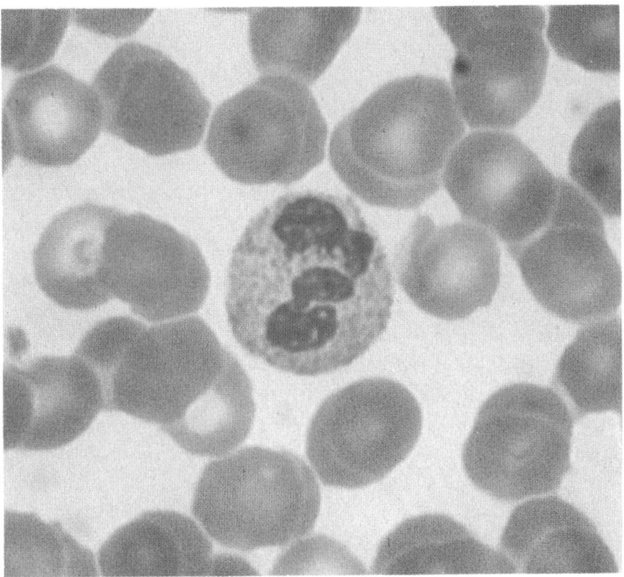

Fig. 2.33 Morphology of the neutrophil. This shows a neutrophil with its characteristic multilobed nucleus and neutrophilic granules in the cytoplasm. Giemsa stain, × 1500.

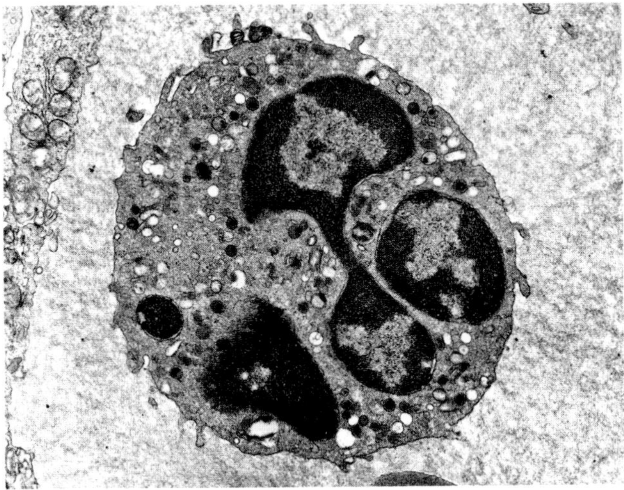

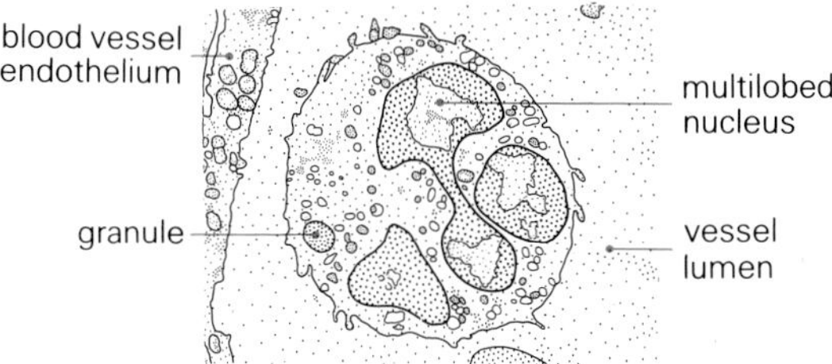

Fig. 2.34 Electronmicrograph showing the ultrastructure of the neutrophil. This mouse neutrophil lies within a skin blood vessel. The neutrophil cytoplasm contains primary and secondary granules of different electron opacity. × 6000. (Courtesy of Dr D. McLaren.)

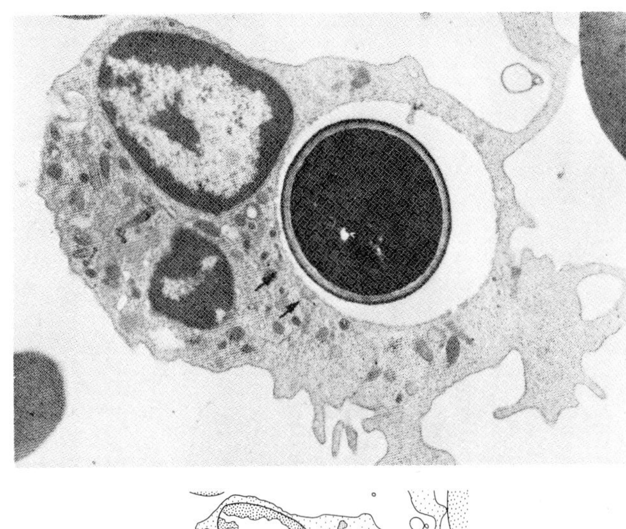

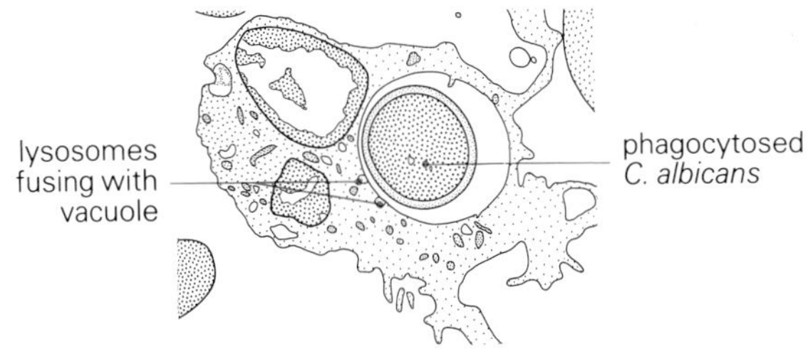

Fig. 2.35 Electronmicrograph showing a neutrophil containing phagocytosed *Candida albicans*. Two lysosomal granules may be seen fusing with the vacuole containing the organism. × 7000. (Courtesy of Dr H. Validimarsson.)

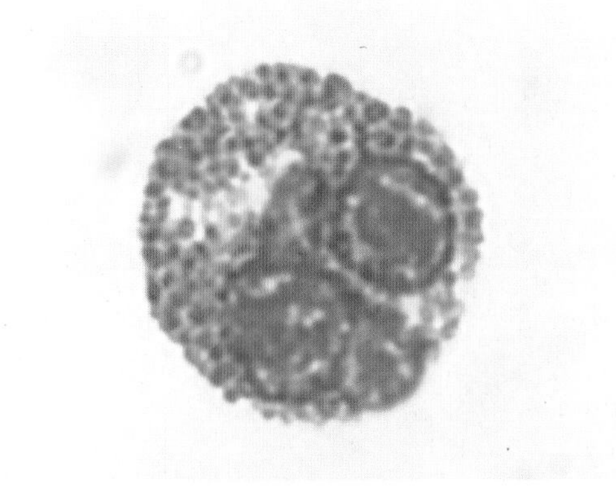

Fig. 2.36 Morphology of the eosinophil. This blood smear enriched for granulocytes shows an eosinophil with a multilobed nucleus and heavily stained cytoplasmic granules. Leishman stain, × 1800.

lactoferrin in addition to lysozyme. These granules can be seen at the ultrastructural level (Fig. 2.34). Ingested organisms are contained within vacuoles termed phagosomes which fuse with the enzyme-containing granules to form phagolysosomes (Fig. 2.35).

Extracellular release of granules and cytotoxic substances may also occur on stimulation with appropriate stimuli, such as Fc of IgG in the form of complexes. This might be an important pathogenic mechanism in immune complex diseases (type III hypersensitivity, see Chapter 21).

EOSINOPHILS

Eosinophils comprise 2–5% of blood leucocytes in healthy, non-allergic individuals (Fig. 2.36). Like neutrophils they appear to be capable of phagocytosing and killing ingested microorganisms, although it is not their primary function. The granules in mature eosinophils are membrane-bound organelles with a 'crystalloid' or 'core' differing in electron opacity from the surrounding matrix (Fig. 2.37). Human blood eosinophils usually have only a bilobed nucleus and many cytoplasmic granules.

Eosinophils (as well as basophils and mast cells described below) can be triggered to degranulate by appropriate stimuli. Degranulation involves fusion of the intracellular granules with the plasma membrane. The contents are released to the outside of the cell. This type of reaction is the only way that these cells can use their 'granule armament' against large targets which cannot be phagocytosed. Eosinophils are thought to play a specialized role in immunity to helminth infections using this mechanism (see Chapter 17)

Eosinophils are attracted by products released from T cells, mast cells and basophils (eosinophil chemotactic factor of anaphylaxis, ECF-A). They bind schistosomulae coated with IgG or IgE, degranulate, and release a toxic protein ('major basic protein'). Eosinophils release histaminase and aryl sulphatase, which inactivate the mast cell products histamine and slow reactive substance of anaphylaxis (SRS-A), respectively.The net effect of these factors is to dampen down the inflammatory response and reduce granulocyte migration into the site of invasion.

BASOPHILS AND MAST CELLS

Basophils are found in very small numbers in the circulation (less than 0.2% of leucocytes) and are characterized by deep violet-blue granules (Fig. 2.38). The mast cell is often indistinguishable from the basophil in a number of its properties and although they are both of bone marrow origin its relationship to the basophil is not completely clear.

There are two different kinds of mast cell; one is mucosa-associated (MMC), and the other is found in the connective tissue (CTMC). MMCs appear to be dependent on T cells for their proliferation, while the CTMCs are T cell independent. Under light microscopy, they can be visualized with Alcian blue (Fig. 2.39).

Mature blood basophils have randomly distributed granules surrounded by membranes (Fig. 2.40). These granules in both basophils and mast cells contain heparin, SRS-A and ECF-A, and these are released on degranulation (Fig. 2.41) initiated by the appropriate stimulus. This is usually an allergen which cross-links specific IgE

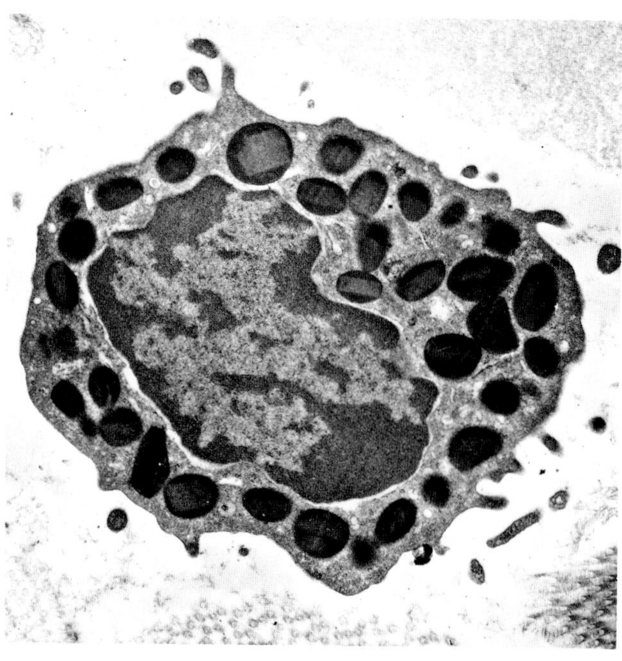

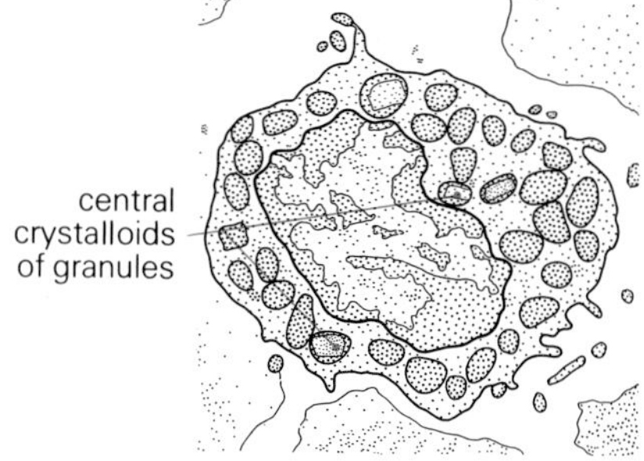

Fig. 2.37 Electronmicrograph showing the ultrastructure of a guinea-pig eosinophil. The mature eosinophil contains granules with central crystalloids. × 8000. (Courtesy of Dr D. McLaren.)

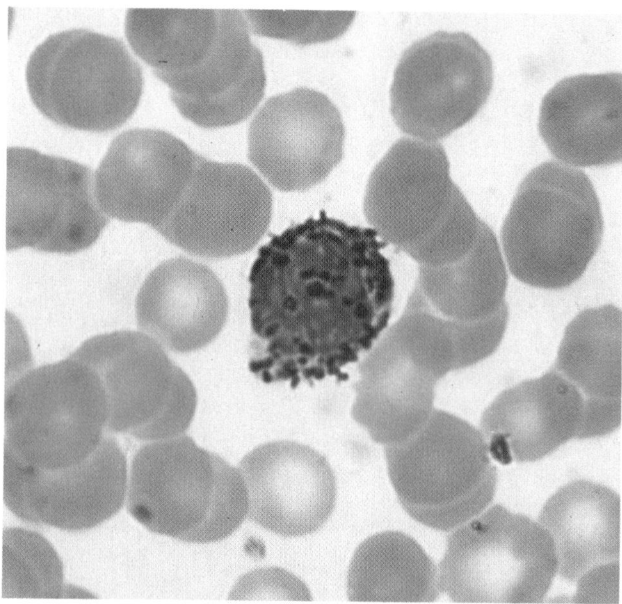

Fig. 2.38 Morphology of the basophil. This blood smear shows a typical basophil with its deep violet-blue granules. Wright's stain, × 1500.

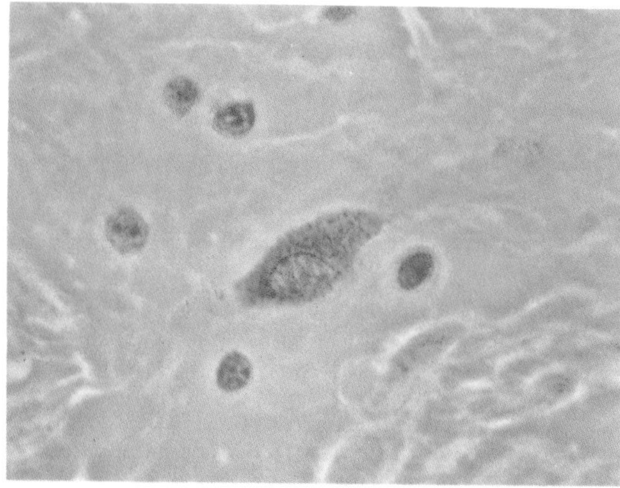

Fig. 2.39 Histological appearance of human connective tissue mast cells. This micrograph shows the dark blue cytoplasm with brownish granules. Alcian blue and Safranin, × 600. (Courtesy of Dr T. S. Orr.)

molecules bound to the surface of the mast cell or basophil via high affinity Fc receptors for IgE. Pharmacological mediators released following degranulation cause the adverse symptoms of allergy but, on the positive side, they may also play a role in immunity against parasites. Granulocyte and mast cell functional markers are summarized in Fig. 2.42.

PLATELETS

The final myeloid cell to be considered here is the blood platelet. Platelets are derived from large megakaryocytes in the bone marrow and contain granules at the ultrastructural level (Fig. 2.43). In addition to their role in blood clotting, platelets are also involved in the immune response, especially in inflammation. They possess class I MHC products and receptors for IgG (FcγRII), and

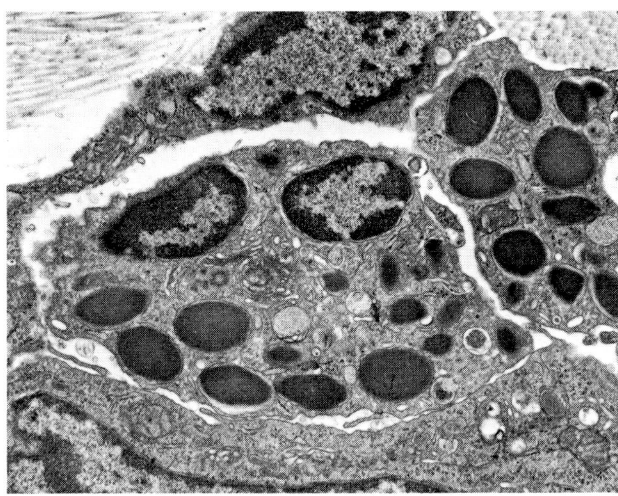

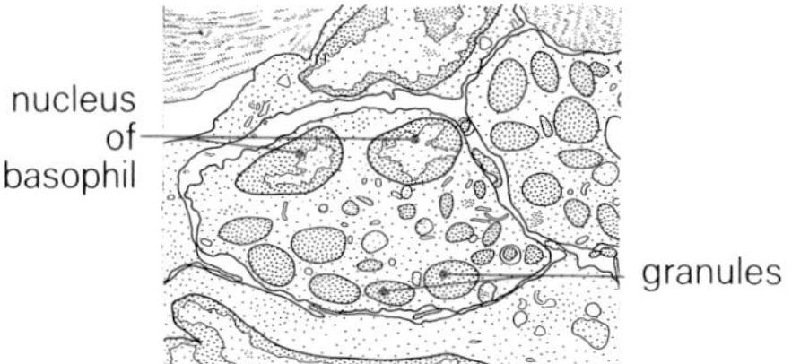

Fig. 2.40 Electronmicrograph showing the ultrastructure of the basophil. Basophils in guinea-pig skin showing the characteristic randomly distributed granules. × 6000. (Courtesy of Dr D. McLaren.)

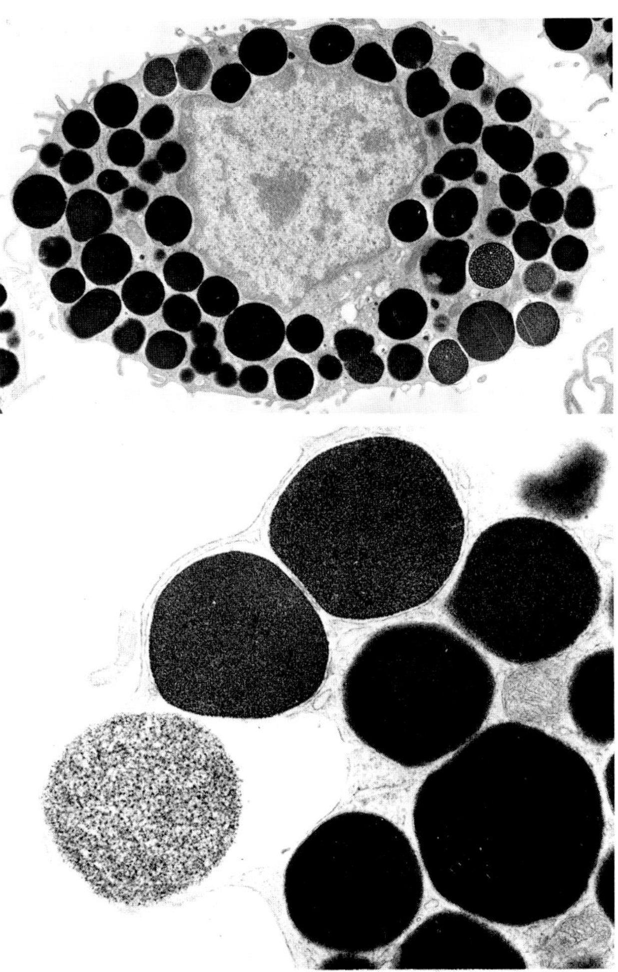

Fig. 2.41 Electronmicrographs of rat peritoneal mast cells. The non-degranulated cell with its electron-dense granules (upper, × 6000) and a granule in exocytosis (lower, × 30,000) are shown. (Courtesy of Dr T. S. C. Orr.)

	FcR IgE (low affinity)	FcR IgE (high affinity)	FcγRIII (CD16)	C5aR	CR1 (CD35)	CR3 (CD11b)	peroxidase	acid phosphatase	alkaline phosphatase
neutrophils	–	–	+	+	+	+	+	+	+
eosinophils	+	–	+	+	+	+	+	+	
basophils	–	+	+	+	+	+	+		
mast cells	–	+	+	+	+	+		+	+

Fig. 2.42 Granulocyte and mast cell functional markers. All cells possess low affinity Fc receptors for IgG (CD16, FcRIII). Only basophils and mast cells have high affinity receptors for IgE. All cells carry receptors for complement components; receptors for C5a are important in chemotaxis; CR1 and CR3 are involved in adhesion and phagocytosis. The granules in different cell types vary qualitatively in their enzyme content. Additional markers that have been defined by monoclonal antibodies include the following: LFA-1, found on all these cell types and clearly shown to be involved in cell adhesion, is made up of an α chain (CD11a) and a β chain (CD18); the CR3 molecule illustrated in the table is made up of an α chain (CD11b) associated with the same β chain (CD18) as for LFA-1. Several other glycoproteins including CD13 and CD14 (weakly expressed) are found on some granulocytes. In addition, glycolipid molecules such as the Le x hapten (CD15) and lactosyl ceramide (CD17) are expressed by these cells.

low affinity receptors for IgE. In addition, megakaryocytes and platelets carry receptors for factor VIII and other molecules important for their function such as Gp 11b/111a (CDw41) and Gp 1b (CDw42). These latter two receptors are important in binding fibrinogen and Von Willebrand factor, respectively. Following endothelial injury, platelets adhere to and aggregate at the endothelial surface releasing permeability increasing substances and factors responsible for activating complement components to attract leucocytes.

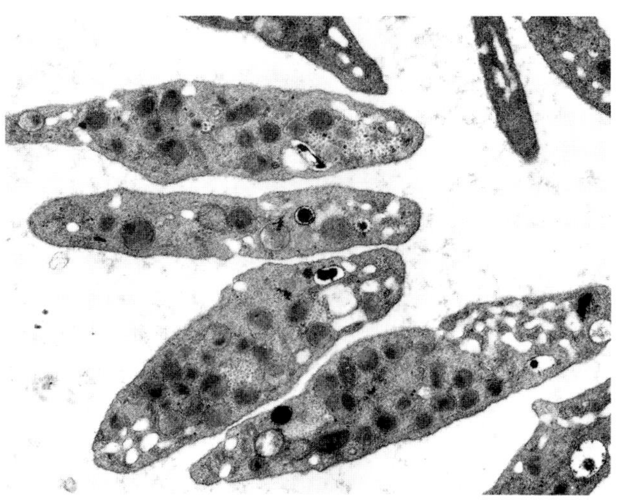

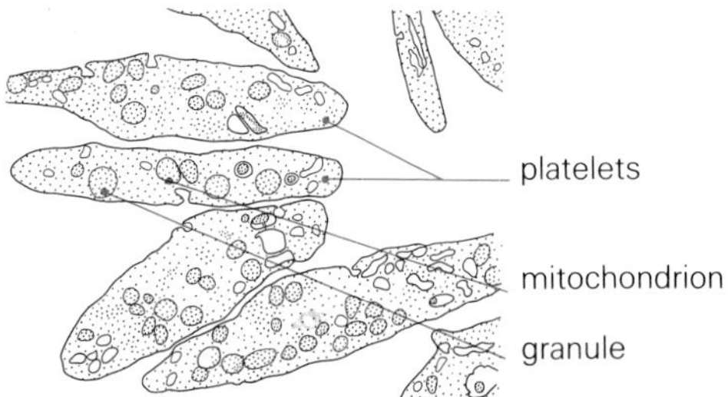

Fig. 2.43 Electronmicrograph showing the platelet ultrastructure. The cytoplasmic organelles, including granules and mitochondria, are randomly dispersed. × 20,000. (Courtesy of Dr J. G. White.)

FURTHER READING

Cohn, Z.A. (ed.) (1988) Innate immunity. *Current Opinion in Immunology*, **1(1)**. London: Current Science Ltd.

Jarrett, E.E.E. & Haig, D.M. (1984) Mucosal mast cells *in vivo* and *in vitro*. *Immunology Today*, **5**, 115.

Lydyard, P.M. (ed.) (1988) Immune response. *Current Opinion in Immunology*, **1(2)**. London: Current Science Ltd.

Lydyard, P.M., Banga, P., Guarnotta, G., Walker, P., Mackenzie, L. & Mackanday, S. (1985) Human lymphocyte antigens – a mini review. *Transactions of the Biochemical Society* (in press).

Playfair, J.H.L. (1984) *Immunology at a Glance*, 2nd edition. Oxford: Blackwell Scientific Publications.

Roitt, I.M. (1984) *Essential Immunology*, 5th edition. Oxford: Blackwell Scientific Publications.

Unanue, E.R. & Allen, P.M. (1987) The basis for the immunoregulatory role of macrophages and other sensory cells. *Science*, **236**, 551.

Zucker-Franklin, D., Greaves, M.F., Grossi, C.E. & Marmont, A.M. (1980) *Atlas of Blood Cells: Function and Pathology*. Milan: Edi. Ermes and Philadelphia: Lea & Febiger.

3 The Lymphoid System

The cells involved in the immune response are organized into tissues and organs in order to perform their functions most effectively. These structures are collectively referred to as the lymphoid system and are illustrated and described below.

PRIMARY AND SECONDARY LYMPHOID TISSUES

The lymphoid system is comprised of lymphocytes, epithelial cells and stromal cells, and is arranged into either discretely capsulated organs or accumulations of diffuse lymphoid tissue. Lymphoid organs contain lymphocytes at various stages of development and are classified into either primary/central lymphoid organs or secondary/peripheral lymphoid organs (Fig. 3.1).

Primary lymphoid organs are the major sites of lymphopoiesis. Here, lymphocytes differentiate from lymphoid stem cells, proliferate and mature into functional cells. In mammals, including man, T lymphocytes are produced in the thymus and B lymphocytes in the fetal liver and bone marrow. In avian species there is a specialized site of B cell generation, the bursa of Fabricius. In the primary lymphoid organs the lymphocytes acquire their repertoire of specific antigen receptors in order to cope with the antigenic challenges the individual receives during its life. They also learn to discriminate between self antigens, which are tolerated, and non-self antigens which are generally not tolerated.

Secondary lymphoid organs include lymph nodes, spleen and mucosa associated tissues, including the tonsils and Peyer's patches of the gut. The secondary lymphoid tissue creates the environment in which lymphocytes can interact with each other and with antigens and disseminates the immune response once generated. These functions are performed by phagocytic macrophages, antigen-presenting cells, and mature T and B lymphocytes in the secondary lymphoid organs.

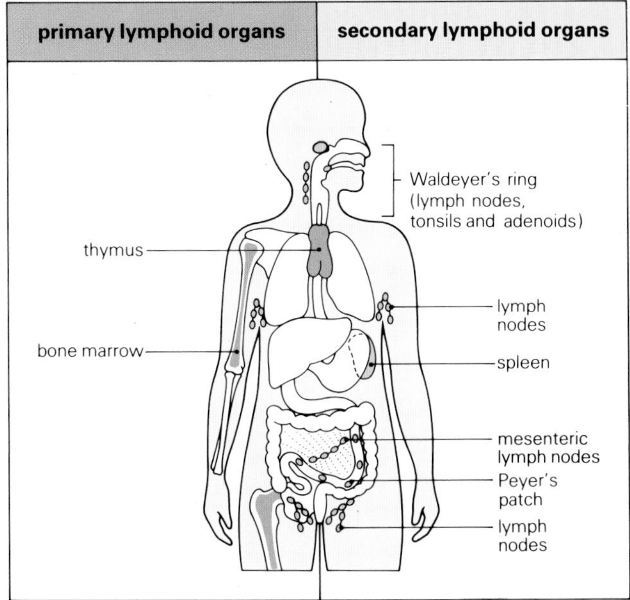

Fig. 3.1 Major lymphoid organs and tissues. The thymus produces T cells and the bone marrow, B cells. The secondary lymphoid organs and tissues contain mature T and B cells and accessory cells. In the mammalian fetus the B cells are initially generated in the liver. In man the adult bone marrow is also a secondary lymphoid organ. Lymph nodes are present throughout the body (only a few are depicted here) and are usually found at the junctions of lymphatic vessels. The group of lymph nodes including the tonsillar and adenoidal lymphoid tissue in the area of the neck and throat is called the Waldeyer's ring of lymphoid tissue. Lymph nodes drain the tissue spaces and the lymphocytes at these sites generally respond to lymph-borne antigens whilst lymphoid cells in the spleen respond to blood-borne antigens. Peyer's patches are unencapsulated masses of lymphoid tissue in the small intestine.

PRIMARY LYMPHOID ORGANS

THE THYMUS

The thymus in mammals is bilobed, located in the thorax and overlies the heart and major blood vessels. Each lobe is organized into lobules separated from each other by connective tissue trabeculae (Fig. 3.2). Within each

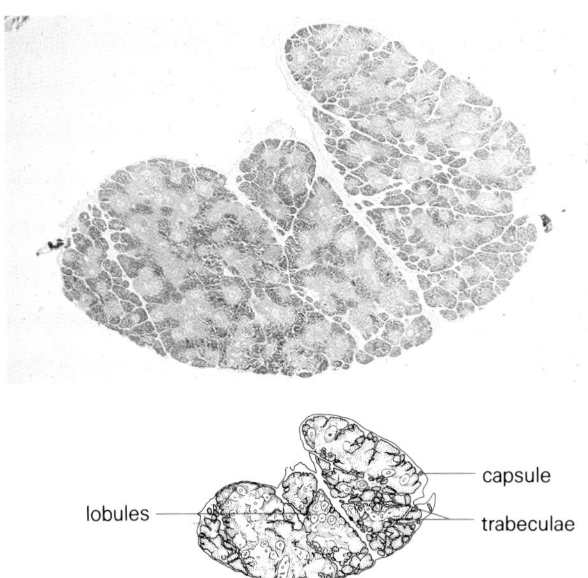

Fig. 3.2 Thymus section showing the lobular structure. This low power cross-section shows a fibrous capsule with the thymocytes (young T lymphocytes) organized into lobules separated from each other by connective tissue trabeculae. H & E stain, × 3.5

lobule the lymphoid cells (thymocytes) are arranged into an outer cortex and an inner medulla (Fig. 3.3). The tightly packed cortex contains the majority of relatively immature proliferating cells whilst the medulla contains more mature cells, implying a differentiation gradient from cortex to medulla. There is a network of epithelial cells throughout the lobules which probably plays a role in the differentiation process from bone marrow stem cells to T lymphocytes. In addition, interdigitating cells (derived from bone marrow) are associated with the epithelial network especially in the medulla. These cells, which are rich in the major histocompatibility (MHC) class II antigens, are thought to be important in the process of learning to recognize self antigens in the thymus (see Chapter 14); MHC class II antigens are important in regulating interactions between cells of the immune system and in determining how antigen is recognized by the helper T cells.

Hassal's corpuscles are found in the thymic medulla. Their function is unknown but they appear to contain degenerating epithelial cells.

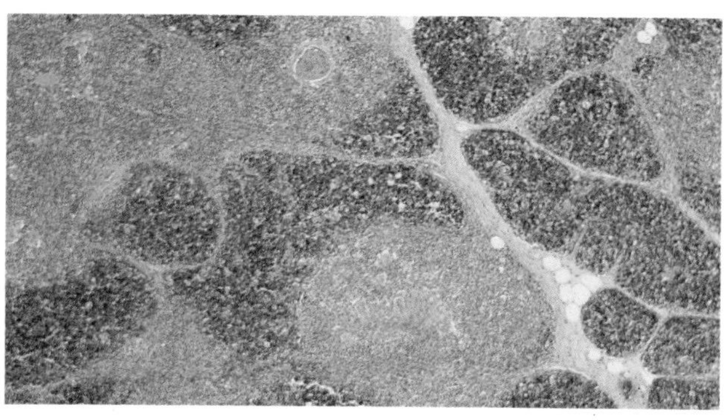

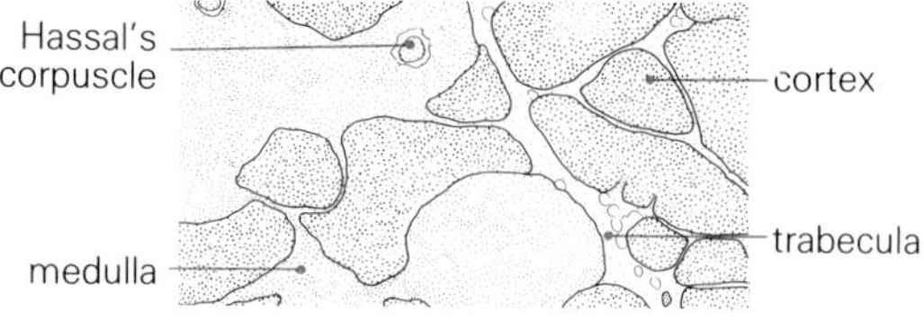

Fig. 3.3 Thymus section showing the lobular organization. This section shows the lobules to consist of two main areas – an outer cortex of rapidly dividing immature cells and an inner medulla of more mature cells. Structures of unknown function called Hassall's corpuscles are found in the medulla. H & E stain. × 25.

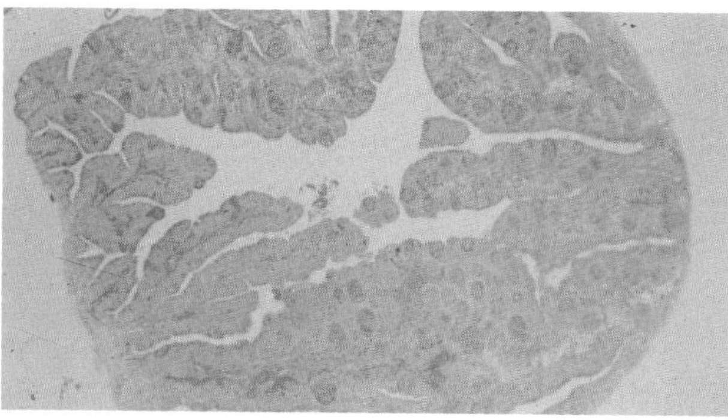

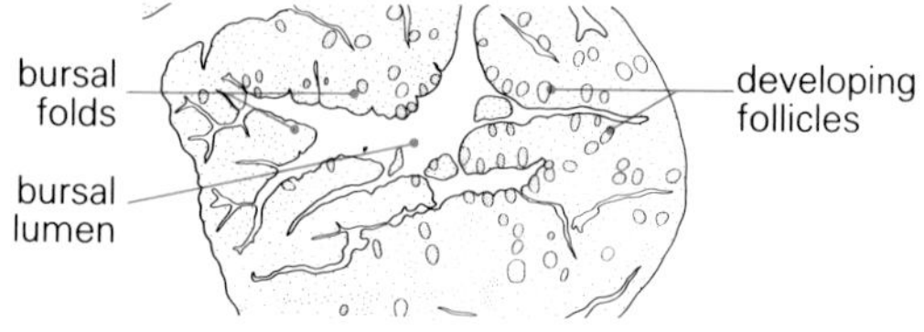

Fig. 3.4 Bursa section showing the follicular structure. The avian bursa of Fabricius is a lympho-epithelial organ (like the thymus) and is found dorsal to the hindgut. The lumen of the bursa opens into the cloaca. The bursa is composed of folds or plicae directed into the central lumen and the follicles are arranged along their surfaces in close contact with the surface epithelium. Like the thymic lobules, bursal follicles are arranged into an outer cortex and inner medulla. The bursa, like the thymus, atrophies with age. H & E stain, × 10.

THE BURSA OF FABRICIUS AND ITS MAMMALIAN EQUIVALENT

In birds, B cells differentiate in the bursa of Fabricius, hence the name 'B' cells. The bursa is like a modified piece of intestine with plicae directed towards a central lumen (Fig. 3.4). The bursal follicles are organized into cortex and medulla and lie along the margins of the plicae. Mammals have no bursa; instead, islands of haemopoietic cells in the fetal liver and in the fetal and adult bone marrow give rise directly to B lymphocytes. As well as being a site of B cell generation, the adult bone marrow contains many mature T cells and plasma cells, that is, in man, it is also an important secondary lymphoid organ.

SECONDARY LYMPHOID ORGANS

The generation of lymphocytes in primary lymphoid organs is followed by their migration into the secondary peripheral organs – 'lymphocyte traffic'. The secondary lymphoid organs include the well organized encapsulated spleen and lymph nodes, and non-encapsulated accumulations of lymphoid tissue throughout the body. Much of this tissue is associated with mucosal surfaces and is referred to as mucosa-associated lymphoid tissue

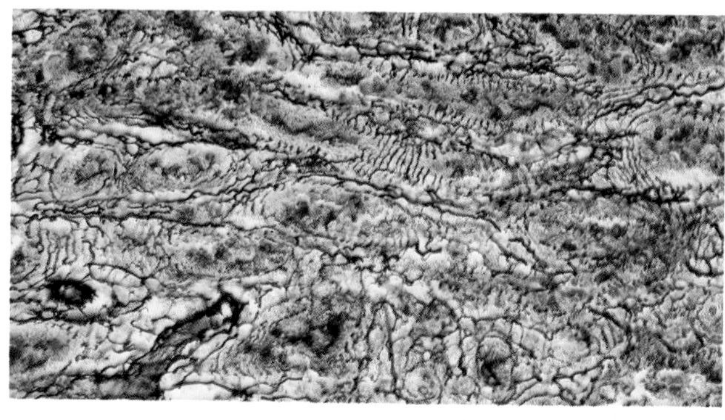

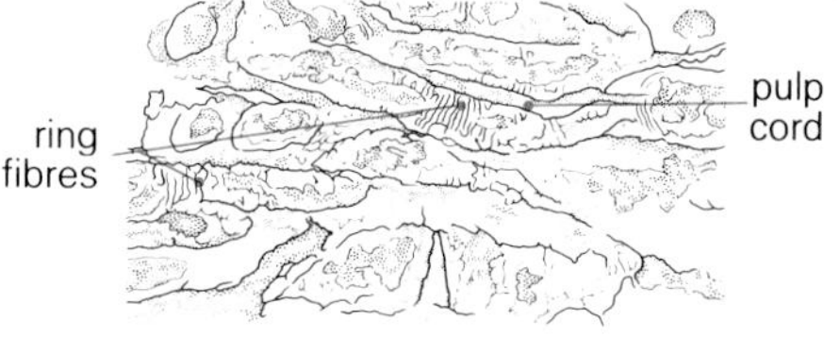

Fig. 3.5 Spleen section showing the connective tissue framework. This section is stained for reticulin and shows the architecture of the red pulp cords and the ring fibres which support the endothelial cells. × 125.

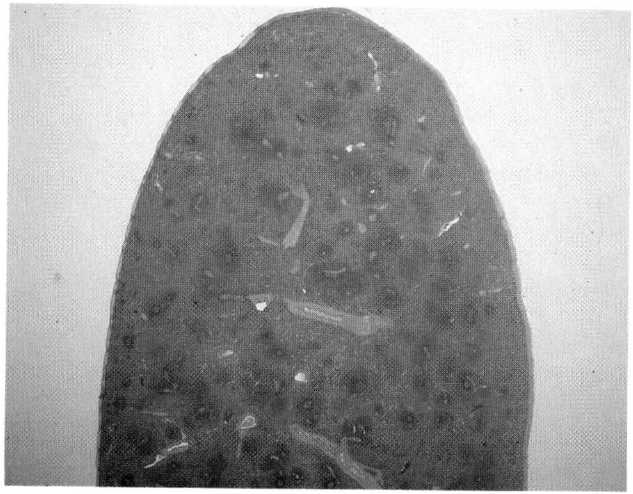

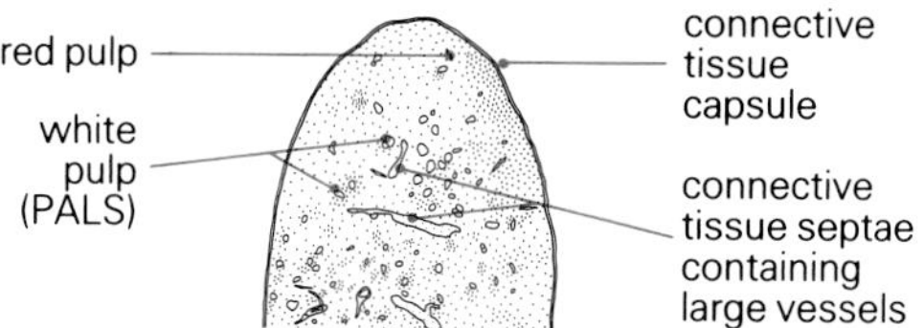

Fig. 3.6 Spleen section showing the tissue organization. This cross section of the spleen shows the lymphoid tissue localized in the white pulp around arterioles. The lymphoid tissue in the periarteriolar lymphoid sheaths (PALS) is easy to distinguish from the red pulp of the spleen. The red pulp is mainly involved in destruction of old erythrocytes, but also contains some lymphocytes and the majority of the plasma cells. H & E stain, × 7.

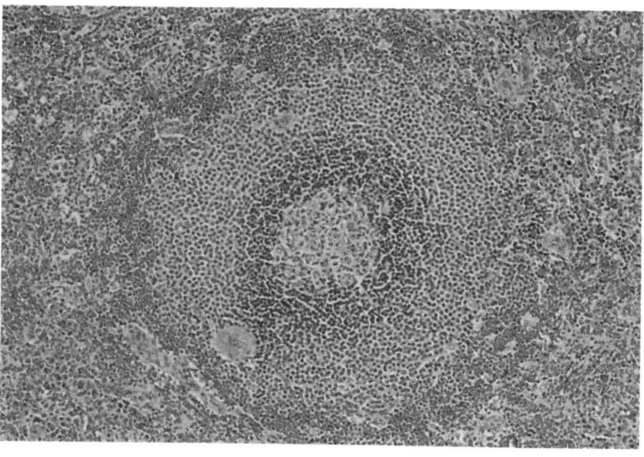

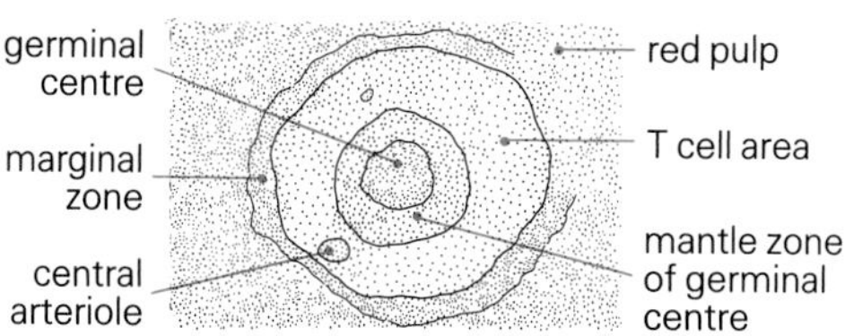

Fig. 3.7 Spleen section showing the periarteriolar lymphoid sheath (PALS). This view shows the lymphoid tissue arranged around an arteriole. The T cells are found close to the central arteriole and the B cell area has a germinal centre. In the 'unstimulated' state the B cell area consists of a primary follicle. The lymphoid tissue is separated from the red pulp by the marginal zone. This contains blood vessels and is the site of entry of blood-borne lymphocytes into the splenic lymphoid areas. H & E stain, × 125.

(MALT) of the gut, respiratory tract and genital tract. It has commonly been called GALT or gut-associated lymphoid tissue when associated with the alimentary tract.

THE SPLEEN

The spleen lies at the upper left of the abdomen behind the stomach and close to the diaphragm. It is surrounded by a collagenous capsule containing smooth muscle fibres, which penetrate into the parenchyma of the organ. These trabeculae, together with the reticular framework support the variety of cells found within the organ (Fig. 3.5). There are two main types of tissue; the red pulp, which is mainly concerned with the destruction of old erythrocytes, and the white pulp, which contains the lymphoid tissue (Fig. 3.6). The bulk of the lymphoid tissue is arranged around a central arteriole – the periarteriolar lymphoid sheath (PALS). The PALS is composed of T and B cell areas, the T cells being found around the central arteriole while the B cells are found beyond this zone. The B cells may be organized into either primary 'unstimulated' follicles, or secondary 'stimulated' follicles which possess a germinal centre (Fig. 3.7). Fig. 3.8 shows a schematic diagram of the spleen.

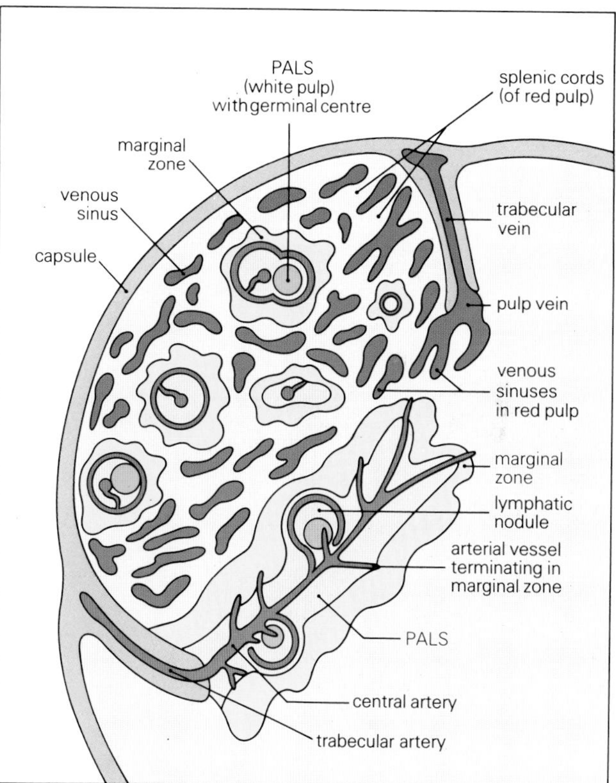

Fig. 3.8 Organization of lymphoid tissue in the spleen. The white pulp is composed of the periarteriolar lymphatic sheaths (PALS) frequently containing germinal centres with mantle zones. The white pulp is surrounded by the marginal zone* . The red pulp contains venous sinuses separated by splenic cords. Blood enters the tissues via the trabecular artery and becomes the central artery which gives rise to many branches; some end in the white pulp, supplying the germinal centres and mantle zones, but most empty into or near the marginal zones. Some arterial branches run directly into the red pulp, mainly terminating in the cords. The venous sinuses drain blood into pulp veins and then trabecular veins.
* Marginal zones contain specialized antigen-presenting cells, macrophages and slowly recirculating B cells.

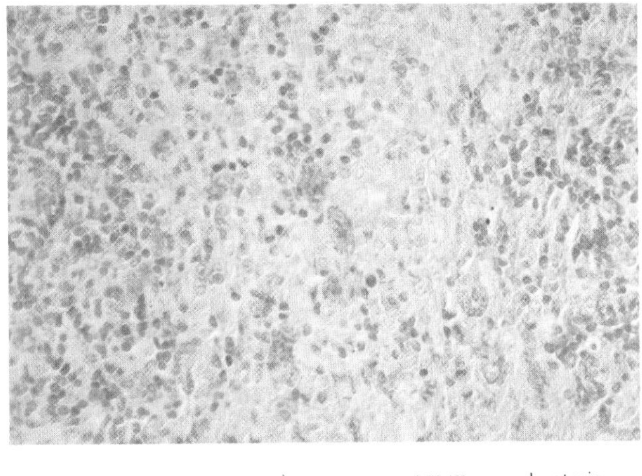

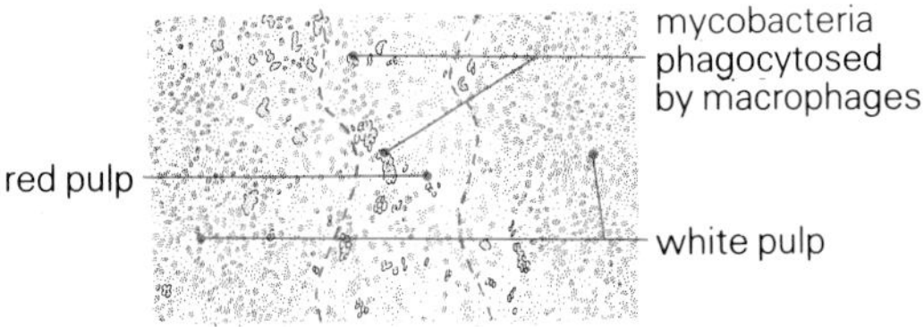

Fig. 3.9 Spleen section showing the red pulp macrophages. Microorganisms in the blood become trapped in the red pulp macrophages of the spleen, which are part of the reticuloendothelial system. This section shows intravenously injected mycobacteria phagocytosed by the red pulp macrophages. Modified Ziehl-Nielsen stain, × 125. (Courtesy of Dr I. Brown.)

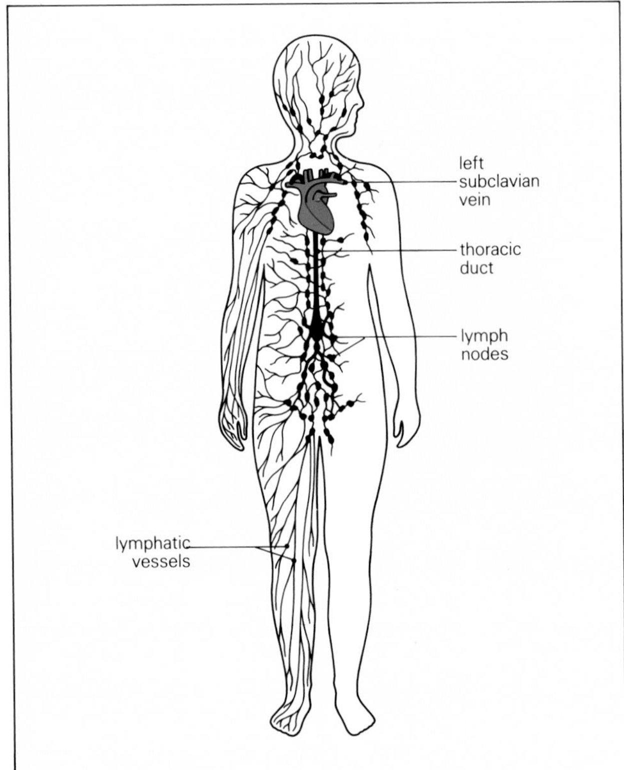

Fig. 3.10 The lymph node network. Lymph nodes are found at junctions of lymphatic vessels and form a complete network draining and filtering lymph derived from the tissue spaces. They are either superficial or visceral, draining the internal organs of the body. The lymph eventually collects in the thoracic duct which drains into the left subclavian vein and thus into the blood circulation.

Follicular dendritic cells and phagocytic macrophages are also found in germinal centres. Specialized macrophages are found in the marginal zone – the area surrounding the PALS. These, together with the follicular dendritic cells of the primary follicles, are the cells which present antigen to B cells. Lymphocytes are free to leave and enter the PALS via capillary branches of the central arterioles in the marginal zone, and both T and B cells are found in this area. Some lymphocytes, especially maturing plasmablasts, can pass across the marginal zone via bridges into the red pulp. The red pulp consists of sinuses and cellular cords containing phagocytic macrophages, platelets, lymphocytes and numerous plasma cells (Fig. 3.9).

LYMPH NODES AND THE LYMPHATIC SYSTEM

Lymph nodes form part of a body network which filters antigen from the tissue fluid and lymph during its passage from the periphery to the thoracic duct (Fig. 3.10). Human lymph nodes are 1–25 mm in diameter, round or kidney shaped and have an indentation, the hilus, where blood vessels enter and leave the node. Lymph nodes frequently occur at branches of the lymphatic vessels. Clusters of lymph nodes are strategically placed in areas such as the neck and axillae, which drain different areas of the body. A particularly large group of lymph nodes occurs in the mesentery, which is well placed to monitor antigens arising from the microbial flora of the gut.

Fig. 3.11 shows a section across a typical lymph node which, like the spleen, is surrounded by a collagenous capsule. The radial trabeculae, together with reticulin fibres, support the various cellular components within the lymph node. The lymph node is composed of a B cell area (cortex), a T cell area (paracortex) and a central medulla containing T cells, B cells and plasma cells. Fig. 3.12 shows the arrangement. The paracortex contains many antigen-presenting cells (interdigitating

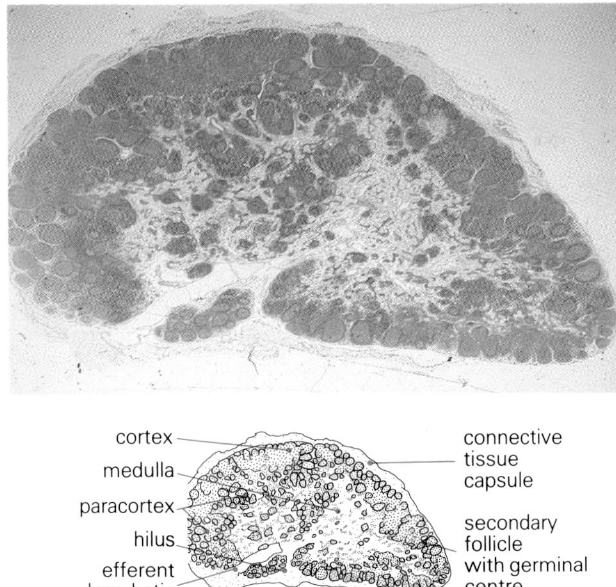

Fig. 3.11 Lymph node section. The lymph node is surrounded by a connective tissue capsule and organized into three main areas – the cortex (B cell area), the paracortex (T cell area) and the medulla, which contains cords of lymphoid tissue (T and B cell area). H & E stain, × 5. (Courtesy of Mr C. Symes.)

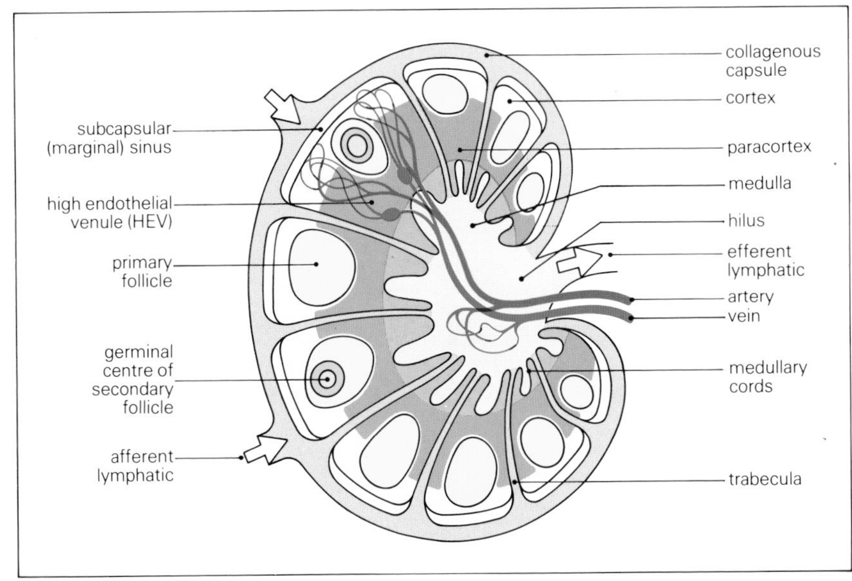

Fig. 3.12 The structure of a lymph node. Beneath the collagenous capsule is the subcapsular sinus which is lined by phagocytic cells. Lymphocytes and antigens (if present) pass into the sinus via the afferent lymphatics from surrounding tissue spaces or adjacent nodes (see section below on lymphocyte traffic). The cortex contains aggregates of B cells (primary follicles) most of which (secondary follicles) have a site of active proliferation (germinal centre). The paracortex contains mainly T cells, many of which are found in close apposition to the interdigitating cells (antigen-presenting cells). Each node has its own arterial and venous supply. Lymphocytes enter the node from the circulation through the specialized high endothelial venules (HEV) in the paracortex. The medulla contains both T and B cells and most of the lymph node plasma cells organized into cords of lymphoid tissue. Lymphocytes can only leave the node through the efferent lymphatics.

cells) which have large quantities of MHC class II antigens on their surface. The bulk of the lymphoid tissue is found in the cortex and paracortex. Some lymphoid tissue extends into the medulla where it is found along strands of connective tissue fibres. These medullary cords are separated by large sinuses and contain most of the plasma cells in the lymph node (Fig. 3.13). In addition, scavenger phagocytic cells are arranged along these sinuses especially in the medulla. During passage of the lymph across the node from the afferent to the efferent lymphatics, particulate antigens are removed by these phagocytic cells (Fig. 3.14).

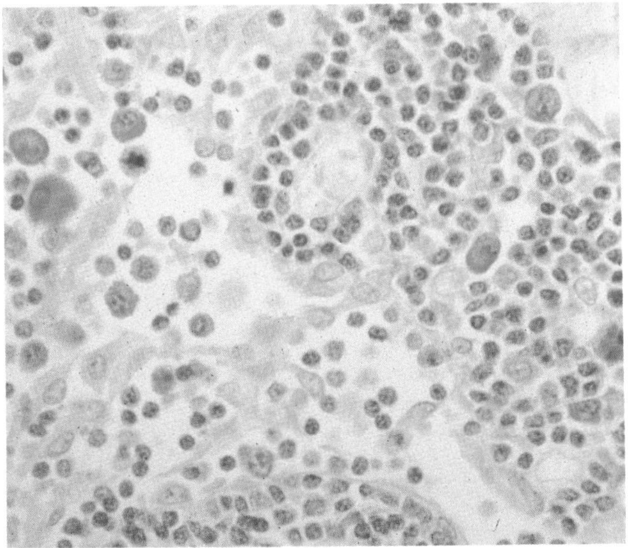

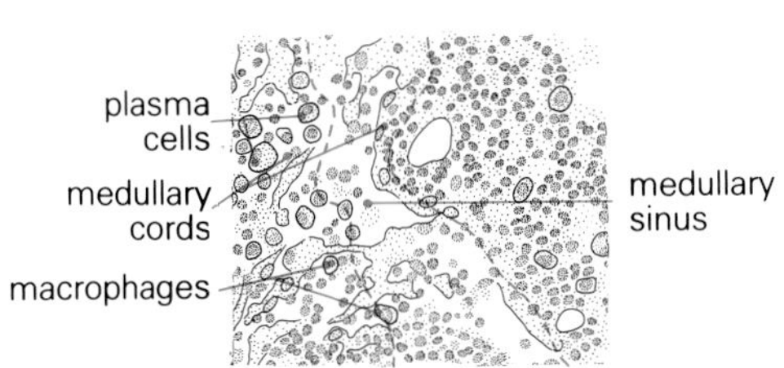

Fig. 3.13 Section of lymph node medulla. This section shows typical plasma cells in the medullary cords and sinuses. The plasma cell cytoplasm stains red with pyronin which binds to RNA. Recirculating macrophages are also seen in this region. Methyl green pyronin stain, × 200.

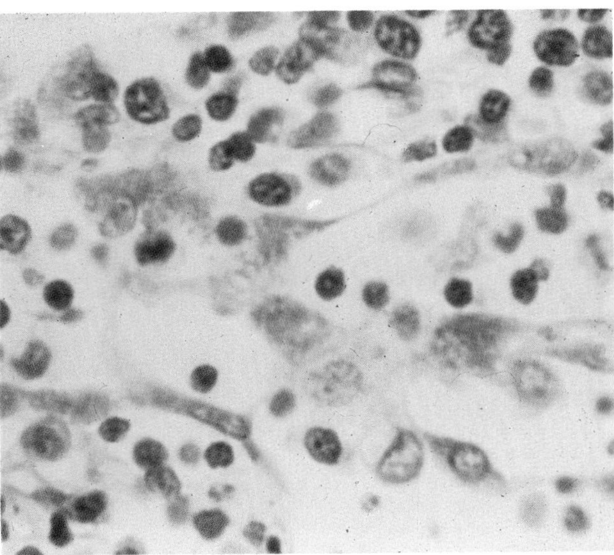

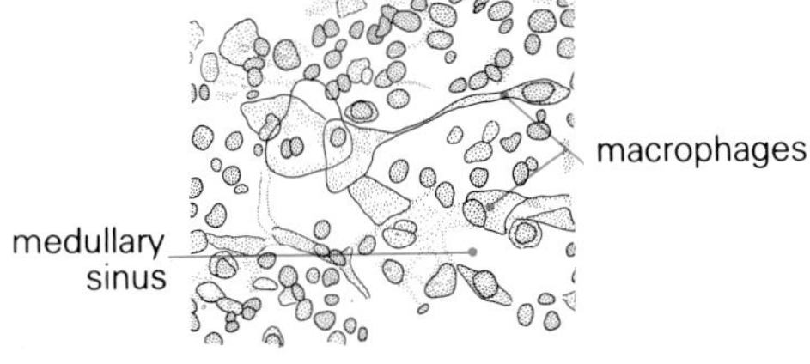

Fig. 3.14 Section of lymph node medulla showing phagocytic macrophages. The macrophages which line the medullary sinuses can be seen following the uptake of the red dye, lithium carmine (counterstained with haematoxylin). × 330.

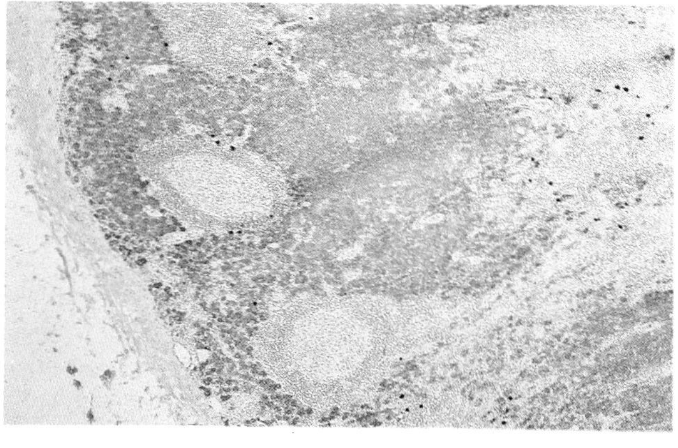

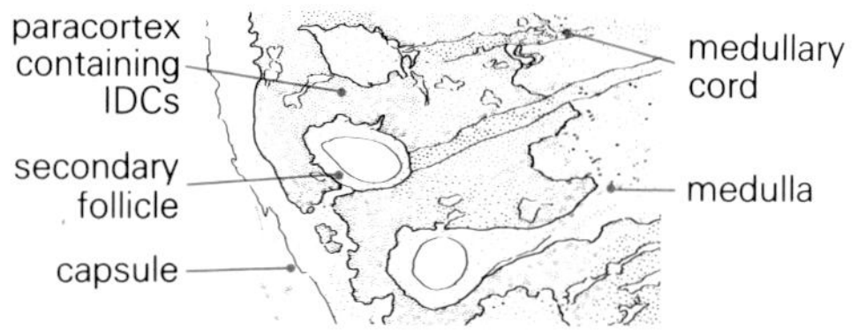

Fig. 3.15 Lymph node section showing paracortical proliferation. This micrograph shows a lymph node draining the skin area of a patient with chronic eczema. Antigens penetrating the skin are carried to draining lymph nodes by antigen-presenting cells which are normally present in the epidermis – Langerhans' cells. These cells are seen as 'veiled' cells in the afferent lymphatics and they settle in the paracortex as interdigitating reticulum cells (IDCs), here stained brown with peroxidase-labelled monoclonal antibody. T cell proliferation in response to specific antigen presented by IDCs results in paracortical expansion. Haematoxylin counterstain, × 40.

The cortex contains aggregates of B cells (primary or secondary follicles), whilst T cells are localized primarily in the paracortex. If an area of skin is challenged by a T-dependent antigen, examination of the lymph nodes draining that area of skin shows active T cell proliferation in the paracortex (Fig. 3.15). On the other hand, patients with congenital thymic aplasia (DiGeorge syndrome) and neonatally thymectomized, or congenitally athymic ('nude') mice or rats have fewer cells in the paracortex than normals (Fig. 3.16).

Germinal centres or secondary follicles are seen in antigen-stimulated lymph nodes. These are similar to the germinal centres seen in the B cell areas of the splenic PALS. The proliferative activity within the germinal centres is dependent on the age of the centre; young centres contain many centroblasts and centrocytes, whilst few are seen in old centres. (Centroblasts and centrocytes are large and small follicle centre cells respectively.) The areas of active proliferation are surrounded by a mantle of lymphocytes (Fig. 3.17). The B lymphocytes in this area are rich in surface antibody of the IgD class, as detected by immunohistochemical staining (Fig. 3.18). In some secondary follicles this thickened mantle or corona is orientated towards the capsule of the node. Secondary follicles contain dendritic antigen-presenting cells and some macrophages in addition to a few $CD4^+$ T cells (Fig. 3.19). These, together with specialized marginal sinus macrophages, appear to play a role in the development of B cell responses and, in particular, of B cell memory, which is probably the primary function of the germinal centres. Proliferating B cells within the germinal centres have a clearly defined nuclear shape (cleaved *vs* non-cleaved) which has been useful in defining malignant lymphoid proliferation.

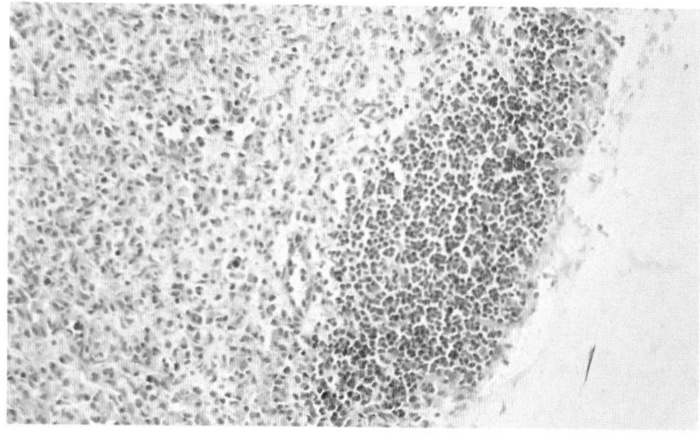

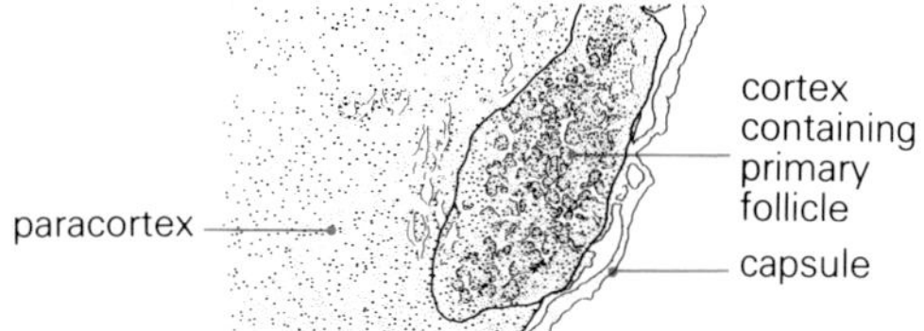

Fig. 3.16 Lymph node section from a congenitally athymic ('nude') mouse showing paracortical depletion. A genetic defect in the nude mouse causes thymic aplasia and failure of T cell development. This section of the lymph node from a 'T-less' mouse shows few cells in the T-dependent paracortex. There are, however, large numbers of interdigitating reticulum cells within the paracortex in this node. The cortex is also poorly developed since T cells are required for the organization of the follicles. H & E stain, × 125. (Courtesy of Dr H. Dockrell.)

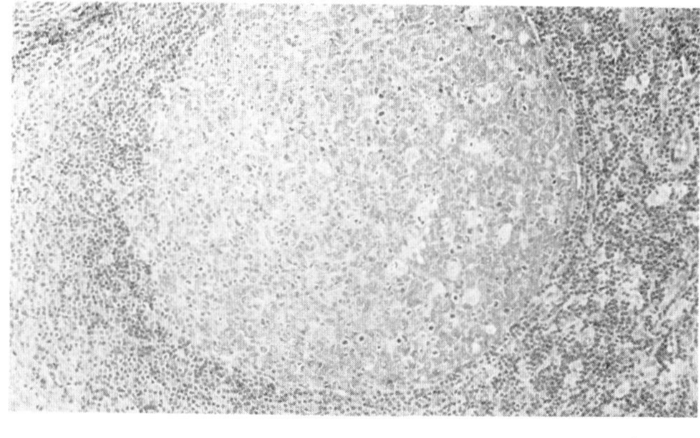

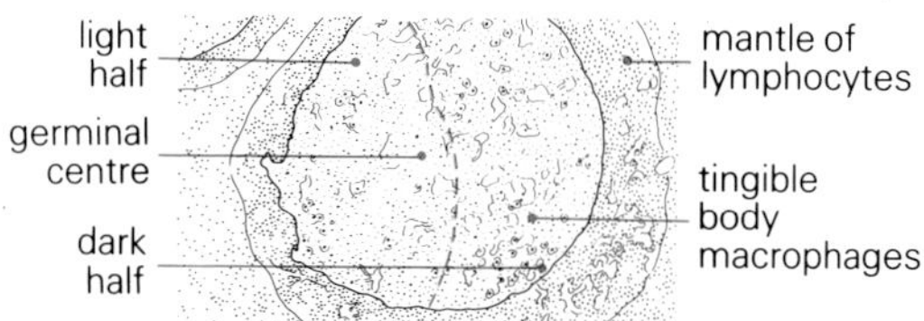

Fig. 3.17 Secondary lymphoid follicle section showing a germinal centre. This human lymph node germinal centre contains actively proliferating B cells. Zoning of this centre may be seen as a light part and a more actively proliferating dark part, which contains the tingible body macrophages. There is a well developed mantle or corona of small resting lymphocytes, which have much less cytoplasm than the lymphoblasts and appear more densely packed. Giemsa stain, × 40. (Courtesy of Dr K. McLennan.)

MUCOSA-ASSOCIATED LYMPHOID TISSUE (MALT)

Dispersed aggregates of non-encapsulated lymphoid tissue are frequently found in a variety of organs, especially in the lamina propria and submucosal areas of the gastrointestinal, respiratory and urogenital tracts. These systems normally provide the main portals of entry into the body for foreign microorganisms. The lymphoid cells are present either as diffuse aggregates or organized into nodules containing germinal centres.

Fig. 3.20 illustrates the diffuse accumulations of lymphoid tissue in the lamina propria of the intestinal wall. The Peyer's patches of the lower ileum are particularly prominent in young animals and frequently contain secondary follicles (Fig. 3.21). The gut epithelium overlying the Peyer's patches is specialized to allow the transport of antigens into the lymphoid tissue. Secretory

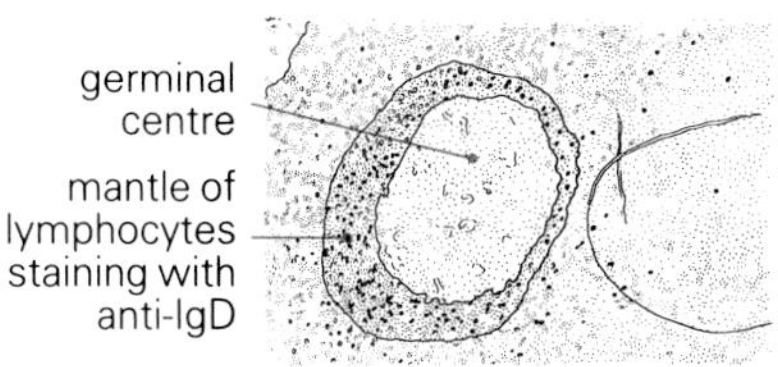

Fig. 3.18 Secondary lymphoid follicle showing the mantle of lymphocytes around the germinal centre. Human lymph node germinal centre stained by anti-human IgD antibody labelled with horse-radish peroxidase. Note that there are few IgD-positive cells in the centre itself; both areas, however, contain IgM-positive cells. × 40. (Courtesy of Dr K. McLennan.)

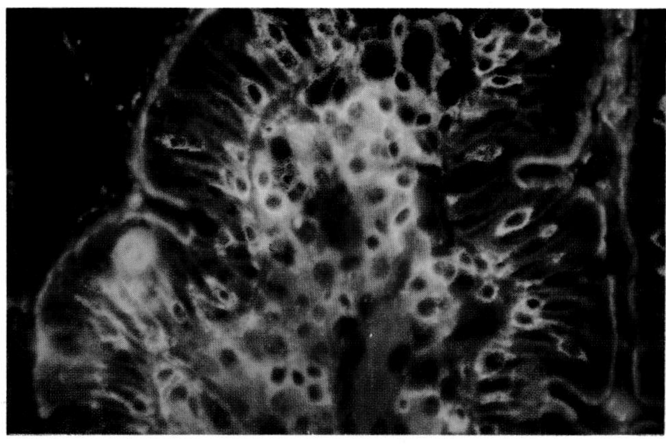

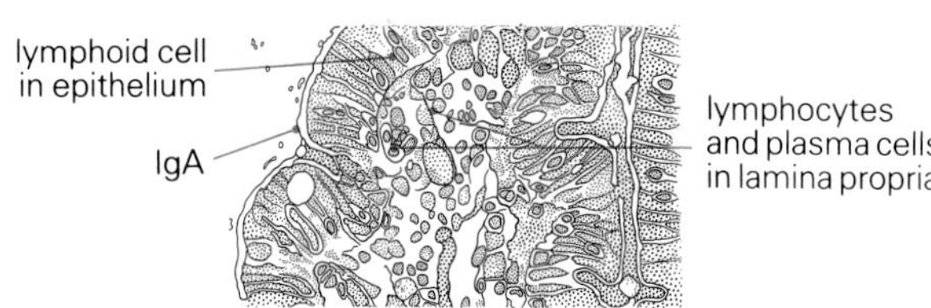

Fig. 3.20 Section of human jejunum showing MALT. This section shows lymphoid cells in the epithelium and lamina propria fluorescing green (using an anti-leucocyte monoclonal antibody, 2D1). Red cytoplasmic staining is obtained with anti-IgA antibody, which detects plasma cells in the lamina propria and IgA in the mucus. (Courtesy of Professor G. Janossy.)

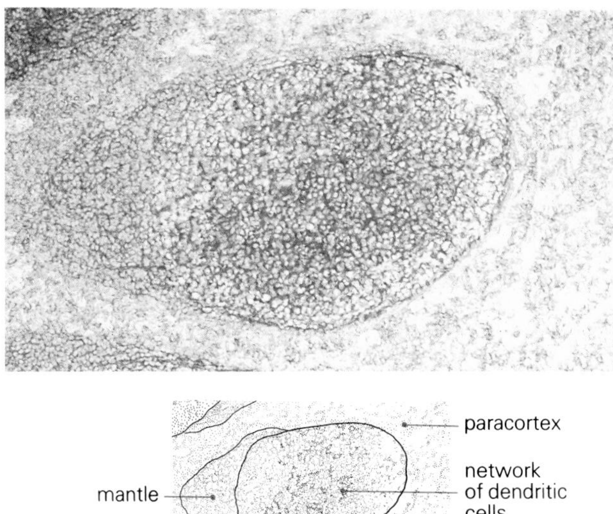

Fig. 3.19 Secondary lymphoid follicle section showing the reticular cell network. This lymph node germinal centre is stained with peroxidase-labelled monoclonal antibody to dendritic cells and macrophages. Note the extension of the network of reticulum cells into the mantle. Haematoxylin counterstain, × 40. (Courtesy of Dr K. McLennan.)

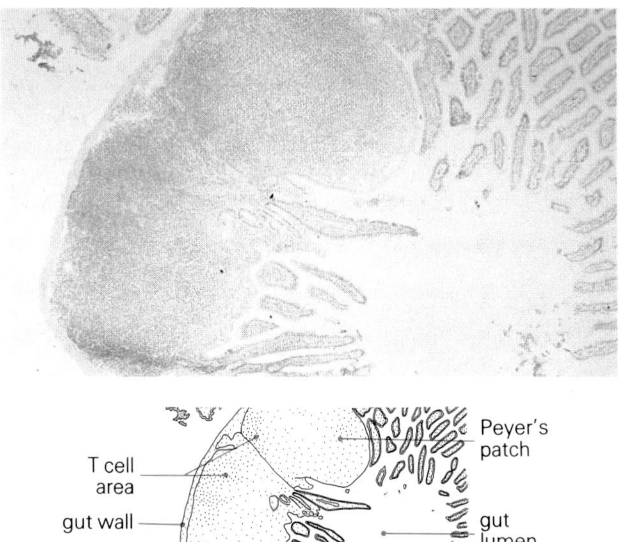

Fig. 3.21 Section of mouse ileum showing Peyer's patches in the MALT. This shows the lymphoid tissue in the intestinal wall organized into Peyer's patches. The T cell areas are stained with peroxidase-labelled monoclonal antibody to the Thy-1 antigen on the T cells. Haematoxylin counterstain, × 40. (Courtesy of Dr E. Andrew.)

IgA is an antibody which can traverse mucosal membranes and prevents entry of infectious microorganisms. The mechanism of IgA transport is shown in Fig.3.22.

In man, the tonsils contain a considerable amount of lymphoid tissue which usually contains many large germinal centres (Fig. 3.23). Similar accumulations of lymphoid tissue are seen lining the bronchi (Fig. 3.24) and along the urogenital tract. MALT is important in the local immune response at mucosal surfaces.

LYMPHOCYTE TRAFFIC

The migration of lymphocytes from the primary to secondary lymphoid tissues has already been described. Once in the secondary tissues the lymphocytes do not simply remain there but many move from one lymphoid organ to another through the blood and lymph. The recirculation routes are shown in Fig. 3.25.

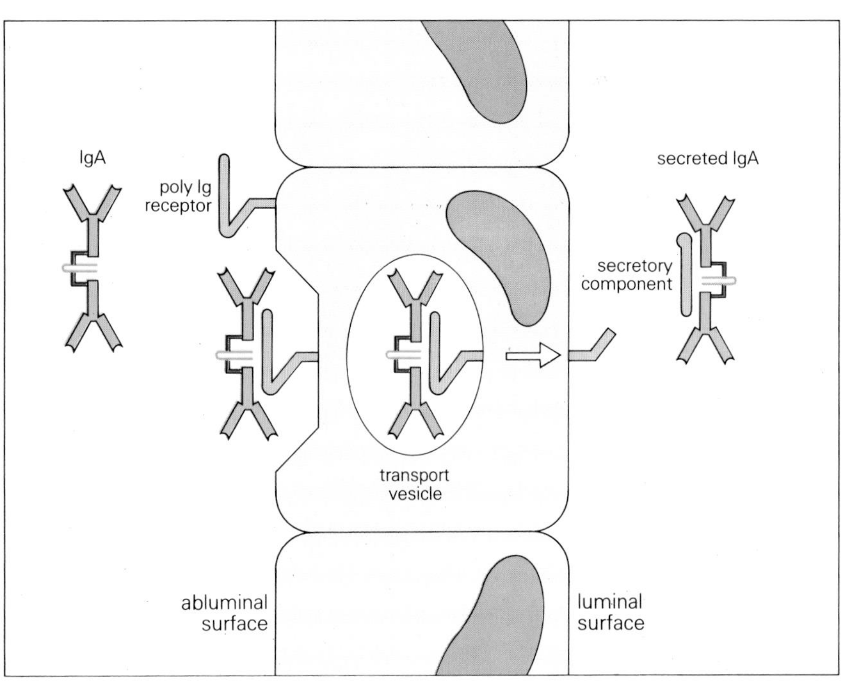

Fig. 3.22 Transport of IgA across the mucosal epithelium. IgA dimers secreted into the interstitial space by plasma cells bind to membrane receptors present on the internal (abluminal) surface of the epithelial cells. The IgA–receptor complex is then endocytosed and transported across the cell, bound to the membrane of transport vesicles. These vesicles fuse with the plasma membrane of the luminal surface, releasing IgA dimers and a secretory component derived from cleavage of the receptor. The dimeric IgA is probably protected from proteolytic enzymes outside the cell by the presence of this secretory component.

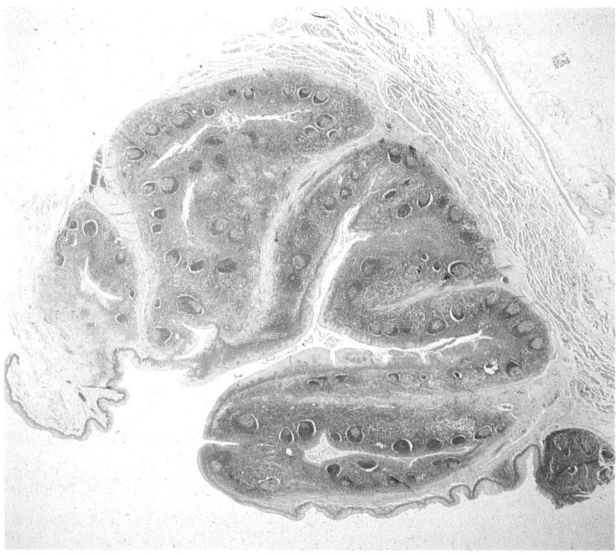

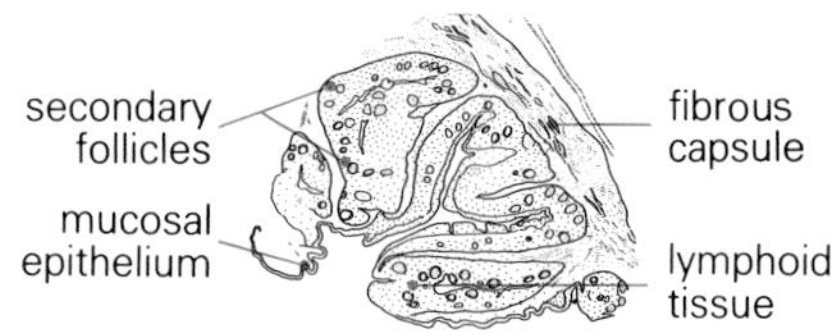

Fig. 3.23 Section of human tonsil showing MALT. This view shows the large number of germinal centres frequently found in tonsillar lymphoid tissue. H & E stain, × 4. (Courtesy of Mr C. Symes.)

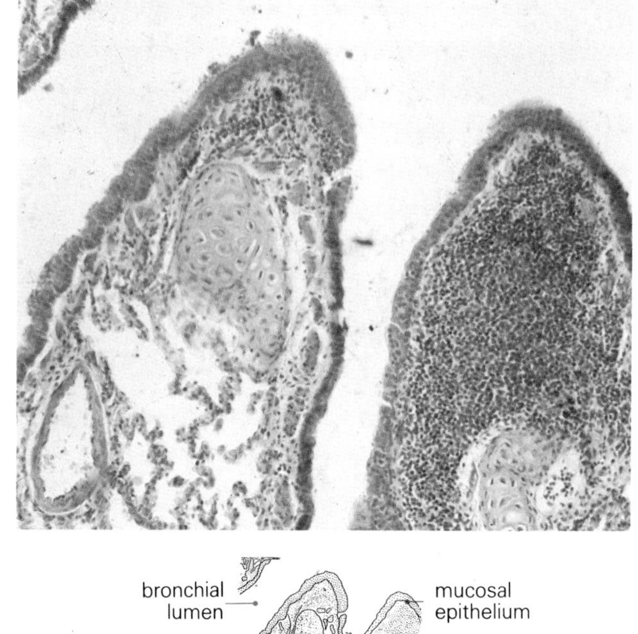

Fig. 3.24 Section of lung showing the MALT. This section shows a diffuse accumulation of lymphocytes in the bronchial wall. H & E stain, × 40.

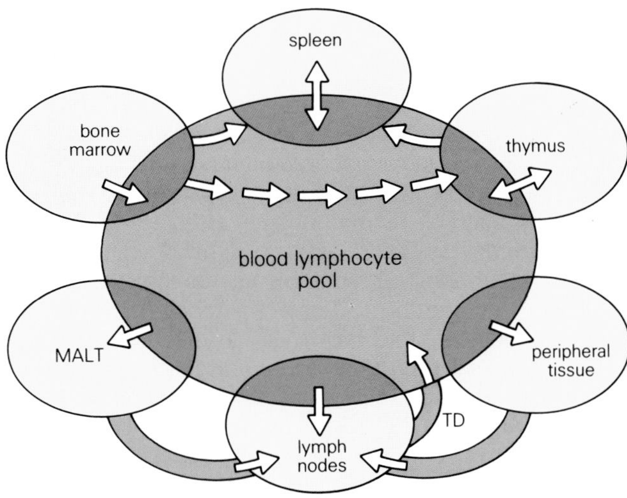

Fig. 3.25 Lymphocyte traffic. The lymphocytes in a mature animal move through the circulation (red) and the lymphatic ducts (orange) between various organs. The lymphocytes can traverse the endothelium (arrows) in particular lymphoid tissues and may become temporarily resident in the various organs which contain accumulations of lymphoid tissue. Newly formed T and B lymphocytes migrate into peripheral tissues and become functionally mature. Lymphocytes leave the vasculature via the high endothelial venule of the MALT, lymph nodes and peripheral tissues. They eventually return to the blood stream via the afferent lymphatics, lymph nodes, efferent lymphatics and ultimately through the thoracic duct (TD) into the venous circulation. Lymphocytes also traffic to some extent across non-specialized endothelium in the periphery and this is greatly enhanced in areas of inflammation.

Although some lymphocytes leave the blood through non-specialized venules, the main exit route in most mammals is through a specialized section of the post-capillary venules known as the high endothelial venule (HEV) (Fig. 3.26). In the lymph nodes these are mainly in the paracortex with some in the cortex; the medulla lacks HEVs. Recirculating lymphocytes interact with the cuboidal high endothelial cells of the HEV and pass through them (Fig. 3.27). These endothelial cells have distinctive cytochemical properties including non-specific esterase activity and production of sulphated molecules. (Fig. 3.28).

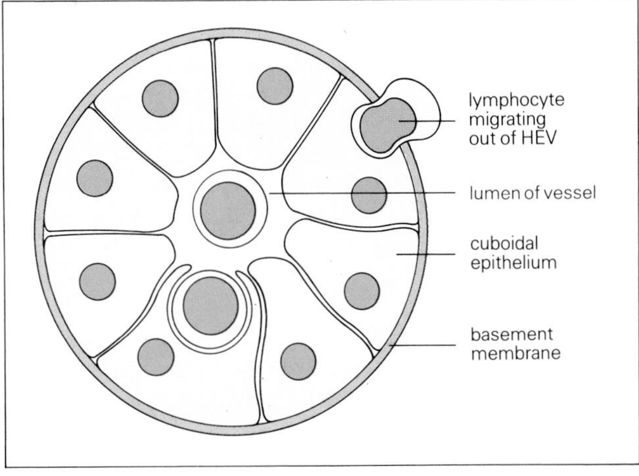

Fig. 3.27 Diagrammatic section of a lymph node post capillary venule. Dark cells are lymphocytes leaving the lumen of the vessel migrating across the endothelial cells. This phenomenon is referred to as emperipolesis.

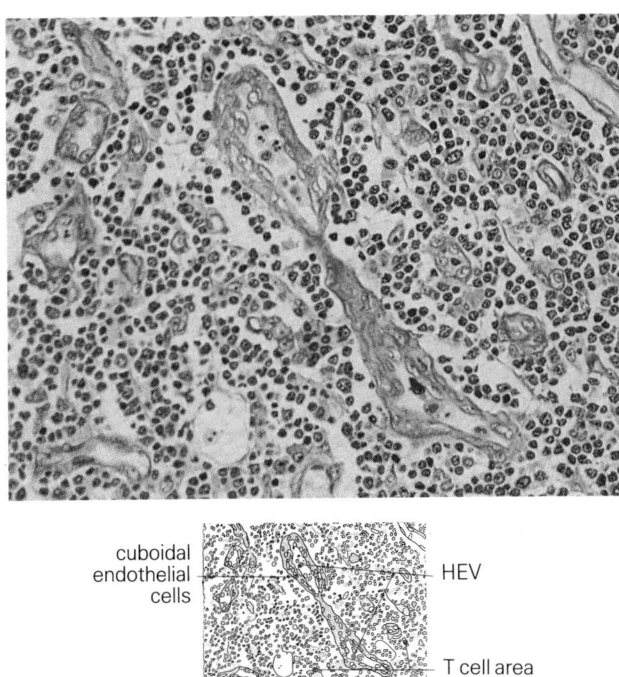

Fig. 3.26 Section of lymph node showing the high endothelial venule (HEV). This section of lymph node paracortex shows the specialized cuboidal-shaped high endothelial cells lining the HEV through which lymphocytes leave the circulation and enter the node. Giemsa stain (resin section), × 180. (Courtesy of Dr K. McLennan.)

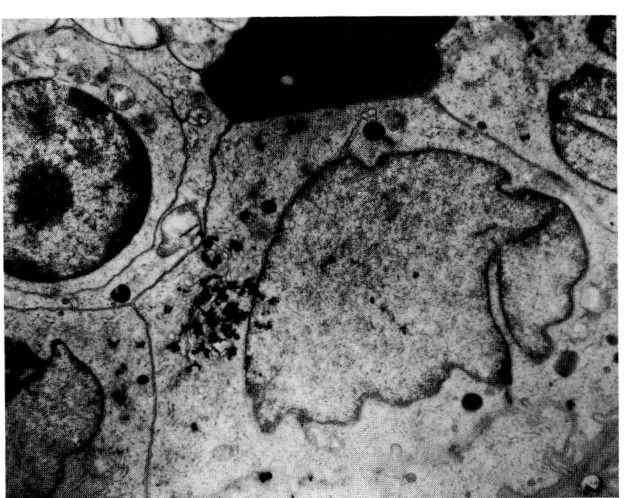

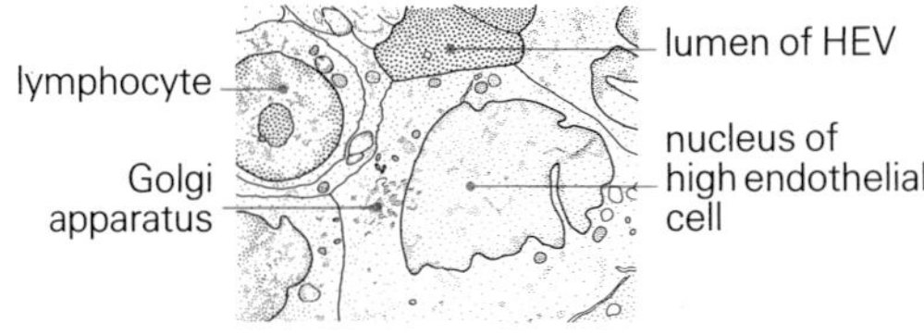

Fig. 3.28 Electronmicrograph showing a high endothelial venule (HEV) in the thymus-dependent area of a lymph node. A lymphocyte can be seen in transit through the specialized capillary wall. The HEV is labelled with ^{35}S and grains occur over the Golgi apparatus. × 5000. (Courtesy of Professor W. L. Ford.)

In the lymph nodes all the lymphocytes return to the circulation by way of the efferent lymphatics which pass via the thoracic duct into the left subclavian vein. Some lymphocytes, primarily T cells, arrive from the drainage area of the node through the afferent lymphatics; this is the main route by which antigen enters the nodes.

Under normal conditions there is a continuous active flow of lymphocyte traffic through the nodes, but when antigen enters the lymph node of an animal already sensitized to that antigen there is a temporary shut down in the traffic which lasts for approximately 24 hours. Thus, antigen-specific lymphocytes are preferentially retained in the lymph nodes draining the source of antigen; in particular, blast cells do not recirculate but appear to remain in one site.

Lymphocytes also enter non-encapsulated lymphoid tissues such as tonsils and Peyer's patches via the HEV and pass into the afferent lymphatics of the draining lymph nodes. The main route of lymphocyte traffic into the spleen from the circulation is via the venous sinuses surrounding the marginal zone of the PALS. They leave through the marginal zone bridging channels into the red pulp sinuses.

Lymphocyte Homing About 1–2% of the lymphocyte pool recirculates each hour. Overall, this process allows a large number of antigen-specific lymphocytes to 'home to' and come into contact with their appropriate antigen in the microenvironment of the peripheral lymphoid organs. This is particularly important since lymphoid cells are monospecific and there is only a finite number of lymphocytes capable of recognizing any particular antigenic conformation. In addition to antigen-specific lymphocyte homing there is now evidence for a non-random migration of lymphocytes to particular lymphoid compartments. For example, lymphocytes with 'gut-homing' properties will migrate preferentially across HEVs in the intestine whilst others will migrate specifically into lymph nodes, and yet others may specifically home to the spleen. Recent data have indicated that both T and B peripheral lymphocytes carry specific adhesion molecules (termed high endothelial binding factors) which allow interaction with 'receptor' structures on HEVs in different anatomical sites. These are only present on a few lymphocytes in primary lymphoid organs. One molecule with a molecular weight of approximately 90 kD and recognized by rat monoclonal antibody MEL 14 is present on mouse T and B cells which 'home' to mesenteric lymph nodes. Other molecules appear to be responsible for homing to Peyer's patches or peripheral lymph nodes. Soluble forms of these molecules have been found in lymph and serum and their interactions with HEVs have been shown to alter the function of these endothelial cells.

Specialized Adhesion Molecules On circulating lymphocytes (and probably on the HEVs themselves) these allow selective (that is, non-random) homing of lymphocyte populations into anatomical sites. This might be particularly important where, for example, lymphocytes stimulated in the gut wall migrate to draining lymph nodes to respond. It would be of importance for 'memory' cells to specifically home back to the intestinal tissue where they would be able to respond to a second antigenic challenge.

Another group of molecules is induced on endothelium at sites of inflammation in response to cytokines and these are partly responsible for the altered traffic of lymphocytes (and other leucocytes) at these sites. In particular, the adhesion molecules LFA-3 and ICAM-1 may be important in this respect, binding to LFA-2 (CD2) and LFA-1 respectively on the lymphocytes. Another member of the LFA-1 family of molecules, CR3, appears to be involved in neutrophil migration into tissues. The diversity of the leucocyte traffic patterns seen in normal individuals and in response to immunopathological stimuli emphasizes the importance of the groups of molecules which control cell traffic.

FURTHER READING

Bos, J.D. & Kapsenberg, M.L. (1986) The skin immune system. *Immunology Today*, **7**, 235.

Hooghe, R. J. & Pink, J. R. L. (1985) The role of carbohydrate in lymphocyte traffic.

Playfair, J.H.L. (1987) *Immunology at a glance*. 4th edition. Oxford: Blackwell Scientific Publications.

Roitt, I.M. (1988) *Essential Immunology*. 6th edition, pp. 85–100. Oxford: Blackwell Scientific Publications.

Stein, H., Gerders, J. & Mason, D.Y. (1982) The normal and malignant germinal centre. In *Clinics in Haematology*. Edited by G. Janossy. London: W.B. Saunders.

Weiss, L. (1972) *The Cells and Tissues of the Immune System: Structure Function Interactions*. New Jersey: Prentice-Hall.

4 Major Histocompatibility Complex

It has long been recognized that successful blood transfusion is dependent on matching the blood groups of donor and recipient red cells. In his Nobel lecture of 1931, Landsteiner suggested that similar 'blood groups' would be involved in the acceptance or rejection of other transplanted tissues. This idea led Gorer to the identification of a group of antigens in mice which, when matched between donor and recipient animals, markedly improved the ability of a graft to survive. The name histocompatibility antigens was coined for these antigens involved in graft rejection. It was also noted that the products of one particular region of the genome were of predominant importance in the rejection process. This region is the major histocompatibility complex (MHC), referred to as H-2 in the mouse and located on chromosome 17. Analogous major histocompatibility systems have been found in all mammalian species studied so far. In man the MHC is the HLA gene cluster on chromosome 6. Recombination between extreme ends of the gene complex occurs at about 1% in human family studies, from which it can be calculated that HLA occupies about 1/3000 of the total genome. This means that there is room for several hundred individual genes. Although the MHC was originally identified by its role in transplant rejection, it is now recognized that proteins encoded in this region are involved in many aspects of immunological recognition, including interaction between different lymphoid cells, as well as between lymphocytes and antigen-presenting cells.

INHERITANCE OF MHC GENES

An individual inherits one maternal and one paternal chromosome 6, that is to say, one HLA haploid genotype (haplotype) is derived from each parent. Since there are a large number of gene loci in the MHC and much polymorphism within the loci, a normal population will have a very large number of different haplotypes. Many of the genetic studies on the MHC have been performed with inbred strains of mice.

INBRED MOUSE STRAINS

In a normal outbred population the chromosome derived from the mother will differ from the same numbered chromosome derived from the father. To simplify the genetic analysis of complicated systems such as the MHC, it is highly desirable to have animals with identical chromosomes from each parent (inbred animals), since progeny from these animals will have identical sets of autosomes (non-sex chromosomes) in all their gametes and therefore their offspring will have a predictable genotype.

It is possible to produce an inbred mouse strain by repeatedly inbreeding a strain by brother × sister matings in successive generations. On average, 50% of the chromosomes in two siblings derived from crossing outbred animals will be identical. If those two F_1 siblings are crossed there is a 25% chance (50% × 50%) that any particular pair of chromosomes in their F_2 progeny will be identical. All the descendants from crossing two such F_2 mice will now have identical pairs of that particular chromosome (Fig. 4.1). Using this method of repeated inbreeding all the chromosome pairs will eventually become identical.

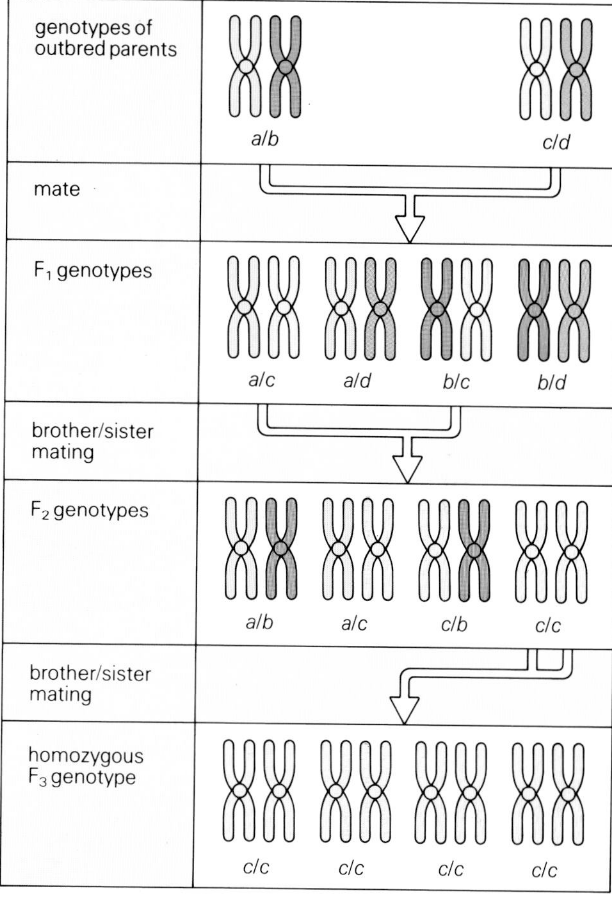

Fig. 4.1 Production of inbred mice from two outbred parents. The parents in the normal outbred population differ at the same chromosome locus, that is, they have different haplotypes (*a/b* and *c/d*). An F_1 individual inherits one haplotype from each parent so that four possible genotypes may occur in the F_1 generation. Mating two F_1 individuals (e.g. *a/c* × *b/c*) will give rise to F_2 offspring, some of which possess identical haplotypes (*c/c*). They are used as parents to produce a population of inbred individuals (F_3), all having identical sets of autosomes – *c/c*. Note that in this simplified scheme only one chromosome has become homozygous – about 20 generations will be required to produce animals identical with respect to all their autosomes.

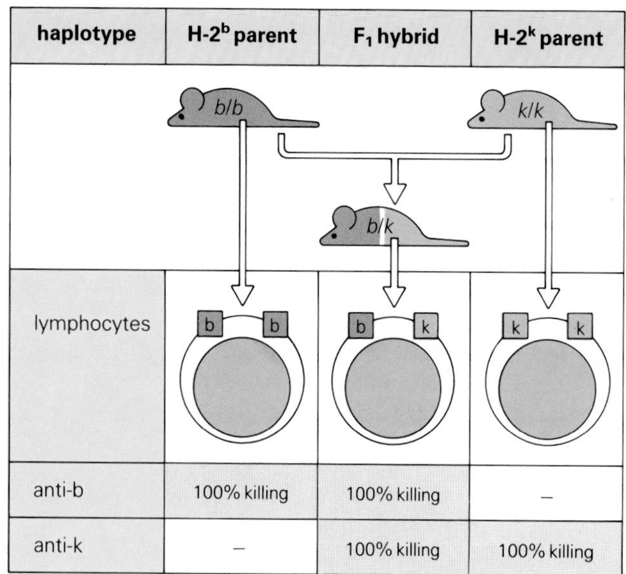

Fig. 4.2 Codominant expression of MHC antigens. Mice of two different genotypes, *b/b* (strain of haplotype H-2^b) and *k/k* (strain of haplotype H-2^k) are crossed. (MHC antigens displayed on the lymphocyte surface are represented by squares.) Antiserum raised to lymphocytes of either parent (anti-b, anti-k) is found to kill lymphocytes of the F_1 hybrid. It is concluded that the F_1 hybrid is of genotype *b/k* and that its cells express the histocompatibility antigens of both parents.

Inbred individuals have identical haplotypes at the H-2 gene loci of both chromosomes. F_1 hybrids between two such inbred strains express (carry) histocompatibility antigens of both parental strains – expression of the MHC antigens is codominant (Fig. 4.2).

ARRANGEMENT OF MHC GENES

The MHC gene complex contains a large number of individual genes. The complex as a whole performs similar functions in different species, but the detailed arrangement of genes within the MHC differs between species.

Three major sets of molecules are encoded within this region: class I, II and III antigens. Class I and class II genes encode molecules involved in immunological recognition. Each class I molecule has one MHC-encoded polypeptide, whereas the class II molecules are formed from two separate MHC-encoded polypeptides – one α and one β chain for each class II molecule. Originally class I and class II molecules were recognized using antibodies and lymphocytes, so they are often referred to as MHC antigens.

Class III genes encode some of the complement components concerned in the cleavage of C3, a central event in the generation of an inflammatory response. There are also a number of other genes in the MHC which are not specifically involved in immune recognition.

Originally the different gene loci of the MHC were identified by functional and serological analysis. These data in association with classical genetic studies allowed the identification of different regions within the MHC, each producing different classes of MHC molecules (Fig. 4.3). More recently, molecular maps have been made of both the mouse and human MHCs which identify the individual genes (Figs 4.4 and 4.5). It has not been possible to identify products of all these genes and some may not be expressed at all (pseudogenes), but the genes for all the MHC molecules discovered by conventional serology have been located.

The human class I genes encode the classical HLA-A, -B and -C antigen heavy chains and a large number of non-classical genes representing the adjacent homologues of the mouse Qa and TLA regions. Southern blotting analysis indicates that more than 20 class I genes lie within this region. The human class II genes are arranged into at least three subregions, DP, DQ and DR, each of which contains at least one α and one β gene. Additional genes are also located in this region and have been called DZα and DOβ, but the protein products of these genes and of the DXα and β genes have not yet been detected. The human class III region comprises the genes for the serum complement components C2 and Factor B, the two genes for the complement component C4 (C4A and C4B) and the two genes for cytochrome P-450 21-hydroxylase (21-OHA and 21-OHB).

The BALB/c mouse MHC region comprises at least 48 class I and class II genes. The proximal (centromeric) end contains the K and I region and comprises two class I and seven class II genes. The distal (telomeric) end contains the D and Qa regions and comprises 13 class I genes, plus the tumour necrosis factor (TNFα) and

Fig. 4.3 MHC genes. Maps of the mouse MHC H-2 and human MHC HLA genes divide them into distinct regions. Each region produces polypeptides of a certain class. The regions shaded emerald code for class I polypeptides; those shaded turquoise code for class II polypeptides; and those coloured light green code for class III molecules. Note that the HLA region encoding class III molecules does not have a particular letter designation.

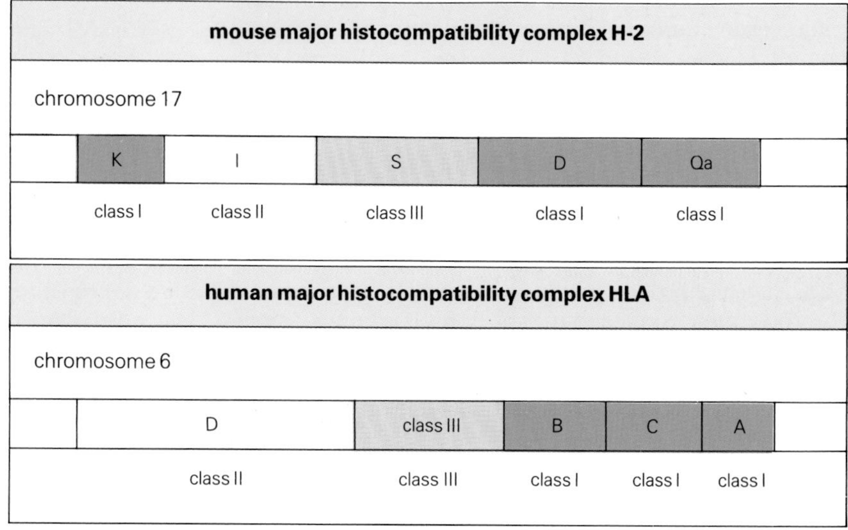

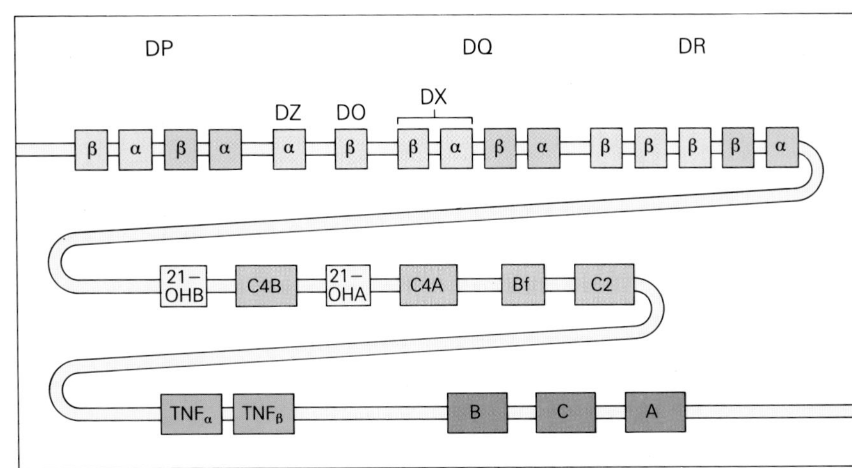

Fig. 4.4 The human MHC. A gene map of the human MHC on chromosome 6. The D region is subdivided into three main regions, DP, DQ and DR, each containing genes for a number of α and β chains. It is not certain that all of these are expressed; the genes which are definitely expressed are shown in dark turquoise. The class III region has genes for C4 (C4A and C4B) and for Factor B (Bf) and C2. Genes for tumour necrosis factor (TNF) lie between class III and the three class I genes, B, C and A.

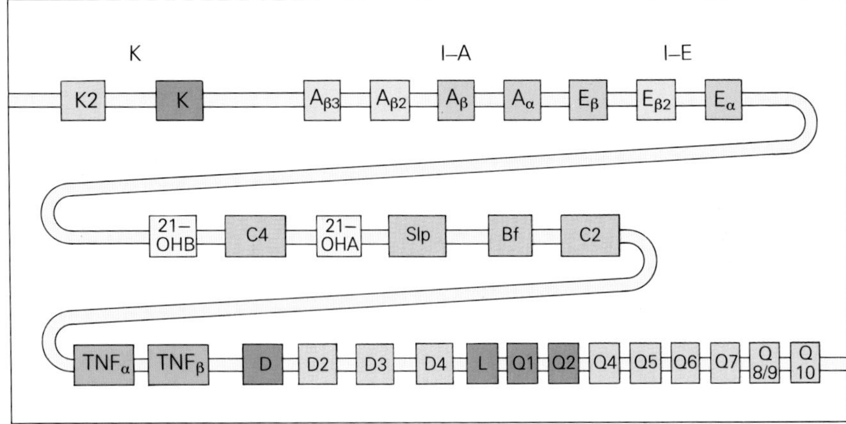

Fig. 4.5 The mouse MHC. A gene map of the mouse MHC on chromosome 17. The I region encoding class II molecules is subdivided into I–A and I–E. Genes for the main class I, II and III molecules are indicated by deeper colours. Gene products for many of the class I genes of the Qa locus have not been identified. The s region (centre) has genes for C4 and its pseudoallele slp (sex-limited protein), as well as for Factor B (Bf) and C2. Genes for tumour necrosis factor (TNF) lie next to the D region. Note the overall resemblance to the human MHC.

lymphotoxin (TNFβ) genes. Between these two regions, the S region comprises the complement and 21-hydroxylase gene clusters. Gene cloning studies have shown a similar orientation for the mouse BALB/c S region to that of the corresponding human region.

The products of the class I genes (class I antigens) comprise a transmembrane glycoprotein heavy chain, encoded by the HLA–A, –B or –C (H-2K, D or L) genes, that is non-covalently associated with the polypeptide β_2-microglobulin which is encoded outside the MHC. Class II proteins consist of two non-covalently associated peptides, referred to as α chains and β chains, both of which are encoded by the MHC. Class III proteins are those complement components which are coded by the MHC. There are additional gene loci outside the H-2 complex (the TLA complex) which also encode class I proteins and these too appear to have immunological functions.

The HLA–A and –B regions in man have analogous functions to K and D in the mouse; they act as cell surface recognition molecules which can be identified by cytotoxic T cells. The D region of man is apparently analogous to the mouse I region and contains genes for class II proteins which are involved in cooperation and interaction between cells of the immune system. Products of the mouse I region are termed Ia antigens, which is also the generic term for antigens encoded by the human D region. The strength of an immune response in mice is partly determined by immune response genes (Ir genes) which map to the H-2I region. There is an enormous degree of structural polymorphism in the MHC of all animals in which it has been studied.

CELLULAR DISTRIBUTION OF MHC ANTIGENS

In man essentially all nucleated cells carry the antigens of the A, B and C regions in varying amounts, but the antigens coded by the D region have a restricted distribution as do the analogous mouse I region antigens which occur only on B lymphocytes, macrophages, monocytes and some epithelial cells. Some activated human T cells also have class II antigens (Fig. 4.6).

MHC subregion		tissue distribution of antigen
H-2	HLA	
K, D, L	A, B, C	all nucleated cells and platelets, erythrocytes (mouse)
I-A I-E	D	B lymphocytes macrophages / monocytes dendritic cells epithelial cells (?) melanoma cells activated T cells (human)

Fig. 4.6 The tissue distribution of MHC antigens. Emerald and turquoise colours are used here as in the previous figures to indicate the analogous functions performed by H-2 and HLA antigens. It should be noted that whereas mouse erythrocytes carry H-2K, D and L antigens, human erythrocytes do not carry the analogous HLA–A, –B and –C antigens. The genes of the mouse I–A and I–E regions encode the class II Ia antigens.

RECOMBINATION BETWEEN INBRED STRAINS

On rare occasions crossing over occurs within the H-2 region of F_1 mice of two parental inbred strains of different haplotype. These variants contain chromosomes with H-2 regions which match each parental strain in some of the regions only. The strains derived from these variants have been valuable in determining the region of H-2 involved in each MHC function, since it is possible for example, to transplant cells into a recipient that differs from the donor at only a small subregion of H-2. Examples of strains resulting from recombination between two inbred parental strains are given in Fig. 4.7.

strain	haplotype	K	I-A	I-E	S	D
B10	H-2^b	b	b	b	b	b
				X		
DBA/2	H-2^d	d	d	d	d	d
				⇩		
B10.GD, D2.GD	H-2^{g2}	d	d	b	b	b
other examples						
B10.A(4R)	H-2^{h4}	k	k	b	b	b
B10.A(2R)	H-2^{h2}	k	k	d	d	b
A.TH	H-2^{t2}	s	s	s	s	d

Fig. 4.7 H-2 regions of some recombinant mouse strains. The haplotype of an inbred strain is designated by a superscript, for example H-2^b, and the polypeptides produced by the MHC regions of a particular strain are designated by the same superscript. Mating F_1 individuals from two inbred strains (H-2^b × H-2^d) may sometimes result in a crossover in the I region, giving rise to a recombinant strain, for example of haplotype H-2^{g2}. Further crossovers involving other inbred strains produce the other examples of recombinant strains shown here.

STRUCTURAL VARIATION IN MHC ANTIGENS– PUBLIC AND PRIVATE SPECIFICITIES

If the antigens of a particular MHC region from different strains are examined they are found to have similar basic structures, but the fine structure of each antigen differs with each haplotype. These fine differences may be assessed by employing alloantisera against the antigens. The antigens produced by an inbred strain will induce antibodies in strains lacking that haplotype and the reaction between the two will be characteristic. A standard panel of antisera has been established covering a wide range of inbred strains. Thus, particular MHC antigens may now be compared and defined with reference to the standard panel of antisera, and using antisera it is possible to recognize antigenic

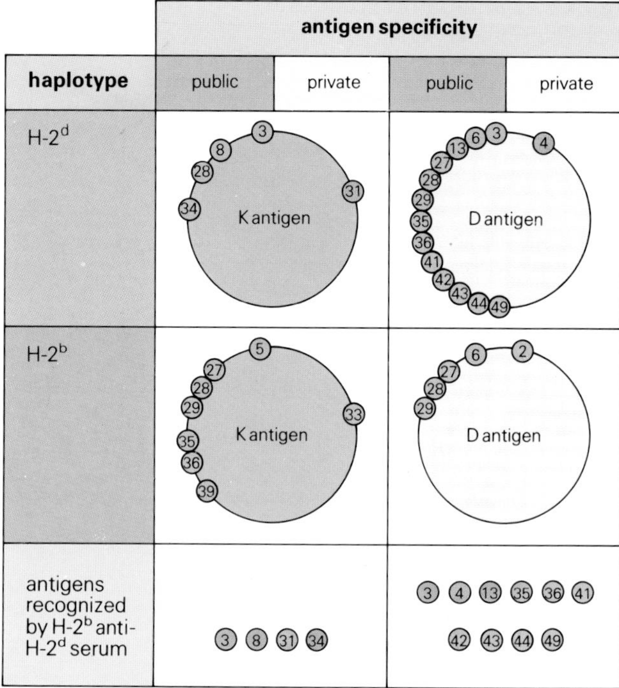

Fig. 4.8 H-2 public and private specificities. In this figure large circles represent K and D antigens and the antigenic specificities carried by these antigens are indicated by circled numbers. Some specificities are shared between antigens and haplotypes, for example specificity 28 is carried on the K and D antigens of both the H-2^d and H-2^b strains. These are known as *public* specificities, shown here all on the left for convenience. A smaller number of specificities are unique to a particular antigen and haplotype and are known as *private* specificities. If an antiserum were raised in the H-2^b strain against antigens of the H-2^d strain it would recognize the private determinants (e.g. 31 on the K antigen) and also the public determinants absent from its own cells (e.g. 3, 8 and 34 on the K antigen) but not public determinants which it shares with the other strain (e.g. 28).

determinants common to several different class I molecules or haplotypes, termed 'public' specificities, and also antigenic determinants unique to a particular molecule and haplotype, termed 'private' specificities. The term specificity is derived from the 'specificity' of the 'tissue typing' antisera which are used to determine and define the antigenic determinants present on cells. An illustration of the difference between public and private specificities is given in Fig. 4.8.

TISSUE TYPING

The technique of using standardized antisera to investigate structural variation between MHC antigens has been mentioned. When such antisera are used in tissue typing (cf. blood typing) the tissue is said to have been typed serologically. This method of tissue typing is performed by applying to the cells to be tested (usually lymphocytes) antisera of defined specificity together with complement and then observing whether the test cells are killed (Fig. 4.9). Other techniques of visualizing antibody binding by cells are used occasionally.

A second method of tissue typing exploits the fact that T lymphocytes are stimulated to grow in the presence of cells carrying foreign histocompatibility class II

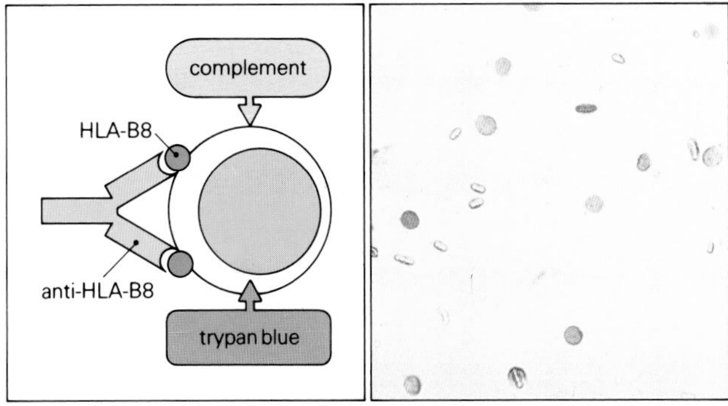

Fig. 4.9 Tissue typing – serological. Tissue typing is performed serologically by adding typing antisera of defined specificity (e.g. anti-HLA–B8), complement and trypan blue stain to test cells on a microassay plate. Cell death, as assessed by trypan blue staining, confirms that the test cell carried the antigen in question (HLA–B8). Dead, trypan blue-stained cells (dark staining) are shown on the right.

antigens, hence the name of the test, the mixed lymphocyte reaction (MLR). In particular, the two types of cell must differ within the I region (mouse) or the HLA–D region (human) for this stimulation to occur. The test lymphocytes are mixed with homozygous typing cells (B lymphocytes with two identical haplotypes at the MHC) of defined specificity. In culture, test cells lacking the specificity of the typing cell recognize it as foreign and so are stimulated to undergo transformation and proliferation (Fig. 4.10).

Proliferation may be detected by the uptake of [^{3}H]-thymidine into DNA and transformed lymphocytes may be distinguished by their characteristic appearance (Fig. 4.11). HLA antigens determined by this technique

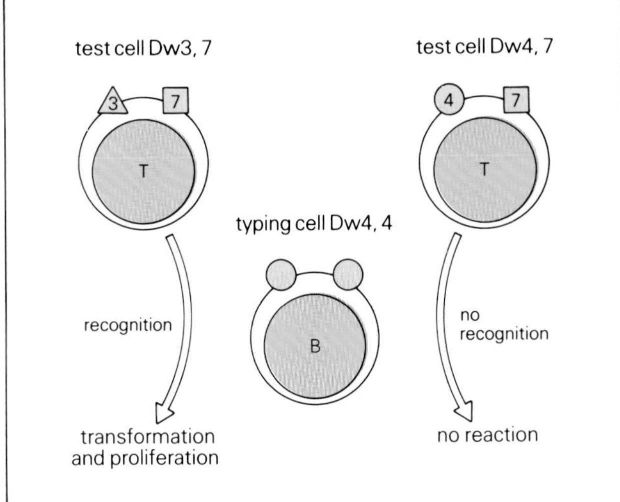

Fig. 4.10 Tissue typing – mixed lymphocyte reaction. In this example the homozygous typing cell is HLA–Dw 4,4 and antigenic specificities are represented by differently numbered shapes. Two different test lymphocytes are shown, Dw 3,7 and Dw 4,7. Dw 4,7 carries the typing cell's specificity (4), does not recognize Dw 4,4 as foreign, and does not react to the typing cell. Dw 3,7 recognizes the typing cell as foreign. This is revealed by the test cell transforming and proliferating. (Typing cells are treated to stop them dividing in response to the test cells.)

are D specificities. Details of the lymphocyte transformation test are given in Chapter 25. It has recently proved possible to detect HLA–D region antigens serologically and these are called DR specificities. When the two typing procedures are apparently detecting identical antigens, identical numbers are given to both D and DR specificities but it is questionable whether the two techniques identify exactly the same part of the molecule. If a particular specificity has not been sufficiently well defined the letter w (for workshop) is added to the designation.

The technique of tissue typing is used to assess the suitability of potential organ donors for transplantation. The aim is to obtain tissue from donors with the closest possible match with the recipient at the MHC, for both class I and class II molecules. A perfect match is often not possible, and other factors, such as the availability of tissues, are equally important considerations. Nevertheless the closer the match, the better the chance of successful transplantation (see Chapter 24).

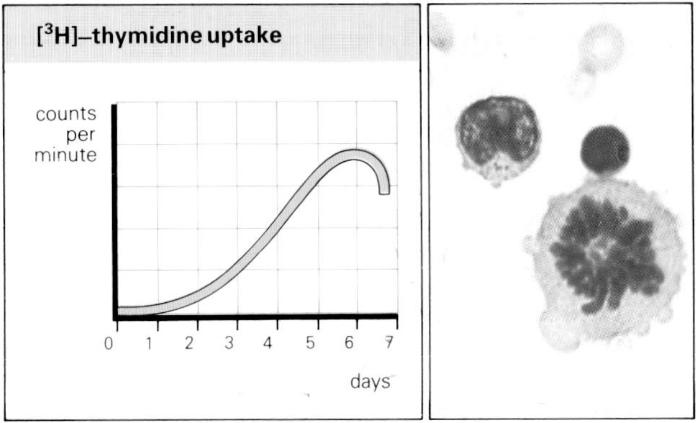

Fig. 4.11 Lymphocyte proliferation and transformation in the MLR typing test. Proliferation of the test lymphocytes may be assessed by the uptake of radioactive thymidine ([^{3}H]-thymidine) into DNA over a period of days (left). The appearance of transformed lymphocytes is shown on the right, with one cell in the process of division.

CURRENTLY RECOGNIZED HLA SPECIFICITIES AND LINKAGE DISEQUILIBRIUM

Many different specificities can be detected at each gene locus in the human population (Fig. 4.12). Since virtually any A region antigen may be linked with any of the B, C or D antigens the number of haplotypes present in the human population is very large and, with two non-identical chromosomes, the total number of possible genotypes is correspondingly enormous. Under ideal conditions (a random breeding population at equilibrium) the frequency with which two specificities occur together in a population is given by the product of the individual gene frequencies. For example, if 16% of the population have a particular HLA–A antigen (A1) and 10% of the population have a particular HLA–B antigen (B8) the chance of finding A1 genetically linked to B8 on the same chromosome is given by the product of their gene frequencies (16% × 10% = 1.6%). In practice this does not always occur. Certain combinations of A and B specificities occur more frequently together than would be expected if their association were random. For example, the combination of

DR		DQ	DP	B		C	A
DR1	Dw1	DQw1	DPw1	Bw4	Bw47	Cw1	A1
DR2	Dw2	DQw2	DPw2	B5	Bw48	Cw2	A2
DR3	Dw3	DQw3	DPw3	Bw6	B49	Cw3	A3
DR4	Dw4		DPw4	B7	Bw50	Cw4	A9
DR5			DPw5	B8	B51	Cw5	A10
DRw6			DPw6	B12	Bw52	Cw6	A11
DR7	Dw7			B13	Bw53	Cw7	Aw19
DRw8	Dw8			B14	Bw54	Cw8	A23
DRw9				B15	Bw55		A24
DRw10				B16	Bw56		A25
DRw11	Dw5			B17	Bw57		A26
DRw12				B18	Bw58		A28
DRw13	Dw6			B21	Bw59		A29
DRw14	Dw9			Bw22	Bw60		A30
DRw52				B27	Bw61		A31
DRw53				B35	Bw62		A32
				B37	Bw63		Aw33
				B38	Bw64		Aw34
				B39	Bw65		Aw36
				B40	Bw67		Aw43
				Bw41	Bw70		Aw66
				Bw42	Bw71		Aw68
				B44	Bw72		Aw69
				B45	Bw73		
				Bw46			

Fig. 4.12 Currently recognized HLA specificities. This table lists the distinct antigenic specificities detected at each HLA subregion. HLA–A, –B, –C and –DR (D-related) antigens are detected serologically. HLA–D specificities are also detected in the MLR. Specificities not yet sufficiently defined are designated by the subscript 'w'.

A1 and B8 is found at a frequency of 8.8% in human populations, compared to an expected frequency of 1.6%. Such paired specificities are said to be in linkage disequilibrium (Fig. 4.13). Two mechanisms may account for linkage disequilibrium.

1. The origin of a specificity has occurred relatively recently and there has been insufficient time for the recombination events which distribute new specificities at random among the chromosomes in the population.
2. Some mechanism, evolutionary or otherwise, favours the association of that pair of genes (although any such mechanism remains obscure).

The phenomenon is not uncommon. For example, of the 300 possible combinations of known A and B locus alleles, eight pairs show significant association. Linkage disequilibria are very common between B locus alleles and the closely genetically linked C locus alleles.

genes	gene frequency (%) observed	expected (pair)	observed (pair)
A1 B8	16 10	1.6	8.8***
A3 B7	13 10	1.3	2.8*
A29 B12	6 17	1.0	3.4***

Fig. 4.13 Examples of linkage disequilibrium. This table gives the frequencies of particular genes observed in European caucasoid populations, the frequency at which pairs of genes would be expected to occur on the same chromosome, and the frequency at which the pairs are actually observed together. The three pairs of genes shown here are more frequently associated than would be expected by chance. χ^2 analysis may be applied to the observed linkages (*=p<5%, ***=p<0.01%).

STRUCTURE OF THE MHC ANTIGENS

Work on the isolated MHC antigens has led to the elucidation of their structure. As might be anticipated for molecules involved in cell–cell recognition, the majority of the cellular MHC antigens are found in the plasma membrane. They are transmembrane glycoproteins and to perform structural analysis on them they must first be

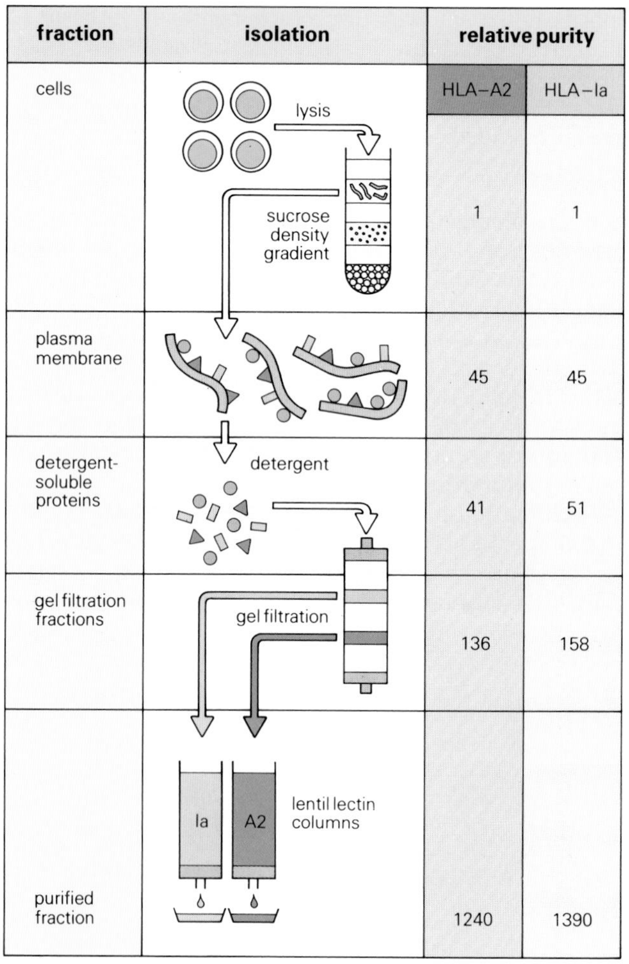

fraction	isolation	relative purity HLA–A2	HLA–Ia
cells	lysis; sucrose density gradient	1	1
plasma membrane		45	45
detergent-soluble proteins	detergent	41	51
gel filtration fractions	gel filtration	136	158
purified fraction	Ia, A2 lentil lectin columns	1240	1390

Fig. 4.14 Biochemical purification of the HLA–A2 (emerald) and Ia (turquoise) antigens from human lymphoblastoid cells. This illustration charts the isolation of the MHC products from cells and gives the relative purity of the antigens at each stage of purification, expressed as specific MHC protein/total protein. The purity increases as MHC antigens are separated from non-MHC proteins (blue) in successive steps. In the first stage the cells are lysed and the subcellular components separated by ultracentrifugation in a sucrose density gradient. The fraction containing the plasma membrane (rich in MHC and other proteins) is treated with detergent (sodium deoxycholate) in order to release the proteins, which are then subjected to gel filtration (on AcA34). The fractions containing HLA–A2 and Ia antigens are further purified on lentil lectin columns which specifically bind the HLA antigens. The antigens are eluted by adding sugar which binds competitively to the lectin.

dissociated from the membrane. This may be achieved in two ways.
1. The intact proteins can be released from the plasma membrane fraction with detergent.
2. The enzyme papain can be used to clip off the section of the MHC molecule exposed at the cell surface.

When the molecules are dissociated enzymatically they are found to differ from the native MHC antigens, since they lack the part of the antigen which traverses the plasma membrane. Purification of the solubilized antigens may be performed by conventional biochemical techniques, including affinity chromatography, using lectins or antisera to the antigens under investigation (Figs 4.14 and 4.15).

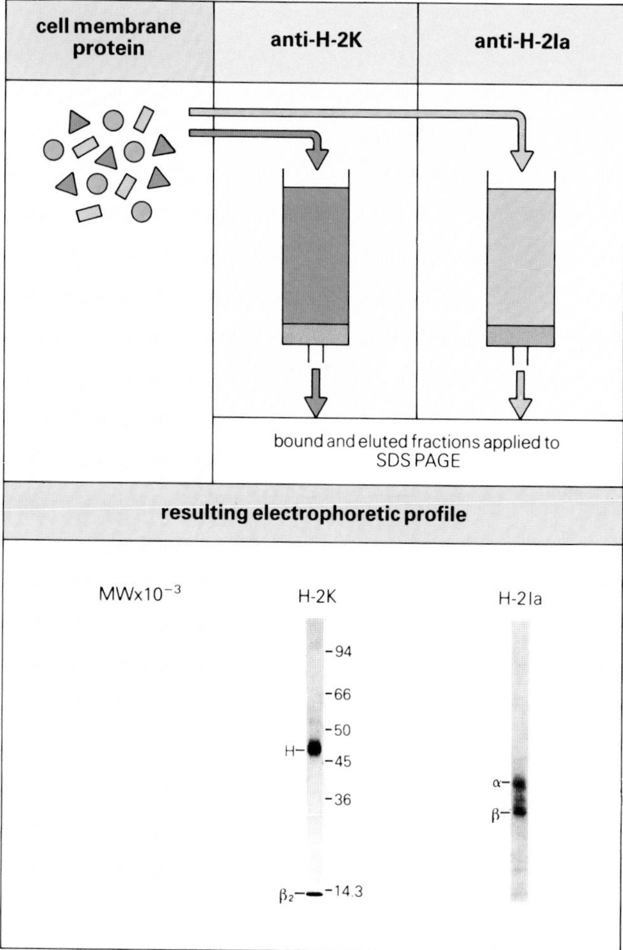

Fig. 4.15 Purification of MHC antigens by affinity chromatography. This technique employs columns carrying antibodies directed against specific MHC antigens. Protein isolated from cell membrane is introduced into columns containing antibody against specific MHC proteins. The columns are washed thoroughly to remove unbound membrane proteins, then specific antigens are eluted from the columns in conditions which dissociate the antigen–antibody interaction. They are then subjected to electrophoresis in reducing conditions (sodium dodecyl sulphate polyacrylamide gel electrophoresis, SDS PAGE). SDS PAGE separates the constituent polypeptides on the basis of molecular weight. The electrophoretic profile reveals that the H-2K and Ia proteins each consists of two subcomponents of different molecular weight (H and β_2, α and β, respectively). Affinity chromatography makes it possible to isolate individual antigens in a single step.

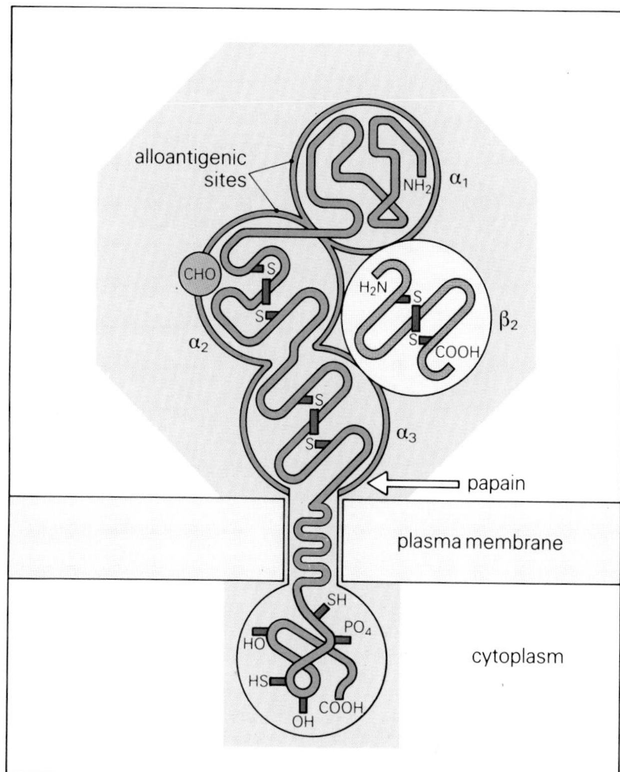

Fig. 4.16 Structure of an intact class I antigen (HLA–A, –B) in plasma membrane. The MHC-encoded chain has three globular domains (termed $\alpha1$, $\alpha2$ and $\alpha3$ shown in green). The $\alpha3$ domain is closely associated with the non-MHC-encoded peptide, β_2-microglobulin (grey). β_2-microglobulin is a small globular peptide (mol. wt 12,000) which is stabilized by an intrachain disulphide bond (red) and has a similar tertiary structure to an immunoglobulin domain. A short hydrophilic section of the MHC-encoded component at the –COOH terminus lies within the cytoplasm. A hydrophobic section traverses the membrane and the majority of the polypeptide, comprising the three globular domains, protrudes from the cell surface. Alloantigenic sites (carrying determinants specific to each individual) occur on the $\alpha1$ and $\alpha2$ domains and there is a carbohydrate unit attached to the $\alpha2$ domain (CHO). Papain cleaves the molecule at the point indicated, close to the outer margin of the plasma membrane.

Purification of MHC antigens by affinity chromatography on monoclonal antibody columns possesses several advantages over biochemical purification techniques. In particular, the 'one-step' nature of the approach results in rapidity, high yield and minimal degradation. Contamination is, however, often a problem due to non-specific adherence of other membrane proteins, in particular actin. This can be overcome by using a combination of the two approaches, for example, by applying a glycoprotein fraction, isolated using lentil lectin chromatography, to a monoclonal antibody column.

The structure of the class I antigens differs from that of the class II antigens. Each class I antigen consists of one glycosylated polypeptide chain of molecular weight about 45,000, non-covalently associated with a non-glycosylated peptide (β_2-microglobulin, about 12,000D) (Fig. 4.16). β_2-microglobulin also occurs free in serum or urine as a small globular peptide which has a similar

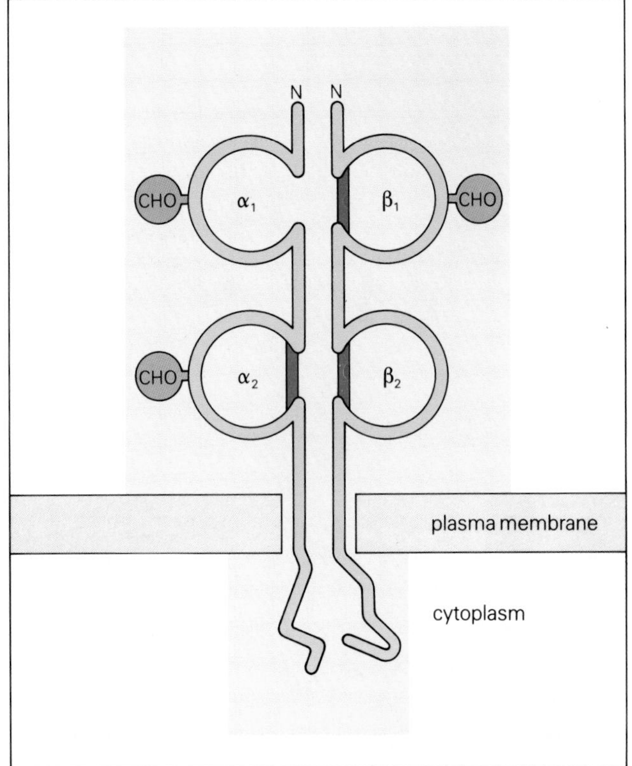

Fig. 4.17 Schematic representation of a class II antigen (HLA–DR). The HLA–DR antigens consist of two non-identical peptides (α and β), non-covalently bound, which traverse the plasma membrane towards the C terminus. Both chains have two globular domains. The membrane-proximal domain of each chain is structurally related to immunoglobulin domains and all except the α1 domain are stabilized by intrachain disulphide bonds (red). Both chains have carbohydrate units attached. The shorter, β chain (mol. wt 28,000) contains the alloantigenic sites although there is also some structural polymorphism in the α chain of some class II molecules.

tertiary structure to an immunoglobulin constant region domain. It is bound non-covalently to the α_3 domain of the class I heavy chain on the outer side of the plasma membrane. Although β_2-microglobulin does not form part of the antigenic site of the HLA molecule, it is necessary for processing and expression of the class I molecules; thus if a cell congenitally lacks β_2-microglobulin, the class I antigenic determinants are not expressed. The gene for β_2-microglobulin lies on a separate chromosome to that containing the MHC gene loci. Comparison of the amino acid sequences from different haplotypes of the human HLA–A and –B antigens and the mouse H-2K and H-2D antigens implies that the alloantigenic sites occur on the α_1 and α_2 domains (see Chapter 12).

The class II antigens consist of two distinct polypeptide chains, the α chain and the β chain. These peptides are held together by non-covalent forces and both chains traverse the plasma membrane. The shorter chain contains the alloantigenic sites, and both chains carry carbohydrate units (Fig. 4.17).

The genetic organization of the mouse H-2I region is better understood than that of the human HLA–D region, and genetic analysis of crossovers within the region H-2I has allowed its subdivision. Although structurally similar molecules are produced by all H-2I region genes so far studied, different subcomponents of the same H-2I molecule are encoded within different subregions (Fig. 4.18).

Examination of the isolated α and β peptides of I-E antigens from mice of different haplotypes indicates that the majority of allotypic variation occurs in the β chain (as is the case with the HLA–D antigen). There is some evidence that limited allotypic variation may also occur in the α chain of the H-2I antigens.

Recently, the HLA–A2 molecule has been crystallized and its structure determined. The α_1 and α_2 domains form the sides of a cleft on the outer surface of the class I molecule. The alloantigenic sites lie on the sides of this cleft, and it is thought that antigenic peptides become non-covalently bound in the cleft, before they are recognized by T cells. It is possible that a small molecule from the host cell normally occupies the cleft and is displaced by the antigenic peptides. This would occur, for example, if the cell became infected with virus, in which case viral peptides would occupy the cleft on the class I molecule. Fig. 4.19 shows the HLA–A2 structure and a model for the class II peptide binding site.

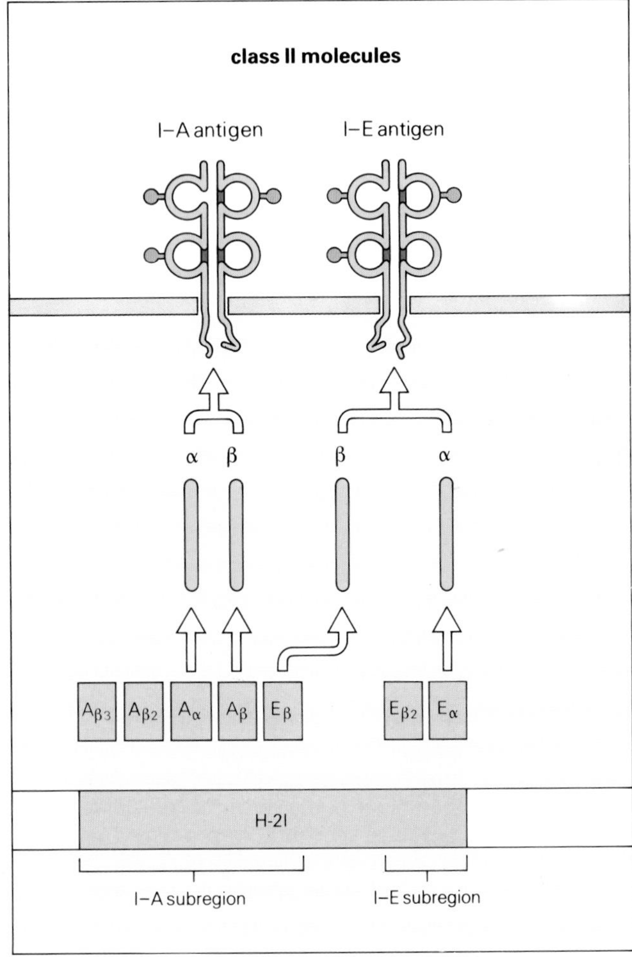

Fig. 4.18 Genetic organization of the mouse H-2I region. The H-2I region codes for antigens consisting of α and β chains. The two types of antigen identified (I–A and I–E) are of similar size but differ in detailed structure. The genes for the Aα and Aβ chains are in the I–A subregion, which also probably includes the gene for Eβ. Another Eβ gene ($E\beta_2$) and the Eα gene are in the I–E subregion.

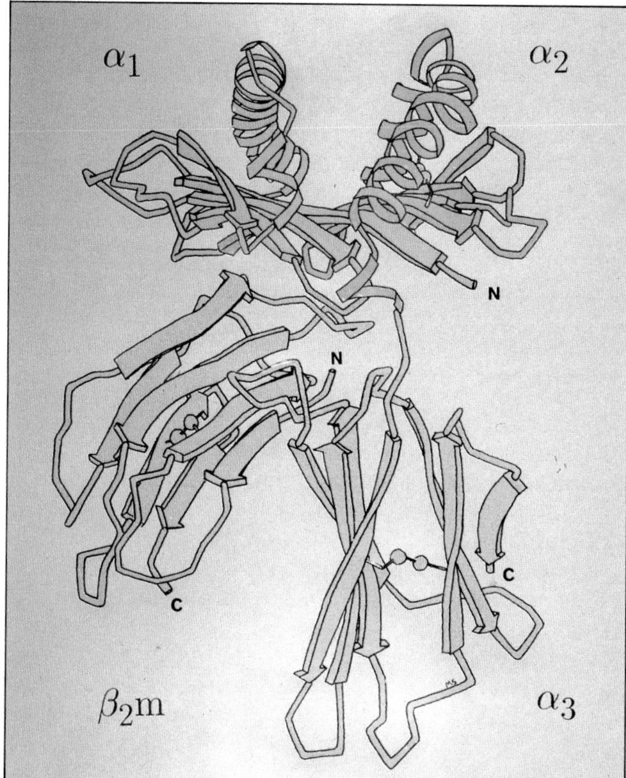

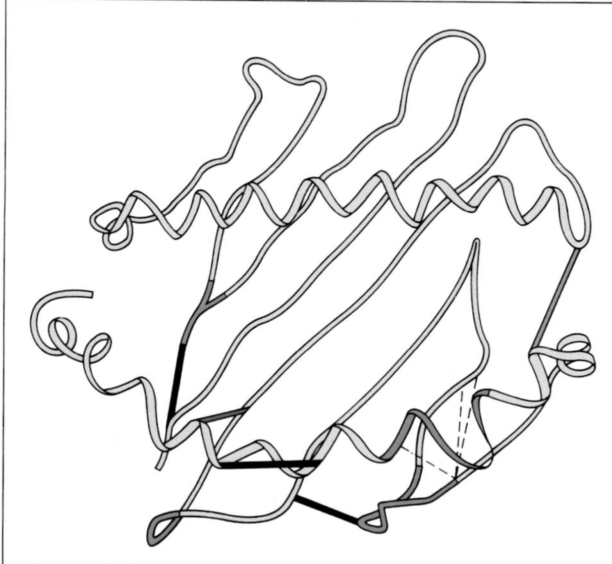

Fig. 4.19 Structure of MHC molecules. The upper figure shows the peptide chain structure of HLA–A2, showing the three domains of the α chain associated with β_2-microglobulin. The α_1 and α_2 domains which are most variable form a cleft lined with α helix and a base of β-pleated sheet which appears to form a site which can bind antigenic peptides. (Courtesy of P. J. Bjorkman, M. A. Sapper, B. Samraoui, W. S. Bennett, J. L. Strominger & D. C. Wiley, reprinted from *Nature*, **329**, 506, with permission.) The lower diagram shows this site viewed from above, and indicates elements of the structure which are conserved in the primary sequences of both class I and class II molecules, suggesting class II molecules may be structurally similar to class I. Conserved regions (darker shade), disulphide bond (red), salt bridges (black bars), hydrophobic region (dashed lines) and conserved secondary bond (blue bar). (Courtesy of J. H. Brown, T. Jardetzky, M. A. Sapper, B. Samraoui, P. J. Bjorkman & D. C. Wiley, adapted from *Nature*, **332**, 845, with permission.)

FUNCTIONS OF THE MHC ANTIGENS

The MHC antigens are essential for reactions of immune recognition. Different MHC antigens are recognized by different T cell types as summarized in Fig. 4.20. Cytotoxic T cells involved in recognition and rejection of virally infected cells and foreign tissue grafts recognize H-2K and H-2D molecules (HLA–A and –B in man) on the foreign cells, and in cooperation with T-helper cells they will cause destruction of the foreign cells. The rejection of foreign tissue has no normal physiological function, but the processes involved in recognition of foreign determinants on cell surfaces are similar to those necessary for recognition of viral antigens on infected cells.

Most virally infected cells display viral antigens on the surface of their plasma membranes which are recognized by cytotoxic T cells. Furthermore it may be demonstrated that cytotoxic T cells recognize the viral antigens in association with their recognition of the H-2K and D antigens present on the surface of the infected cells. In this way cytotoxic T cells of a particular H-2 haplotype from an animal infected with a virus are

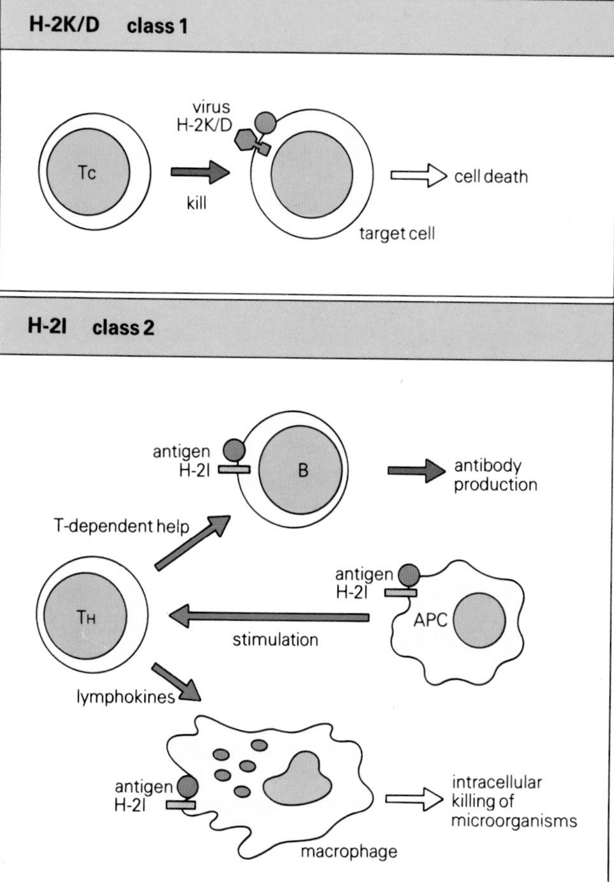

Fig. 4.20 Functions of the MHC in the mouse.
H-2K/D. Cytotoxic T cells (Tc) recognize foreign antigen (e.g. virus) when associated with either H-2K or H-2D products.
H-2I. Helper T cells (TH) recognize foreign antigen in association with H-2I gene products on antigen-presenting cells (APC). TH cells can cooperate with B cells to induce antibody production and they can also release lymphokines, which help macrophages to kill intracellular microorganisms.

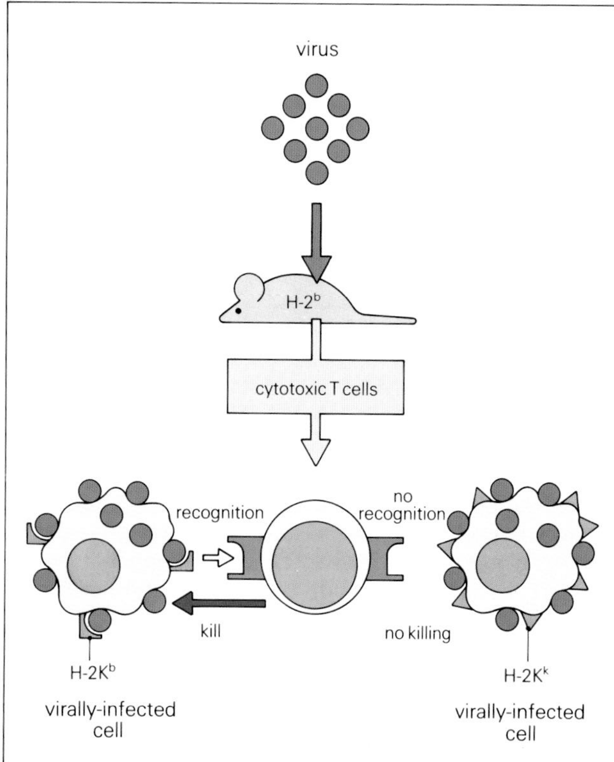

Fig. 4.21 Killing of virally infected target cells and haplotype restricted killing. A mouse of the H-2^b haplotype is primed with virus, and the cytotoxic T cells thus generated are then isolated. These T cells are then tested for their ability to kill cells of the H-2^b and H-2^k haplotypes infected with the same virus. The Tc cells kill H-2^b infected cells but not infected cells of a different haplotype, H-2^k. It is concluded that the T cell is recognizing a specific structure resulting from the association between the H-2K (or H-2D) product and viral antigen (e.g. a virus/H-2K complex). The association between antigen and MHC protein is most probably at the molecular level. (As a control measure, both groups are treated with anti-viral antibody, which does not exhibit haplotype restriction: infected cells of both haplotypes are killed by anti-viral antibody and complement.)

primed to kill cells infected with that virus. However, it is found that they will not kill cells of a different haplotype infected by the same virus. This phenomenon is referred to as haplotype-restricted killing. Since the cytotoxic T cells have been primed by a combined recognition of H-2 and viral antigens, they can only subsequently kill cells carrying both antigen types. In effect the H-2 molecules on the surface of the virally infected cell act as a code, guiding the cytotoxic T cell to its target, and allowing it to differentiate the target cell from other tissues carrying the viral antigens (Fig. 4.21). Similar principles of haplotype restriction apply to T-helper cells which recognize antigen on macrophages and B cells in association with H-2I region molecules. In this case the I region molecules act as recognition signals between antigen-presenting cells and the lymphocyte. Genetically restricted interactions of this kind are characteristic of immune reactions involving MHC molecules.

One rationalization for the evolution of a joint recognition system for MHC antigen plus viral antigen is that by recognizing viral antigen in association with MHC antigen, receptors on cytotoxic T cells do not become saturated with free virus: saturation would inhibit the cytotoxic T cells from killing virally infected cells.

Many functions of the MHC will be discussed more fully in connection with other aspects of the immune system since the MHC is involved in most reactions of immune recognition. Indeed recent evidence suggests that the MHC and other molecules involved in immune recognition share sequence homologies.

THE IMMUNOGLOBULIN SUPERFAMILY

Members of the so-called immunoglobulin superfamily all share an immunoglobulin-like domain, about 100 amino acid residues long and characterized by a centrally placed disulphide bridge that stabilizes a series of antiparallel β strands into an immunoglobulin-like fold. Members of the superfamily can share homology with either immunoglobulin variable or constant domains. Superfamily members expressed by cells of the immune system are shown in Fig. 4.22 and include both multigene (for example, MHC class I and class II) and single gene (for example, CD4 and CD8) members. Other

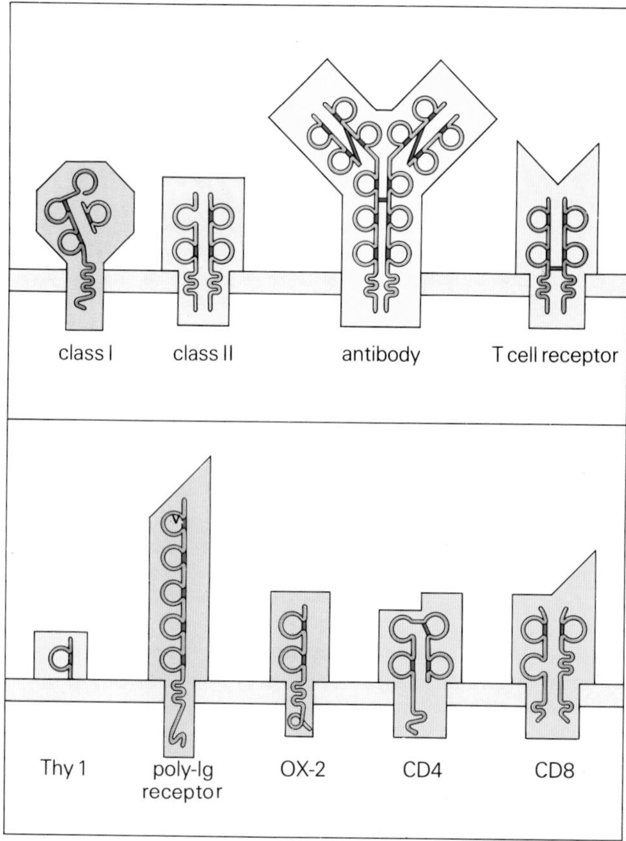

Fig. 4.22 The immunoglobulin supergene family. Many cell surface molecules have polypeptide chains folded into domains related to the domain first identified in antibody. These include molecules involved in immune recognition (top) and others involved in recognition. Thy-1 is expressed on T cells and brain cells. The poly-Ig receptor binds IgA and transports it across epithelial cells. OX-2 is a marker of B cells but is also found on brain cells and thymocytes. CD4 and CD8 are markers of T-helper and T-suppressor cells, respectively, and are involved in interactions with MHC molecules.

lymphocyte cell surface molecules, such as CD3γ, δ and ε polypeptides and the CD2 antigen, share weaker, although nonetheless significant, homology with immunoglobulin domains and may, therefore, be distantly related members of this family.

Immunoglobulin superfamily members are not confined to the immune system; the brain in particular possesses several members. It is possible that the primordial immunoglobulin homology unit mediated cell–cell interactions through homophilic associations and that its descendants all mediate cell interactions in the immune and other systems by this type of association.

FUNCTION OF ALLOTYPIC VARIATION

It is pertinent at this point to speculate on the enormous amount of allotypic variation observed in the MHC region antigens. The development of new MHC specificities can be seen in different but related species (Fig. 4.23). The reason for the great variation is not known, but it has been suggested that possession of a large number of different MHC molecules makes it less likely that a microbe could evade the body's immune system by imitating one of the recognition molecules of the system. Moreover when seen at a population level the self/non-self recognition systems of different individuals are all different, though working on the same principle. Since the immune system of each individual is different, the 'perfect pathogen' cannot evolve to spread through a population. Despite this, it is known that the possession of particular MHC antigens renders that individual more susceptible to particular diseases, some examples of which are given in Fig. 4.24.

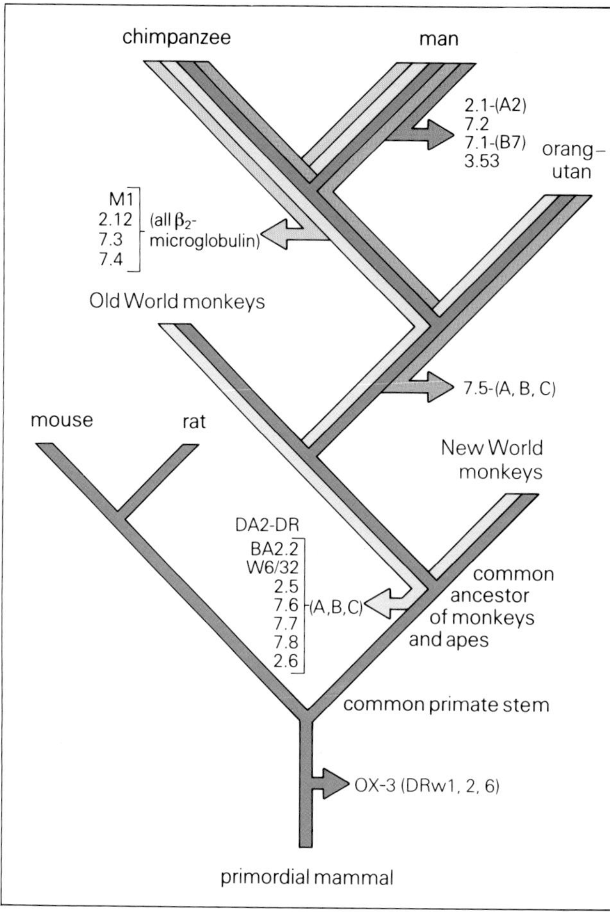

Fig. 4.23 Development of MHC specificities. This evolutionary tree traces the appearance of new MHC determinants. It should be emphasized that the shape of the tree is not derived from the MHC determinants but is based on other considerations. The older specificities shown are named after the monoclonal antibodies employed to detect them. Thus OX-3 is a monoclonal antibody recognizing rat Ia antigens and also a cross-reacting determinant on HLA–DR1, 2,6. W6/32 is a monoclonal antibody which recognizes a determinant common to the HLA–A, –B, –C antigens and transplantation antigens of Old World monkeys. The colours show the representation of the various determinants in different species. The molecules recognized are bracketed.

disease	antigen	frequency of antigen		
		control	patients	relative risk
Ankylosing spondylitis	B27	8	90	87.8
Reiter's disease	B27	9	80	35.9
Rheumatoid arthritis	DRw4	31	64	4.0
Multiple sclerosis	A3	21	33	1.8
	B7	18	35	2.0
	Bw2	21	74	1.9
	DRw2	22	42	3.8
Myasthenia gravis	B8	16	39	3.4
	DRw3	17	40	3.0
Psoriasis	A1	26	39	2.1
	B13	6	21	8.7
	Bw37	2	4	8.1
	Cw6	23	70	4.3
Addison's disease	Dw3	21	70	8.8
Graves' disease	B8	18	44	2.5
	Bw35	20	57	5
	Dw3	53	18	5.5
Coeliac disease	B8	20	67	8.6
	Dw3	27	96	73.0
Haemochromatosis	A3	20	71	9.0
Active chronic hepatitis	B8	16	36	9.2
	DRw3	7	79	4.6

Fig. 4.24 Disease associations of HLA antigens in European caucasoids. This table lists some diseases which are associated with particular HLA antigens. The extent to which an individual carrying the antigen is more likely to contract the disease, relative to an individual without the determinant, is given in the relative risk column. (The Bw 35 association is based on a study in Japan.)

FURTHER READING

Bjorkman, P. J., Saper, M. A., Samaroui, B., Bennett, W. S., Strominger, J. L. and Wiley, D. C. (1987) Structure of the human class I histocompatibility antigen, HLA-A2. *Nature*, **329**, 506–512.

Brown, J. H., Jardetzky, Saper, A., Samaroui, B., Bjorkman, P. J. and Wiley, D. C. (1988) A hypothetical model of the foreign antigen binding site of class II histocompatibility molecules. *Nature*, **332**, 845–850.

Germain, R. N. & Malissen, B. (1986) Analysis of the expression and function of class-II major histocompatibility complex-encoded molecules by DNA-mediated gene transfer. *Annual Review of Immunology*, **4**, 281–315.

Hood, L., Steinmotz, M. & Malissen, B. (1983) Genes of the major histocompatibility complex of the mouse. *Annual Review of Immunology*, **1**, 529–568.

Strominger J. L. *et al* (1980). In *The Role of the Major Histocompatibility Complex in Immunobiology*. Edited by B. Benacerraf & M. Dorf. New York: Garland Publishing Inc.

Zinkernagel, R. M. & Doherty, P. C. (1979) MHC-restricted cytotoxic T cells: studies on the biological role of polymorphic major transplantation antigens determining T-cell restriction – specificity, function and responsiveness. *Advances in Immunology*, **27**, 51–177.

5 Molecules which Recognize Antigen

The recognition of foreign antigen is the hallmark of the specific adaptive immune response. It is now clear that two distinct types of molecule are involved in this process – the immunoglobulins and the T cell antigen receptors. Diversity and heterogeneity are characteristic features of each family and there are further similarities at the genetic level in that both show evidence of extensive gene rearrangements in order to generate different immunoglobulins or cell surface receptors able to recognize many different antigens.

The immunoglobulins, or antibodies, are a group of glycoproteins present in the serum and tissue fluids of all mammals. They are produced in large amounts by plasma cells which have developed from precursor B lymphocytes. Such lymphocytes carry membrane bound immunoglobulin of the same binding specificity as that produced by the terminally differentiated plasma cell. Contact between these B lymphocytes and foreign antigen is required for the induction of antibody formation.

The T cell receptors are expressed exclusively on the membrane surface of T lymphocytes and there is no comparable production of soluble molecules analogous to the circulating antibodies. T cell recognition of antigen through the T cell receptor is the basis of a range of immunological phenomena including T cell helper and suppressor activity, cytotoxicity and possibly NK (natural killing) activity.

The two families of molecules, which are considered separately in the following sections, are compared schematically in Fig. 5.1.

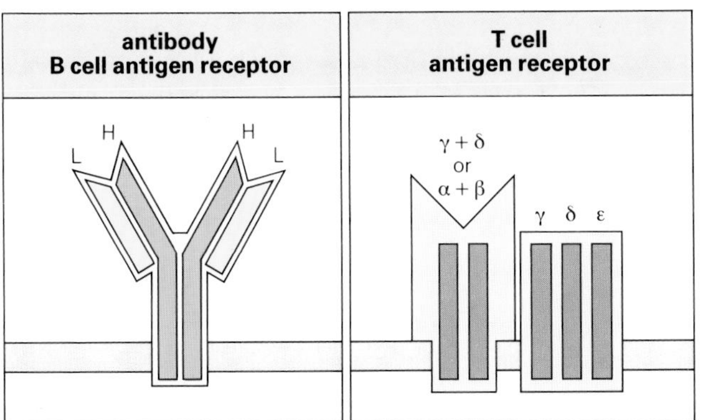

Fig. 5.1 Antigen recognition molecules. The antigen receptors of T and B lymphocytes are probably derived from a common ancestor and both belong to the immunoglobulin supergene family. Antibody consists of two identical heavy (H) chains and two identical light (L) chains. The T cell receptor has an antigen-binding portion consisting of an α and a β chain (or a γ and a δ chain) which are associated with three other transmembrane polypeptides (γ, δ, and ε), structurally distinct from the chains of the receptor. Circulating antibodies are structurally identical to B cell antigen receptors but lack the transmembrane and intracytoplasmic sections

THE IMMUNOGLOBULINS

Five distinct classes of immunoglobulin molecule are recognized in most higher mammals, namely IgG, IgA, IgM, IgD and IgE (Fig. 5.2). These differ from each other in size, charge, amino acid composition and carbohydrate content.

present nomenclature	shorthand	previous nomenclature
immunoglobulin G	IgG	γG globulin 7S γ-globulin
immunoglobulin A	IgA	γA globulin β_2A-globulin
immunoglobulin M	IgM	γM globulin 19S γ-globulin, γ-IM γ-macroglobulin
immunoglobulin D	IgD	—
immunoglobulin E	IgE	reagin, IgND

Fig. 5.2 Nomenclature of the five immunoglobulin classes recognized in most higher mammals.

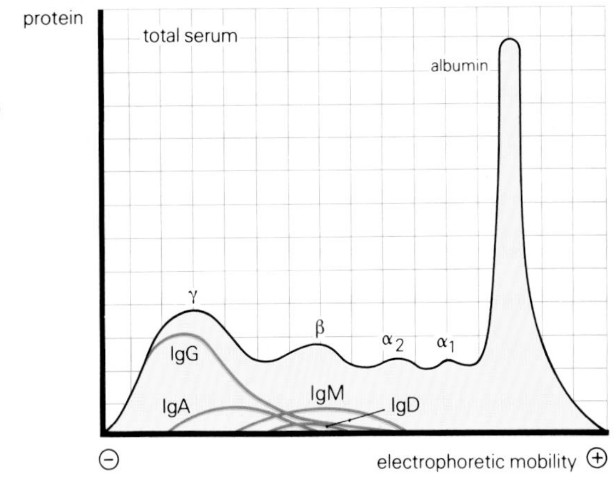

Fig. 5.3 Electrophoresis of human serum showing the distribution of the four major immunoglobulin classes. Serum proteins are separated according to their charge in an electric field, and classified as α_1, α_2, β, and γ, depending on their mobility. (The IgE class has a similar mobility to IgD but cannot be represented quantitatively because of its low level in serum.) IgG exhibits most charge heterogeneity, the other classes having a more restricted mobility in the slow β and fast γ regions.

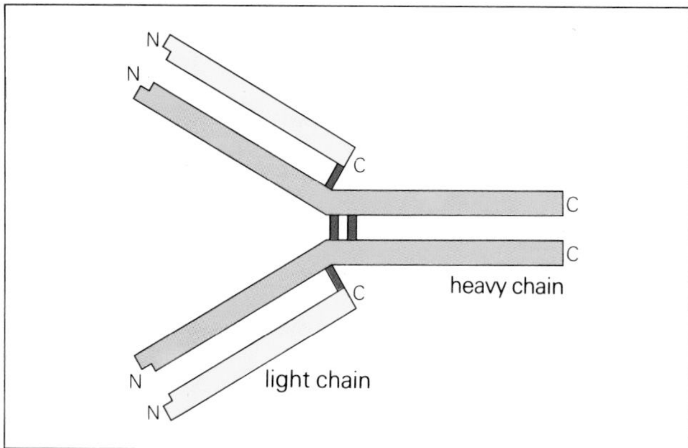

Fig. 5.4 The basic immunoglobulin structure. The unit consists of two identical light polypeptide chains and two identical heavy polypeptide chains linked together by disulphide bonds (red). Note the position of the amino (*N*)- and carboxy (*C*)-terminal ends of the peptide chains.

In addition to the differences between classes, the immunoglobulins within each class are also very heterogeneous. Electrophoretically the immunoglobulins show a unique range of heterogeneity which extends from the γ to the α fractions of normal serum. In general it is the IgG class which exhibits most charge heterogeneity, the other classes having a more restricted mobility in the slow β and fast γ regions (Fig. 5.3). These fractions suffer marked depletion following absorption with antigen suggesting a role for them in the immune response. The basic four-chain polypeptide structure of the immunoglobulin molecule is represented in Fig. 5.4.

ANTIBODY FUNCTION

Essentially each immunoglobulin molecule is bifunctional; one region of the molecule is concerned with binding to antigen while a different region mediates binding of the immunoglobulin to host tissues, including various cells of the immune system, some phagocytic cells, and the first component (C1q) of the classical complement system.

IMMUNOGLOBULIN CLASSES AND SUBCLASSES

The basic structure of all immunoglobulin molecules is a unit consisting of two identical light polypeptide chains and two identical heavy polypeptide chains linked together by disulphide bonds. The class and subclass of an immunoglobulin molecule is determined by its heavy chain type. Thus the four human IgG subclasses (IgG1, IgG2, IgG3 and IgG4) have heavy chains called γ_1, γ_2, γ_3 and γ_4 which differ only slightly, although all are recognizably γ heavy chains. The differences between subclasses within a class are less than those between the different classes; thus IgG1 is more closely related to IgG2, 3, or 4 than to IgA, IgM, IgD or IgE.

The four subclasses of human IgG (IgG1, IgG2, IgG3 and IgG4) occur in the approximate proportions of 66%, 23%, 7% and 4%, respectively. There are also known to be subclasses of human IgA (IgA1 and IgA2), but none have been unambiguously described for IgM, IgD and IgE.

Immunoglobulin subclasses appear to have arisen after speciation and the human subclasses cannot be compared with, for example, the four known subclasses of IgG which have been identified in the mouse.

GENERAL PROPERTIES OF IMMUNOGLOBULINS

All immunoglobulins appear to be glycoproteins but the carbohydrate content ranges from 2–3% for IgG to 12–14% for IgM, IgD and IgE. The physicochemical properties of the immunoglobulins are summarized in Fig. 5.5.

IgG is the major immunoglobulin in normal human serum accounting for 70–75% of the total immunoglobulin pool. IgG is a monomeric protein with a sedimentation coefficient of 7S and a molecular weight of 146,000. However, studies of IgG subclasses have indicated that IgG3 proteins are slightly larger than the other subclasses; this is due to the slightly heavier γ_3 chain. The IgG class, which is distributed evenly between the intravascular and extravascular pools, is the major antibody of secondary immune responses and the exclusive antitoxin class.

IgM accounts for approximately 10% of the immunoglobulin pool. The molecule has a pentameric structure in which individual heavy chains have a molecular weight of approximately 65,000 and the whole molecule has a molecular weight of 970,000. IgM is largely confined to the intravascular pool and is the predominant 'early' antibody frequently seen in the immune response to antigenically complex infectious organisms.

immunoglobulin	IgG1	IgG2	IgG3	IgG4	IgM	IgA1	IgA2	sIgA	IgD	IgE
heavy chain	γ_1	γ_2	γ_3	γ_4	μ	α_1	α_2	α_1 or α_2	δ	ε
mean serum concentration (mg/ml)	9	3	1	0.5	1.5	3.0	0.5	0.05	0.03	0.00005
sedimentation constant	7S	7S	7S	7S	19S	7S	7S	11S	7S	8S
molecular weight	146,000	146,000	170,000	146,000	970,000	160,000	160,000	385,000	184,000	188,000
half-life (days)	21	20	7	21	10	6	6	?	3	2
distribution (% intravascular)	45	45	45	45	80	42	42	trace	75	50
carbohydrate (%)	2–3	2–3	2–3	2–3	12	7–11	7–11	7–11	9–14	12

Fig. 5.5 Physicochemical properties of human immunoglobulin classes. Each class possesses a characteristic type of heavy chain. Thus IgG possesses γ chains; IgM, μ chains; IgA, α chains; IgD, δ chains and IgE, ε chains. Variation in heavy chain structure within a class gives rise to immunoglobulin subclasses. For example, the human IgG pool consists of four subclasses reflecting four distinct types of heavy chain. The physicochemical properties of the immunoglobulins vary between the different classes. Note that in secretions IgA occurs in a dimeric form (sIgA) in association with a protein chain termed the secretory piece.

IgA represents 15–20% of the human serum immunoglobulin pool. In man more than 80% of IgA occurs as the basic four-chain monomer, but in most mammals the IgA in serum is mainly polymeric, occurring most commonly as a dimer. IgA is the predominant immunoglobulin in seromucous secretions such as saliva, colostrum, milk, tracheobronchial and genito-urinary secretions.

Secretory IgA (sIgA), which may be of either subclass, exists mainly in the 11S, dimeric form and has a molecular weight of 385,000. sIgA is abundant in seromucous secretions where it is associated with another protein – the secretory component.

IgD accounts for less than 1% of the total plasma immunoglobulin but is known to be present in large quantities on the membrane of many circulating B lymphocytes. The precise biological function of this class is not known but it may play a role in antigen-triggered lymphocyte differentiation.

IgE, though a trace serum protein, is found on the surface membrane of basophils and mast cells in all individuals. This class of immunoglobulin may play a role in active immunity to helminthic parasites, but in developed countries it is more commonly associated with immediate hypersensitivity diseases such as asthma and hay fever.

The diversity of the structure of the different classes suggests that they perform different functions, in addition to their primary function of antigen binding, but in spite of this diversity all antibodies have a common basic structure.

ANTIBODY STRUCTURE

In 1962 Rodney Porter proposed a basic four-chain model for immunoglobulin molecules as shown in Fig. 5.4, based on two distinct types of polypeptide chain. The smaller (light) chain has a molecular weight of 25,000 and is common to all classes, whereas the larger (heavy) chain has a molecular weight of 50,000–77,000 and is structurally distinct for each class or subclass. The polypeptide chains are linked together by covalent and non-covalent forces to give a four-chain structure based on pairs of identical heavy and light chains. IgG, IgD and IgE occur only as monomers of the four-chain unit, IgA occurs in both monomeric and polymeric forms, and IgM occurs as a pentamer with five four-chain subunits linked together.

The light chains of most vertebrates have been shown to exist in two distinct forms called kappa (κ-type) and lambda (λ-type). They may be distinguished by their behaviour as antigens – antisera may be raised to one type which do not react with the other. Either of the light chain types may combine with any of the heavy chain types, but in any one molecule both light chains are of the same type and hybrid molecules do not occur naturally.

Hilschmann, Craig and others in 1965 established that when light chains of the same type are sequenced they are found to consist of two distinct regions. The carboxy-terminal half of the chain (approximately 107 amino acid residues) is constant except for certain allotypic and isotypic variations (see below) and is called the C_L (Constant:Light chain) region, whereas the amino-terminal half of the chain shows much sequence variability and is known as the V_L (Variable:Light chain) region.

The IgG molecule may be considered as a typical example of the basic antibody structure. As shown in Figs 5.6 and 5.7, IgG has two intrachain disulphide bonds in the light chain – one in the variable region and one in the constant region. Similarly, there are four such bonds in the heavy (γ) chain, which is twice the length of a light chain. Each disulphide bond encloses a peptide loop of

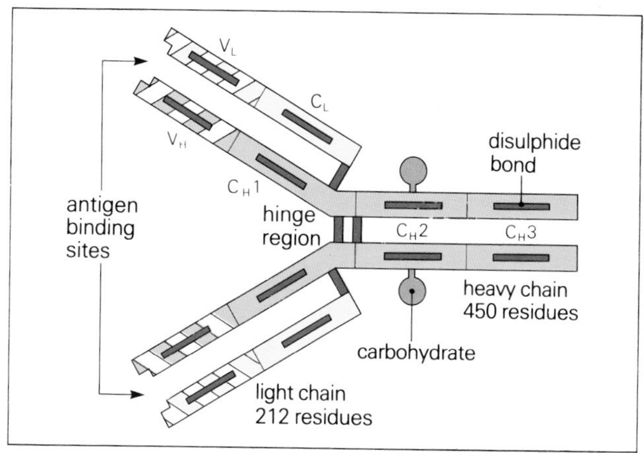

Fig. 5.6 The basic structure of IgG. The amino-terminal end is characterized by sequence variability (V) in both the heavy and light chains, referred to as the V_H and V_L regions respectively. The rest of the molecule has a relatively constant (C) structure. The constant portion of the light chain is termed the C_L region. The constant portion of the heavy chain is further divided into three structurally discrete regions: C_H1, C_H2 and C_H3. These globular regions, which are stabilized by intrachain disulphide bonds, are referred to as 'domains'. The sites at which the antibody binds antigen are located in the variable domains. The hinge region is a segment of heavy chain between the C_H1 and C_H2 domains. Flexibility in this area permits the two antigen-binding sites to operate independently. There is close pairing of the domains except in the C_H2 region (see Fig. 5.8). Carbohydrate moieties (blue) are attached to the C_H2 domains.

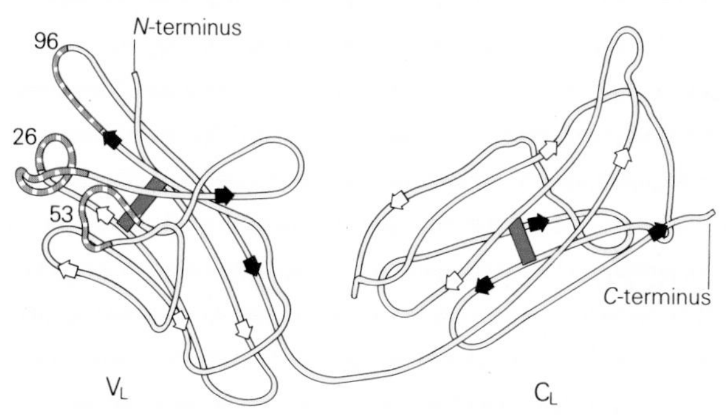

Fig. 5.7 The basic folding pattern of the variable and constant domains of the light chain. The domains are essentially comprised of two layers of polypeptide chain; one is composed of four segments (arrowed white) and the other of three segments (arrowed black). The segments of these layers, which are joined by disulphide bonds (red), run in opposite directions. Folding of the V_L domains causes the hypervariable regions to become exposed in three separate but closely disposed loops. One numbered residue from each hypervariable region is identified.

60–70 amino acid residues and if the amino acid sequences of these loops are compared a striking degree of homology is revealed. Essentially this means that each immunoglobulin peptide chain is composed of a series of globular regions with very similar secondary and tertiary structure (folding). The peptide loops enclosed by the disulphide bonds represent the central portion of a 'domain' of about 110 amino acid residues. In the light chain these domains (V_L and C_L) correspond to the variable and constant regions respectively (Fig. 5.7). In the heavy chain, the *N*-terminal region is called the V_H domain and in γ, α and δ chains there are three domains in the constant part of the chain C_H1, C_H2 and C_H3. In both μ and ε chains there is an additional domain after C_H1. Thus, the carboxy-terminal domains in the μ and ε chains (referred to as $C_\mu4$ and $C_\varepsilon4$) are homologous to $C_\gamma3$.

A specific nomenclature may be used to describe the domains of different classes; for example Cγ1, Cγ2 and Cγ3 for IgG and Cμ1, Cμ2, Cμ3 and Cμ4 for IgM. With this additional information about domain structure it is possible to refine the basic model presented in Fig. 5.6 into one which more closely approximates the structure of the actual molecule (Fig. 5.8).

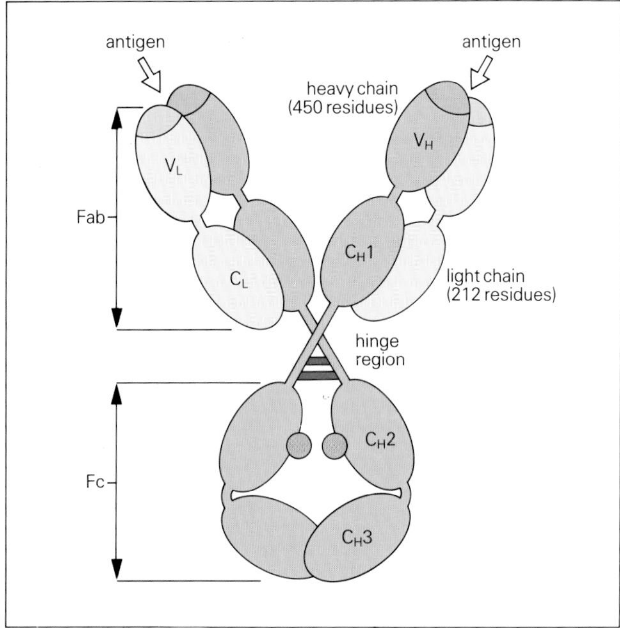

Fig. 5.8 Structure of IgG. A model of IgG indicating the globular domains of heavy (H) and light (L) chains. Note the apposition of the C_H3 domains and the separation of the C_H2 domains. The carbohydrate units lie between the C_H2 domains. In this and subsequent figures the interchain disulphide bonds between H and L chains are not shown.

IgG Although the four-chain structure of human IgG1 shown in Fig. 5.8 is a useful model for all immunoglobulins there are differences of detail in every class. Even with human IgG, no two subclasses are identical in the number and distribution of interchain disulphide bonds. Indeed, the light–heavy chain bonds in IgG2, 3 and 4 are linked to the junction between the variable and constant regions of the heavy chains and this pattern is the one most frequently observed in other classes. Similarly the number of inter-heavy chain bonds may be two (IgG1 and Ig4), four (IgG2), or fifteen (IgG3) (Fig. 5.9).

IgM IgM is a pentamer of the four-chain basic structure common to all immunoglobulin classes, consisting of two μ heavy chains and two light chains (Fig. 5.10). The μ chains differ from γ chains in amino acid sequence and in the number of constant region domains. The subunits are held together by disulphide bonds between the Cμ3 domains. The complete molecule consists of a densely packed central region with radiating arms. This structure is clearly seen in many electronmicrographs of IgM molecules. Photographs of IgM antibodies binding to bacterial flagella show molecules cross-linking two flagella, as well as molecules adopting a 'staple' configuration (Fig. 5.11). The latter suggests that flexion readily occurs between the Cμ2 and Cμ3 domains although this region is not structurally homologous to the IgG hinge.

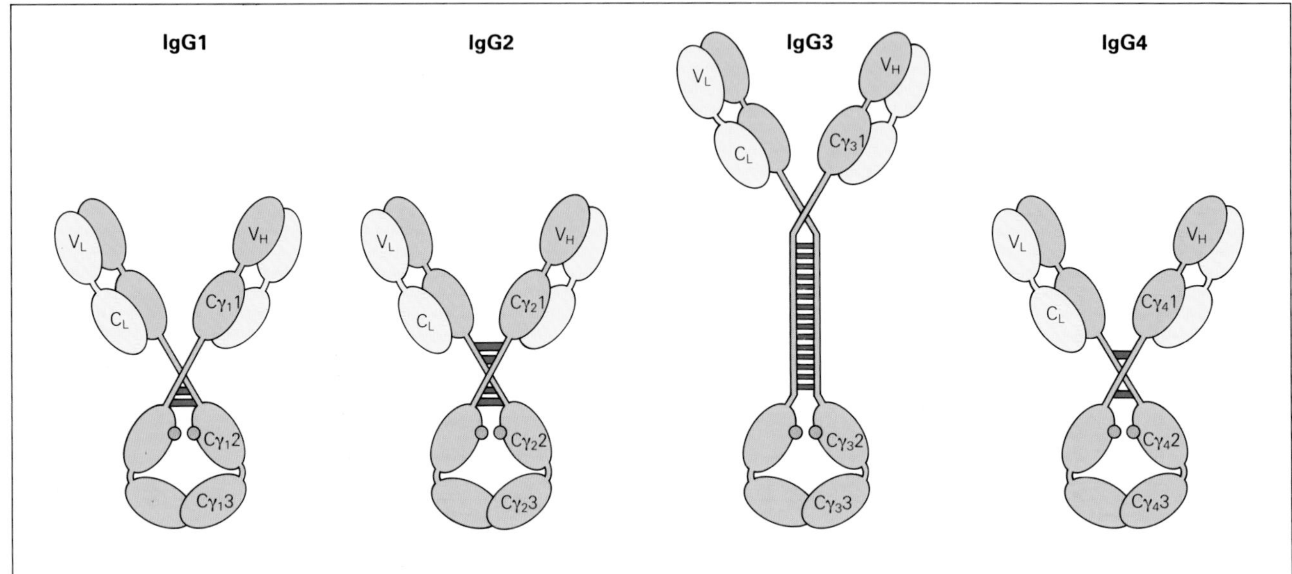

Fig. 5.9 Polypeptide chain structure of the four human IgG subclasses. The subclasses have different numbers and arrangements of the interchain disulphide bonds.

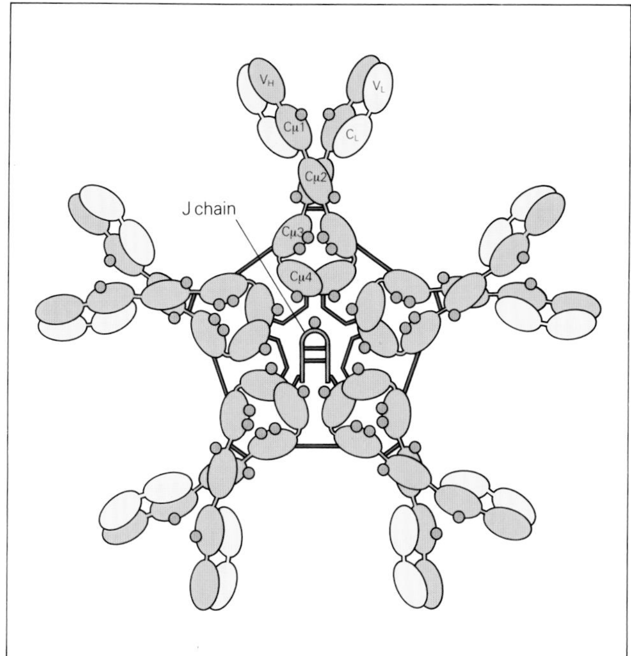

Fig. 5.10 Pentameric polypeptide chain structure of human IgM. IgM heavy chains have five domains with disulphide bonds cross-linking adjacent $C\mu3$ and $C\mu4$ domains of different units. Also shown are the carbohydrate side-chains and possible location of the J chain. There are no hinge regions in the monomeric subunits.

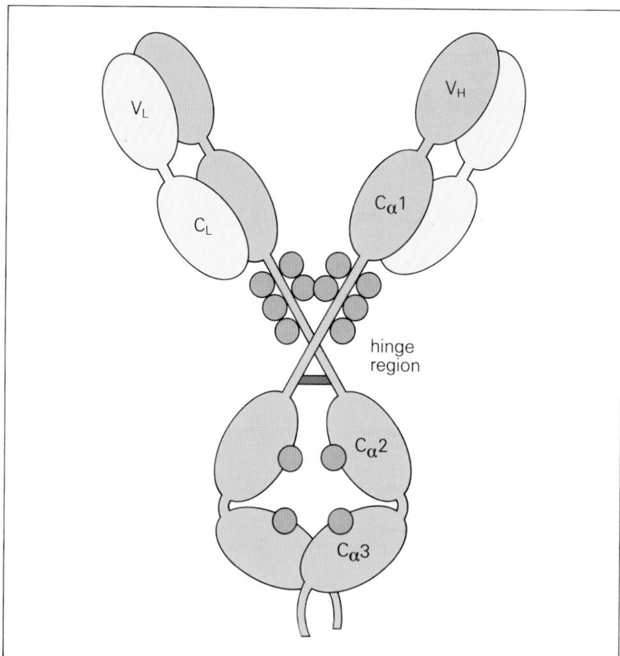

Fig. 5.12 Structure of human IgA1. This diagram shows the domain structure and the possible location of carbohydrate units. Note the presence of the *C*-terminal octadecapeptide 'tail' (a feature shared with IgM) and a hinge region.

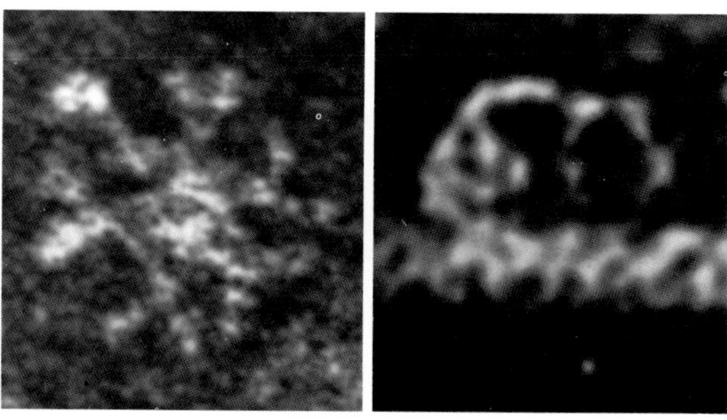

Fig. 5.11 Electronmicrographs of IgM molecules. In free solution adopting the characteristic star-shaped configuration (left, $\times 5.2 \times 10^6$; courtesy of Dr R. Dourmashkin), and a crab-like or staple configuration due to cross-linkage with a single flagellum (right, $\times 5.2 \times 10^6$; courtesy of Dr A. Feinstein).

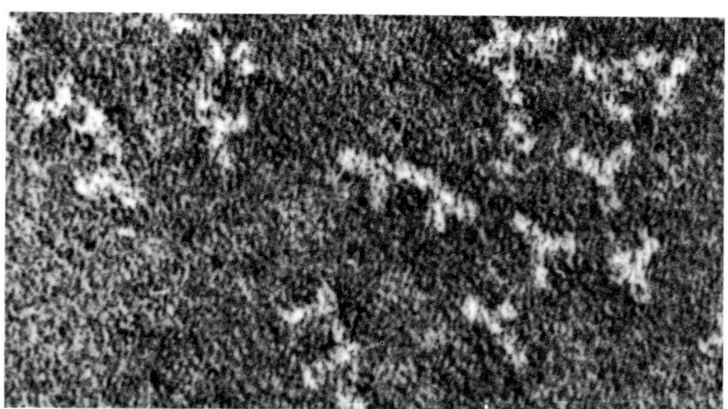

Fig. 5.13 Electronmicrograph of a human dimeric IgA myeloma protein. The double Y-shaped appearance suggests that the monomeric subunits are linked end to end through the *C*-terminal $C\alpha3$ domain. $\times 1.6 \times 10^6$. (Courtesy of Dr R. Dourmashkin).

Two other features characterize the IgM molecule; an abundance of oligosaccharide units associated with the μ chain and an additional peptide chain, the J (joining) chain, thought to assist the process of polymerization prior to secretion by the antibody-producing cell. One J chain (a cysteine-rich peptide of 137 amino acid residues) is incorporated into the IgM structure by disulphide bonding to the penultimate cysteine residues of two μ chains from two separate monomeric subunits.

IgA Polymeric serum IgA and all secretory IgA molecules also contain the J chain; this peptide is not associated with IgG, IgD or IgE. The primary structure of 3 human IgA1 molecules have been determined. The 472 amino acid residues of the α chain are arranged in four domains, V_H, $C\alpha1$, $C\alpha2$ and $C\alpha3$. (Fig. 5.12). A feature shared with IgM is the presence of an additional *C*-terminal octadecapeptide with a penultimate cysteine residue, which is able to bind covalently to the J chain in polymeric molecules. The $C\alpha1$ and $C\alpha2$ domains possess an additional intrachain disulphide bond and in each $C\alpha2$ domain there are two cysteine residues of unknown function. Electronmicrographs of IgA dimers show double Y-shaped structures which suggest that the monomeric subunits are linked end to end through the *C*-terminal $C\alpha3$ regions (Fig. 5.13).

Secretory IgA (sIgA) exists mainly in the form of a molecule sedimenting at 11S and having a molecular weight of 380,000. The complete molecule is made up of two four-chain units of IgA, one secretory component

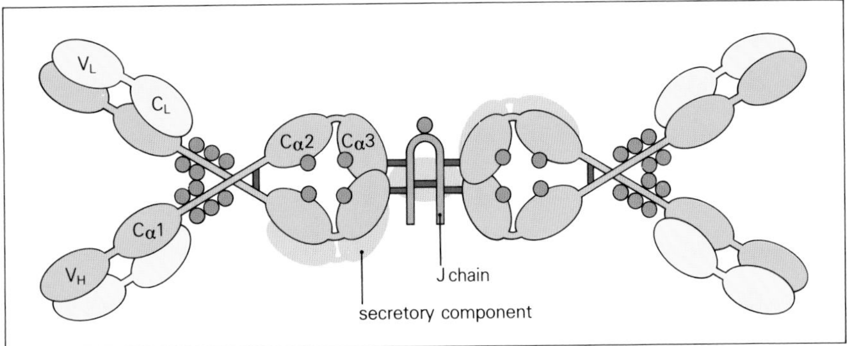

Fig. 5.14 Structure of human secretory IgA (sIgA). The secretory component is probably wound around the sIgA dimer as shown and attached by disulphide bonds to the Cα2 domain of each IgA monomer. The J chain is required for the joining of the two subunits.

(molecular weight 70,000) and one J chain (molecular weight 15,000) (Fig. 5.14). It is not clear how the various peptide chains are linked together. In contrast to the J chain, secretory component is not synthesized by plasma cells but by epithelial cells. IgA held in dimer configuration by a J chain and secreted by submucosal plasma cells actively binds secretory component as it traverses epithelial cell layers. Bound secretory component facilitates the transport of sIgA into secretions as well as protecting it from proteolytic attack. Although IgA1 is the predominant subclass in serum there is relatively more IgA2 present in secretions, possibly related to the fact that many microorganisms present in the respiratory and gastrointestinal tracts appear to release proteases capable of cleaving the IgA1 subclass.

IgD IgD is a trace immunoglobulin in serum (less than 1% of the total). This protein is more susceptible to proteolysis than IgG1, IgG2, IgA or IgM and has a tendency to undergo spontaneous proteolysis. IgD has a structure similar to that shown in Fig. 5.15. There appears to be a single disulphide bond between the δ chains and a high content of carbohydrate distributed in multiple oligosaccharide units. One of these units is rich in *N*-acetylgalactosamine, a sugar which also occurs in IgA1, but in no other known immunoglobulin.

IgE Despite the low serum concentration of IgE the complete amino acid sequence of the human molecule is available following work on various IgE myeloma proteins. The higher molecular weight of the ε chain (72,500) is explained by the larger number of amino acid residues (approximately 550) distributed over five domains (V_H, $C_ε1$, $C_ε2$, $C_ε3$ and $C_ε4$). When IgE is cleaved by the proteolytic enzyme, papain, a 5S fragment of molecular weight 98,000 is released. This fragment (Fc), which contains many of the IgE specific determinants of the whole molecule and binds to the mast cell surface, also shares some antigenic determinants with the $F(ab')_2$ fragment produced when the molecule is cleaved by another proteolytic enzyme, pepsin. A fragment corresponding to the region of overlap (Fc'') of these two fragments has also been isolated but does not retain mast cell binding activity (Fig. 5.16).

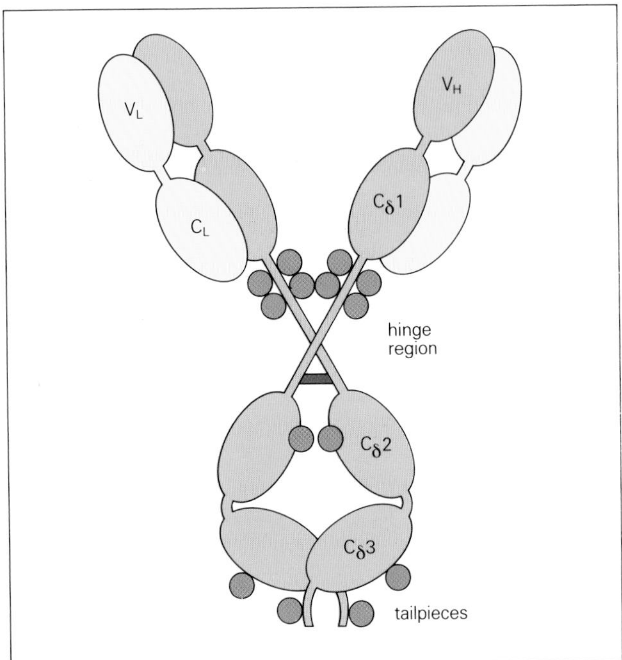

Fig. 5.15 Polypeptide chain structure of human IgD. This diagram shows the domain structure and a characteristically large number of oligosaccharide units. Note also the presence of a hinge region and short octapeptide tailpieces.

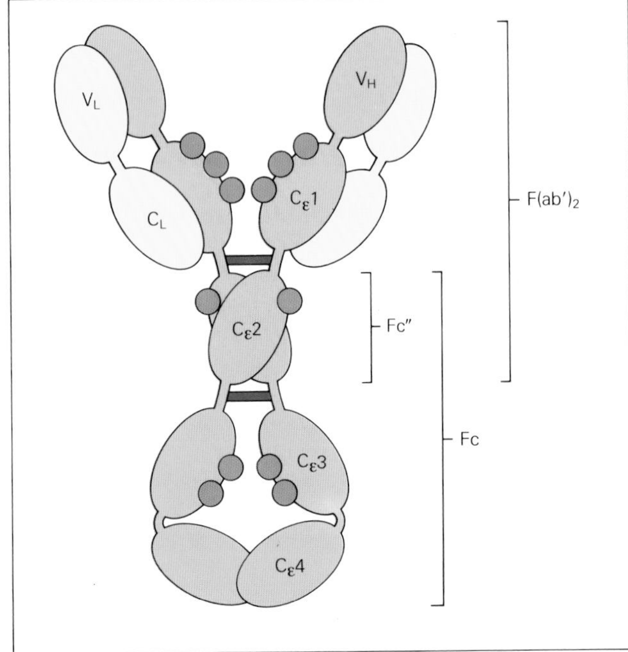

Fig. 5.16 Polypeptide chain structure of human IgE. The four constant region domains, the inter-heavy chain disulphide bonds and the location of oligosaccharide units are shown. IgE can be cleaved by enzymes to give the fragments $F(ab')_2$, Fc and Fc''. Note the absence of a hinge region.

THE GENETIC BASIS OF ANTIBODY HETEROGENEITY

The mRNA for an immunoglobulin polypeptide is made by splicing together sections of mRNA coding for different parts of the polypeptide. For example, the production of light chain mRNA involves the splicing together of 2 mRNA segments – for the V domain and the C domain. The segment of DNA coding for the V genes is, in turn, produced by recombination of two germ-line genes (see Chapter 6). Since a single polypeptide is produced from several genes this creates problems in analysing its genetic variability. Nevertheless the variability of antibodies can be divided into three types, which are described below and summarized in Fig. 5.17.

Isotypic Variation The genes for isotypic variants are present in all healthy members of a species. For example, the genes for γ1, γ2, γ3, γ4, μ, α1, α2, δ, ε, ϰ and λ chains are all present in the human genome and these are therefore isotypes.

Allotypic Variation This refers to genetic variation within a species involving different alleles at a given locus. Not all healthy members of a species have a particular allotype (cf. allelic forms in blood groups). For example, the variant of IgG3 called G3m(b°), which is an allotype characterized by having phenylalanine at position 436 of the γ3 heavy chain, is not found in all people and is therefore an allotype. Allotypes occur mostly as variants of heavy chain constant regions.

Idiotypic Variation Variation in the variable domain, particularly in the highly variable segments known as hypervariable regions, produces idiotypes. Idiotypes are usually specific for the individual antibody clone (private idiotypes), but are sometimes shared between different antibody clones (public, cross-reacting or recurrent idiotypes). The precise genetic basis of idiotypic variability is only partially understood.

ANTIBODY EFFECTOR FUNCTIONS

The primary function of an antibody is to bind the antigen but, aside from those cases where this has a direct neutralizing effect, for example, on bacterial toxin or viral penetration of cells, such interactions would generally be without significance if secondary 'effector' functions did not then become manifest (Fig. 5.18).

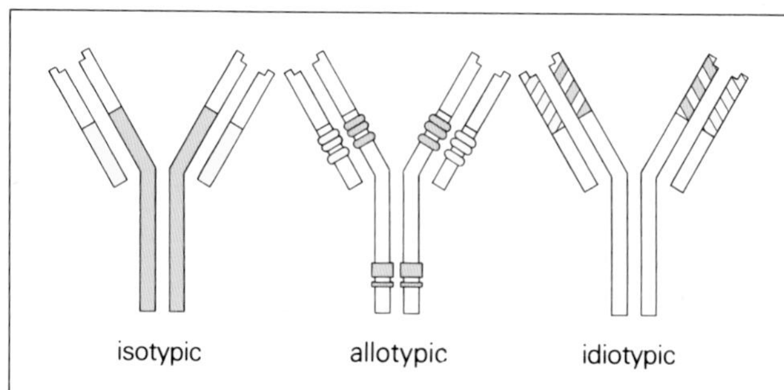

Fig. 5.17 Antibody variants. Isotypic variation refers to the different heavy and light chain classes and subclasses: the variants produced are present in all healthy members of a species. Allotypic variation occurs mostly in the constant region: not all variants are present in all healthy individuals. Idiotypic variation occurs in the variable region only and idiotypes are specific to each antibody molecule.

properties of human immunoglobulins

immunoglobulin	IgG1	IgG2	IgG3	IgG4	IgM	IgA	IgD	IgE
complement fixation	++	+	+++	–	+++	–	–	–
placental transfer	+	±	+	+	–	–	–	–
reactivity with staphylococcal protein A	+	+	–	+	–	–	–	–

Fig. 5.18 Major properties of human antibody classes and subclasses. Classes and subclasses differ in their ability to fix complement, cross the placenta and react with staphylococcal protein A. (Staphylococcal protein A is a cell wall protein of staphylococci which binds to the Fc region of certain immunoglobulins and as such is a natural receptor for antibody.) These properties are determined by the Fc region.

selected cell binding functions of human immunoglobulins

immunoglobulin		IgG1	IgG2	IgG3	IgG4	IgM	IgA1	IgA2	sIgA	IgD	IgE
mononuclear cells	FcRI	+++	–	+++	+	–	–	–	–	–	–
	FcRII	+++	+	+++	+	–	–	–	–	–	–
	FcRIII	++	–	++	–	–	–	–	–	–	–
	$Fc_{\varepsilon}RII$*	–	–	–	–	–	–	–	–	–	++
neutrophils	FcRII▲	+++	+	+++	+	–	–●	–●	–	–	–
	FcRIII▲	++	–	++	–	–	–●	–●	–	–	–
mast cells/ basophils	$Fc_{\varepsilon}RI$	–	–	–	–	–	–	–	–	–	+++

* This receptor is also expressed on eosinophils, platelets and T/B lymphocytes.
▲ These receptors are also expressed on eosinophils.
● An IgA-specific receptor has been isolated from neutrophils.

Fig. 5.19 Some cell binding functions of human immunoglobulins. Cell binding ability varies between the different classes and subclasses.

The activation of the complement system is one of the most important effector mechanisms of IgG1 and IgG3 molecules. The complement system is a complex group of serum proteins which mediate inflammatory reactions. Having bound to antigen, IgM, IgG1 and IgG3 may activate the complement enzyme cascade. IgG2 appears to be less effective in activating complement, while IgG4, IgA, IgD and IgE are ineffective in this respect.

In man IgG molecules of all subclasses cross the placenta and confer a high degree of passive immunity to the newborn. In other species in which maternal immunoglobulin reaches the offspring postnatally, for example the pig, it is IgG derived from the maternal milk which selectively crosses the gastrointestinal tract.

The immunoglobulins display a complex pattern of interactions with various cell types and some of these are tabulated in Fig. 5.19. Some of this data is controversial and further clarification may follow from improved definition of cell subpopulations.

IgG STRUCTURE IN RELATION TO FUNCTION

The plant protease papain cleaves the IgG molecule in the hinge region between the Cγ1 and Cγ2 domains to give two identical Fab fragments and one Fc fragment. These fragments generated by papain have been of enormous value in structure/function studies on the antibody molecule. It has been noted that the Fab region is concerned with binding to antigen, while the Fc region mediates effector functions such as complement fixation, monocyte binding and placental transmission.

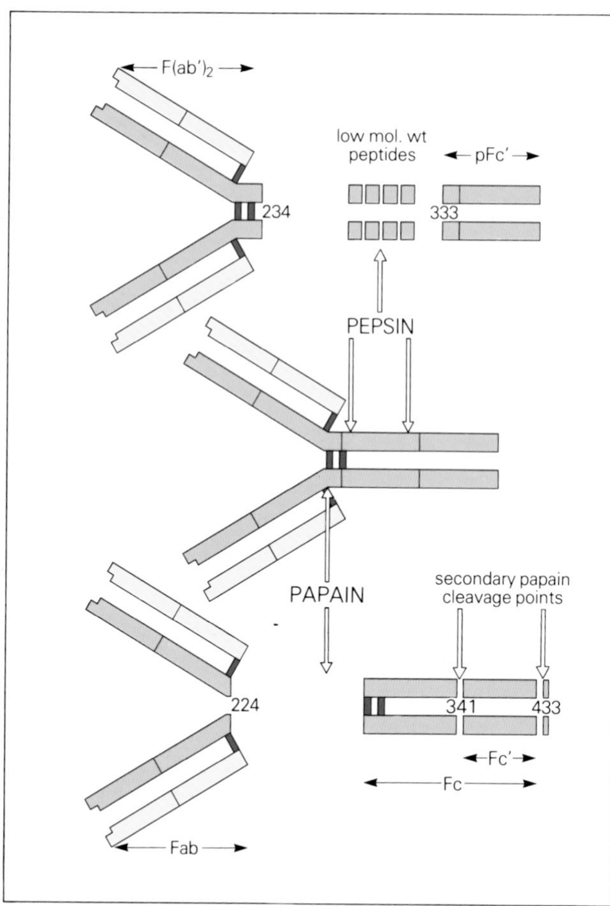

Fig. 5.20 Enzymic cleavage of human IgG1. Pepsin cleaves the heavy chain at the amino acid residues, 234 and 333, to yield the F(ab')$_2$ and pFc' fragments. Further action reduces the central fragment to low molecular weight peptides. Papain splits the molecule in the hinge region (at residue 224) yielding two Fab fragments and the Fc fragment. Secondary action on the Fc fragment at residues 341 and 433 gives rise to Fc'.

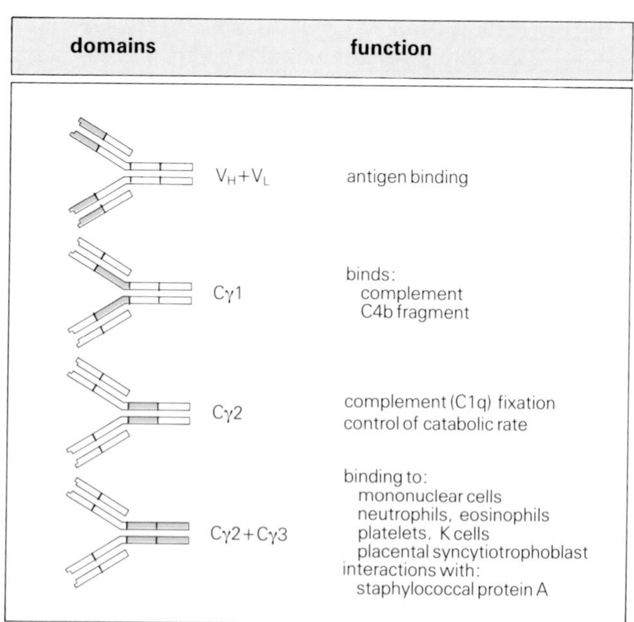

Fig. 5.21 Functions of IgG domains. The relevant domains are shown shaded, together with the functions they perform.

Another useful enzyme for structure/function studies is pepsin which generates two major fragments: the F(ab')$_2$ fragment which broadly encompasses the two Fab regions linked by the hinge region, and the pFc' fragment, which corresponds to the Cγ3 domain of the molecule. Papain also generates, after prolonged digestion, a degraded fragment of the Cγ3 region which is called the Fc' fragment. Some of these major points of enzymic cleavage are shown in Fig. 5.20.

Many other enzymes are known to cleave the immunoglobulin molecule. Brief trypsin digestion of acid-treated Fc fragment yields the Cγ2 domain; isolation of this fragment has permitted structural and functional comparison with other subfragments such as pFc'.

The recognition of immunoglobulin domains as functional subunits led Edelman in 1970 to suggest that each had evolved to subserve a specific function. There was already clear evidence that the V_H and V_L domains interact to form the antigen-binding surfaces of the antibody molecule, and subsequent crystallographic work (see Fig. 5.24) has amply confirmed this prediction. Edelman suggested that the other domains would be shown to mediate the other (effector) functions of immunoglobulin. Precise structural location of these other sites has still to be achieved but there is good evidence that the C1q component of complement interacts with the Cγ2 domain in the case of IgG. Recently, residues 318 (glu), 320 (lys), and 322 (lys) have been implicated in the binding of C1q. Other studies suggest that residue 235 (leu) in the $C_\gamma2$ region is an important determinant in FcRI interactions. However, in this case the closely paired $C_\gamma3$ domains probably have a stabilizing role. Other sites, such as that for interaction with staphylococcal protein A, are known to span the two Fc domains ($C_\gamma2$ and $C_\gamma3$) and critically involve a histidine residue at position 435. Functions of IgG domains are shown in Fig. 5.21.

STRUCTURE IN RELATION TO ANTIGEN BINDING

When the primary amino acid structure of a large number of light and heavy polypeptide chains is examined it is found that the variability between their V domains is not distributed evenly throughout the length of these regions. Some short polypeptide segments show exceptional variability and these segments are termed hypervariable regions. In both heavy and light chains such hypervariable regions are located near positions 30, 50 and 95 (Fig. 5.22). It is now generally accepted that such hypervariable regions are involved directly in the formation of the antigen-binding site. Hypervariable regions are sometimes referred to as Complementarity Determining Regions (CDR) and the intervening peptide segments as Framework Regions (FR). In both light and heavy chain V regions there are three CDRs (CDR1–CDR3) and four FRs (FR1–FR4).

When sequences are examined for evidence of homology the variable regions of κ, λ and heavy chains may each be divided into subgroups depending on their framework amino acid sequences. The numbers of such recognizable subgroups differ from species to species; in man there are four major κ chain subgroups, six λ chain subgroups and three heavy chain subgroups.

Within the past decade the three-dimensional structure of immunoglobulins has been investigated by X-ray diffraction techniques. Such studies have shown that the immunoglobulin domains share a basic folding pattern with several straight segments of polypeptide chain lying parallel to the long axis of the domain. These sections are arranged in two layers running in opposite directions with many hydrophobic amino acid side-chains between the layers. One of the layers is composed

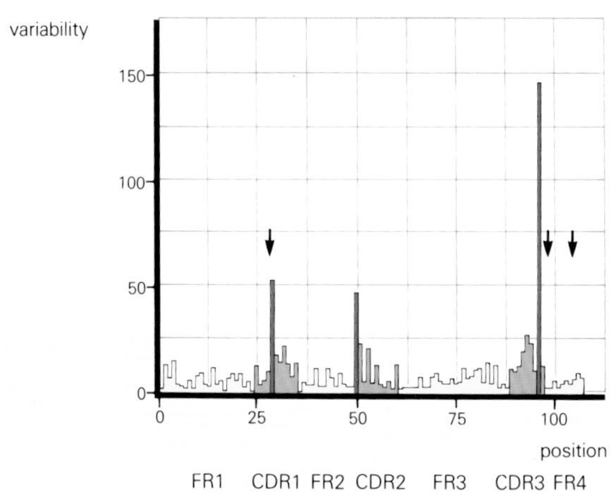

Fig. 5.22 Amino acid variability in the variable region of immunoglobulin light chains. Variability is calculated by comparing the sequences of many individual chains and, for any position, is equal to the ratio of the number of different amino acids found at that position to the frequency of the most common amino acid. The areas of greatest variability, of which there are three in the V_L domain, are the hypervariable regions. In some sequences studied, extra amino acids are found but these have been excluded here to enhance comparison and their positions are indicated by arrows. The areas shaded orange denote regions of hypervariability (CDR), and the most hypervariable positions are shaded red. The four framework regions (FR) are shown in yellow. (Courtesy of Professor E.A. Kabat.)

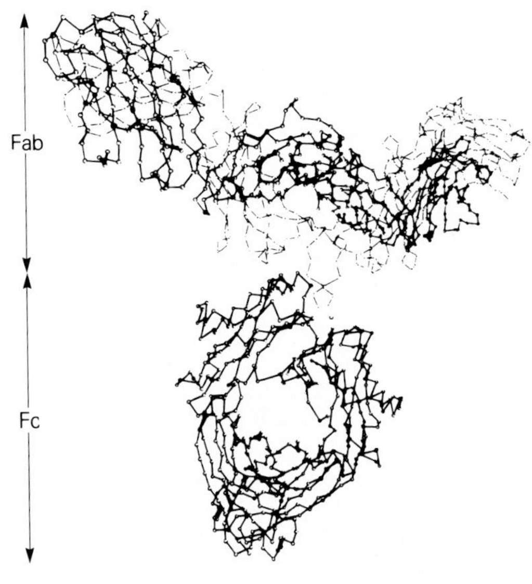

Fig. 5.23 Model of the α-carbon backbone of human IgG1. This model is based on X-ray crystallography studies which reveal that the polypeptide is folded into globular domains forming a Y-shaped structure. The antigen-binding surfaces formed between the variable regions of the light and heavy chains are located at the tips of the arms. The model clearly shows the hinge region between the Fab and Fc regions, as well as suggesting weak interaction between the Cγ2 domains and strong interaction between the Cγ3 domains (Courtesy of Professor R. Huber.)

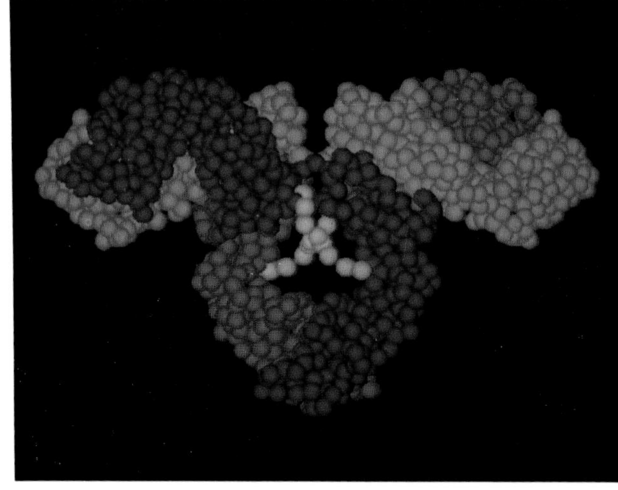

Fig. 5.24 Computer generated model of the hinge-deleted human IgG1 protein Dob. One heavy chain is show in blue and one in red with two light chains being depicted in green. Carbohydrate bound to the Fc portion of the molecule is shown in turquoise. The structure of this immunoglobulin, which lacks a hinge region, was determined by David R. Davies *et al. (Proc. Nat. Acad. Sci. USA,* 1977; **74**). The figure was generated by computer graphics using the system developed by Richard J. Feldmann at the National Institutes of Health.

of four segments, the other has three segments and both are linked by a single disulphide bridge (see Fig. 5.7).

Homologous domains of the light and heavy chains are paired in the Fab regions as are the Cγ3 domains of the γ heavy chains; Cγ2 domains tend to be separated by the carbohydrate moieties. Despite the structural similarities between domains there are striking differences at the level of domain interaction. For example, the variable domains associate with each other through their three segment layers, whereas the constant domains associate through the four segment layers. A further difference between the constant and variable domains is the presence of additional loops of peptide, each bearing a hypervariable segment, in the variable regions. The variable regions of the light and heavy chains are folded in such a way that the regions of hypervariability are brought together to create the surface structure which binds antigen. As shown in Fig. 5.7, these regions are, in the main, associated with bends in the peptide chain.

X-ray crystallography is now yielding structural data on complete IgG molecules and it is possible to construct both an α-carbon back-bone and computer generated atomic models for this class of immunoglobulin (Figs 5.23 and 5.24). These show the general Y-shaped structure with three limbs which has also been visualized by electron microscopy. An appropriate analogy of the antigen–antibody interaction is shown in Fig. 5.25.

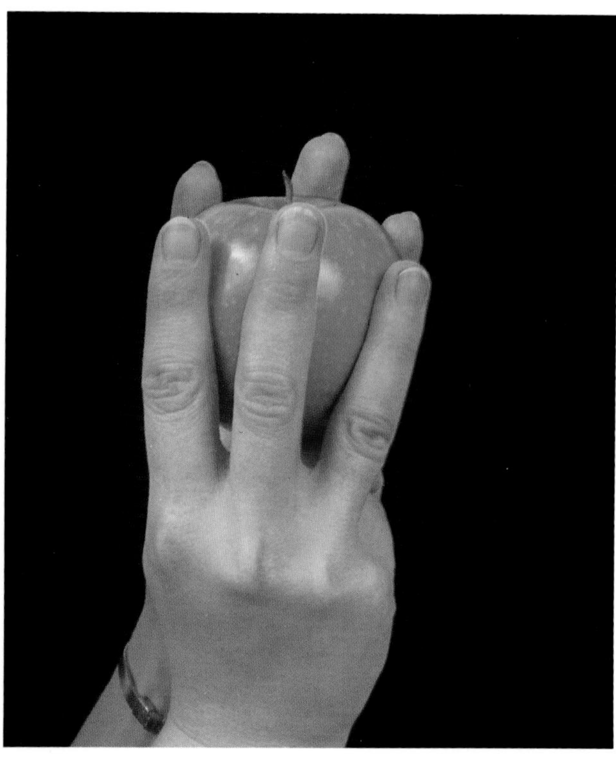

Fig. 5.25 Analogy for antigen–antibody binding. In this analogy, binding of antigen to antibody is represented by an apple (antigen) being held by the fingers of two hands (heavy and light chains) representing hypervariable loops formed into a cleft (the antigen-binding site). If the apple were still attached to the tree it might also serve to illustrate the point that there are usually many such antigenic determinants displayed on the surface of even simple microorganisms.

THE T CELL RECEPTORS

It has emerged that the T cell receptors fall into two main groups defined by the nature of the heterodimeric receptor chains (γδ or αβ) expressed (see Fig. 5.1). A provisional designation of TCR1 and TCR2 has been proposed by Janeway *et al.* (1988) since the γ and δ genes are rearranged and expressed before the α and β genes in ontogeny. The most recent data suggest that cells expressing the αβ receptor and those expressing γδ are on separate lineages.

THE TCR1 SUBUNIT

The characterization of the TCR1 subunit and the organization of the relevant genes is still the subject of much research, but the overall protein structure of the γδ heterodimer is believed to be similar to that of the αβ heterodimer described in detail below. The genetics of the γ and δ genes have been studied in the mouse. The γ genes are located in a cluster on chromosome 13 and include four sets of J region and C region genes and seven sets of V region genes. The δ chain genes (which are close to the Vα region on chromosome 14) are at present less well characterized. A precise functional role for cells bearing the TCR1 subunit has yet to be described but may include regulation of the differentiation of T cells with the TCR2 receptor.

THE TCR2 SUBUNIT

The T cell antigen receptor (TCR2) is a heterodimer with a molecular weight of 90,000. It comprises two peptide chains, an α chain (molecular weight 45 kD) encoded by a cluster of genes on chromosome 14 in both man and mouse, and a β chain (molecular weight 40 kD) encoded by a gene cluster on chromosome 7 (man) or chromosome 6 (mouse). As shown in Fig. 5.26, each chain has a distinct constant (C) region and a distinct variable (V) region. Each of these regions is characterized by an intrachain disulphide bridge and some sequence homology with the immunoglobulin domains.

The α and β peptide chains are themselves linked by a single interchain disulphide bridge in an extracellular region of connecting peptide. Despite the paucity of proline residues this may correspond to the hinge regions of immunoglobulins. Both chains pass through the cell membrane and terminate with short intracytoplasmic tails.

The amino acid sequences of the T cell receptor α and β chains places the TCR2 subunit in the immunoglobulin superfamily. By comparison with immunoglobulins there are fewer genes encoding the different V domains for the T cell receptor, consequently it is more difficult to identify areas of hypervariability. Nevertheless, there appear to be regions equivalant to the CDR1, CDR2 and CDR3 of immunoglobulins. Furthermore, by analogy to the arrangement of CDRs in the immunoglobulin antigen binding site Davis and Bjorkman (1988) have recently proposed a model for the alignment of three CDRs of the T cell receptor. This envisages the CDR3 of the α chain and the CDR3 of the β chain interacting closely with each other and making close contact with antigenic peptide held in the binding site of an MHC molecule. In this model the CDR1 and CDR2 regions of the TCR interact with the α1 and β2 domains of the MHC molecule.

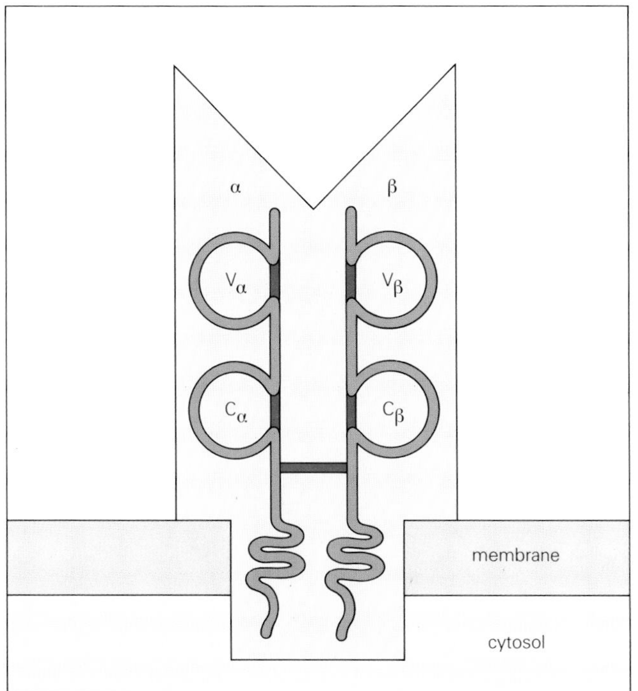

Fig. 5.26 The TCR2 receptor. This T cell receptor is a heterodimer of α and β peptide chains. Each peptide chain comprises a constant region and a variable region with sequence homology to the immunoglobulin domains. The α and β chains are disulphide-linked near the membrane.

Genetic studies suggest that the random association of Vα and Jα genes could generate approximately 2500 mature α chain genes whereas similar interactions of the β chain gene elements would generate at least 4000 different β chain sequences. The combinatorial product for the αβ heterodimer is greater than 10^7 different sequences.

Functionally the α and β chains of the TCR2 subunit appear to have co-evolved to recognize antigen in association with MHC-encoded molecules on the surface of cells.

THE CD3 (T3) SUBUNIT

Both helper T cells and cytoxic T cells express their T cell antigen receptor (TCR) in a molecular complex involving three other polypeptide chains. These three chains comprise the CD3 subunit (previously identified with monoclonal antibodies as T3 and Leu 4) in man. The three chains of CD3 are the γ chain (molecular weight 25 kD), the δ chain (molecular weight 20 kD) and the ε chain (molecular weight 20 kD). These chains are non-covalently associated with each other and the αβ heterodimer of the TCR (Fig. 5.27). Each chain is a transmembrane peptide and approximately one third of the γ chain is intracytoplasmic. All appear to have an extracellular domain; they may be members of the immunoglobulin supergene family.

The intracytoplasmic tails of the γ and δ chains of mouse and man are highly conserved structures and there is evidence that they are closely related since there is 65% sequence homology between them.

There are active phosphorylation sites on the intracytoplasmic portions of the γ chain and it is widely believed that the CD3 complex mediates signal transduction when T cells are activated by antigen binding to the TCR.

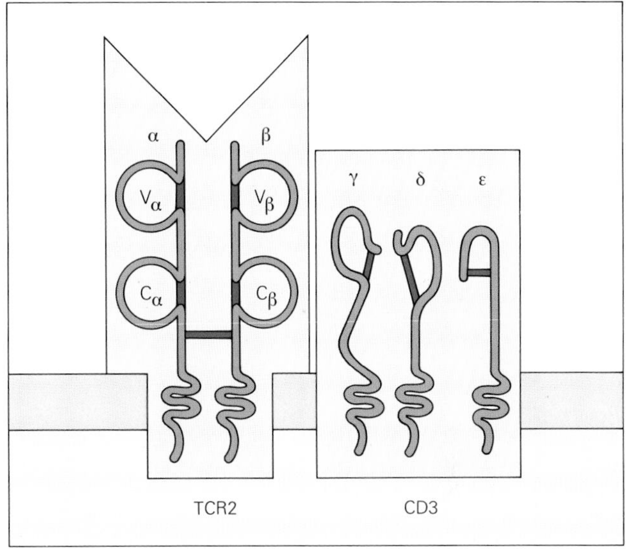

Fig. 5.27 The CD3 (T3) subunit. This subunit is closely associated with both the TCR1 and TCR2 receptors. It comprises three peptide chains (γ, δ and ε) each of which has a transmembrane orientation. The subunit is believed to be involved in mediating signal transduction when T cells are activated by antigen.

FURTHER READING

Allison, J.P. & Lanier, L.L. (1987) Structure, function and serology of the T-cell antigen receptor complex. *Annual Review of Immunology*, **5**, 503–540.

Capra, D. & Edmundson, A.B. (1977) The antibody combining site. *Scientific American*, **236**, 50.

Davies, D.R. & Metzger, H. (1983) Structural basis of antibody function. *Annual Review of Immunology*, **1**, 87–117.

Davis, M.M. & Bjorkman, P.J. (1988) T-cell antigen receptor genes and T-cell recognition, *Nature*, **334**, 395-402 and *Nature*, **335**, 744 (corrigendum).

Hahn, G.S. (1982) Antibody structure, function and active sites. In *Physiology of Immunoglobulins: Diagnostic and Clinical Aspects*. Edited by S.E. Ritzmann. New York: Alan Liss Inc.

Janeway Jr, C.A., Jones, B. & Hayday, A. (1988) Specificity and function of T cells bearing $\gamma\delta$ receptors. *Immunology Today*, **9**, 73–76.

Mestecky, J. & McGhee, J.R. (1987) Immunoglobulin A (IgA): molecular and cellular interactions involved in IgA biosynthesis and immune response. *Advances in Immunology*, **40**, 153–245.

Möller, G. (ed.) (1977) Immunoglobulin D: structure, synthesis, membrane representation and function. *Immunological Reviews*, **37.**

Möller, G. (ed.) (1978) Immunoglobulin E. *Immunological Reviews*, **41.**

Möller, G. (ed.) (1984) T-cell receptors and genes. *Immunological Reviews*, **81.**

Nisonoff, A. (1984) *Introduction to Molecular Immunology*. 2nd edition. Baltimore: Sinauer Associates Inc.

Turner, M.W. (1977) Structure and function of immunoglobulins. In *Immunochemistry: An Advanced Textbook*. Edited by L.E. Glynn & M.W. Steward. Chichester: John Wiley & Sons.

Turner, M.W. (1983) Immunoglobulins. In *Immunology in Medicine. A Comprehensive Guide to Clinical Immunology*. 2nd edition. Edited by E.J. Holborow & W.G. Reeves. London: Grune & Stratton.

Underdown, B.J. & Schiff, J.M. (1986) Immunoglobulin A: Strategic defence initiative at the mucosal surface. *Annual Review of Immunology*, **4**, 389–417.

6 The Generation of Diversity

The ability of the immune system to recognize antigens depends on the antibodies generated by B cells and on the antigen receptors expressed by T cells. Although the ways in which T cells and B cells recognize antigen is quite different, both cell populations are capable of recognizing a wide range of antigens. This chapter is concerned with the ways in which the immune system generates a great diversity of antibodies and T cell antigen receptors, of different antigenic specificities. In spite of the differences between antibodies and T cell receptors, the cellular and molecular processes which generate diversity are very similar for each type of molecule.

Antibodies are remarkably diverse; not only must they provide enough different combining sites to recognize the millions of antigenic shapes in the environment, but also each class of antibody has a different effector region such that, for instance IgE can bind to Fc receptors on mast cells whilst IgG can bind similarly to phagocytes. It has been estimated that an individual produces more different forms of antibody than all the other proteins of the body put together. Looked at another way, we produce more types of antibody than there are genes in our genome. How then can all this diversity be generated? Ideas about the formation of antibodies have changed considerably over the years but it is perhaps surprising how close Ehrlich came with his side-chain hypothesis at the beginning of this century (Fig. 6.1). His idea of antigen-induced selection is close to our present view of clonal selection except that he placed several different receptors on the same cell.

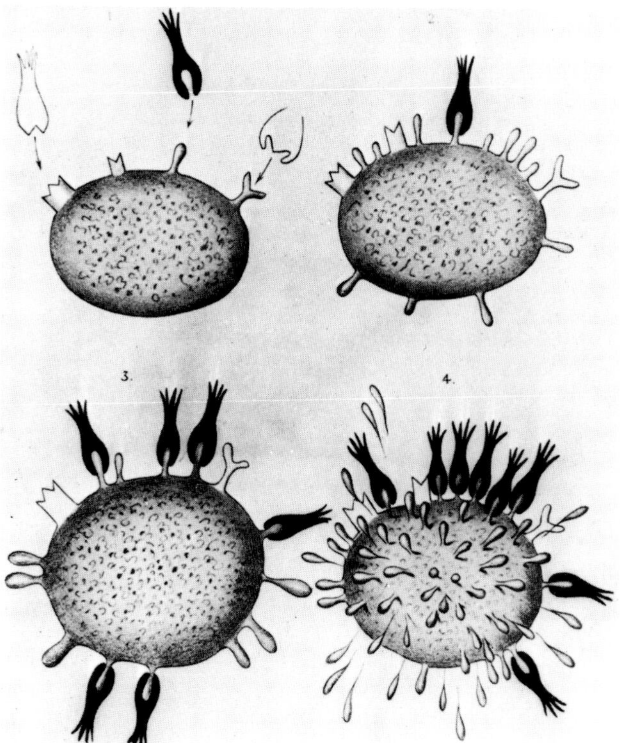

Fig. 6.1 Ehrlich's side-chain theory. Ehrlich proposed that the combination of antigen with a preformed B cell receptor (now known to be antibody) triggered the cell to produce and secrete more of those receptors. Although the diagram indicates that he thought a single cell could produce antibodies to bind more than one type of antigen, it is evident that he anticipated both the clonal selection theory and the idea that the immune system could generate receptors before contact with antigen.

THEORIES OF ANTIBODY FORMATION

After Ehrlich the situation became complicated. The problem was that many new organic chemicals were now being synthesized and Landsteiner was showing that the immune system could react with the production of specific antibody for each new compound. It was simply not thought possible that the immune system could have maintained genes for all these antibodies directed at novel, artificial compounds, by natural selection. This led to the development of the instructive hypothesis which suggested that a flexible antibody molecule is induced by antigen to form a complementary binding site. With the spectacular progress in molecular biology in the 1950s and 1960s the instructive hypothesis became untenable. The circle turned, and selective theories came back into favour with Jerne and Burnet independently putting forward the idea of clonal selection—each lymphocyte produces one type of immunoglobulin only, and the antigen selects and stimulates cells carrying that immunoglobulin type.

This still leaves the problem of antibody diversity. At its simplest we can propose the existence of a separate gene for each antibody specificity (Fig. 6.2). This immediately presents a problem: if we consider the structure of a light chain, half the chain is variable in amino acid sequence but the other half is constant. Similarly with heavy chains, a quarter of the chain is variable while the rest is constant. How, if there are many genes, is it possible to maintain this constancy of sequence in the constant regions? Dreyer and Bennett proposed a solution to this problem by suggesting that the constant and variable portions of the chains are coded for by separate genes with one or only a few genes coding for the constant region and many genes coding for the variable region. Thus this germ line theory now only had to account for the multiple variable regions! A second solution of the diversity problem was suggested by the idea of somatic mutation. A relatively few germ line genes would give rise to many mutated genes during the lifetime of the individual. Furthermore, it has been

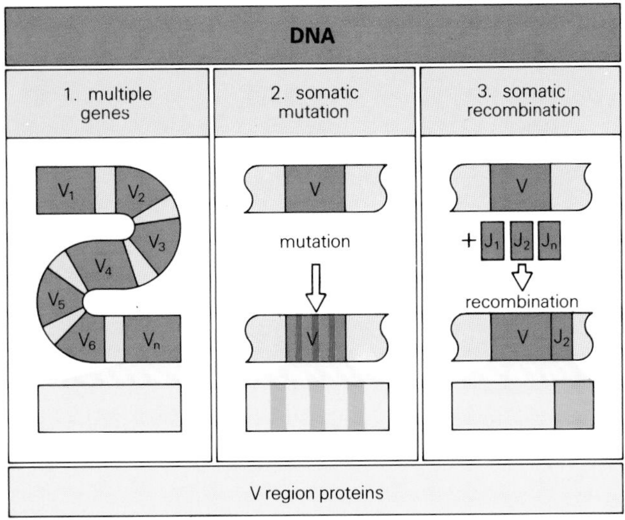

Fig. 6.2 Generation of antibody diversity. Three mechanisms are proposed by which the immune system could generate different V regions on the immunoglobulin H and L chains.
1. Multiple genes. There are a large number of separate genes (V_1–V_n) each encoding one V region domain.
2. Somatic mutation. A primordial V gene mutates during B cell ontogeny to produce different genes in different B cell clones.
3. Somatic recombination. A number of gene segments (J_1–J_n) recombine to join the main part of the V region gene. This occurs during B cell ontogeny and results in a protein containing elements coded for by different gene segments. It is known that all three mechanisms are involved in the generation of antibody diversity.

peptide	mouse	human
IgH	12	14
λ	16	22
ϰ	6	2
TCR α	14	14
TCR β	6	7
TCR γ	13	7
TCR δ	14	14
MHC	17	6
β_2-microglobulin	2	15

Fig. 6.3 Chromosome location of MHC and antigen receptor genes. The numbers refer to the chromosomal location of the genes for the various peptides in man and mouse. Note that all of the loci are completely separate, with the single exception of the T cell receptor (TCR) δ chain which lies within the TCR α gene loci.

suggested that a number of gene segments could recombine to give a complete V gene. This gives three possible solutions to the problem of generating diversity:
1. multiple V region genes in the germ line
2. somatic recombination between elements forming a V region gene
3. somatic mutation.

It is now known that mammals use all three mechanisms to generate diversity. Interestingly however sharks rely on having a large number of antibody genes, and do not use somatic recombination, while birds have small numbers of antibody genes which undergo a very high level of somatic recombination (see Chapter 15).

IMMUNOGLOBULIN VARIABILITY

Immunoglobulins are composed of heavy and light chains, the light chains being either ϰ or λ. Since virtually any light chain can combine with any heavy chain the number of possible combining sites is the product of the number of heavy and light chains. Part of the variability in immunoglobulin structure is derived from the interaction of these separate polypeptide chains. For example, if there are 10^4 different light chains each capable of binding with any of 10^4 different heavy chains, then theoretically, 10^8 different antibody specificities may be produced. Separate diversification mechanisms exist for each of the chains as they are coded for on separate chromosomes (Fig. 6.3) Polymorphic forms of immunoglobulins derive from variation in many parts of the molecule (Fig. 6.4).

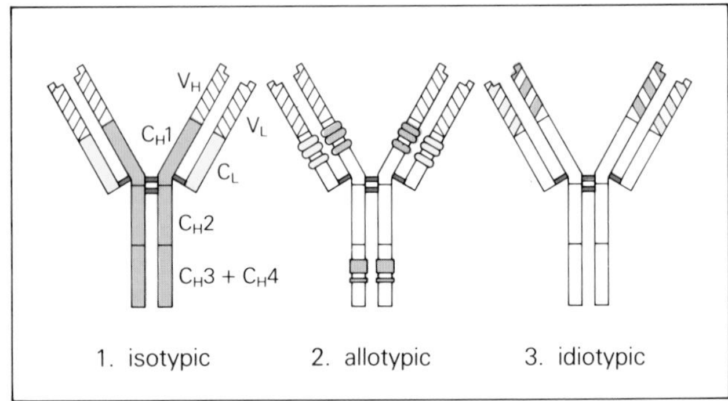

Fig. 6.4 Variability of immunoglobulin structure. All immunoglobulins have the basic four-chain structure. The variability of different immunoglobulins is of three types.
1. Isotypic variation is present in the germ line of all members of a species, producing the heavy (μ, δ, γ, ε, α) and light chains (ϰ, λ), and the V region frameworks (subgroups).
2. Allotypic variation is intraspecies allelic variability.
3. Idiotypic variation refers to the diversity at the binding site and in particular relates to the hypervariable segments of the antibody-combining site (paratope).

It is the idiotypic variability, which pertains to the generation of the antigen-combining site, with which we shall first be concerned. Kabat and Wu analysed the amino acid sequences of many light and heavy chains. When the variable regions from light chains derived from myelomas (monoclonal B cell tumours producing antibody) were compared it was clear that the variability in amino acid sequence was concentrated in three hypervariable regions surrounded by relatively invariant framework residues. These hypervariable regions

position
0
25
50
75
100
base changes from λ prototype sequence
myeloma protein
SAPC 178
4
HOPC 2020
2
SAPC 176
1
RPC 20
1
Y 5606
1
Y 5444
1
PC 5060
1
variability
150
100
50
0
position

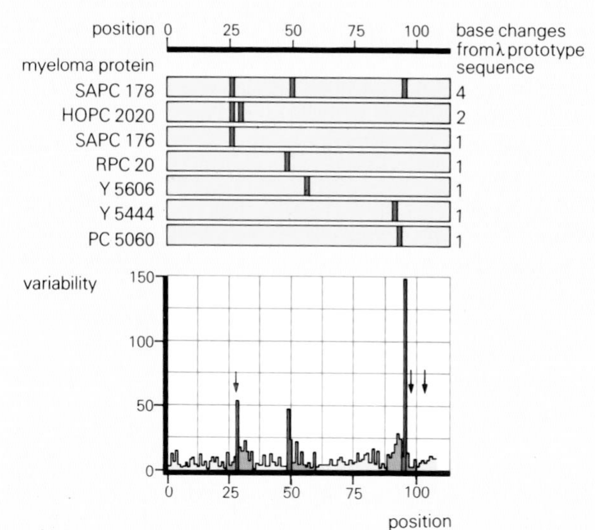

Fig. 6.5 Variability of lambda light chains. The amino acid sequences of seven λ1 myeloma proteins are represented. Positions in yellow indicate identity to the prototype sequence (MOPC 104E), positions in red indicate differences. The number of base changes in the DNA required to produce the given alteration in amino acid structure is given on the right. Below is a Kabat and Wu plot of light chain variability as described in Chapter 5. Arrows indicate extra bases in some sequences.

heavy chain variability
150
100
50
0
0
20
40
60
80
100
120
position

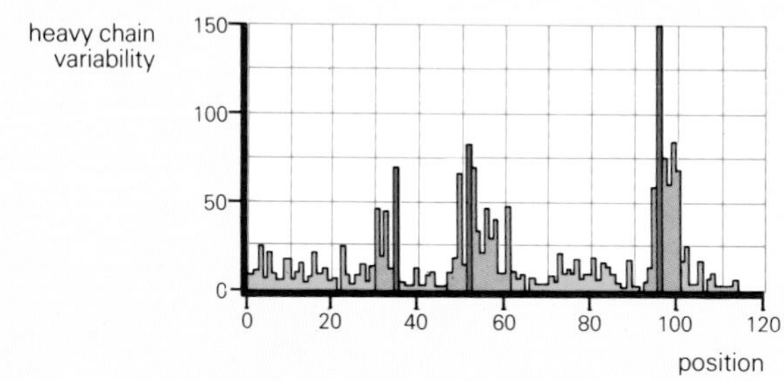

Fig. 6.6 Variability of heavy chains. This Kabat and Wu plot shows variability concentrated in three regions of the variable region of heavy chains. The method for determining variability is described in Chapter 5.

were shown to be the regions which made contact with the antigen (complementarity determining regions, CDRs). In the mouse less than 5% of the antibodies possess λ light chains and diversity is correspondingly less. Out of 19 λ1 light chain sequences examined, 12 were found to be identical, with the other 7 differing from each other and the prototype sequence by only a few residues (Fig. 6.5).

The variability in the heavy chain is similarly concentrated in three hypervariable regions with background variability on each side of the CDRs (Fig. 6.6). The heavy chain frameworks can be arranged into groups on the basis of similarity and in some cases identity of framework sequences (Fig. 6.7).

LIGHT CHAIN GENE RECOMBINATION

With the advent of recombinant DNA techniques in the 1970s it became possible to attempt analysis of the genes responsible for coding for antibodies. Because of its lesser heterogeneity, work started on the λ1 system using restriction endonucleases to digest the DNA. It was found that two separate segments of DNA coded for the constant and variable regions and also, in cells not producing antibody, that these gene segments are far apart on the chromosome, whereas in antibody-forming cells they are brought closer together. Even in a fully differentiated B cell these two gene segments do not join directly, but remain about 1500 base pairs apart. Between the V and C segments and joined onto the V segment in the rearranged chromosome is an extra short section of DNA known as the J segment.

Basically the V segment codes for the V region of the light chain up to and including amino acid 95 and the J segment gene codes for the rest of the V region (Fig. 6.8). In the mouse λ light chain system there are four C genes, each with its own J gene, and two V genes. Each V segment gene is preceded by a signal or leader sequence coding for a short hydrophobic sequence that is responsible for the transport of the antibody molecule through the membrane of the endoplasmic reticulum during translation. This leader sequence is then cleaved away after synthesis of the chain. The J segments which form part of the V domains are completely different from the J chain present in IgM and dimeric IgA.

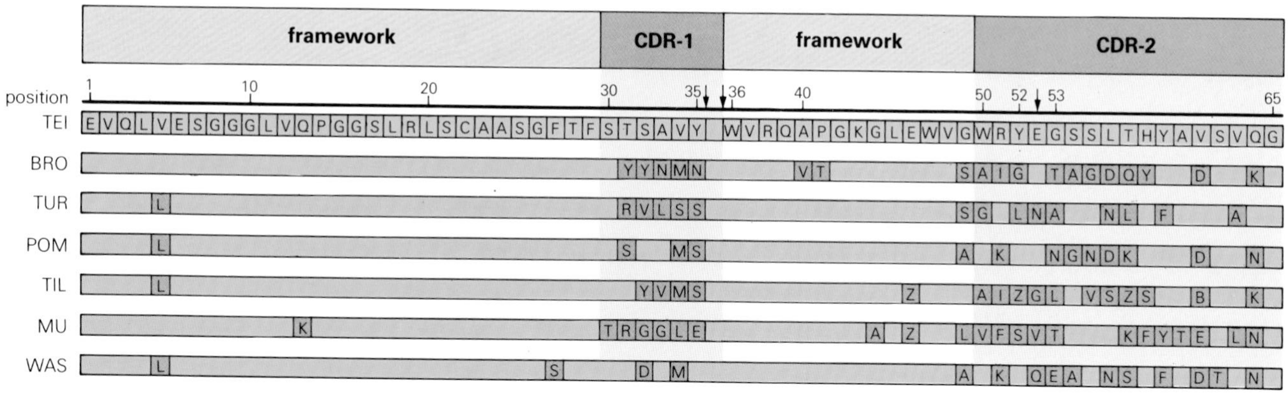

framework
CDR-1
framework
CDR-2
position
1
10
20
30
35
36
40
50
52
53
65
TEI EVQLVESGGGLVQPGGSLRLSCAASGFTFSTSAVY WVRQAPGKGLEWVGWRYEGSSLTHYAVSVQG
BRO YYNMN VT SAIG TAGDQY D K
TUR L RVLSS SG LNA NL F A
POM L S MS A K NGNDK D N
TIL L YVMS Z AIZGL VSZS B K
MU K TRGGLE A Z LVFSVT KFYTE LN
WAS L S D M A K QEA NS F DT N

Fig. 6.7 Heavy chain group V_HIII: human. The 65 *N*-terminal amino acids of six human myelomas falling into the V_HIII group are compared diagrammatically to the prototype sequence TEI. Amino acids identical to those in TEI are shown in yellow, amino acids which differ from those at the same position in TEI are orange. The majority of the differences within a single group occur within the complementarity determining regions CDR-1 and CDR-2.

The ϰ chain system is more heterogeneous because there are more V segment genes but only one constant region gene (Fig. 6.9). In an embryonic or non-lymphoid cell the V segment genes, of which there are about 350, are again at some distance on the chromosome from the C gene. In the mouse these V segment genes appear to be organized in sets comprising about seven genes / set. In between and closer to the C gene are five J genes; one of the J genes is a pseudogene and is never expressed. During differentiation of lymphoid cells there is a rearrangement of the DNA such that one of the V segment genes is joined to a J segment gene. Thus the number of possible ϰ chain variable regions that can be produced is approximately 1400 (350 × 4). There is still a gap or intron between the J segment genes and the gene for the C region. This whole stretch of DNA, including introns, from the leader to the end of the C gene is then transcribed into heterogeneous nuclear RNA, that is, unprocessed messenger RNA (mRNA). A process of RNA splicing then removes the introns, leaving RNA which is finally translated into protein. This splicing out of introns can be revealed by heteroduplex analysis, where the mRNA is mixed with denatured single-stranded DNA from the antibody-forming cell, allowed to reanneal and then examined by electron microscopy. Hybridization of V and C regions readily occurs revealing the intron that lies between them (Fig. 6.10).

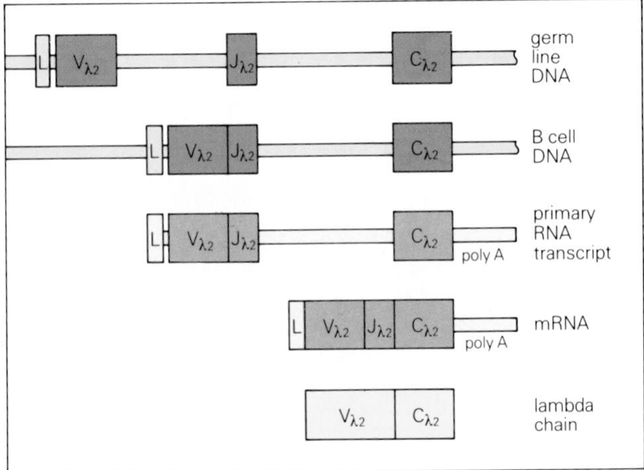

Fig. 6.8 Lambda chain production: mouse. During B cell differentiation one of the germ line V_λ genes ($V_{\lambda 2}$) recombines with its J segment ($J_{\lambda 2}$) to form a VJ combination. The V gene is preceded by an appropriate signalling leader sequence (L). The rearranged gene is transcribed into a primary RNA transcript complete with introns (DNA occurring between the genes), exons (which code for protein) and a poly A tail. This is spliced to form messenger RNA (mRNA) with loss of the introns and is in turn translated into protein. Note that the gene segments which encode the final polypeptide are indicated in a darker shade, DNA in red, RNA in green and immunuoglobulin peptides in yellow. The λ2 gene illustrated is only one of a small number of different λ genes arranged in tandem on the same chromosome.

HEAVY CHAIN GENE RECOMBINATION

The heavy chain is also encoded by V and J segment genes. Additonal diversity is provided by a third gene segment, the D segment gene (Fig. 6.11). If one examines the family of monoclonal antibodies which bind dextran, the gene segment for the V_H domain appears to end at codon 99 while the gene segment for the J_H segment starts at codon 102. This leaves two codons in between not accounted for by either V or J segments, and these form the additional D or diversity segment. This section is highly variable both in the sequences of the codons

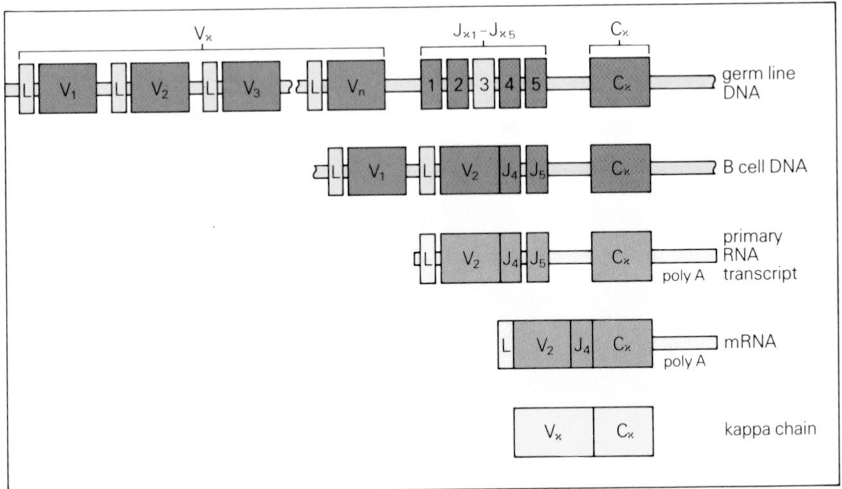

Fig. 6.9 Kappa chain production: mouse. During differentiation of the pre-B cell one of several $V_ϰ$ genes on the germ line DNA (V_1-V_n) is recombined and apposed to a $J_ϰ$ segment ($J_{ϰ1}-J_{ϰ5}$). Each $V_ϰ$ gene is preceded by a leader sequence (L). The B cell transcribes a segment of DNA into a primary RNA transcript which contains a long intervening sequence of additonal J segments and introns. This transcript is processed into mRNA by splicing the exons together and is translated by ribosomes into kappa chains. Note that the J3 gene lacks the necessary base sequences to allow it to recombine and is therefore effectively an intron. The rearrangement illustrated is only one of the many possible recombinations.

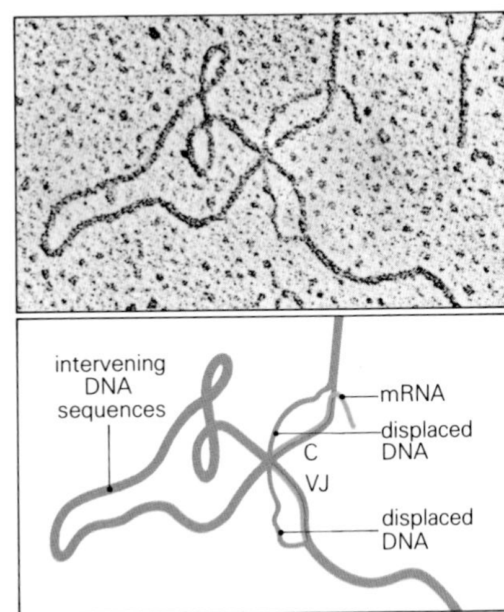

Fig. 6.10 Heteroduplex analysis of a kappa VC region. The mRNA for a kappa gene is incubated with denatured single-stranded germ line DNA of a plasmacytoma producing the heteroduplex above, as seen under the electron microscope. There is a large intron in the DNA between VJ and C but no intron between V and J in this active B cell.

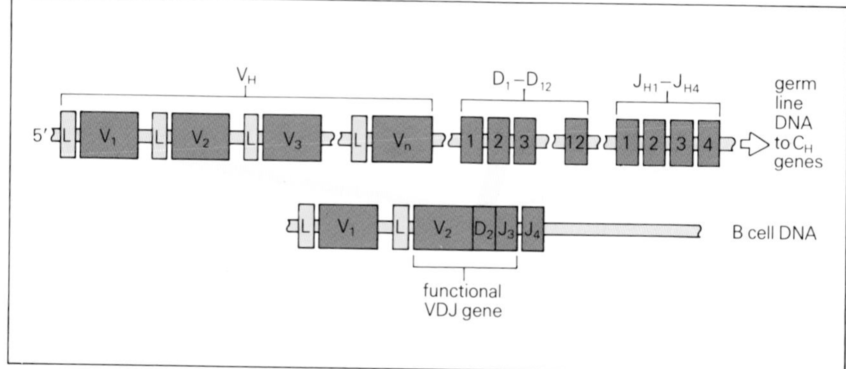

Fig. 6.11 VDJ recombination: mouse. The heavy chain gene loci combine three segments to produce the exon (VDJ gene) which will code for the V_H domain. One of several hundred V genes recombines with one of twelve D segments, and one of four J segments, to produce a functional VDJ gene, in the B cell. The rearrangement illustrated is only one of the many thousands possible.

and in their number. In antibodies binding dextran this section comprises two amino acids, but in those binding phosphorylcholine up to eight amino acids are inserted, while in anti-levan antibodies this section is completely missing. So far 12 germ line D segments have been identified by DNA sequence and Southern blotting analysis, together with 100–200 different V_H segments and four functional J segments, but solution analysis has now indicated that there may be more than 1000 murine V_H segments. The combination of V, D and J segments in the heavy chain make up the third complementarity determining region, which forms an essential part of the antigen-binding site. In fact in some systems, such as the family of anti-dextran antibodies, the differences between antibodies are nearly all situated in this region.

RECOMBINATION SEQUENCES

A key feature then of the generation of a functional gene for both light and heavy chain variable regions is the recombination of gene segments. The precise mechanism by which this recombination is brought about is unknown but specific base sequences that appear to act as joining signals have been identified (Fig. 6.12). On the J or downstream side of each V and D segment gene (in the direction of the J gene) are found two signal sequences, each of which is highly conserved.

The first is composed of seven nucleotides, a heptamer CACAGTG or its analogue, followed by a spacer of unconserved sequence, and then a nonamer ACAAAAACC, or its analogue. Immediately preceding all germ line D and J segments are again two signal sequences, first a nonamer and then a heptamer, again separated by an unconserved sequence. The heptameric and nonameric sequences following a V_L, V_H or D segment are complementary to those preceding the J_L, D or J_H segments with which they recombine. All functional V_κ J_λ and D spacers are 12 base pairs long, while all functional V_λ, V_H and J_H spacers are 22–24 base pairs long. This has led to the suggestion that the recombination may be brought about by a recombinase enzyme containing two DNA binding proteins, one recognizing the

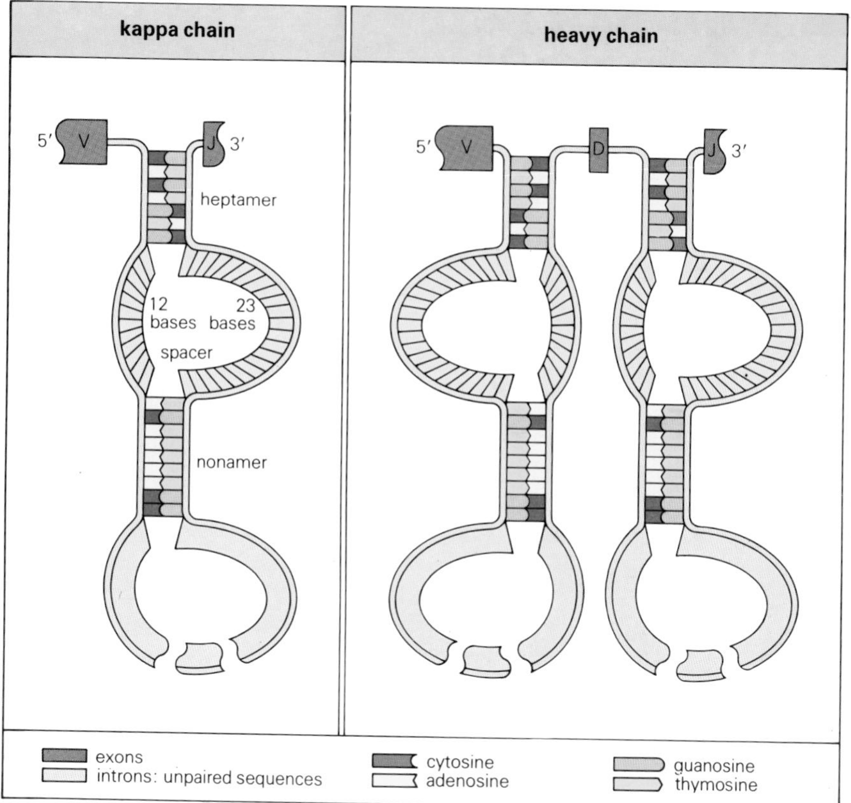

Fig. 6.12 Recombination sequences. This diagram shows the sequences of introns next to the V and J genes (kappa light chains) and V, J and D genes (heavy chains) which are involved in recombination of these genes. The recombinational events involved in VJ splicing and VDJ splicing are facilitated by the base sequences of the introns following the 3' end of V and D matching up with the bases preceding the 5' end of J and D. Base pairing between these sequences apposes the exons. Note that individual base pair sequences may vary slightly from the stated ones but the heptamer/spacer/nonamer pairing patterns remain. It is thought that enzymes related to those involved in DNA repair effect the join.

heptamer and nonamer with a 12 base pair spacer and the other recognizing them with a 23 base pair spacer. Alternatively, base pairing may occur directly between heptamers and nonamers, and the recombining enzyme(s) then recognize the overall paired structure.

ADDITIONAL DIVERSITY

VARIABLE RECOMBINATION

As if the diversity generated by simple recombination were not enough, the precise place at which V and J segment genes join may vary slightly. The 95th residue of the ϰ light chain is coded for by the last codon of the V segment gene; the 96th is frequently coded by the first $J_\varkappa$ triplet. Sometimes, however, the 96th amino acid is coded for by a composite triplet formed by the second and third, or third base alone, of the first $J_\varkappa$ triplet with the other bases of the triplet being supplied by additional bases from the intron 3′ from the V segment gene (Fig. 6.13). This will lead to variations in amino acid sequence at this point. Obviously to produce a functional light chain the correct reading frame must be preserved but it is possible for the gene segments to join out of phase leading to non-functional lymphocytes.

Similar imprecision in joining occurs on the heavy chain chromosome between the D and J_H segment genes and can extend over as many as 10 nucleotides (Fig. 6.14). Furthermore, a few nucleotides may be inserted between D and J_H and between V_H and D without the need for a template by means of the enzyme terminal deoxynucleotidyl transferase. The addition of these novel nucleotides is known as N-region diversity.

SOMATIC MUTATION

The idea that somatic mutations during the lifetime of an individual could increase the diversity of antibodies has been strongly argued for many years. As seen earlier (Fig. 6.5) most V_λ sequences are identical, with a few variations in the complementarity determining regions giving eight sequences in all, but as only one $V_{\lambda 1}$ gene segment has been found per haploid genome and as this corresponds to the main shared prototype sequence, all the variant sequences must be generated by somatic mutations. All the variants could be produced by single base changes. Similar somatic mutants have been identified in ϰ light chains and in heavy chains.

The family of antibodies binding phosphorylcholine has been extensively investigated. Nineteen V_H segments from antibodies binding phosphorylcholine have been fully sequenced. Ten of these have an identical sequence while the other nine differ by one to eight residues. The germ line genome from sperm was examined to see if each of these sequences was encoded by a separate DNA sequence. In fact, only DNA coding for the main prototype sequence could be found, indicating that the other sequences must have arisen by somatic mutation (Fig. 6.15). Strikingly, all the mutated forms were in the IgA and IgG classes suggesting that the mutation event might even be associated with immunoglobulin class switching. Presumably those somatic variants with a better fit for antigen are selected for, and certainly the somatic variants binding phosphorylcholine are of higher affinity than the germ line coded antibodies.

There is some evidence that the region of DNA encoding the variable region may be particularly susceptible to mutation. For example, examination of the nucleotide

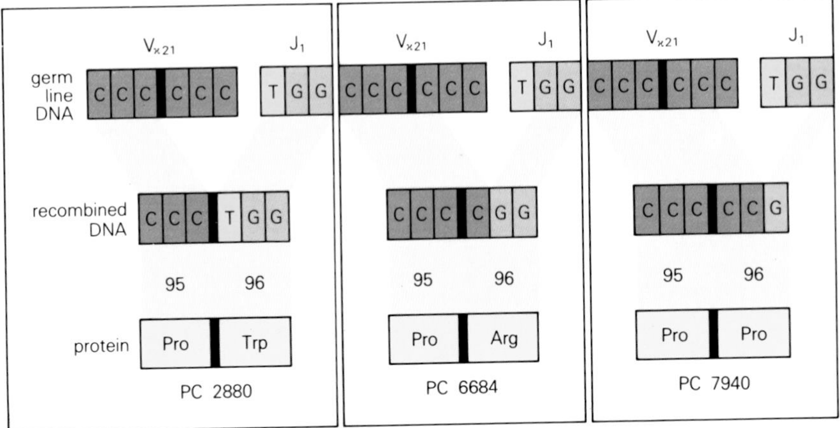

Fig. 6.13 Light chain diversity created by variable recombination. The same $V_{\varkappa 21}$ and J_1 sequences of the germ line genes create three different amino acid sequences in the proteins PC 2880, PC 6684 and PC 7940 by variable recombination. PC 2880 has proline and tryptophan at positions 95 and 96, caused by recombination at the end of the CCC codon. Recombination one base further down produces proline and arginine in PC 6684 and recombination two bases down from the end of $V_{\varkappa 21}$ produces proline and proline in PC 7940.

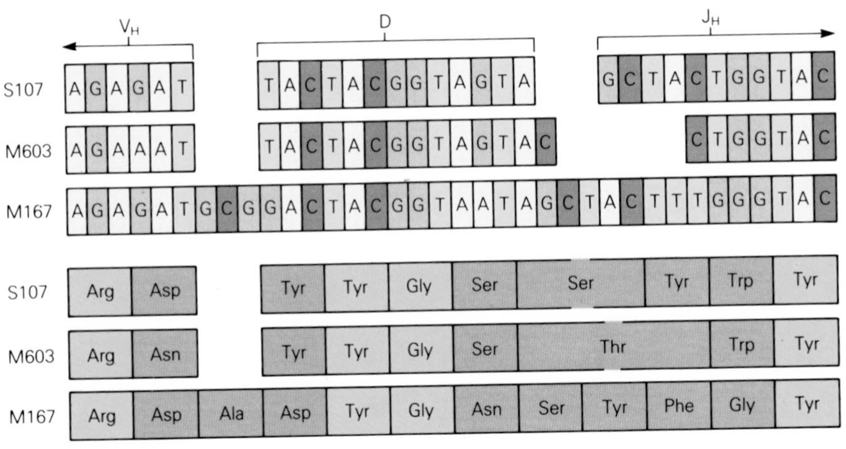

Fig. 6.14 Heavy chain diversity created by variable recombination. The DNA sequence (above) and amino acid sequence (below) of three heavy chains of anti-phosphorylcholine are shown. Variable recombination between the germ line V, D, and J regions causes variation (red) in amino acid sequences. In some cases (e.g. M167) there appear to be additional inserted codons, however, these additions do not alter the overall reading frame.

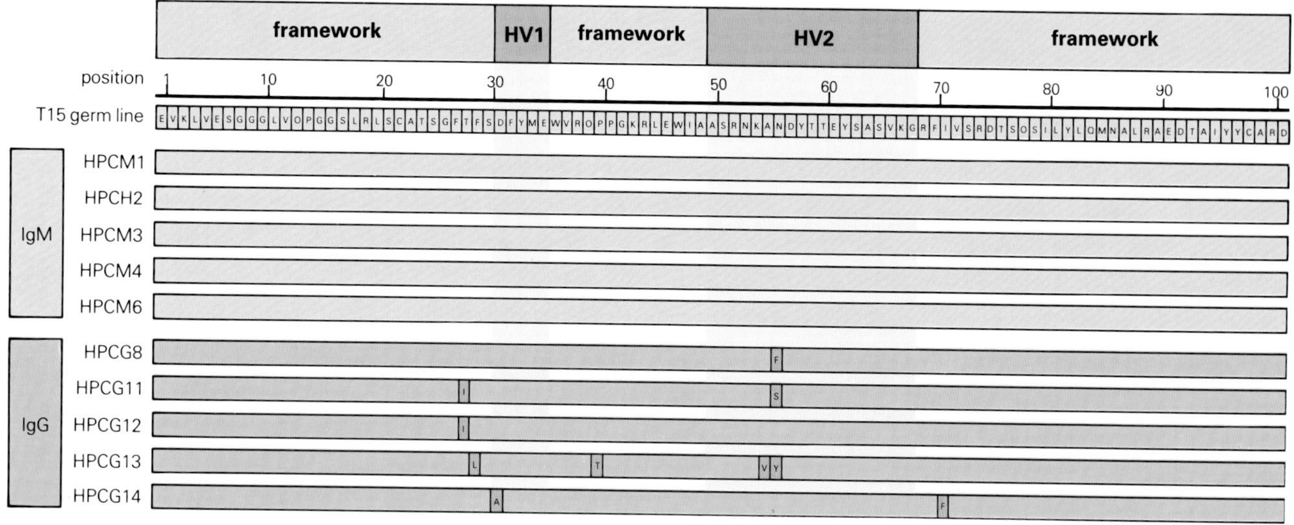

Fig. 6.15 Somatic mutation. The amino acid sequences of five IgM and five IgG hybridoma anti-phosphorylcholine antibody V_H regions are compared to the primary amino acid structure of the T15 germ line DNA, as identified by sequencing sperm cell DNA. Positions which correspond to the germ line sequence are shown in yellow; points at which different amino acids occur are shown in red. Areas of hypervariability (HV1, HV2) are also indicated. Mutations have only occurred in the IgG molecules and the mutations are seen in both hypervariable and framework segments.

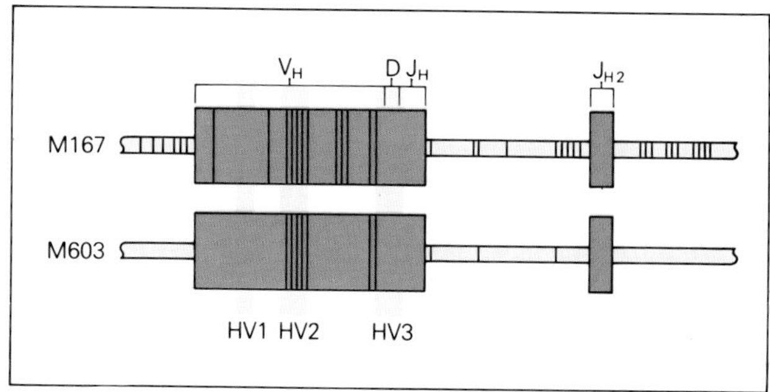

Fig. 6.16 Mutations in the DNA of two V_H T15 genes. The DNA of two anti-phosphorylcholine antibodies with the T15 idiotype is shown (black lines indicate positions where the genome has mutated from the germ line sequence). There are large numbers of mutations in the introns and the exons of both genes, but particularly in the second hypervariable region, HV2. By comparison, no mutations are detectable in the genes coding for the constant regions.

generation of immunoglobulin diversity

1. multiple germ line V genes
2. VJ and VDJ recombinations
3. recombinational inaccuracies
4. somatic point mutation
5. assorted heavy and light chains

Fig. 6.17 Five mechanisms for the generation of antibody diversity. Since each mechanism can occur with any of the others the potential for increased diversity multiplies at each step of immunoglobulin production.

sequences of two anti-phosphorylcholine antibodies (T15 idiotype) shows them to have numerous mutations from the germ line sequence (3·8% of bases are mutated in the protein M167). These mutations occur in both introns and exons of the region implying that the whole region of DNA is particularly mutable, by comparison with adjoining regions of DNA, where mutations have not been found (Fig. 6.16).

Antibody diversity thus arises at several levels. First there are the multiple variable region genes recombining with J and D segments. Then above this the imprecision with which recombination occurs achieves further variation. At this level the structures of the first and second hypervariable regions are coded for entirely by germ line genes while the third complementarity determining region is largely the result of recombination. Additionally, point mutations are added throughout the variable region to give fine variations in specificity. As virtually any light chain may pair with any heavy chain the combinatorial binding of heavy and light chains amplifies the diversity enormously (Fig. 6.17)

HEAVY CHAIN CONSTANT REGION GENES

All classes of immunoglobulin use the same set of variable region genes. When the class is changed all that is switched is the constant region of the heavy chain, as shown by the sharing of heavy chain variable region subgroups on different classes and by the analysis of double myelomas, where two monoclonal antibodies are present in the serum at the same time. IgM and IgG antibodies from a patient with multiple myeloma have been found to have identical light chains and V_H regions; only the constant regions were switched from μ to γ. Often IgM and IgD are found on the lymphocyte surface at the same time. Capping these receptors with

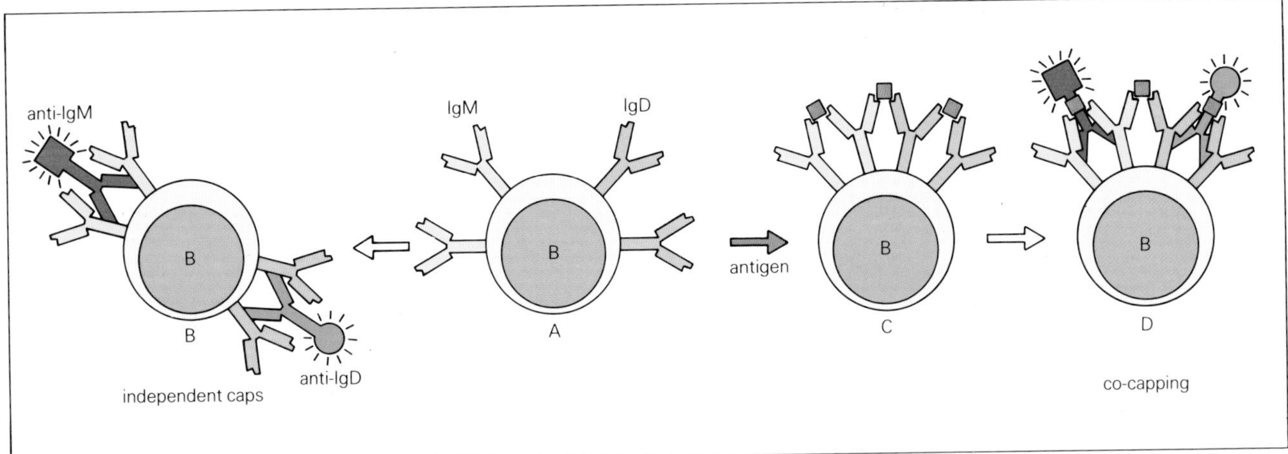

Fig. 6.18 Co-capping of IgM and IgD with antigen. Some B cells have both IgM and IgD on their surface (A). This can be demonstrated by treating the cells with rhodaminated anti-IgM (red) and fluoresceinated anti-IgD (green) in which case the conjugated antibodies separately aggregate the surface IgM and IgD causing a red and green cap to occur on the cell (B). If the experiment is repeated by first treating the cells with antigen (blue) as in (C) and then with the anti-IgM and anti-IgD, both the red anti-IgM and green anti-IgD caps appear together on the cell, that is, they cocap. This implies that IgM and IgD on the cell surface were cross-linked by antigen (D). This can only occur if the IgM and IgD have the same antigen binding specificity and is therefore evidence that different constant regions (μ and δ) can be linked to the same V region.

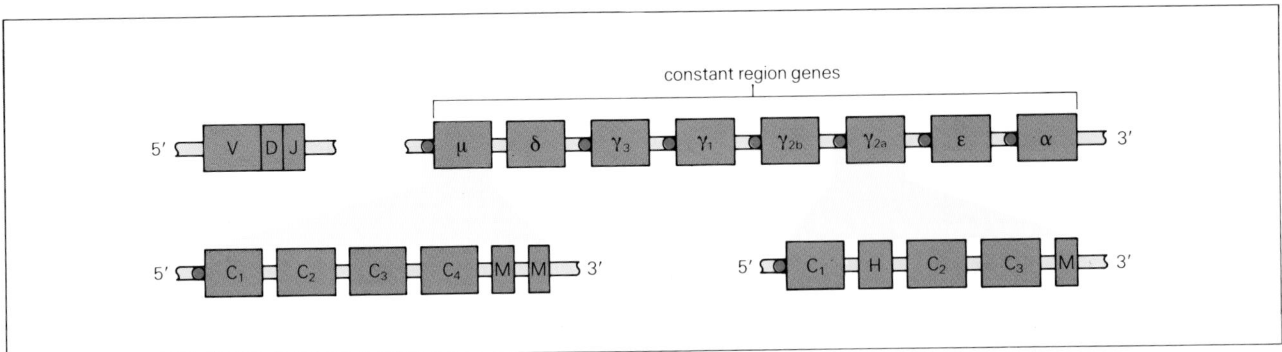

Fig. 6.19 Constant region genes: mouse. The constant region genes of the mouse are arranged 6.5 kilobases downstream from the recombined VDJ segment. Each C gene except that for δ has a switching sequence at its start (red circles) which corresponds to a sequence at the 5′ end of the μ gene. This allows any of the C genes to recombine with VDJ. δ genes appear to use the same switching sequences as μ but the μ gene is lost in RNA processing to produce IgD. The C genes (expanded below for μ and γ_{2a}) contain introns separating the exons for each domain (C1, C2, etc.). The γ genes also have separate exon coding for the hinge (H) and all the genes have one or more exons coding for membrane bound immunoglobulin (M). All the introns are lost during RNA processing.

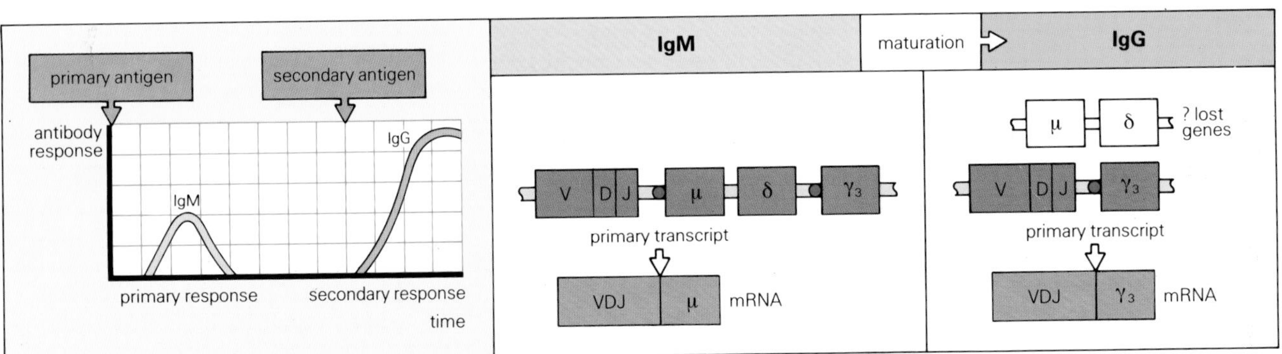

Fig. 6.20 Maturation of the immune response and class switching. As shown in the graph, following a primary antigen injection there is an antibody response which consists mostly of IgM whereas the response following a secondary challenge is mostly IgG. The underlying cellular mechanism for this class switch is shown on the right. In the primary response the VDJ region is transcribed with a μ gene and, after removal of introns during processing, mRNA for secreted IgM is produced. During maturation, which involves T cell help, and possibly also the activation of a mutation mechanism for the VDJ segment, another C gene (here illustrated as Cγ3) is brought up to exchange with the μ gene at its switch region (red). The μ and δ genes are probably lost; transcription and processing produce mRNA for IgG3.

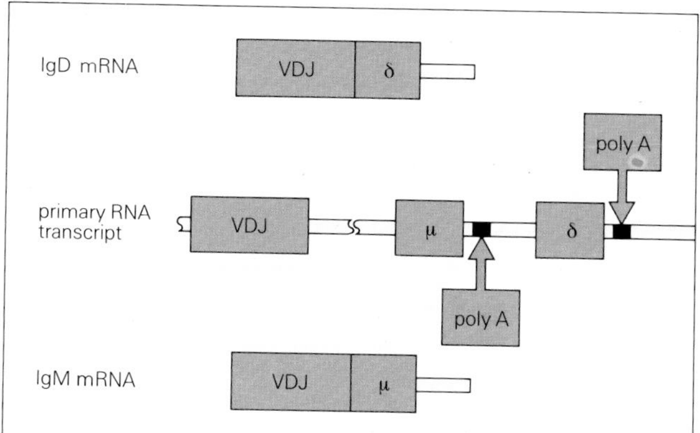

Fig. 6.21 Isotype switching by differential RNA splicing. Single B cells can produce more than one antibody isotype from a single long primary RNA transcript. In this diagram, a transcript containing μ and δ is shown but longer ones with other C genes are possible. Polyadenylation can occur at different sites (black squares), leading to different forms of splicing, producing mRNA for IgD (top) or IgM (bottom). In fact there are additional polyadenylation sites even within this region, which determine whether membrane immunoglobulin or secreted immunoglobulin is formed.

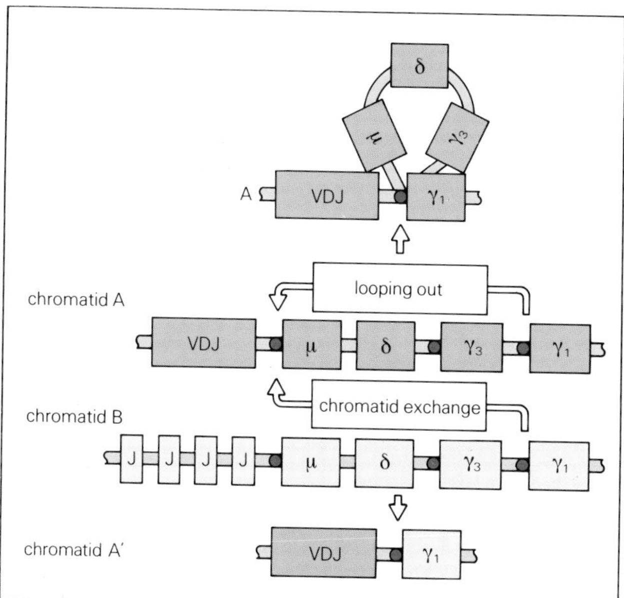

Fig. 6.22 Lost genes: hypotheses. Two hypotheses explain the loss of genes during class switching (here illustrated as an IgM→IgG1 switch). A and B are chromatids of the chromosome section for the immunoglobulin genes. Chromatid A contains the rearranged VDJ segment. According to the looping out hypothesis, a section of C genes (μ, δ, γ_3) loop out and are lost. According to the chromatid exchange hypothesis the similarities in the switching sequences permit unequal somatic recombination between maternal and paternal chromatids. The A chromatid recombines with another part of the unrearranged B chromatid. The loss of gene segments giving rise to the IgM→IgG1 switch shown is A'. The 'lost' intervening C genes are found on the other, non-functional chromatid B' (not shown), which now contains two copies of several C genes (i.e. unrearranged V, D, J, μ, δ, γ_3, μ, δ, γ_3, γ_1, etc.).

antigen has revealed that the IgM and IgD have the same specificity for antigen, indicating similarity of V_H regions on the two classes (Fig. 6.18).

All the constant region genes are arranged downstream from the J segment genes. In the mouse there is one gene for each of the μ, δ, ε and α isotypes and one γ gene for each of the four different IgG isotypes (Fig. 6.19). In man the constant region genes are more complicated, and it appears that one section of this region has undergone gene duplication and diversification. In man the ordering of genes is μ, δ, [γ3,γ1, ε1,α1], γ,[γ2, γ4, ε, α2]. The two sets within square brackets indicate the possible area of reduplication. The genes ε1 and γ are pseudogenes and are not expressed . Just upstream (5′) to the μ gene is a switch sequence (S) which is repeated 5′ to each of the other constant region genes except δ. This S region is a recombination site which allows class switching to the other constant region genes (Fig. 6.20). Class switching is important in the maturation of the immune response and may be accompanied or preceded by somatic mutation. Initially a complete section of DNA, including the recombined V_H region through the δ and μ constant regions, is transcribed; then by differential splicing, two messenger RNA molecules are produced each with the same V_H but having either μ or δ constant regions. It is suggested that sometimes much larger stretches of DNA are also transcribed together, with differential splicing giving other immunoglobulin classes sharing V_H regions (Fig. 6.21). This has been observed in cells simultaneously producing IgM and IgE. More often class switching appears to be mediated by a recombination between S recombination sites allowing a looping out and deletion of DNA and bringing another C region gene close to the VDJ gene (Fig. 6.22). A further possibility has been suggested involving exchange between sister chromatids.

MEMBRANE AND SECRETED IMMUNOGLOBULIN

The membrane immunoglobulin produced by a cell as its antigen receptor and the immunoglobulin that it secretes are identical except for a stretch of amino acids at the C-terminus of the heavy chains. Membrane immunoglobulins are larger than their secreted counterparts; their additional amino acids traverse the cell membrane to anchor the molecule. This can be seen in membrane IgM where a section of hydrophobic (lipophilic) amino acids are sandwiched between hydrophilic residues which lie on either side of the membrane (Fig. 6.23); the hydrophobic residue is thought to form a stretch of α helix within the membrane. Membrane immunoglobulins do not form polymers of the basic four-chain unit.

The production of the two forms of immunoglobulin is brought about by differential transcription of the germ line C region gene which can be transcribed in two different ways (Fig. 6.24). It is thought that the poly A sequence is important in determining which RNA transcript is produced, but how this is controlled is uncertain.

Evidently the way the cell regulates which immunoglobulin it produces is complicated. The first step is the heavy chain rearrangement of D to J, followed by addition of V; μ chain stimulates the kappa locus to attempt VJ rearrangement, followed by the lambda locus if necessary. It is postulated that this occurs repeatedly in both maternal and paternal chromosomes until a functionally recombined gene is produced or the genetic material is exhausted and the cell is aborted. Once the V regions of that cell are determined they remain essentially unaltered thereafter (except for any somatic mutation). However there is still switching in the C_H genes to produce different isotypes and a change to production of secreted immunoglobulin following cell activation. A compilation of facts and hypotheses is shown in Fig. 6.25.

PRODUCTION OF IMMUNOGLOBULIN

Before the antibody protein is synthesized it is first necessary to splice the introns out of the primary RNA transcript. It is found that the beginning and end of each intron have particular forms of RNA base sequences referred to as donor and acceptor junctions. It is thought that the junctions interact with each other and with ribonucleoproteins in the nucleus to remove the introns and splice the joins back together again to form mRNA. It is, of course, essential that this is done accurately so that the reading frame of the mRNA is unaltered.

Messenger RNA for immunoglobulins is translated across the membranes of the endoplasmic reticulum, after which the H and L chains associate (Fig. 6.26). Cellular immunoglobulins and secreted immunoglobulins are processed differently to arrive at their correct locations, by mechanisms which are unknown at present.

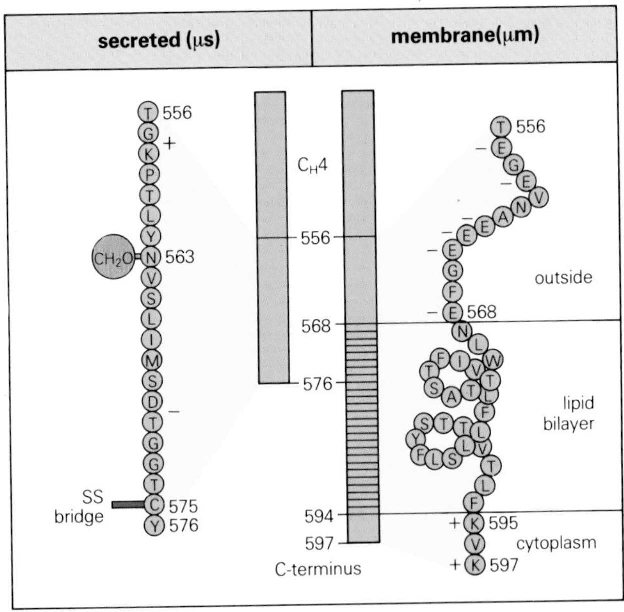

Fig. 6.23 Membrane and secreted IgM: mouse. This diagram shows the *C*-terminal amino acid sequences of the IgM molecule for the secreted and membrane-bound molecules. The structures of both molecules are identical up to residue 556. Secreted IgM has 20 further residues. Residue 563 (asparagine) has a carbohydrate unit attached to it while residue 575 is a cystine involved in the formation of interchain disulphide bonds. Membrane IgM has 41 residues beyond 556. A stretch of 26 residues between 568 and 595 contains hydrophobic amino acids sandwiched between sequences containing charged residues. It has been proposed that this hydrophobic portion traverses the cell membrane as two turns of α helix. A short, positively charged section lies inside the cytoplasm.

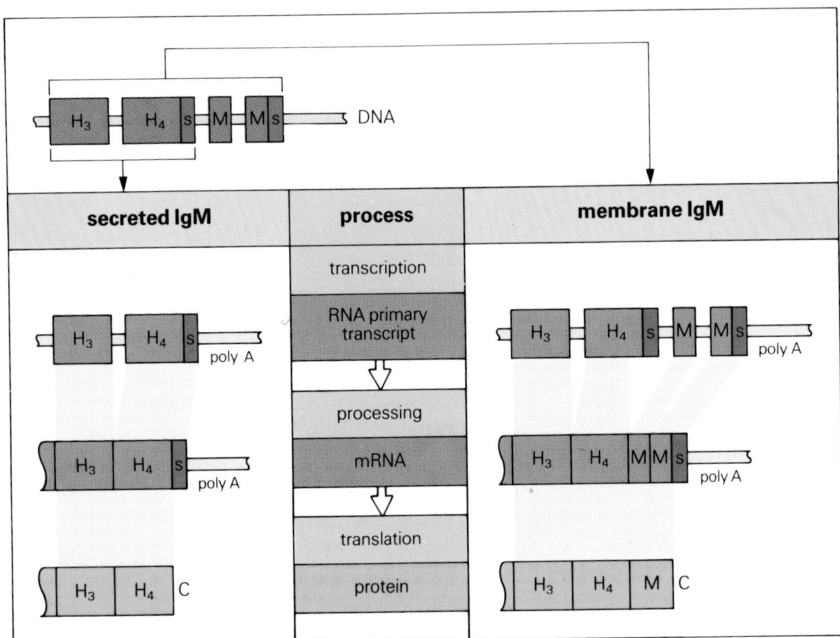

Fig. 6.24 Membrane and secreted IgM. Part of the DNA coding for IgM is shown diagrammatically. The exons for the μ3, and μ4 domains (H_3 and H_4) and the intramembranal segment of membrane IgM (M) are indicated. Translation stop sequences (s) are present at the end of the H_4 and second membrane segments. The DNA can be transcribed in two ways. If transcription stops after H_4 the transcript with a poly A tail is processed to produce mRNA for secreted IgM. If transcription runs through to include the membrane segments, processing removes the codons for the terminal amino acids and the stop signal of H_4 so that translation yields a protein with a different C-terminus.

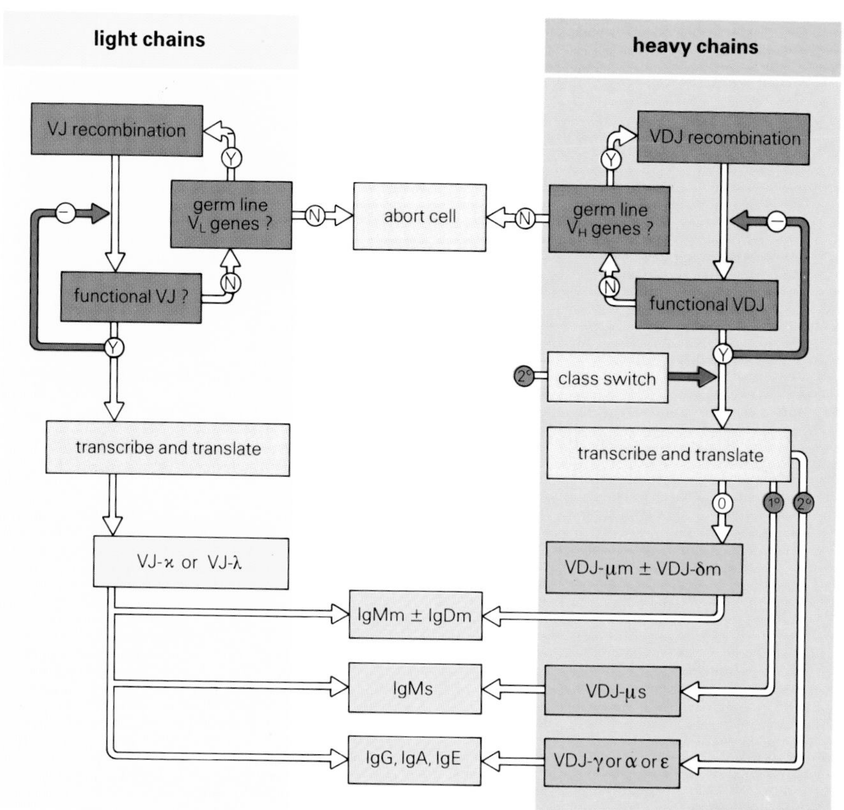

Fig. 6.25 Summary scheme of immunoglobulin production. This diagram is based on a series of steps at which different outcomes may occur. Pre-B cells attempt to recombine a VJ from the germ line genes (left). If functional (Y) it is transcribed and translated to form a light chain. Once a cell has produced a functional recombination, feedback (−) prevents further rearrangements. If the VJ is not functional (N) the cell makes another attempt. If a cell exhausts its store of germ line gene segments then it is aborted. A similar process occurs for heavy chains (right) so that the early B cell (right) expresses IgMm±IgDm. This occurs with no antigen stimulation (O). After primary antigen stimulation (1°), the transcriptional process changes so that secreted IgM is released. After secondary antigen stimulation (2°) and with T cell help there is DNA rearrangement, resulting in a class switch, possibly also with mutation in V_H and V_L. The end products are cells bearing and secreting IgG, IgA or IgE.

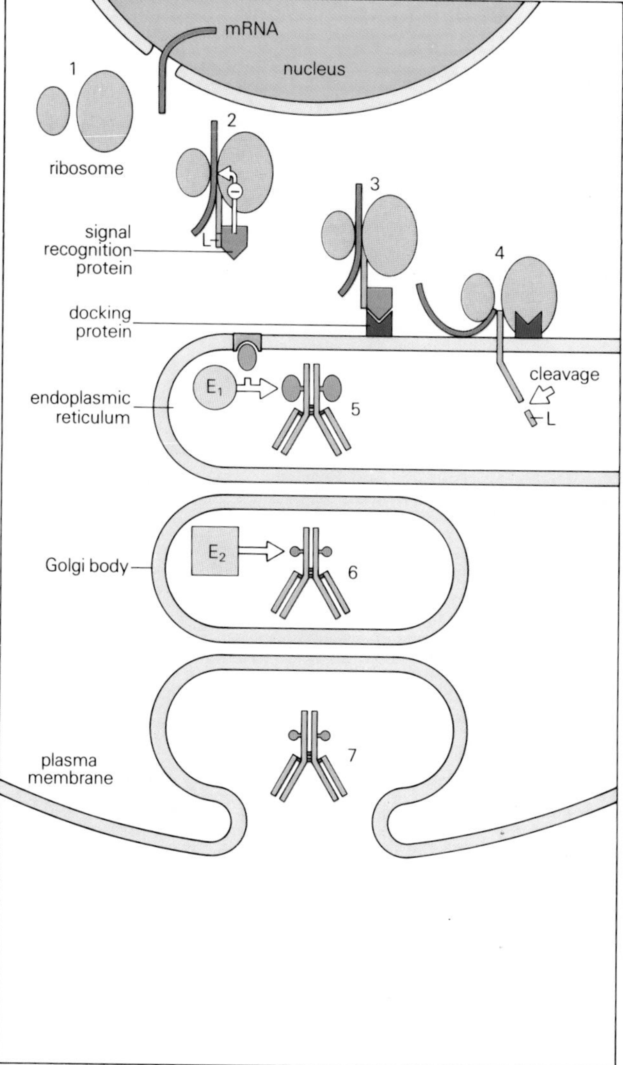

Fig. 6.26 Production of secreted immunoglobulin. Messenger RNA for a secreted heavy chain leaves the nucleus and enters the cytoplasm where it is bound by a ribosome (1). The leading sequence (L) is translated and this binds to signal recognition protein (SRP) which blocks further translation (2). The SRP ribosome complex migrates to the endoplasmic reticulum (ER) where the SRP binds to the docking protein at a vacant site on the ER (3). Translation may now proceed and the synthesizing chain traverses the membrane into the ER (4). The leader sequence is removed and the chain combines with other H and L chains to form the immunoglobulin subunit (5). Enzymes (E_1) add carbohydrate (blue) as the ER pinches off to form the Golgi body (6). In the Golgi body further enzymes (E_2) modify the carbohydrate before the completed molecule is secreted to the outside by reverse pinocytosis (7).

GENES OF THE T CELL ANTIGEN RECEPTOR

There are four different sets of genes which generate the antigen/MHC binding portion of the T cell receptor. These are the α and β gene sets which are expressed in the majority of peripheral T cells and the γ and δ genes which are expressed in a subpopulation of thymic T cells and also in a minor population of peripheral T cells. These chains become associated with the γ, δ, and ε chains of the CD3 molecule to form the complete T cell receptor as indicated in Chapter 5.

The general arrangement of T cell receptor genes is remarkably similar to that of immunoglobulin heavy chains. Fig. 6.27 illustrates the arrangement of the mouse α and β genes. Interestingly the δ genes for the T cell receptor lie in the middle of the α genes, with their own sets of D, J and C segments.

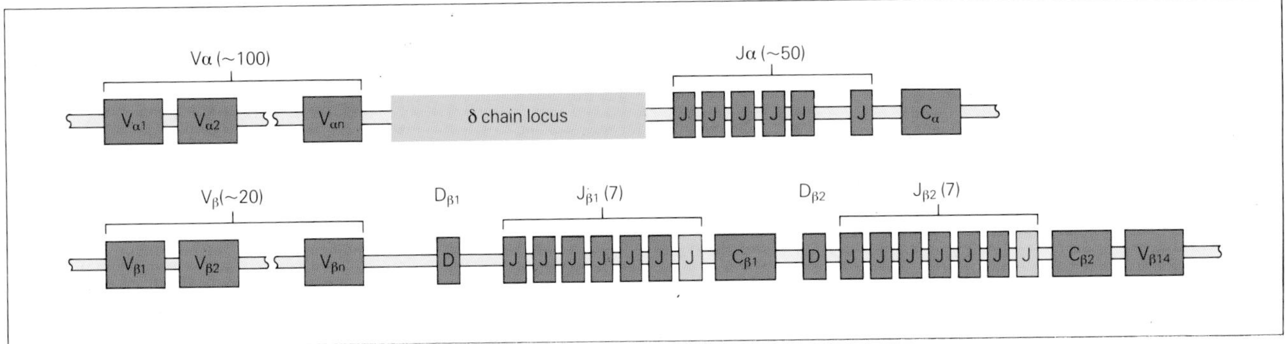

Fig. 6.27 T cell receptor genes. The genes of the murine T cell receptor α and β polypeptides are shown. Note the location of the δ loci embedded within the α loci and the tandem duplication which has occurred in the β chain loci. The last of each set of J_β genes is a pseudogene.

RECOMBINATION OF T CELL RECEPTOR GENES

Diversification of the T cell receptor genes occurs by recombination between V, D, and J segments, with minor variations in detail for each locus.

The α chain is superficially simple, except for the complication of the δ chain embedded between V and J loci. As in the κ locus a complete variable region is produced by rearrangement of a V_α segment to a J_α segment. Diversity is markedly increased by the unusually large number of J segments.

The β locus includes two sets of D, J and C genes. Most of the V_β genes are grouped together, but one ($V_{\beta 14}$) is present at the extreme 3′ end of the locus. The tandem duplication of D_β, J_β, C_β, must have occurred early in the evolution since it is present in both mice and men. Extensive diversity is generated in the joining process as not only are VDJ arrangements possible, but also VJ and VDDJ joins. The D segments are used in all three reading frames, adding even further to β chain diversity.

The γ chain locus is rather differently arranged in mice and men. The murine locus bears a striking similarity to the light chain locus, with four C_γ genes (one a pseudogene) each of which is associated with one J_γ genes and one to four V_γ genes. There are no D genes. In man there are eight V_γ genes followed upstream (5′) by three J_γ and the first C_γ; then there are two additional J_γ genes before $C_\gamma 2$. Imprecise joining of V with J, together with insertions in the joins is important in generating diversity.

The δ locus was discovered during studies on the α locus. Although relatively simple, with only five V_δ, two D_δ and six J_δ genes, it has been calculated that 10^{14} different δ chains could be generated by imprecision in joining, insertion of additional residues and usage of the D genes in all three reading frames.

The mechanisms by which T cell receptor gene recombination occurs, appear to be similar to those of B cells, since the genes have similar patterns of heptamer, 12 or 23 base pair spacer, nonamer sequences flanking them. Although somatic mutation is an important mechanism in generating immunoglobulin diversity, it does not occur in T cell receptor genes. This is probably linked with the necessity to maintain tolerance to self and recognition of MHC by T cells.

FURTHER READING

Alt, F.W., Blackwell, T.K., DePinho, R.A., Reth, M.G. & Yancopoulos, G.D. (1986) Regulation of genome rearrangement events during lymphocyte differentiation. *Immunological Reviews,* **89**, 5.

Baltimore, D. (1981) Somatic mutation gains its place among the generators of diversity. *Cell,* **26**, 295.

Brack, C., Hirama, M., Lenhard-Schuller, R. & Tonegawa, S. (1978) A complete immunoglobulin gene is created by somatic recombination. *Cell,* **15**, 1.

Cushley, W. & Williamson, A.R. (1982) Expression of immunoglobulin genes. *Essays in Biochemistry,* **18**, 1.

Davis, M.M. & Bjorkman, P.J. (1988) T-cell antigen receptor genes and T-cell recognition. *Nature,* **334**, 395.

Elliot, J.F., Rock, E.P., Patten, P.A., Davis, M.M. & Chien, Y-h. (1980) The adult T-cell receptor delta chain is diverse and distinct from that of fetal thymocytes. *Nature,* **331**, 627.

Gearhart, P.J. (1982) Generation of immunoglobulin variable gene diversity. *Immunology Today,* **3**, 107.

Honjo, T. (1983) Immunoglobulin genes. *Annual Review of Immunology,* **1**, 499.

Hood, L., Kronenberg, M. & Hunkapiller, T. (1985) T-cell antigen receptors and the immunoglobulin supergene family. *Cell,* **40**, 225.

Owen, M.J. & Lamb, J.R. (1988) *Immune Recognition.* Oxford: IRL Press.

Radbruch, A., Burger, C., Klem, S. & Muller, W. (1986) Control of immunoglobulin class switch recombination. *Immunological Reviews,* **89**, 69.

Saito, T., Weiss, A., Miller, J., Norcross, M.A. & Germain, R.N. (1987) Specific antigen-Ia activation of transfected human T-cells expressing murine Ti αβ-human T3 receptor complexes. *Nature,* **325**, 125.

Siu, G., Clark, S.P., Yoshikai, Y., Mailissen, M., Yanagi, Y., Strauss, E., Mak, T.W. & Hood, L. (1984) The human T-cell antigen receptor is encoded by variable, diversity, and joining gene segments that arrange to generate a complete V gene. *Cell,* **37**, 393.

Tonegawa, S. (1983) Somatic generation of antibody diversity. *Nature,* **302**, 573.

Williamson, A.R. & Turner, M.W. (1987) *Essential Immunogenetics.* Oxford: Blackwell Scientific Publications.

Yanagi, Y., Yoshikai, Y., Legett, K., Clark, S., Aleksander, I. & Mak,T. (1984) A human T cell-specific cDNA clone encodes a protein having extensive homology to immunoglobulin chains. *Nature,* **308**, 145.

7 Antigen Recognition

Antibody and the T cell antigen receptor have many features in common. They both have variable (V) and constant (C) domains, and the process of gene recombination which produces the variable domains from V, D and J gene segments is also similar for each type of receptor. Nevertheless the ways in which B cells and T cells recognize antigen is quite different: antibody recognizes antigens in solution or on cell surfaces in their native conformation, while the T cell receptor sees antigen in association with MHC molecules on cell surfaces. Frequently, antigens recognized by T cells are degraded or processed in some way, so that the determinant recognized by the T cell antigen receptor is only a small fragment of the original antigen.

Another difference between antibody and the T cell antigen receptor is that antibody may be produced in two forms, either as the B cell antigen receptor or as secreted antibody, whereas the T cell antigen receptor is an integral membrane protein. Secreted antibody is essentially a bifunctional molecule in which the V domains are primarily concerned with antigen binding and the C domains interact with receptors on host tissues.

This chapter describes the ways in which the V domains of antibody and the T cell antigen receptor form an antigen binding site and how they then interact with their specific antigens or antigen/MHC. These interactions underlie the specificity of the adaptive immune response.

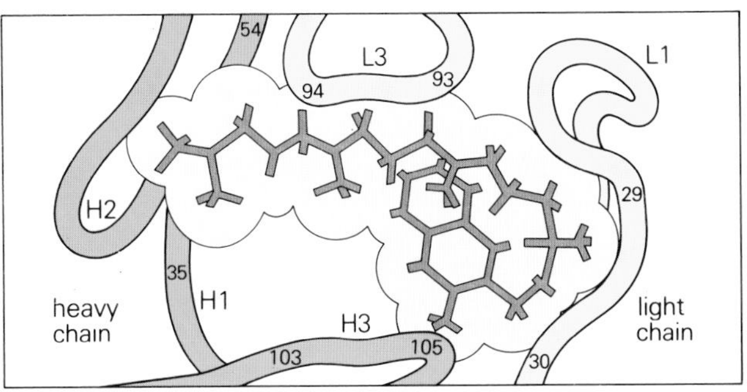

Fig. 7.1 The antibody combining site. The antigen molecule nestles in a cleft formed by the antibody combining site. The example shown is based on X-ray crystallography studies of human IgG (the myeloma protein NEW) binding γ-hydroxyl vitamin K. The antigen makes contact with 10–12 amino acids in the hypervariable regions of both heavy and light chains. The numerals refer to amino acids identified as actually making contact with the antigen.

ANTIGEN–ANTIBODY BINDING

X-ray crystallography of antibody V domains shows that the hypervariable regions are clustered at the end of the Fab arms, and it is particular residues in these regions which interact specifically with antigen (Fig. 7.1). The framework residues do not usually form bonds with the antigen but are essential for producing the folding of the V domains and maintaining the integrity of the binding site.

The binding of antigen to antibody takes place by the formation of multiple non-covalent bonds between the antigen and amino acids of the binding site. Although the attractive forces (namely, hydrogen bonds, electrostatic, Van der Waals and hydrophobic) involved in these bonds are individually weak by comparison with covalent bonds, the multiplicity of the bonds leads to a considerable binding energy.

The non-covalent bonds are critically dependent on the distance (d) between the interacting groups. The force is proportional to $1/d^2$ for electrostatic forces and to $1/d^7$ for Van der Waals forces; thus the interacting groups must be close in molecular terms before these forces become significant (Fig. 7.2). The consequence of this is

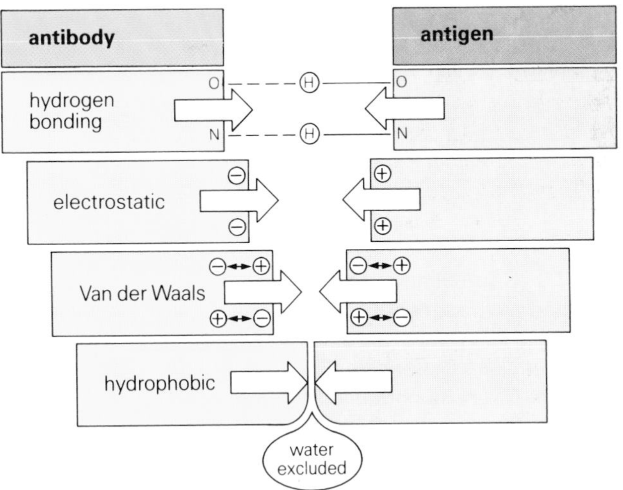

Fig. 7.2 The intermolecular attractive forces binding antigen to antibody. These forces require the close approach of the interacting groups.
Hydrogen bonding results from the formation of hydrogen bridges between appropriate atoms.
Electrostatic forces are due to the attraction of oppositely charged groups located on two protein side chains.
Van der Waals bonds are generated by the interaction between electron clouds (here represented as induced oscillating dipoles).
Hydrophobic bonds (which may contribute up to half the total strength of the antigen–antibody bond) rely upon the association of non-polar, hydrophobic groups so that contact with water molecules is minimized.
The distance of separation between the interacting groups which produces optimum binding varies for the different types of bond.

that an antigenic determinant and the antigen combining site must have complementary structures to be able to combine, meaning that:

1. there must be suitable atomic groupings on opposing parts of the antigen and antibody
2. the shape of the combining site must fit the antigen, so that several non-covalent bonds can form simultaneously.

If the antigen and the combining site are complementary in this way, there will be sufficient binding energy to resist thermodynamic disruption of the bond. However, if electron clouds of the antigen and antibody overlap, steric repulsive forces come into play which are inversely proportional to the twelfth power of the distance between the clouds ($F \alpha 1/d^{12}$). These forces play a vital role in determining the specificity of the antibody molecule for a particular antigen and its ability to discriminate between antigens, since any variation from the ideal complementary shape will cause a fall in the total binding energy through increased repulsive forces and decreased attractive forces. Examples of a good fit and a poor fit between antigen and antibody are illustrated in Fig. 7.3.

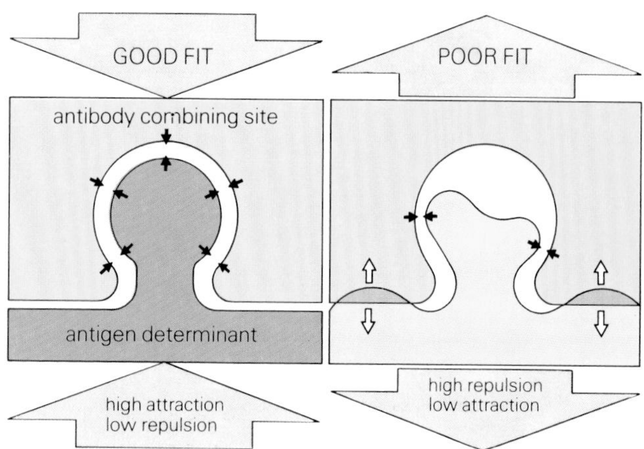

Fig. 7.3 Good fit and poor fit between antigen and antibody. A good fit between the antigenic determinant and the binding site of the antibody will create ample opportunities for intermolecular attractive forces to be created and few opportunities for repulsive forces to operate. Conversely, when there is a poor fit the reverse is true, that is, when electron clouds overlap high repulsive forces are generated, which dominate any small forces of attraction.

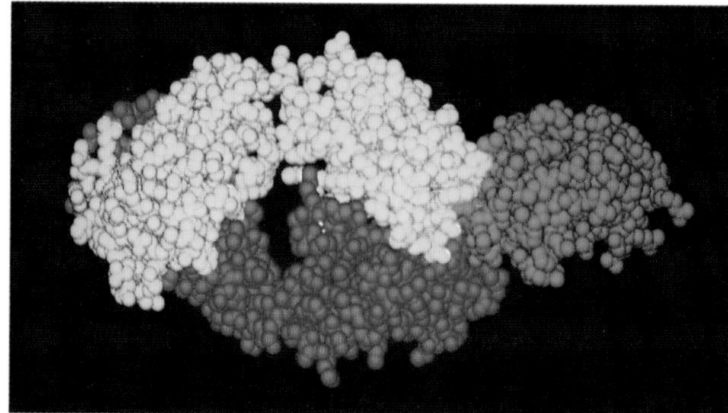

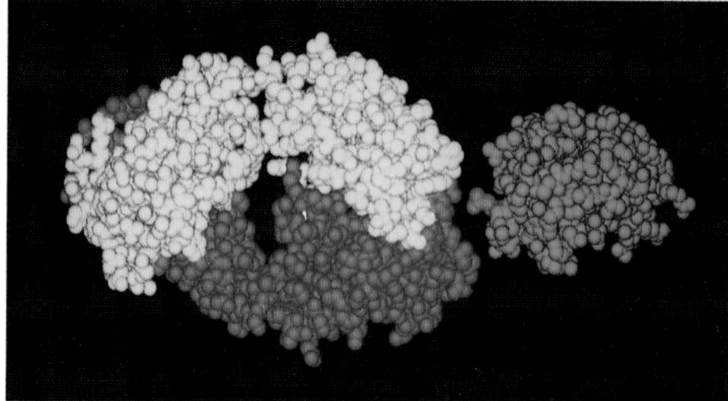

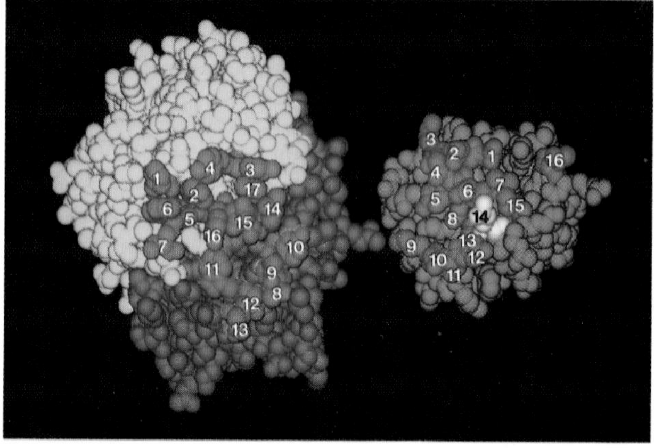

Fig. 7.4 The Fab–lysozyme complex. The upper figure shows lysozyme (green) binding to the hypervariable regions of the heavy (blue) and light (yellow) chains of the Fab fragment of antibody DI.3. The centre panel shows the complex separated with Glu 121 (red) visible. This residue fits into the centre of the cleft between the heavy and light chains. The lower panel shows the molecules rotated forward 90° to show the contact residues which contribute to the antigen–antibody bond. (Courtesy of Dr R.J. Poljak; permission from *Science* 1986, **233**, 747–753. Copyright 1986 by the AAAS.)

Recent studies have shown how protein antigens interact with specific antibodies. For example, an examination of the interaction between the antigen lysozyme and the Fab of an antibody to lysozyme shows that the antigen epitope and the binding site have complementary surfaces and that these extend even beyond the hypervariable regions. In this example, 17 amino acid residues on the antibody were in contact with 16 residues on the antigen (Fig. 7.4). All of the hypervariable regions contributed to the antibody binding site, although the third hypervariable region formed by the VDJ join in the heavy chain gene appeared to be most important. This may be related to the greater variability generated by recombination of the V, D, and J segments.

ANTIBODY AFFINITY

The strength of a single antigen–antibody bond is the antibody affinity; it is produced by summation of the attractive and repulsive forces described above (Fig. 7.5). Interaction of the antibody combining site with antigen can be investigated thermodynamically. To measure the affinity of a single combining site it is necessary to use a monovalent antigen or even a single isolated antigenic determinant – a hapten. Since the non-covalent bonds between antibody and hapten are dissociable, the overall combination of an antigen and antibody must also be reversible; thus the Law of Mass

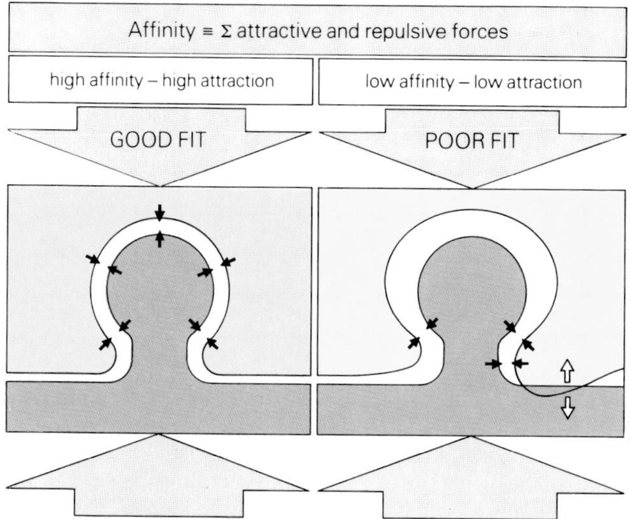

Fig. 7.5 Antibody affinity. The affinity with which antibody binds antigen results from a balance between the attractive and repulsive forces. A high affinity antibody implies a good fit and conversely, a low affinity antibody implies a poor fit.

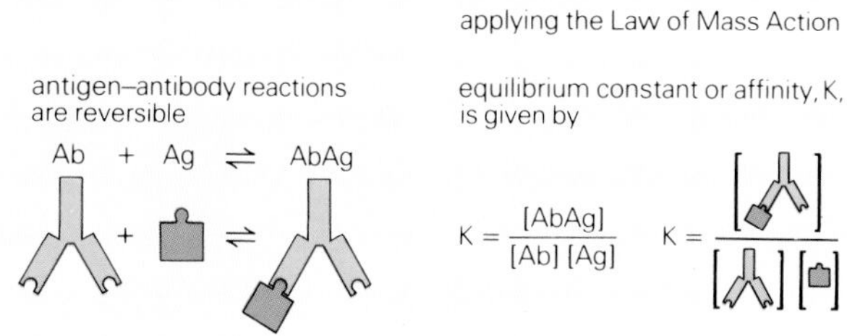

Fig. 7.6 Reversibility of the antigen–antibody bond and the calculation of antibody affinity. All antigen–antibody reactions are reversible and the Law of Mass Action has been applied, from which antibody affinity (given by the equilibrium constant, K) can be calculated at equilibrium. (Square brackets refer to the concentration of the reactants.)

Action can be applied to the reaction and the equilibrium constant, K, can be determined. This is the affinity constant (Fig. 7.6).

AFFINITY AND AVIDITY

Since each antibody unit of four polypeptide chains has two antigen binding sites, antibodies are potentially multivalent in their reaction with antigen. In addition, antigen can also be monovalent or multivalent. A hapten has only one antigenic determinant and can therefore react with only one antigen combining site; thus it is monovalent. Many molecules however, have more than one antigenic determinant. Microorganisms have a large number of antigenic determinants exposed on their surfaces, hence they are all multivalent. When a multivalent antigen combines with more than one of an antibody's combining sites, the binding energy between the two is considerably greater than the sum of the binding energies of the individual sites since all the antigen–antibody bonds must be broken simultaneously before the antigen and antibody dissociate.

The strength with which a multivalent antibody binds a multivalent antigen is termed avidity, to differentiate it from the affinity of the bond between a single antigenic determinant and an individual combining site. Thus, the avidity of an antibody for its antigen is dependent on the affinities of the individual combining sites for the determinants on the antigen, but is greater than the sum of these affinities if both antigen and antibody are multivalent (Fig. 7.7). In normal physiological situations avidity is likely to be more relevant than affinity since naturally occurring antigens are multivalent; however, the precise measurement of hapten–antibody reactions is more likely to give an insight into the immunochemical nature of the antigen–antibody reaction.

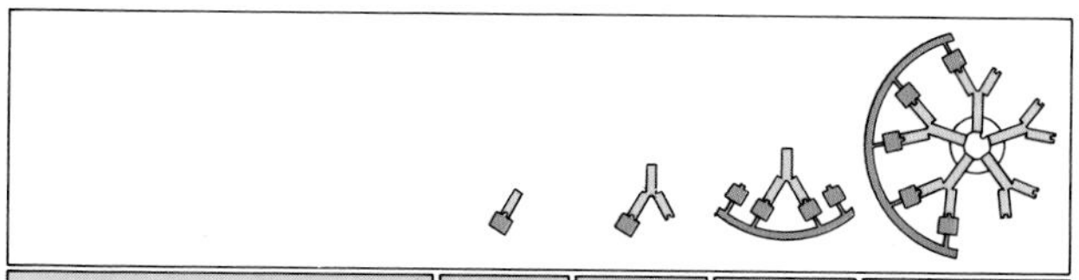

antibody	Fab	IgG	IgG	IgM
effective antibody valence	1	1	2	up to 10
antigen valence	1	1	n	n
equilibrium constant (L/M)	10^4	10^4	10^7	10^{11}
advantage of multivalence	–	–	10^3-fold	10^7-fold
definition of binding	affinity	affinity	avidity	avidity
	intrinsic affinity		functional affinity	

Fig. 7.7 Affinity and avidity. Multivalent binding between antibody and antigen (avidity or functional affinity) results in a considerable increase in stability as measured by the equilibrium constant, compared to simple monovalent binding (affinity or intrinsic affinity, here arbitrarily assigned a value of 10^4 L/M). This is sometimes referred to as the 'bonus effect' of multivalency. Thus there may be a 10^3-fold increase in the binding energy of IgG when both valencies (combining sites) are utilized, and a 10^7-fold increase when IgM binds antigen in a multivalent manner.

ANTIBODY SPECIFICITY

Antigen–antibody reactions can show a high level of specificity. For example, antibodies to a virus like measles will bind to the measles virus and confer immunity to this disease, but will not combine with, or protect against, an unrelated virus such as polio. The specificity of an antiserum is the result of the summation of the actions of the various antibodies in the total population each reacting with a different part of the antigen molecule and even different parts of the same determinant (Fig. 7.8). However, when some of the determinants of an antigen, A, are shared by another antigen, B, then a proportion of the antibodies directed to A will also react with B. This phenomenon is termed cross-reactivity. The specificity and cross-reactivity expressed by an antiserum are properties which result from the antibody molecules within the serum.

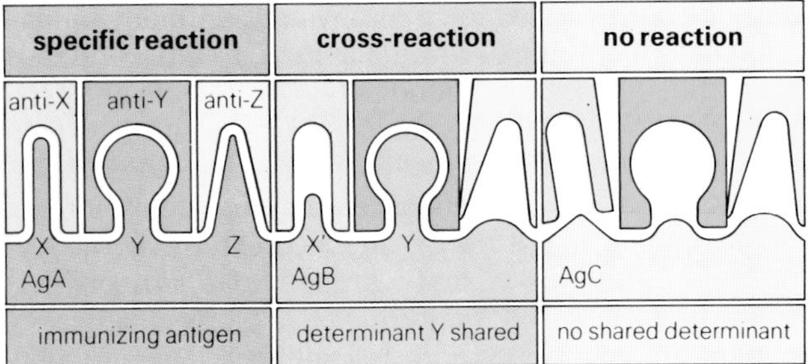

Fig. 7.8 Specificity, cross-reactivity and non-reactivity. Antiserum specificity results from the action of a population of individual antibody molecules (anti-X, anti-Y, and anti-Z) directed against different determinants (X,Y,Z) on the antigen molecule. Antigen A (AgA) and antigen B (AgB) share determinant Y in common. Antiserum raised against AgA (anti-XYZ) not only reacts specifically with AgA but cross-reacts with AgB (through recognition of shared determinant Y and weak recognition of determinant X'). The antiserum gives no reaction with AgC (no shared determinants).

radical (R)	sulphonate	arsonate	carboxylate
	tetrahedral	tetrahedral	planar
ortho	+ +	–	–
meta	+ + +	+	±
para	±	–	–

Fig. 7.9 An example of specificity and cross-reactivity. An antiserum is raised to the meta isomer of aminobenzene sulphonate (the immunizing antigen). This antiserum is then reacted with the ortho and para isomers of aminobenzene sulphonate and also with the three isomers (ortho, meta, para) of two different but related antigens: aminobenzene arsonate and aminobenzene carboxylate. The antiserum reacts specifically with the sulphonate group (which has a tetrahedral structure) in the meta position but will give a cross-reaction (though weaker) with sulphonate in the ortho position. Further, but weaker, cross-reactions are possible when this antiserum is reacted with either the tetrahedral arsonate group or the planar carboxylate group in the meta, but not in the ortho or para position. The arsonate group is larger than sulphonate and has an extra H atom, while the carboxylate is smaller and planar. These results suggest that the overall configuration of the antigen is as important as the individual chemical groupings.

antiserum	antigen		
	p-aminophenol α glucoside	*p*-aminophenol β glucoside	*p*-aminophenol β galactoside
anti-α glucoside	+ + +	+ +	–
anti-β glucoside	+ +	+ + +	–
anti-β galactoside	–	–	+ + +

Fig. 7.10 Configurational specificity–I. Antibody was raised to each of three different, but very similar antigens: *p*-aminophenol α glucoside, *p*-aminophenol β glucoside and *p*-aminophenol β galactoside and the ability of each antibody to cross-react with the other two antigens was assessed.

antiserum	antigen		
	lysozyme	isolated 'loop' peptide	reduced 'loop'
anti-lysozyme	+ +	+	–
anti-'loop' peptide	+	+ +	–

Fig. 7.11 Configurational specificity–II. The lysozyme molecule possesses an intrachain bond (red) which produces a loop in the peptide chain. Antisera may be raised against either whole lysozyme (anti-lysozyme) or the isolated loop (anti-'loop' peptide) and are found to distinguish between the two. Neither antiserum reacts with the isolated loop in its linear, reduced form. This demonstrates the importance of tertiary structure in determining antibody specificity.

There is evidence that antibody recognizes the overall configuration of the antigen rather than its chemical composition and it is envisaged that antibodies are directed against particular three-dimensional electron cloud shapes rather than specific chemical structures (Fig. 7.9).

Antibodies are capable of expressing remarkable specificity and are able to distinguish between small differences in the primary structure of the antigen, and differences in charge, optical configuration and steric conformation. Further examples of antibody specificity are illustrated in Figs 7.10 and 7.11. One of the consequences of this specificity is that many antibodies will only bind to native antigens, or fragments of antigens which retain sufficient structure to make the multiple interactions required for antigen–antibody bond formation.

Over the past few years research has suggested that an antibody molecule may be complementary to several dissimilar antigens. The binding of these antigens is competitive, and it appears that there are specially separated positions within the combining site (Fig. 7.12).

On this basis the specificity of a population of antibodies would not necessarily arise because all the antibodies have the same exclusive specificity. However, if a large number of different polyfunctional antibodies all had a site which could combine with a particular antigen A, the net reactivity of those antibodies would be high to A but low to all other antigens. Thus specificity would be a population phenomenon, an average characteristic of all the antibodies in an antiserum (Fig. 7.13).

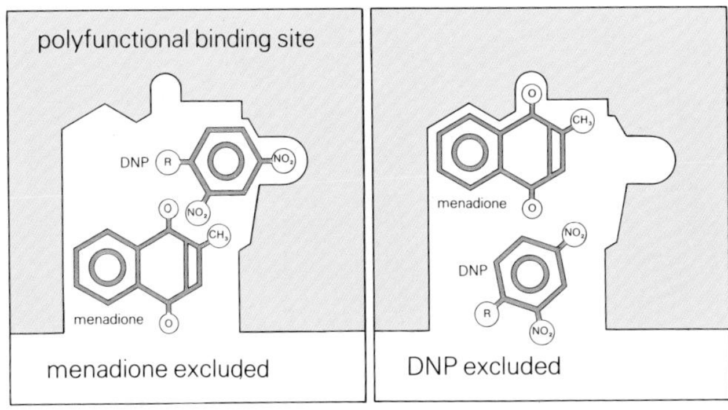

Fig. 7.12 Competitive binding. The antibody combining site may bind more than one antigenic determinant. For example, antibody 460 has two different sites in the binding cleft which are 1.2–1.4 nm apart. The antibody binds the haptens menadione and DNP competitively, that is, the binding of one excludes binding of the other. Binding sites capable of specifically binding more than one antigenic determinant are termed polyfunctional binding sites.

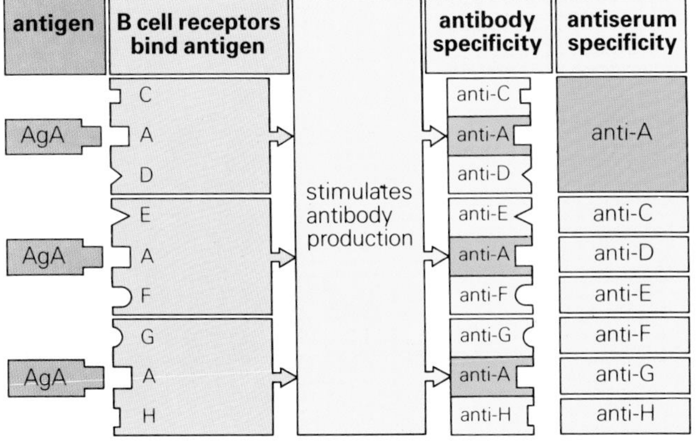

Fig. 7.13 Polyfunctional binding sites – specificity as a population phenomenon. A single antigen (AgA) may bind to the antibody molecules of different B cells which are specific not only for A but also for other antigens (C, D, E, F, etc.), that is, the receptors possess polyfunctional binding sites. Each B cell stimulated by AgA produces antibody specific not only to AgA but also to the other antigens. Since all the B cells stimulated are AgA specific, but not all are specific to the other antigens, the concentration of antibody would be high to AgA but low to the other antigens.

THE PHYSIOLOGICAL SIGNIFICANCE OF HIGH AND LOW AFFINITY ANTIBODIES

The determination of antibody affinity and avidity has provided considerable information on the nature of the antigen–antibody bond, and it has become clear that binding affinity is not merely a matter of theoretical interest, since affinity and avidity affect the physiological and pathological properties of the antibodies.

High affinity antibody is superior to low affinity antibody in a number of biological reactions (Fig. 7.14). Antibody affinity may also have immunopathological significance since, in experimental animals, antigen–antibody complexes containing low affinity antibody persist in the circulation, localize on the glomerular basement membrane of the kidney and impair renal function. High affinity complexes are more rapidly removed from the circulation, localize in the mesangium of the kidney, and have little effect on renal function.

haemagglutination

haemolysis

complement fixation

passive cutaneous anaphylaxis

immune elimination of antigen

membrane damage

virus neutralization

protective capacity against bacteria

enzyme inactivation

Fig. 7.14 Biological reactions in which high affinity antibody is superior to low affinity antibody.

DETERMINATION OF AFFINITY AND AVIDITY

Since the affinity of an antibody can affect its action, it is often necessary, for research purposes, to determine this parameter.

A number of methods are available for the determination of affinity and avidity. In each procedure a system is set up in which antigen and antibody are allowed to come to equilibrium: Ab + Ag $\rightleftarrows$ Ab Ag. The quantities of free antigen and complexed antigen are then measured without disturbing the equilibrium. There are several ways of doing this, including separation of free antigen from bound antigen by physical methods such as dialysis, gel filtration, centrifugation and selective precipitation, or by utilization of changes in the fluorescence properties of the complexed antigen or antibody. Data from these systems can be analysed by application of the Law of Mass Action to give the equilibrium constant, K, which is a measure of antibody affinity since:

$K = \dfrac{[AbAg]}{[Ab][Ag]}$, where [AbAg] is the concentration of complexed antigen, [Ag] is the concentration of free antigen and [Ab] is the concentration of free binding sites at equilibrium. When half the binding sites are occupied by antigen, [Ab] = [AbAg] and it follows that K = 1/[Ag]. In other words, a high affinity antibody only requires a low antigen concentration to achieve binding of antigen to half its combining sites.

ANTIBODY AFFINITY HETEROGENEITY

When enzymes interact with their substrate, the equilibrium constant (K value) for the reaction at different substrate concentrations is invariant. The reaction between an antigen and an antiserum differs from this: K varies with antibody concentration reflecting the heterogeneity

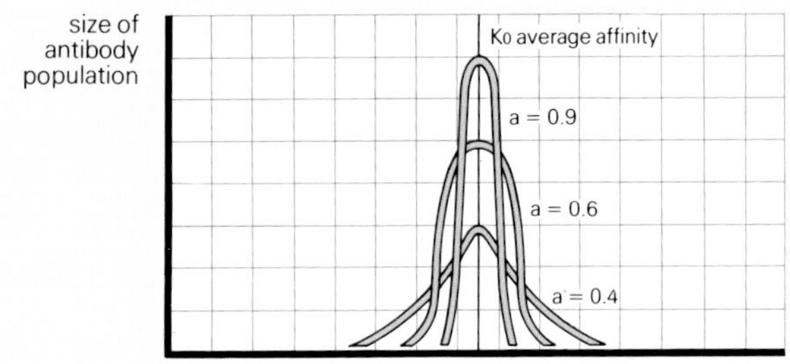

Fig. 7.15 Gaussian distribution of affinities. The heterogeneity of affinity has been assumed to be described by a normal, Gaussian, distribution (that is, equal distribution of affinities around the average affinity, K_0). The peak of the curve represents K_0. With an assumed Gaussian distribution of affinities, the heterogeneity index (a) represents the distribution of affinities around K_0. Thus a perfectly homogeneous antiserum would have a heterogeneity index of 1, as may be seen with monoclonal antibodies.

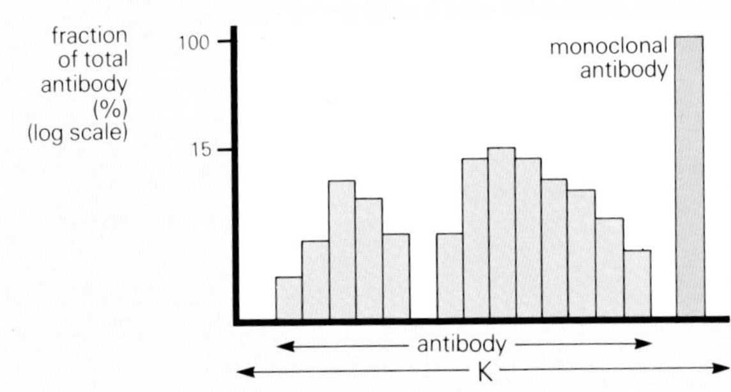

Fig. 7.16 Affinity heterogeneity. This histogram shows a typical distribution of antibody affinities (K) in an antiserum to an antigenic determinant, compared to the single affinity with which a monoclonal antibody binds its antigenic determinant. Note that the antibody affinities do not have a normal distribution.

of a normal antibody population. For many years it was assumed that in any particular population of antibodies, the affinities would have a Gaussian (normal) distribution (Fig. 7.15). Average affinity (K_0) is defined as the reciprocal of the free antigen concentration at equilibrium when half of the total antigen binding sites are occupied: $K_0 = \frac{1}{[Ag_{free}]}$. When the equilibrium constant for the reaction between an antiserum and antigen is analysed using different antigen concentrations however, a non-Gaussian range of K values (affinities) is obtained (Fig. 7.16).

This distribution creates problems in determining the average affinity of an antiserum. This finding is not surprising however, given that even with a simple hapten, antibodies may be raised against different parts of the hapten's structure and possibly to varying parts of the carrier protein surrounding the amino acid to which the hapten is coupled. The binding affinities of the antibodies will depend upon the number and type of secondary bonds formed between antigen and antibody, as discussed earlier in this chapter.

THE STRUCTURE OF ANTIGENS

The number of possible antibodies which may be produced to an antigen is high because antigens are three dimensional structures and present many different configurations to the antibody producing cells. Moreover different antibodies to an antigen often bind to epitopes which overlap on the antigen surface. In this way different antibodies can bind to a particular antigenic region of the molecule, without binding to exactly the same antigenic determinant (epitope).

Although it is possible to produce antibodies to almost any part of an antigen, this does not normally happen in an immune response. It is usually found that certain areas of the antigen are particularly antigenic, and that the majority of antibodies bind to these regions. These regions, which are referred to as the immunodominant regions of the antigen, are often at exposed areas on the outside of the antigen, particularly where there are loops of polypeptide that lack a rigid tertiary structure. In some cases, the immunodominant regions of the antigen correspond to the most mobile surface areas of the molecule. This observation has led immunologists to suspect that the interaction between antibody and antigen is not a rigid fit with perfect complementarity between the shape of the antibody and antigen, but that there is some flexibility, both in the antigen epitope and the hypervariable loops of the antigen, which allows the optimum binding energy to be achieved. This proposal has been amply confirmed by X-ray crystallographic analysis of the complex between Fab and the antigen neuraminidase.

T CELL ANTIGEN RECOGNITION

Although the antigen receptors on T cells and B cells have many structural similarities, antigen recognition by T cells differs from the simple paratope–epitope interaction described above.

Even before T cells and B cells had been differentiated,

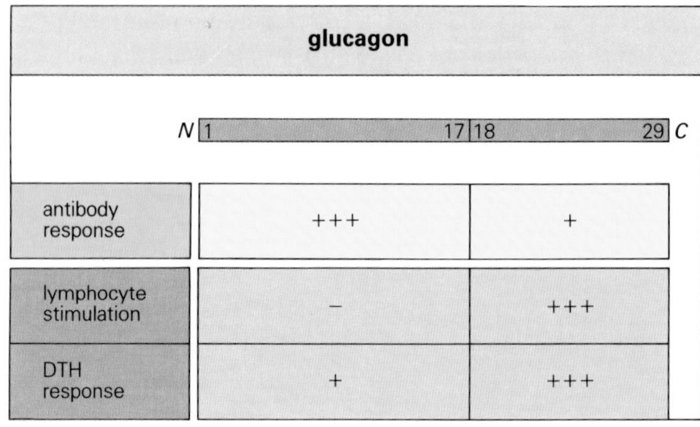

Fig. 7.17 T cell and B cell epitopes are distinct. The immune response to two peptides of the antigen glucagon are shown. Antibody (B cell response) is primarily directed to epitopes at the *N*-terminus, while the *C*-terminal peptide 18–29 stimulates T cell responses – lymphocyte stimulation *in vitro* and the delayed type hypersensitivity (DTH) response *in vivo*.

Fig. 7.18 Antigen recognition by B cells and T cells. Animals were immunized with the hapten 2,4 DNP coupled to mycobacteria (Myc-2,4 DNP). Their T and B cell responses to four related antigens were then assessed. Myc-4 NP and Myc-2,4,6 TNP are recognized by both T and B cells. Myc-2,6 DNP is recognized poorly by T and B cells, indicating the importance of the 4 NP group in recognition. Using a spacer molecule, ala.gly.gly. between the carrier and the 2,4 DNP hapten allows antibody binding but does not stimulate T cells.

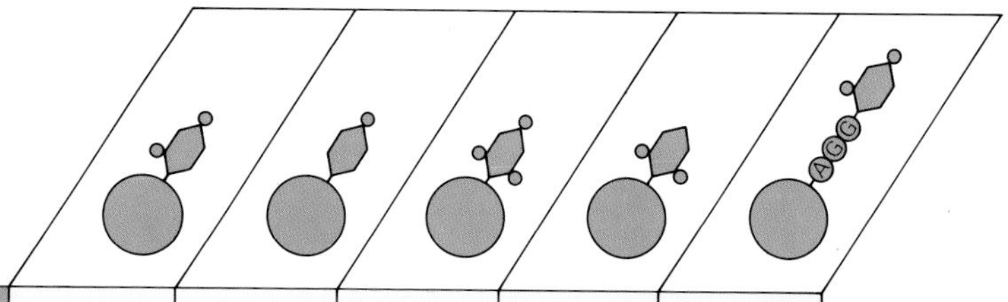

antigen	Myc-2,4DNP	Myc-4NP	Myc-2,4,6TNP	Myc-2,6DNP	Myc-spacer 2,4DNP
T cell response	++++	+++	+++	weak	–
B cell response	+++	+++	+++	weak	++++

Gell and Benacerraf had demonstrated that antibody responses and cell-mediated immune reactions were directed against different determinants on an antigen. When they compared the antibody responses and delayed type hypersensitivity (DTH) to native or denatured protein antigens, they found that DTH could be elicited with either native or denatured antigen, whereas the antibody response was specific for the undenatured immunizing antigen. This finding suggested that the structures seen by antibodies are tertiary, while the cells giving rise to the DTH responses recognize primary sequences. This suggestion has been confirmed by many subsequent studies and it has been shown that T cells and B cells recognize different regions of antigens. For example, mouse B cells recognize an epitope at the *N*-terminus of glucagon, whereas the T cells recognize determinants near the *C*-terminus (Fig. 7.17). In other instances it can be shown that the precise conformation of a particular antigenic determinant will affect its ability to generate T cell or B cell responses (Fig. 7.18).

T CELLS RECOGNIZE PROCESSED ANTIGEN PLUS MHC

T cells do not see free antigen. They recognize it on the surface of other cells, which may be either specialized antigen-presenting cells (APCs), capable of stimulating T cell division, or any virally infected cells within the body, which then become a target for cytotoxic T cells. It can be shown that APCs actually take up the antigens that they will present. For example, if APCs, such as dendritic cells, are pulsed with antigen, they can subsequently stimulate T cell division, even though no free antigen is present. Furthermore the great majority of antigens require some form of internal processing before they can be presented to the T cells in an immunogenic form (Fig. 7.19). If internal degradation of the antigen is blocked, APCs are unable to present the antigen. For example, if macrophages are treated with chloroquine before being pulsed with antigen they are unable to stimulate T cells. If however the chloroquine is added after the antigen pulse, the macrophages have already processed sufficient antigen to present to T cells and induce T cell activation.

In Chapter 4, it was shown that cytotoxic T cells specific for a particular virus, will only recognize that virus on infected cells of their own MHC haplotype. The interaction between the T cells and the targets is said to be genetically restricted; this is a common feature of immune reactions involving T cells. The principle also

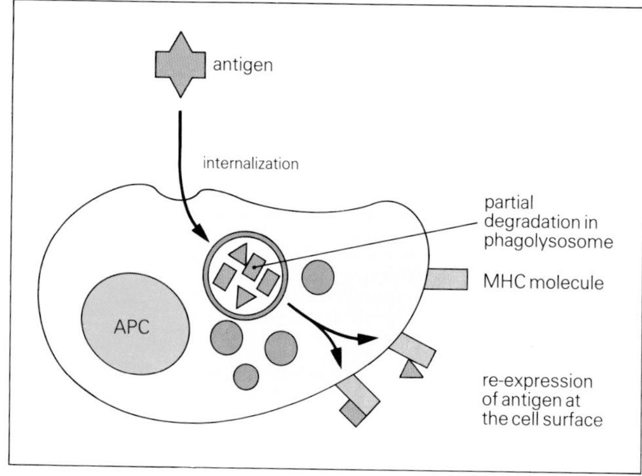

Fig. 7.19 Antigen processing. Antigens are internalized by antigen-presenting cells (APCs) and are then degraded by proteolytic enzymes in the phagolysosomes. Some of the material is only partly degraded and is re-expressed at the cell surface, where it comes to be associated with MHC molecules.

applies to T-helper cells (usually $CD4^+$), which recognize antigen on APCs of their own haplotype. Since antigen recognition by T cells is genetically MHC restricted, this implies that the T cell can in some way recognize both the antigen and the MHC molecules on other cells.

When MHC restriction was first discovered, there were two major theories to explain the observations: either the T cells could separately recognize MHC molecules and antigen on the other cells, or there was a single T cell receptor which recognized an MHC–antigen combination. The evidence now overwhelmingly favours the second theory, that is, the T cell antigen receptor recognizes MHC molecules plus processed antigen.

It appears that the processed antigen is physically associated with the MHC molecules. This has led to models of T cell antigen recognition such as that shown in Fig. 7.20. In these theories, processed antigens interact with MHC molecules and with the T cell antigen receptor via different amino acid residues. The part of the antigen which interacts with MHC molecules is the 'agretope' (Antigen's REcognition -tope); the part which interacts with the T cell antigen receptor is the epitope. In this scheme the part of the MHC molecule which interacts with the antigen is the desetope (DEterminant

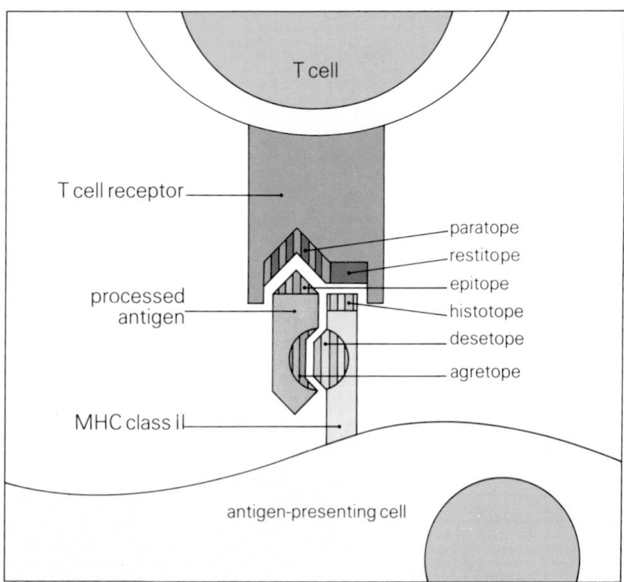

Fig. 7.20 T cell antigen recognition. T cell antigen recognition involves a 3-way interaction involving the T cell receptor, MHC molecule and processed antigen. To facilitate understanding of the interaction, the various interacting parts are named as shown. The antigen's agretope binds to the MHC desetope while its epitope binds to the T cell receptor paratope. The MHC molecule and T cell receptor may also interact separately via their histotope and restitope.

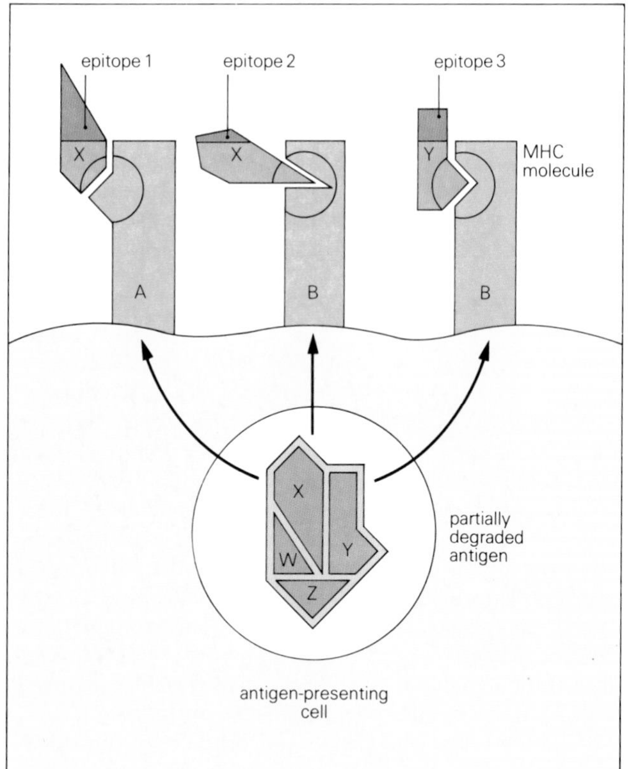

Fig. 7.21 MHC haplotype controls antigen presentation. Fragments W, X, Y and Z are produced by partial proteolysis of an antigen. Fragment X associates with an MHC molecule of haplotype A exposing epitope I. A different MHC molecule (B) binds to a different agretope on X thus exposing a different epitope. Alternatively, haplotype B may bind preferentially to a different fragment Y, again presenting a different epitope to that presented by A.

SElection -tope), and the part which interacts with the T cell antigen receptor is the histotope. This nomenclature provides a convenient way of describing the types of interaction which may be involved in T cell antigen/MHC recognition, but it is not certain how the tripartite interaction takes place. For example, the antigen, T cell receptor and MHC molecule may each interact with the others, or the MHC molecule may link to the antigen in such a way that a particular set of amino acids are available for recognition by the T cell antigen receptor. In both cases, parts of the antigen interact with both the T cell antigen receptor and the MHC molecule. Whichever of these mechanisms is correct, it is easy to see how the interaction is genetically restricted. MHC molecules of different haplotypes will have different desetopes. Consequently they will bind to different agretopes on the antigen, and this will result in different epitopes becoming exposed to the T cell antigen receptor in animals of different MHC haplotype (Fig. 7.21). It has been possible to demonstrate that immunogenic peptides of antigens such as lysozyme associate directly with MHC class II molecules on the cell surface, which confirms the validity of the model outlined above.

Another consequence of MHC restriction is that different portions of an antigen may be immunogenic for T cells in animals of different MHC haplotype. An example of this is the immune response elicited by the molecule, myelin basic protein, in mice or rats of different H-2 haplotype (Fig. 7.22). Even within a single MHC haplotype there are usually several different class I and class II gene loci. Each MHC molecule will probably interact with antigen in a slightly different way, and some MHC molecules will interact more effectively than others. This means that an individual's MHC molecules determine the part of an antigen which the T cells can recognize, and hence the nature and strength of that individual's immune response to the antigen. The ways in which MHC molecules determine the ability to mount an immune response is discussed further in Chapter 11.

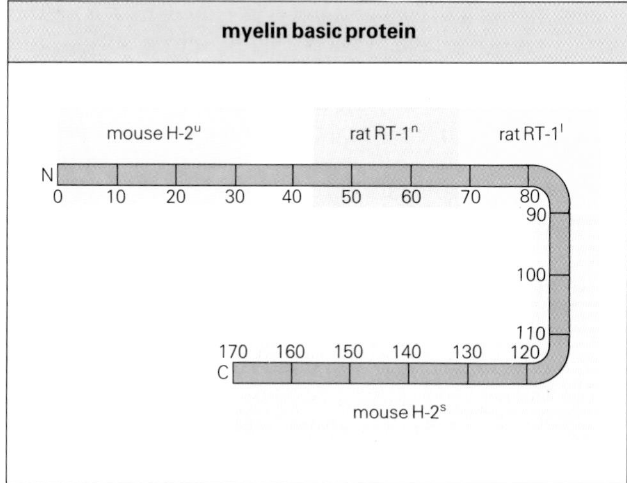

Fig. 7.22 T cell response to antigen peptides. The T cell response in rats and mice to myelin basic protein is illustrated. Mice of haplotype H-2^u respond to determinants at the *N*-terminus (0–32), while SJL mice (H-2^s) respond to a determinant in the peptide 90–170. Lewis rats (RT-1^l) respond to peptide 68–88, while Brown Norway (RT-1^n) respond strongly to 43–88, less strongly to 43–67 and not at all to 68–88, indicating a determinant in 43–67. (RT-1 is the rat MHC).

ANTIGENIC STRUCTURES RECOGNIZED BY T CELLS

In considering which amino acids of an antigen interact with T cells, one useful technique has been to prepare immunogenic peptides from protein antigens, which can stimulate T cells when presented on appropriate APCs. Different amino acids are then substituted in the peptides, which are then tested for immunogenicity. Failure of the modified peptide to stimulate peptide-specific T cells when correctly presented implies that the substituted residues were essential for either the MHC–antigen interaction, or the T cell receptor antigen interaction. This technique can be taken further using peptides which bind to MHC molecules. It is possible to substitute amino acids on these peptides, so that they no longer bind to the MHC molecule; thus the amino acids involved in binding to the MHC molecule and those binding to the T cell receptor can be differentiated.

An analysis of binding residues on the immunogenic peptide 52–61 of lysozyme suggests that this adopts an α-helical configuration, with three amino acid residues contacting the MHC molecule and three other residues contacting the T cell antigen receptor (Fig. 7.23). In some cases, the residues of immunogenic peptides appear to adopt a β-sheet structure with adjoining residues contacting the MHC molecule or T cell receptor.

In several instances the immunogenic portions of proteins coincide with amphipathic regions of the molecule, that is regions where there is a mixture of hydrophilic and hydrophobic residues. This can be seen in peptide 132–146 of myoglobin, where the T cell receptor contacting residues are hydrophilic and are ranged on one side of the α-helix, while the class II contacting residues are hydrophobic and lie on the opposite side (Fig. 7.24). Several proteins have been examined to correlate amphipathicity with immunogenic regions. In one study 18 out of 23 amphipathic regions overlapped with immunogenic peptides, suggesting that amphipathic regions are good T cell stimulators (Fig. 7.25).

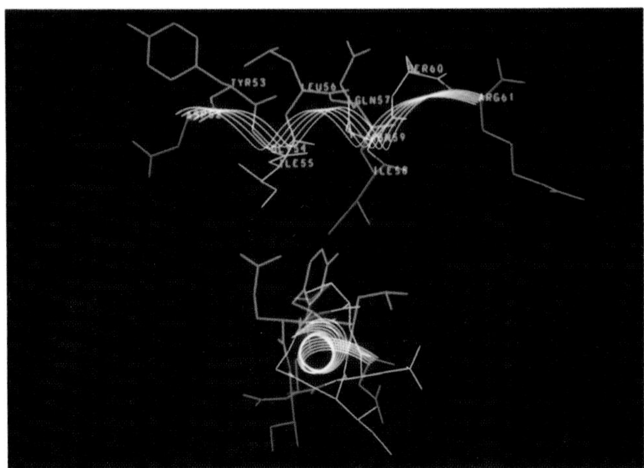

Fig. 7.23 T cell receptor and class II contact residues. Peptide 52–61 of hen egg-white lysozyme modelled in an α-helix viewed from the side (above) and end (below) with the *N*-terminus to the left (T cell receptor contact residues in red, class II contact residues in blue, other residues in yellow. The α-helix is shown as a white ribbon). Residues of the epitope tend to occur on one side of the antigen and of the agretope on the other. (Courtesy of Professor P.M. Allen; reprinted by permission from *Nature*, **327**, 714. © Copyright 1987 Macmillan Magazines Ltd.)

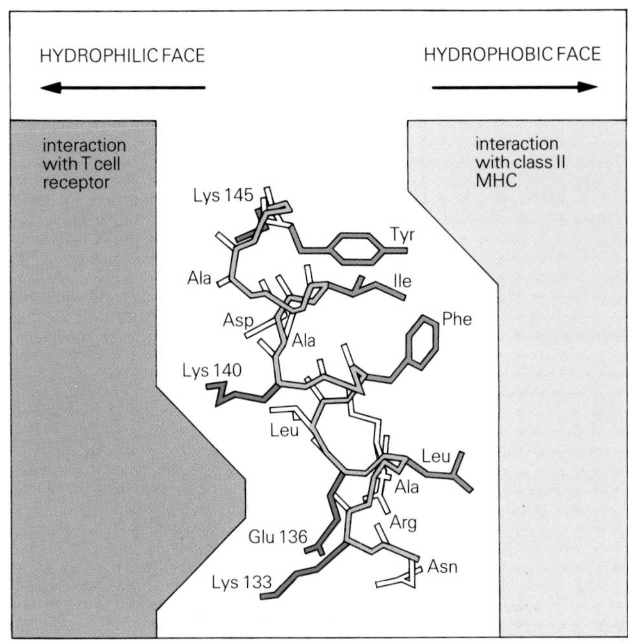

Fig. 7.24 Amphipathic T cell epitope of myoglobin. Peptide 132–146 of myoglobin is shown in α-helical configuration. The helix (blue) presents hydrophilic residues (red) on one face, which are known to be required to interact with the T cell receptor, while a group of hydrophobic residues (purple) are expressed on the opposite face. (Structure based on data of Berkower.)

	known T cell stimulating peptide	amphipathic regions (AMPHI program)
myoglobin	69–78 102–118 132–145	64–78 99–117 128–145
flu haemagg.	109–119 130–140 302–313	97–120 – 291–314
hepatitis B surface Ag	38–52 95–109 140–154	36–49 – –
hepatitis B pre s	120–132	121–135
FMDV VPI	141–160	148–165
rabies spike precursor	32–44	29–46

* 6 other proteins also studied in this way: 18 of 23 known sites predicted

Fig. 7.25 Correlation of T cell sites with amphipathic regions. The table compares known T cell stimulating peptides with regions of amphipathicity within the protein antigen predicted by a computer programme. Although T cell stimulating peptides frequently coincide with amphipathic areas this is not always so and other regions may also be immunogenic. (Data of Margalit *et al* 1987.)

ROLE OF CD2, CD4, CD8 AND LFA-1

Antigen recognition by T cells is MHC restricted, but not all T cells recognize the same MHC products. In general, most helper T cells express the CD4 surface marker and recognize antigen in association with class II MHC molecules, while most cytotoxic cells express CD8 on their surface and recognize antigen in association with class I molecules. This delineation is not absolute however, since there are cytotoxic cells which express CD4 and recognize antigen with class II. Cells which recognize antigen plus class I are said to be class I restricted, while cells recognizing antigen plus class II are class II restricted.

There are many ways in which class I and II restriction can be demonstrated. For example, class I restricted cytotoxic T cells which recognize virus A on haplotype H-2^k target cells will not recognize the virus on H-2^d targets, nor will they recognize infected target cells from a recombinant strain which has class II molecules of H-2^k haplotype and class I molecules of H-2^d haplotype. In other words, the T cells only recognize antigen associated with class I molecules of the correct haplotype.

Class I and class II restriction makes sense from an evolutionary viewpoint. Cytotoxic cells, which are required to destroy virally infected targets in any tissue, recognize antigen plus class I molecules, which are expressed on all nucleated cells. Class II restricted helper cells, which regulate and amplify the immune response, recognize antigen plus the class II molecules, which are present on antigen-presenting cells and B cells. There is a very strong correlation between:

1. class II restriction and CD4 expression
2. class I restriction and CD8 expression.

Moreover class I restricted cytotoxic reactions can be blocked with either anti-class I antibody or anti-CD8, while class II restricted reactions can be blocked with either anti-class II or anti-CD4. This has led to the suggestion that CD4 interacts with class II molecules, and CD8 with class I molecules. In this hypothesis, CD4 and CD8 would interact with invariant framework portions of MHC molecules, while the T cell antigen receptor would recognize the antigen associated with a polymorphic part of the MHC molecule (Fig. 7.26).

Recent studies have shown that the CD4 molecule does indeed have a weak affinity for MHC class II molecules. These observations support the idea that antigen recognition by T cells involves the formation of a complex of the T cell antigen receptor and CD4 or CD8 on the T cell which recognizes antigen plus MHC on another cell. In this scheme, the normally weak interactions involving the CD4 and CD8 molecules would help to stabilize the specific immune recognition reaction.

There are a number of other molecules which are involved in antigen non-specific interactions. These include the receptors which interact with endothelium and control lymphocyte homing to different tissues, as well as the lymphocyte function antigens LFA-1, LFA-2 and LFA-3 (Fig. 7.27). These were originally described as molecules involved in cell adhesion, cooperation, and some cytotoxic interactions. LFA-1 and LFA-2 are present on lymphocytes, whereas LFA-3 is more widely distributed. LFA-2, now known to be CD2, interacts with LFA-3 on other cells. The ligand for LFA-1 is an intercellular adhesion molecule termed ICAM-1. The relationship of these adhesion molecules to the T cell receptor, CD4 and CD8 is still under investigation.

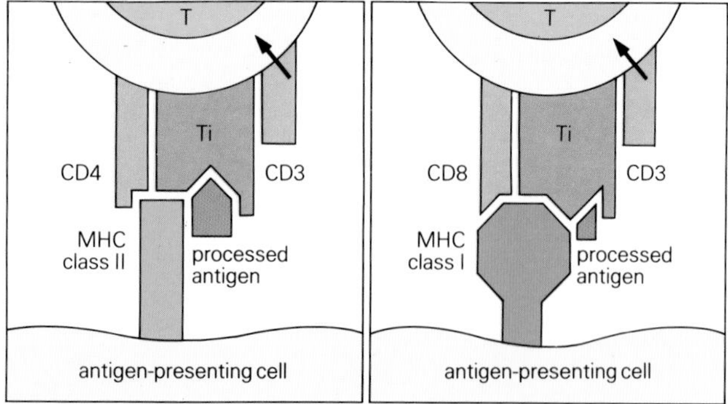

Fig. 7.26 Role of CD4 and CD8. CD4 present on class II restricted cells, interacts with class II molecules on other cells and with the T cell receptor complex. This has led to the proposal that T cell recognition is stabilized by interactions between CD4 and class II molecules, or CD8 and class I.

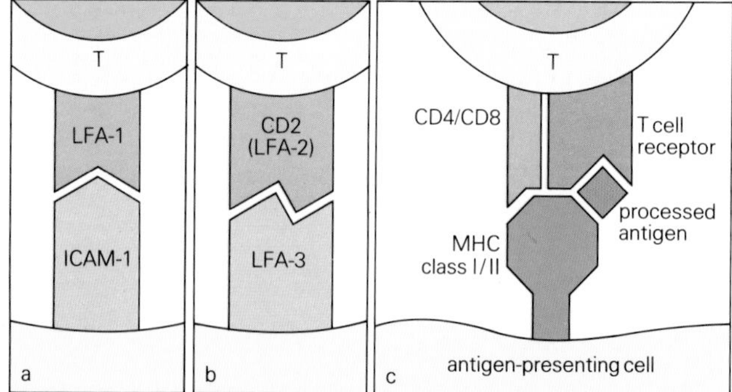

Fig. 7.27 Structures in T cell interactions. The diagram summarizes the molecules involved in T cell-mediated interactions. One ligand for LFA-1 is ICAM-1 which is widely distributed on non-haemopoietic cells. LFA-3 is also widely distributed on haemopoietic and non-haemopoietic tissue.

FURTHER READING

Day, E. D. (1972) *Advanced Immunochemistry*. Baltimore: Williams & Wilkins.

Karush, F. (1962) Immunologic specifity and molecular structure. *Advances in Immunology*, **2**, 1–40.

Steward, M. W. (1983) *Antibodies: their structure and function*. London: Chapman and Hall.

Steward, M. W. & Steensgaard, J. (1983) *Antibody affinity: Thermodynamic aspects and biological significance*. Boca Raton, Florida: C. R. C. Press.

Weir, D. M. (ed.) (1986) *Handbook of Experimental Immunology*, Vol.I. 4th edition. Oxford: Blackwell Scientific Publications.

8 Cell Cooperation in the Antibody Response

When an individual first encounters an antigen the cells of the immune system recognize the antigen and either produce an immune reaction to it or become tolerant to it depending on the circumstances. The immune reaction can take the form of cell-mediated immunity or may involve the production of antibodies directed towards the antigen, the type of reaction depending on the way in which the antigen is presented to the lymphocytes: many immune reactions display both kinds of response. On second and subsequent encounters with the antigen the type of response is largely determined by the outcome of the first antigenic challenge, but the quantity and the quality of the response are different.

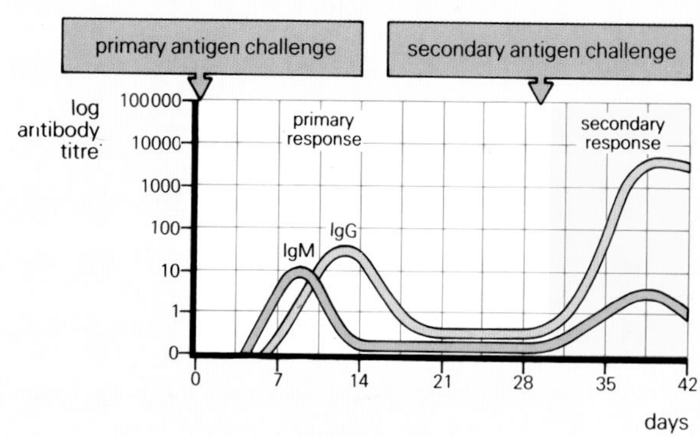

Fig. 8.2 Primary and secondary antibody responses. In comparison with the antibody response following primary antigenic challenge, the antibody level following secondary antigenic challenge in a typical immune response:
1. appears more quickly and persists for longer
2. attains a higher titre
3. consists predominantly of IgG.
In the primary response the appearance of IgG is preceded by IgM.

PRIMARY AND SECONDARY ANTIBODY RESPONSES

Following primary antigenic challenge with an antigen such as sheep erythrocytes injected into a mouse there is an initial lag phase when no antibody can be detected. This is followed by phases in which the antibody titre rises logarithmically to a plateau and then declines again as the antibodies are naturally catabolized or bind to the antigen and are cleared from the circulation (Fig. 8.1). Examination of the responses following primary and secondary antigenic challenge shows that the responses differ in four major respects.

1. Time course. The secondary response has a shorter lag phase and an extended plateau and decline.

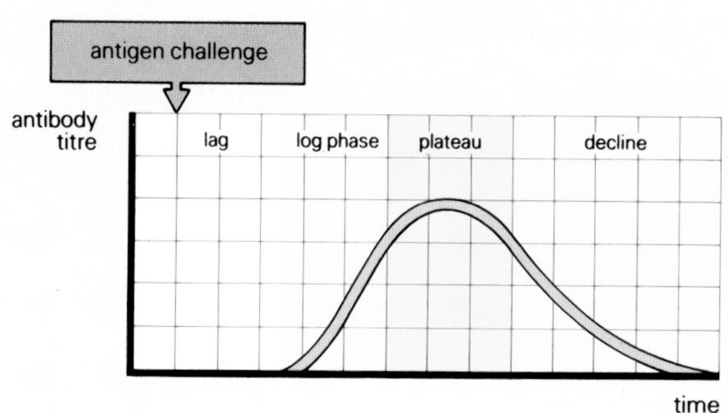

Fig. 8.1 The four phases of a primary antibody response. Following antigen challenge the antibody response proceeds in four phases:
1. a lag phase when no antibody is detected
2. a log phase when the antibody titre rises logarithmically
3. a plateau phase during which the antibody titre stabilizes
4. a decline phase during which the antibody is cleared or catabolized.
The actual time course and titres reached will depend on the nature of the antigenic challenge and the responder.

2. Antibody titre. The plateau levels of antibody are much greater in the secondary response, typically 10-fold or more than plateau levels in the primary response.
3. Antibody class. IgM antibodies form a major proportion of the primary response, whereas the secondary response consists almost entirely of IgG.
4. Antibody affinity. The affinity of the antibodies in the secondary response is usually much greater. This is referred to as 'affinity maturation'.

The characteristics of primary and secondary antibody responses are compared in Fig. 8.2.

It is possible to detect antibody-forming cells in the spleen following antigen challenge, using plaque forming cell assays (see Chapter 25). Studies show that the appearance of antibody-forming cells in the spleen precedes the rises in serum antibody titres by about 1 day (Fig. 8.3).

IMMUNOLOGICAL MEMORY

The second and subsequent responses to an antigen are different in both nature and magnitude from the primary response. The capacity to mount a secondary response is based on 'immunological memory' and is the rationale behind the process of vaccination.

The cellular basis of memory is the expansion of populations of antigen-specific lymphocytes during the primary response, so that there is an increased frequency of B and T cells capable of responding to that antigen. Memory B cells differ qualitatively from unprimed B cells, as they are prone to make IgG earlier and they

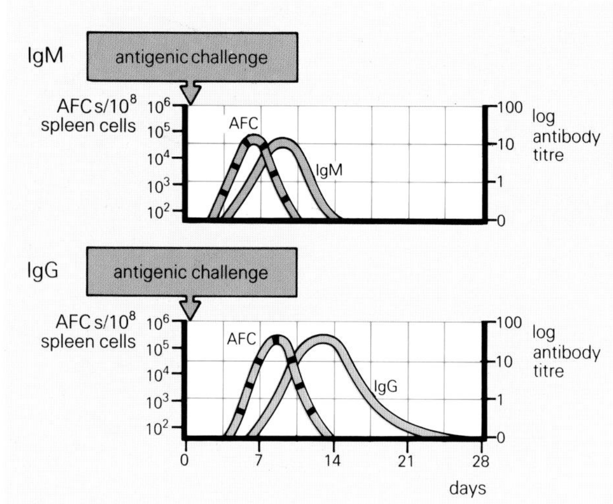

Fig. 8.3 The kinetics of IgM and IgG antibody production. Specific serum antibody concentration is compared with the number of specific antibody-forming cells (AFCS)/10^8 spleen cells in mice following antigenic challenge. The rise in serum antibody levels occurs approximately 1 day after the rise in AFCs. IgM-producing cells appear before those producing IgG.

usually have higher affinity antigen receptors, due to selection during the primary response. It is not known whether memory T cells have higher affinity receptors than unprimed T cells, as methods for measuring the affinity of T cell receptors are not available, but memory T cells can respond to lower doses of antigen, implying that their receptors are more efficient.

HAPTENS AND CARRIERS

To obtain the optimum secondary response to an antigenic determinant, for example a hapten, which is not immunogenic by itself, it is usually necessary to immunize the animal with the same antigen in both the primary and the secondary challenge. It is not sufficient that the antigens share a common antigenic determinant recognized by the B cells; the determinant must also be attached to the same carrier molecule. This is referred to as the carrier effect. A carrier is a molecule which renders a hapten linked to it able to stimulate antibody production. The carrier effect implies that the cells involved in making the antibody response recognize at least two parts of the antigen (Fig. 8.4).

The requirement for priming lymphocytes to the carrier can be circumvented in the response to a hapten–carrier conjugate if the animal has been previously primed to the carrier alone, or receives spleen cells from a donor primed to that carrier (Fig. 8.5). Furthermore, it may be demonstrated, by removing T cells from the carrier-primed donor spleen cells, that the T cells are responsible for recognizing carrier determinants on the antigen and delivering help to the B cells which recognize the hapten (Fig. 8.6). In these two experiments, antigen-primed cells are injected into X-irradiated recipient mice to determine their immunological activity – the X-irradiated mice act in this instance as 'living test tubes'. A more detailed analysis of the T cells responsible for this helper effect in the mouse shows that they are $CD4^+$, $CD8^-$ T-helper cells.

These results have led to the basic scheme for cell interactions in the antibody response set out in Fig. 8.7. It is proposed that antigen entering the body is processed by antigen-presenting cells which present the antigen in a highly immunogenic form to the T-helper cells and B cells. The T cells recognize separate determinants on the antigen to those recognized by the B cells, but

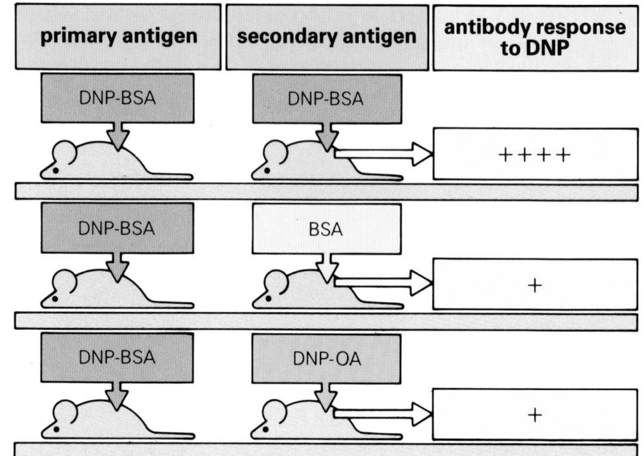

Fig. 8.4 The carrier effect. Three groups of mice were immunized (primary antigen) with dinitrophenylated bovine serum albumin (DNP-BSA) and rechallenged (secondary antigen) with either DNP-BSA, BSA, or dinitrophenylated ovalbumin (DNP-OA). The antibody response to the DNP hapten was then measured. The optimal antibody response to DNP was obtained with animals immunized twice with the same antigen. The BSA acts as a specific carrier for the antibody response to DNP.

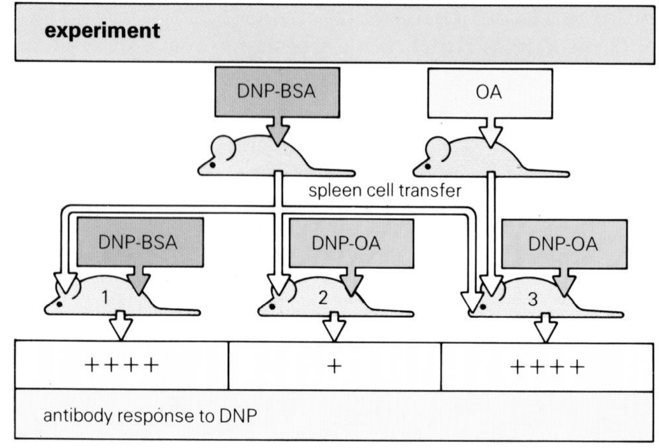

Fig. 8.5 Carrier priming. Three groups of X-irradiated mice were reconstituted with antigen-primed spleen cells and challenged with antigen. Group 1 received DNP-BSA primed cells and when challenged with DNP-BSA produced a strong antibody response to DNP. Group 2 received DNP-BSA primed cells and were challenged with DNP-OA. This group produced a weak antibody response, demonstrating the carrier effect. Group 3 received cells primed to both DNP-BSA and to OA: they were then challenged with DNP-OA. This group made a strong response to DNP, demonstrating that the requirement for carrier priming can be circumvented by supplying carrier-primed spleen cells.

they deliver help to the appropriate B cells which are stimulated to differentiate and divide into antibody-forming cells. This has led to the concept that two types of signal are required to activate a B cell:

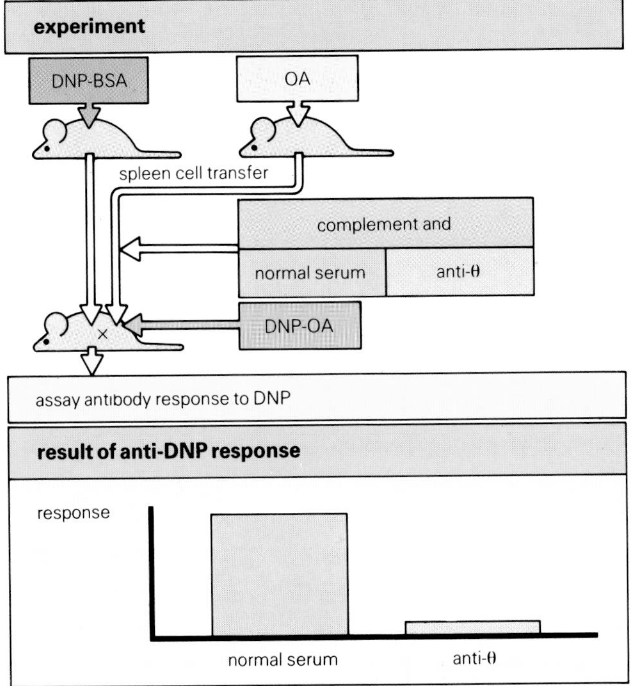

Fig. 8.6 T cell recognition of carrier (OA). An X-irradiated mouse, if reconstituted with spleen cells primed to the OA carrier and to DNP-BSA will, on subsequent challenge with DNP-OA produce a normal antibody response to DNP. This response is unaffected if the OA-primed cells are previously treated with normal serum and complement. However, if the OA-primed cells are treated with anti-T cell serum (anti-θ) and complement, which destroys T cells, the anti-DNP response is abrogated. This indicates that T cells recognize the carrier and give help to the hapten-primed B cells.

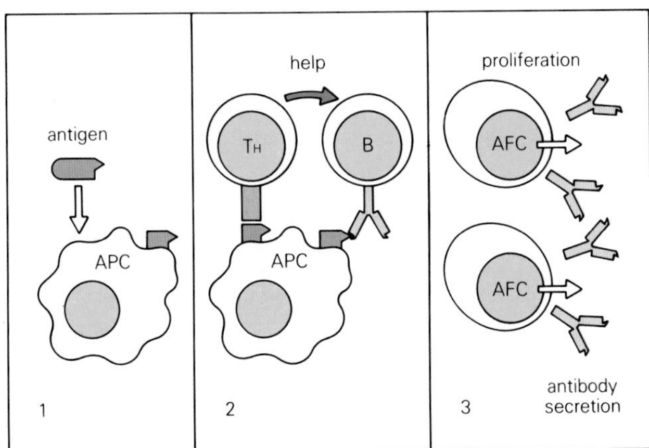

Fig. 8.7 Simplified overview of the immune response.
1. Antigen encountering the immune system is processed by antigen-presenting cells (APCs) which retain fragments of the antigen on their surfaces.
2. T-helper cells (T_H) recognize the antigen via their surface receptors and provide help to B cells (B) which also recognize antigen by their surface receptors (immunoglobulin).
3. The B cells are stimulated to proliferate and divide into antibody-forming cells (AFCs) which secrete antibody.

1. antigen interacting with B cell immunoglobulin receptors
2. a second signal(s) from T-helper cells. (A variety of T cell stimuli are needed for optimal growth and differentiation of B cells.)

T-DEPENDENT AND T-INDEPENDENT ANTIGENS

According to the evidence presented so far the response to an antigen depends on both T cells and B cells recognizing that antigen. This type of antigen is called T-dependent (T-dep). There are, however, a small number of antigens capable of activating B cells independently of T cell help, referred to as T-independent antigens (T-ind). T-ind antigens share a number of common properties (Fig. 8.8); in particular they are all large polymeric molecules with repeating antigenic determinants, and many possess the ability, at high concentrations, to activate B cell clones other than those specific for that antigen, that is, polyclonal B cell activation. At a lower concentration they activate only B cells with specific antigen receptors for them. Many T-ind antigens are particularly resistant to degradation. Primary antibody responses to

antigen	polymeric	polyclonal activation	resistance to degradation
lipopolysaccharide (LPS)	+	+++	+
Ficoll	+++	–	+++
dextran	++	+	++
levan	++	+	++
poly-D amino acids	+++	–	+++
polymeric bacterial flagellin	++	++	+

Fig. 8.8 T-independent antigens. The major common properties of some of the main T-independent (T-ind) antigens are listed. (Note: both poly *L*-amino acids and monomeric bacterial flagellin are T-dependent (T-dep) antigens.)

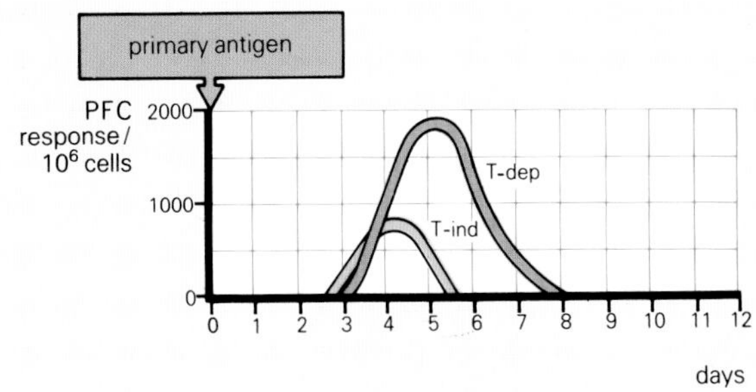

Fig. 8.9 Comparison of primary immune responses to T-dependent and T-independent antigens *in vitro*. The primary response as assessed by plaque forming cell (PFC) assay, to a T-dependent (T-dep) antigen and a T-independent (T-ind) antigen is shown. The response to T-ind antigens is weaker than to T-dep antigens and peaks earlier.

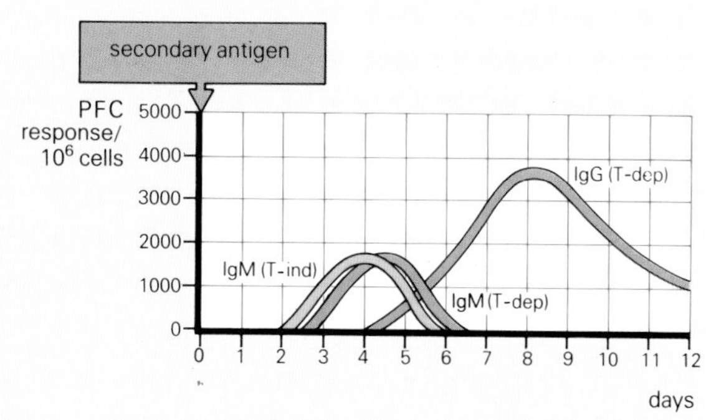

Fig. 8.10 Comparison of the secondary immune responses to T-dependent and T-independent antigens *in vitro*. The IgM plaque forming cell (PFC) response is similar for T-dependent (T-dep) and T-independent (T-ind) antigens but only T-dep antigens produce an IgG PFC response.

T-ind antigens in *vitro* are generally weaker than those to T-dep antigens and peak fractionally earlier (Fig. 8.9).

The secondary response in *vitro* also differs between T-dep and T-ind antigens. The secondary response to T-ind antigens resembles the primary response, by being weak and almost entirely confined to IgM production, whereas the secondary response to T-dep antigens is far stronger and appears earlier (Fig. 8.10). It appears therefore that T-ind antigens do not usually induce the maturation of a response involving class switching to IgG and increase in affinity which is seen with T-dep antigens. Memory induction is also relatively poor. The mechanism by which T-ind antigens trigger B cells without requiring T-helper cells will be discussed later in this chapter.

DEVELOPMENT OF THE ANTIBODY RESPONSE

AFFINITY MATURATION

It has been noted that the antibodies produced in a secondary response to a T-dependent antigen have higher average affinity than those produced in the primary response. This is associated with the switch from IgM to IgG production, since there is no maturation in the affinity of the IgM response. Moreover, the degree of affinity maturation is dependent on the antigen dose administered. High antigen doses produce poor maturation and a lower affinity response than low antigen doses (Fig. 8.11). A plausible hypothesis to account for this observation is as follows: in the presence of low antigen concentrations only B cells with high affinity receptors bind sufficient antigen and are triggered to divide and differentiate. However, in the presence of high antigen concentrations there is sufficient to bind and trigger both high and low affinity B cells (Fig. 8.12).

Although individual B cells do not change their overall specificity, the affinity of the antibody produced by a clone may be altered as a result of somatic hypermutation acting on the recombined antibody genes as mentioned above. It appears then, that two processes are involved in affinity maturation.

1. The generation of higher affinity clones of B cells by slight alterations in the antibody structure which occur late in the primary response to a T-dependent antigen.
2. The selective expansion of high affinity clones driven by antigen.

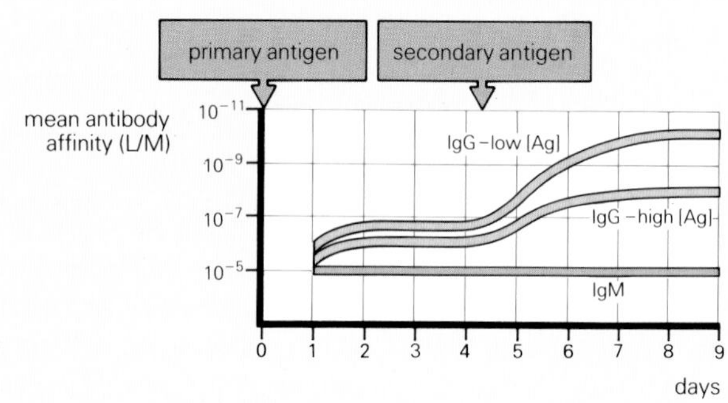

Fig. 8.11 Affinity maturation. The average affinity of the IgM and IgG antibody responses following primary and secondary challenge with a T-dependent antigen are shown. The affinity of the IgM response is constant throughout. The affinity maturation of the IgG response depends on the dose of the antigen. Low antigen doses (low [Ag]) produce higher affinity immunoglobulin than high antigen doses (high [Ag]).

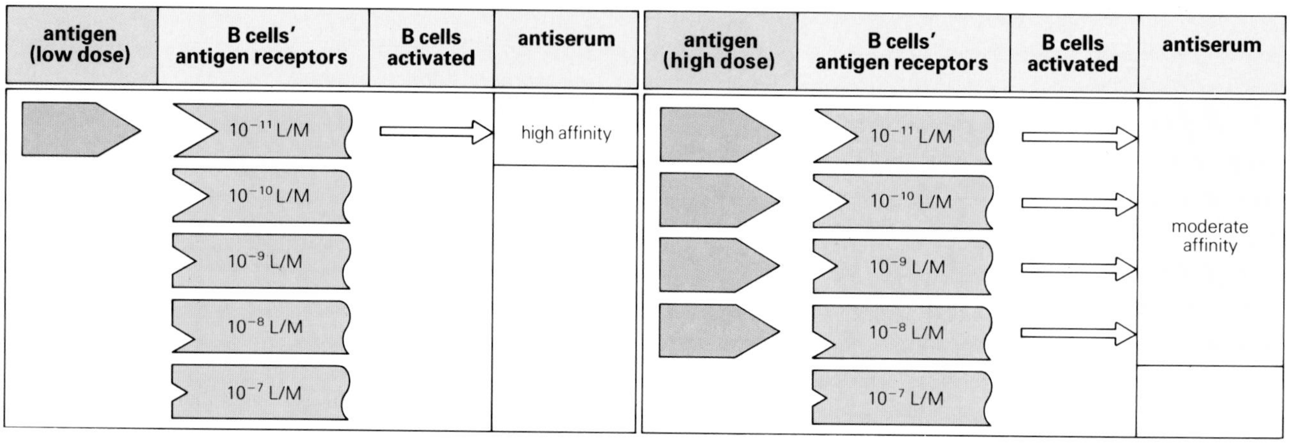

antigen (low dose)	B cells' antigen receptors	B cells activated	antiserum
▶	10^{-11} L/M	⇨	high affinity
	10^{-10} L/M		
	10^{-9} L/M		
	10^{-8} L/M		
	10^{-7} L/M		

antigen (high dose)	B cells' antigen receptors	B cells activated	antiserum
▶	10^{-11} L/M	⇨	moderate affinity
▶	10^{-10} L/M	⇨	
▶	10^{-9} L/M	⇨	
▶	10^{-8} L/M	⇨	
	10^{-7} L/M		

Fig. 8.12 Postulated mechanism of affinity maturation. Low antigen doses (left) bind to, and trigger only those B cells with high affinity receptors, whereas high antigen doses (right) allow triggering of more B cell clones and therefore produce antibody responses with lower average affinity.

ISOTYPE SWITCHING

During a T-dependent immune response there is a progressive switch in the predominant immunoglobulin class of the specific antibody produced. This is in contrast to T-independent responses when the predominant immunoglobulin usually remains IgM.

Isotype switching from IgM to IgG is not a random event. The IgG subclasses produced depend on the stimulus. Thus in the mouse, complete Freund's Adjuvant yields predominantly IgG2 antibodies, whereas alum-precipitated protein antigens result in a predominantly IgG1 response. Switching to IgA or IgE also occurs and cells producing these isotypes are concentrated in the appropriate mucosal areas.

Evidence has accumulated which explains the molecular mechanisms, of isotype switching (see Chapter 6), and although there is universal agreement that T cells are important in controlling this phenomenon, the signals which control the switch are less well understood. Interleukin-4 (IL-4), formerly known as B cell stimulatory factor 1, is a T cell derived protein important in the production of IgG1 and IgE. Interleukin-5 (IL-5), formerly known as T cell replacing factor, is important in the switch to IgA production, and interferon-γ (IFNγ) favours the production of IgG2a in mice.

MUTATION AND PROGRESSION OF THE IMMUNE RESPONSE

Somatic hypermutation is a common event in antibody-producing B cells during T-dependent responses which selectively affects the immunoglobulin genes, and is important in the generation of high affinity antibody-forming cell precursors. In this context it is a normal and beneficial event. However, certain mutations can yield high affinity IgG autoantibodies, such as anti-DNA, and may be highly deleterious. This type of mutation has been demonstrated experimentally in long term tissue culture, but its role in the development of common autoimmune diseases is not known. It has been demonstrated in mouse anti-DNA hybridomas.

ANTIGEN PRESENTATION

The preceding section has described the course of events in the development of an antibody response and the evidence that both B and T cells are normally required for responses to T-dependent antigens. These constitute the majority of the antigens encountering the immune system. One of the crucial stages in the development of the immune response has been mentioned only briefly – the way in which antigen encountering the immune system is presented to the lymphocytes which react to it. *In vivo* this phase is complicated by the structural organization of the lymphoid tissue. Thus antigen from the periphery moves via the lymphatics to the local lymph nodes. The antigen may be carried free in solution or on the surface of the antigen-presenting cells (APCs). On reaching the lymph node, different antigens move selectively to different areas and are thus capable of stimulating different populations of lymphocytes. Some antigens remain within the lymph node for long periods providing a constant source of antigenic stimulation; others are fairly rapidly degraded or lost via efferent lymphatics (Figs 8.13 and 8.14).

area	antigen-presenting cells	antigen	persistence
subcapsular (marginal) sinus	marginal zone macrophages	polysaccharides Ficoll (T-ind)	++++
follicles and B cell areas	follicular dendritic cells	antigen/antibody complement fixing complexes	+++
medulla	classical macrophages	most antigens	+
T cell areas	interdigitating dendritic cells	most antigens	++

Fig. 8.13 Localization of antigen in lymph nodes. A lymph node represented schematically (above, left) shows afferent and efferent lymphatics, follicles, the outer cortical B cell area and the paracortical T cell area. Different antigen-presenting cells predominate in these areas (though the demarcation is not absolute) and selectively take up different types of antigen which then persist on the surface of the cells for variable periods. Thus antigen–antibody complexes are preferentially taken up by follicular dendritic cells via their C3 and Fc receptors and may persist for months or years, whereas antigens on recirculating (classical) macrophages in the medulla may last for only a few days or weeks. Note that recirculating 'veiled' cells (Langerhans' cells), which are thought to arise from the skin, change their morphology to become interdigitating dendritic cells within the lymph node. Both these cells and the follicular dendritic cells have long processes which are in intimate contact with lymphocytes. The persistence of the different antigens varies between species.

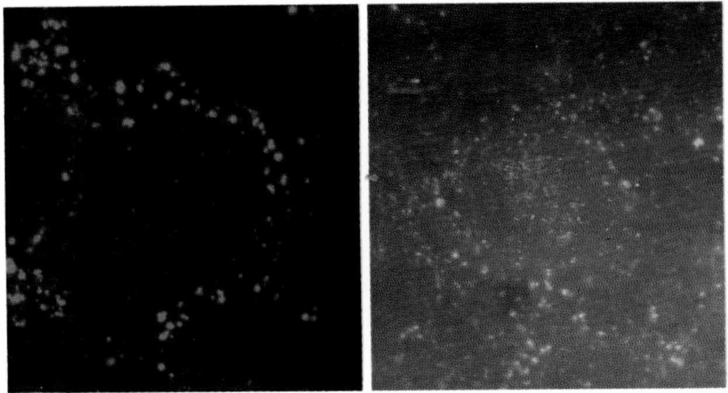

Fig. 8.14 Localization of antigen in the spleen. T-independent antigens (here TRITC-Ficoll) preferentially locate on the marginal zone macrophages (red, left), while T-dependent antigens (FITC antigen – antibody complexes) locate on the follicular dendritic cells (green, right). (Courtesy of Professor J. Humphrey.)

As T cells recognize antigen fragments in association with MHC molecules on the surface of other cells, it follows that antigen presentation to T cells is MHC restricted (see Chapters 4 and 7). Although all cells express class I MHC molecules, class II expression is confined to APCs. These cells are potentially capable of presenting antigen to the class II restricted T-helper cells which control the development of an immune response. Thus the expression of class II MHC molecules is the key to antigen presentation. Some cells constitutively express MHC class II and may be thought of as professional or constitutive APCs, but many cell types can be induced to express class II and present antigen if suitably stimulated; these are referred to as facultative APCs. The relative importance of these different types of APC depends on whether a primary or a secondary immune response is involved, and on the location of the response.

There is a large number of different APCs in the body (Fig. 8.15); the best studied are macrophages, interdigitating dendritic cells and follicular dendritic cells. These are the classical APCs of the lymphoid organs. However, their importance in antigen presentation may at times be less than that of B cells, which are able to bind antigen efficiently and present it to T cells. The relative importance of B cells in antigen presentation is highest with primed and activated B cells in secondary antibody responses. In primary responses, the B cell receptors are of lower affinity and are therefore not as efficient at capturing antigen. There is also a range of APCs in non-lymphoid tissues. In the skin at the junction of the epidermis and dermis, there is a continuous sheet of Langerhans' cells, which are of vital importance in maintaining the integrity of the body, as the skin is a common route of infection. In other organs, there are both macrophages, sometimes in large numbers, for example Kupffer cells lining the liver sinusoids, and dendritic type cells, which are found in virtually all tissues except brain parenchyma. In pathological states, other cells may also function as APCs, for example, thyroid follicular cells may present antigen in autoimmune thyroiditis.

The essential feature of these different APCs is that they can take up antigen, either specifically, or non-specifically, and present it in an MHC class II restricted fashion to T-helper cells (Fig. 8.16). Since the T cell antigen receptor recognizes processed antigen (see Chapter 7), APCs must partly degrade the antigens before they become associated with the MHC molecules.

ANTIGEN PROCESSING

APCs perform a number of closely linked functions, which result in the activation of T lymphocytes, including antigen processing, during which large antigen moieties, cells or proteins are degraded to fragments more recognizable by T cells. These fragments are peptides which associate with either class I or class II MHC molecules. Exactly how antigen processing takes place, where in the cell it occurs and which enzymes are involved, is not known in detail. Phagocytosis is not essential, as non-phagocytic cells, such as the interdigitating dendritic cells can process antigens as large as red blood cells or *Mycobacteria*. Thus it is possible that processing may take place in a number of sites at the cell surface, or following pinocytosis or phagocytosis in endosomes or phagolysosomes. It is critical that processing does not proceed to completion and yield amino acids, as the optimal size of peptides for antigen presentation is

	phagocytosis	type	location	class II expression
phagocytes (monocyte/macrophage lineage)	+	monocytes	blood	(+) → + + + inducible
		macrophages	tissues	
		marginal zone macrophages	spleen and lymph node	
		Kupffer cells	liver	
		microglia	brain	
non-phagocytic constitutive antigen-presenting cells	–	Langerhans' cells	skin	+ + constitutive
		interdigitating dendritic cells	lymphoid tissue	
		follicular dendritic cells	lymphoid tissue	–
lymphocytes	–	B cells and T cells	lymphoid tissues and at sites of immune reactions	– → + + inducible
facultative antigen-presenting cells	+	astrocytes	brain	– → + + inducible
	–	follicular cells	thyroid	
		endothelium	vascular and lymphoid tissue	
		fibroblasts	connective tissue	
		other types in appropriate tissue		

Fig. 8.15 Antigen-presenting cells.

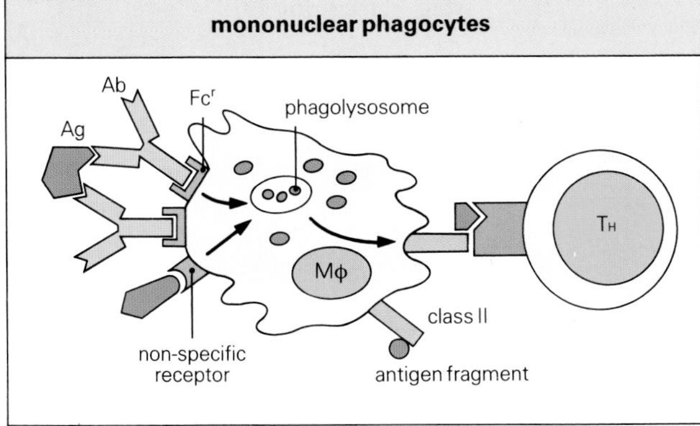

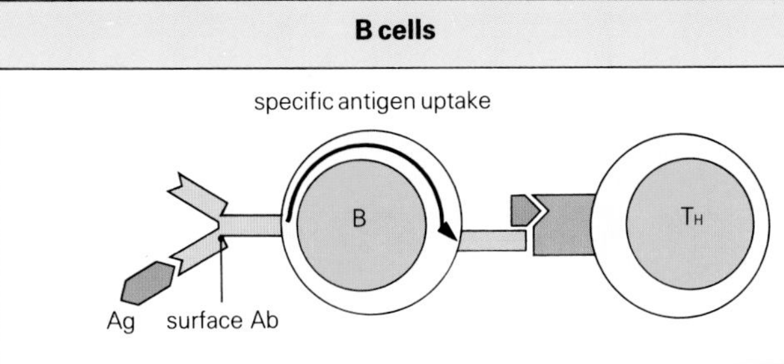

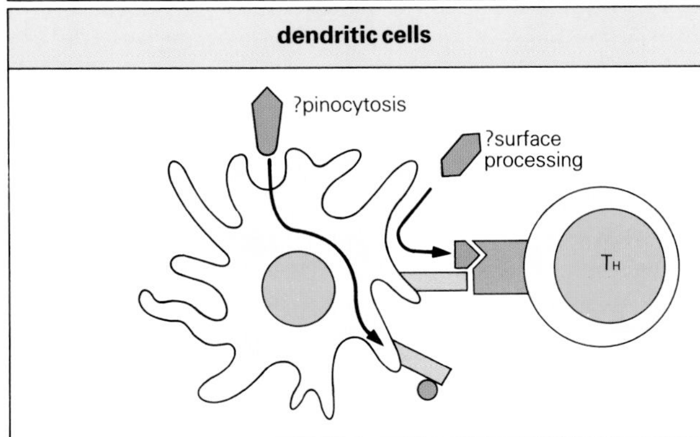

approximately 8–24 amino acids; this size fits into the grooves of HLA molecules (see Chapter 4).

It is not clear whether association of antigenic peptide with MHC molecules takes place inside the cell or at the cell surface. Conceivably, it may occur in both locations. There is evidence that class I MHC molecules are more commonly associated with intracellular parasites, for example viruses, than class II molecules; thus, perhaps class I association with peptides occurs intracellularly, while class II association occurs extracellularly.

INTERLEUKIN-1 AND ITS ROLE IN LYMPHOCYTE ACTIVATION

As well as processing antigen, APCs produce molecules which are involved in the activation of lymphocytes, particularly T cells. The best characterized of these is interleukin-1 (IL-1). There are two related molecules of IL-1, IL-1α (acidic pI ≃ 5) and IL-1β (pI ≃ 7), which have exactly the same function, because they bind to the same receptor at similar affinities. IL-1 has many other actions apart from activation of lymphocytes and these are summarized in Figs 8.17 and 8.18.

Fig. 8.16 Antigen presentation. Mononuclear phagocytes (top), B cells (centre) and dendritic cells (bottom) can all present antigen to MHC class II restricted T-helper (T$_H$) cells. Macrophages take up antigen via non-specific receptors or as immune complexes, and probably process it internally before returning fragments to the cell surface in association with class II molecules. Activated B cells can take up antigen via their surface antigen receptor and this may be the basis of antigen-specific T cell–B cell cooperation. Dendritic cells constitutively express class II MHC molecules, but are not phagocytic; it is therefore presumed that they either take up antigen by pinocytosis or process it at the cell surface.

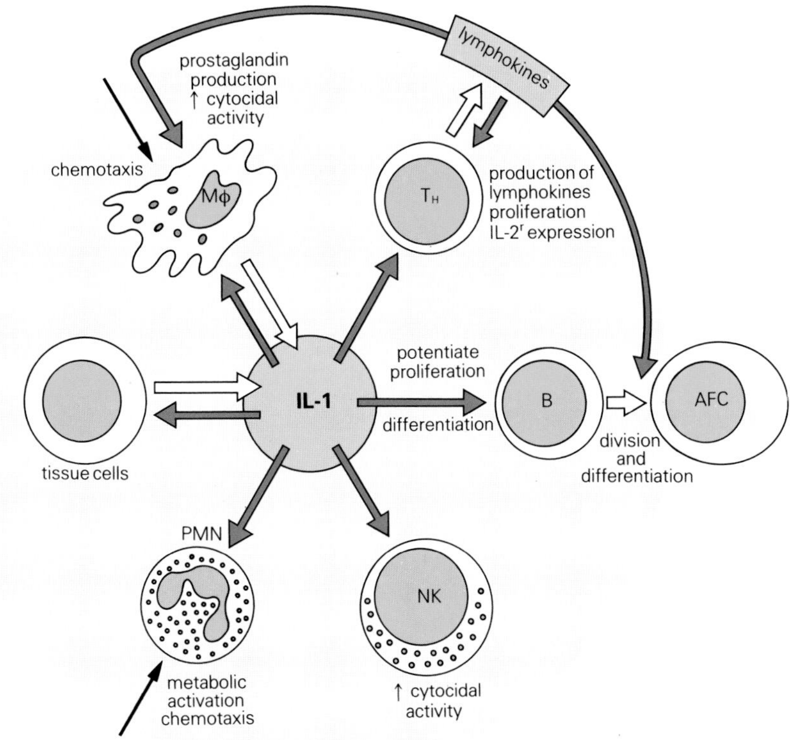

Fig. 8.17 Actions of interleukin-1 (IL-1) on cells of the immune system. IL-1 is produced by many cell types in response to damage, infection or antigens, and acts on T cells and B cells to potentiate their responses to other lymphokines. It also activates natural killer (NK) cells, and macrophages, either directly or indirectly, via lymphokines, such as interferon-γ.

tissue/cell type	prostaglandin synthesis	proliferation	protein synthesis	other effects
brain	+	astrocyte tumours		fever somnolence anorexia
synovial cells	+		collagenase	proteolytic enzyme release
bone/osteoclasts			collagenase	
cartilage/ chondrocytes	+		collagenase plasminogen activator	
muscle cells	+			proteolysis
fibroblasts	+	+	collagenase	
endothelium	+	+	procoagulant activity	↑ macrophage and neutrophil adhesion
epithelial cells		+	type IV collagen	
liver/ hepatocytes			acute phase proteins	

Fig. 8.18 Actions of interleukin-1. Interleukin-1 (IL-1) acts on many cell types other than those of the immune system in its role as an inflammatory mediator. On many cell types IL-1 induces the production of other cytokines, for example TNF, GM-CSF, M-CSF.

One of the important actions of IL-1 is to induce production of other cytokines, such as TNF from macrophages and endothelium, IL-6 from fibroblasts, GM-CSF from T cells; thus, there is a cytokine network.

Both resting T and B lymphocytes have receptors for IL-1. Occupation of receptors when the antigen specific receptors are activated, leads to the induction of both T and B cells. T cells then express receptors for IL-2 (previously known as T cell growth factor) and start to produce IL-2; thus T cell growth is initiated. Other lymphokines are also required for B cell growth and activation. The properties and functions of IL-2 are summarized in Fig. 8.19.

INTERFERON γ AND ITS ROLE IN THE ANTIGEN PRESENTING PROCESS

APCs have one feature in common; they have MHC class II antigens on their surface. The expression of these class II antigens is not a fixed process, but is under complex regulation.

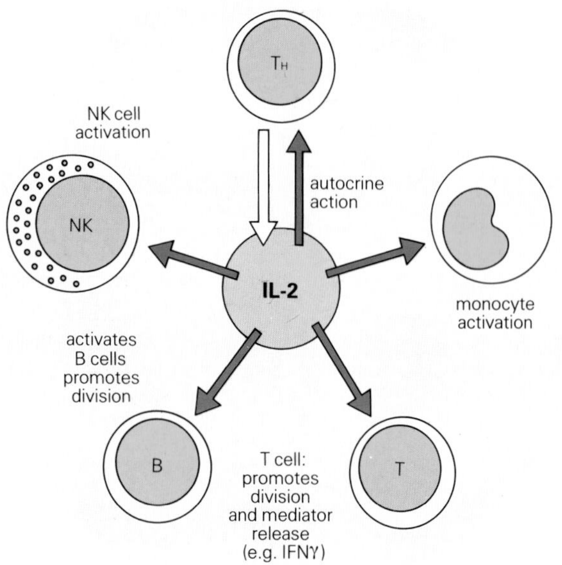

Fig. 8.19 Actions of interleukin-2. Interleukin-2 (IL-2) is generated by T-helper cells. In addition to its essential role in promoting T cell division, IL-2 also potentiates B cell growth and the activation of monocytes and natural killer (NK) cells. In clinical practice, high doses of IL-2 (1000 U/ml) are used to activate NK precursors into lines of so-called 'lymphokine-activated killer, (LAK) cells which are used in experimental cancer therapy.

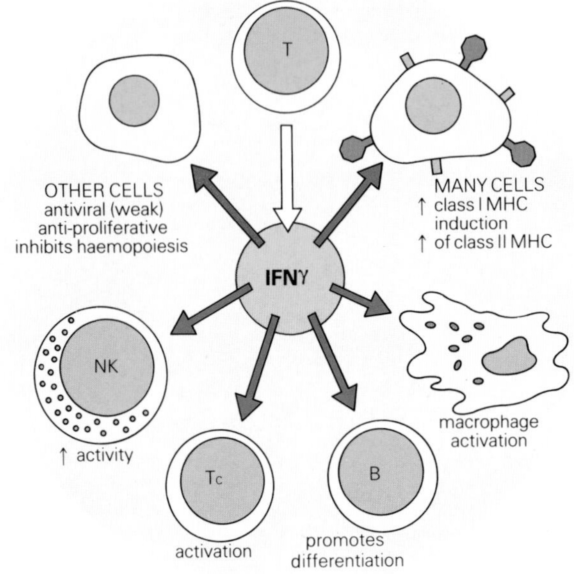

Fig. 8.20 Actions of interferon-γ. Interferon-γ (IFNγ) has numerous immunoregulatory actions. Its antiviral and antiproliferative activities are less potent than those of IFNα and IFNβ, and it is not as effective as IFNα at inducing natural killer (NK) cells. It is, however, the most potent inducer of class II molecules on tissue cells, and in this and other functions it synergizes with tumour necrosis factor-α and-β.

Interdigitating dendritic cells appear to be constitutive expressors of class II antigens, but other APCs for example monocytes, macrophages, endothelial cells and astrocytes, require the presence of inducing signals such as interferon-γ (IFNγ). B cells have moderate amounts of class II antigens on their surface, which are increased by IL-4 and inhibited by IFNγ. Thus, IFNγ has a critical role in the antigen presenting function of macrophages, astrocytes, microglia, astroglia and endothelium.

IFNγ is produced by activated T cells and natural killer (NK) cells. A degree of immune activation therefore, leads to the production of IFNγ and an increase in APC function, and the potential to activate T cells further. Thus, IFNγ acts as a positive feedback signal. IFNγ also activates macrophages in general, and probably enhances their capacity to take up and process antigens. The properties of IFNγ are summarized in Fig. 8.20.

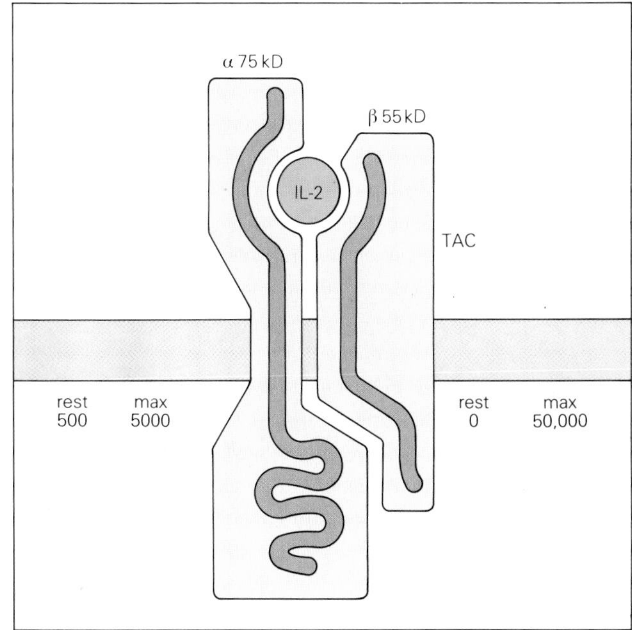

Fig. 8.21 Structure of the high affinity interleukin-2 receptor. The high affinity interleukin-2 (IL-2) receptor consists of two chains, each of which can bind IL-2 weakly. Resting T cells (rest) do not express the β chain, but following activation, they may express up to 50,000/cell (max) some of which associate with the α chain to form the high affinity IL-2 receptor. A monoclonal antibody (anti-TAC) recognizes the β chain. Numbers indicate molecules of each chain/cell.

LYMPHOCYTE ACTIVATION

Most lymphocytes are in the resting phase, not having encountered the appropriate activating antigen for a considerable period of time, if ever, the cells are small and quiescent. However, on encountering antigen on appropriate antigen presenting cells (APCs), lymphocytes with appropriate receptors become activated. These lymphocytes acquire new receptors, enlarge, and become more metabolically active as a prelude to mitosis.

The selective but transient activation of lymphocytes and their subsequent clonal expansion to provide enough cells to mount an effective immune response to a given pathogen permits the immune system to maintain a wide repertoire of specificities within a relatively small number of cells.

THE ACTIVATION OF T CELLS

The activation of T-helper cells marks the beginning of an effective immune response, and the successful completion of antigen presentation by an APC. During the activation process, the surface of T cells alters; the most important change is the acquisition of receptors for interleukin-2 (IL-2). Other surface changes include increased numbers of IL-1 receptors, and the acquisition, on human T cells, of HLA class II antigens. Subsequently, transferrin receptors also appear as iron is essential for cell growth.

IL-2 Receptors Receptors for IL-2 have been closely studied with the help of monoclonal antibodies. It is now recognized that two polypeptides (α chains and β chains) form the IL-2 receptors.

Resting T cells have small numbers (≃500) of α chains (molecular weight 75 kD) and essentially no β chains (molecular weight 55 kD). β chains are recognized by the use of anti-TAC monoclonal antibody. After activation, the β chains are actively produced and the α chains less so, resulting in approximately 5000 α chains and up to 50,000 β chains on each activated T cell. The high affinity receptors for IL-2 (Kd ≃ 10 pM) are α–β heterodimers (Fig. 8.21), which are effective at driving T cell growth. The low affinity receptors are the β chains (Kd ≃ 10 nM); these do not activate cells. The α chain alone is an IL-2 receptor of intermediate affinity (≃ 1 nM) and can be involved in activation in the presence of high concentrations of IL-2, for example 1000 units/ml, particularly on NK cells which can possess 5000 α chains at rest.

Once induced, IL-2 receptors remain on the cell surface for only about 1 week, unless their surface expression is re-induced by T cell activation. When appropriately triggered, T cells secrete IL-2, which interacts with IL-2 receptors to mediate growth. This may be in an 'autocrine' manner, with the T cell releasing IL-2 which it then takes up via its IL-2 receptors, or in a 'paracrine' manner, with one T cell producing IL-2 which is then taken up by neighbouring cells. There is no evidence for an 'endocrine' action (that is, secretion into the blood and action on distant target cells), as IL-2 is not detectable in the blood.

T Cell Growth Factors Although it was thought that IL-2 was the only T cell growth factor, it is now known that IL-4 and also IL-1 are T cell growth factors as well though they are not as potent as IL-2.

IL-2 is only transiently produced by T cells after activation with synthesis stopping after 2–3 days. This, together with the transient expression of IL-2 receptors, provides a built-in brake to limit T cell growth and clonal expansion.

In the past few years it has been possible to grow T-helper and killer cells long term and to clone them in the presence of IL-2, with periodic stimulation. Such studies have verified practically the principles of T cell growth control.

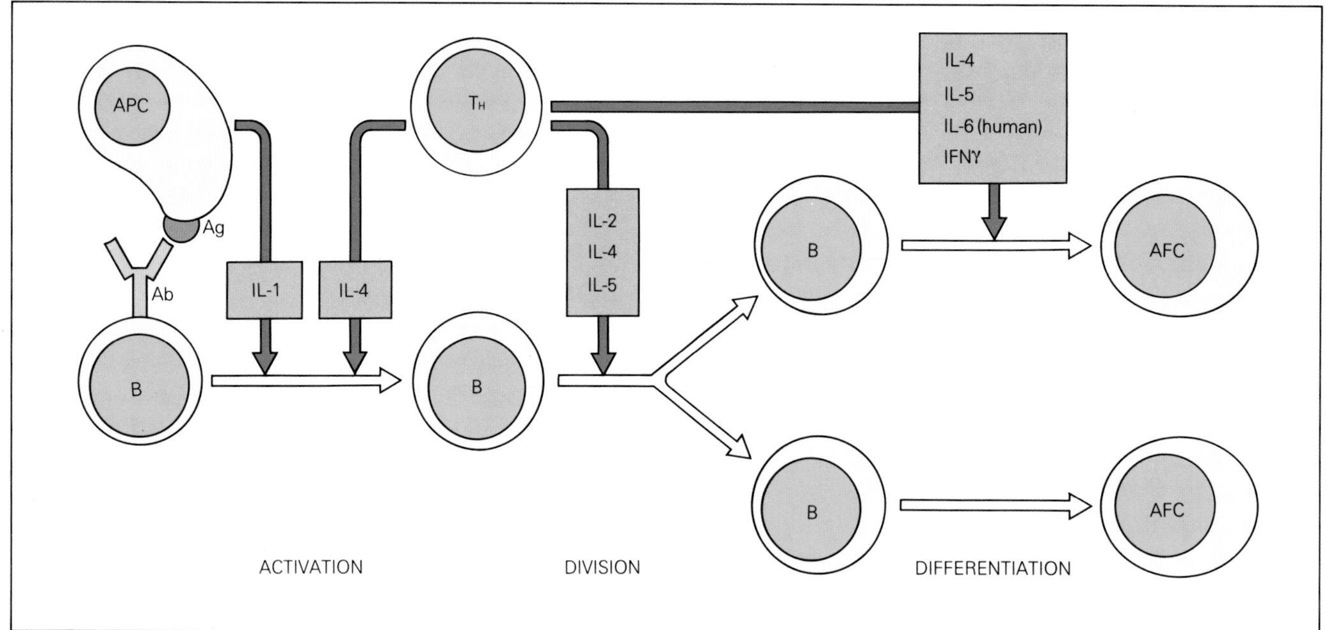

Fig. 8.22 Stages in B cell activation and development. B cells are activated by antigen on antigen-presenting cells (APCs) in the presence of IL-4 and IL-1. This causes expression of receptors for IL-2 and other lymphokines. IL-2, IL-4 and IL-5 (in mouse) drive cell division. Only one cycle of cell division is illustrated although many cycles will usually occur. Differentiation into antibody-forming cells (AFCs) is effected by IL-4, IL-5, IL-6 (in man) and IFNY.

B CELL ACTIVATION

B cell activation may take place in the absence of T cells, with T-independent antigens. However, the full development of B cells takes place only in the presence of T cells and their products.

Resting B cells, like T cells, respond to IL-1. The first T cell product to act on resting B cells is IL-4 (formerly known as B cell stimulating factor-1). B cells stimulated by antigen, IL-1 and IL-4, enlarge and enter the cell cycle. Subsequently, activated B cells encounter a T cell-derived molecule, IL-5 (previously and erroneously termed T cell replacing factor), which is involved in the growth of B cells and the production of immunoglobulin. The next characterized T cell-produced molecule required by B cells for high rate immunoglobulin production is IL-6 (previously known as B cell stimulatory factor-2). The precise requirements for B cell growth may vary between species.

The regulation of B cell growth factor by T cell products is complex. Activated B cells transiently express receptors for IL-2 which can act on B cells as a potent growth and differentiation factor.

IFNY also acts as a B cell differentiation factor. A scheme of B cell growth and differentiation is illustrated in Fig. 8.22, but is probably not complete as, unlike T cells, it is not yet possible to clone B cells or grow them long term in the non-transformed state.

ANTIGEN – RECEPTOR INTERACTIONS

It has been noted that polymeric T-independent antigens activate B cells, but if depolymerized, the same antigens do not; this implies that cross-linking of receptors is important in B cell activation. The capacity of antibodies to immunoglobulin to recognize antigen-specific receptors on B cells has made it possible to study directly how receptors on B cells function. B cells can be activated by intact anti-immunoglobulin, but not by the Fab fragments. Anti-immunoglobulin cross-links receptors into 'patches' and subsequently 'caps' them, whereas anti-Fab does not. These observations suggest that receptor cross-linking is a necessary step in B cell activation, and this conclusion is supported by many other lines of evidence (Fig. 8.23).

The antigen–receptor interactions of T cells are not so easy to study, but it is probable that antigen presentation also acts to cross-link receptors at the surface of the T cell and the APC.

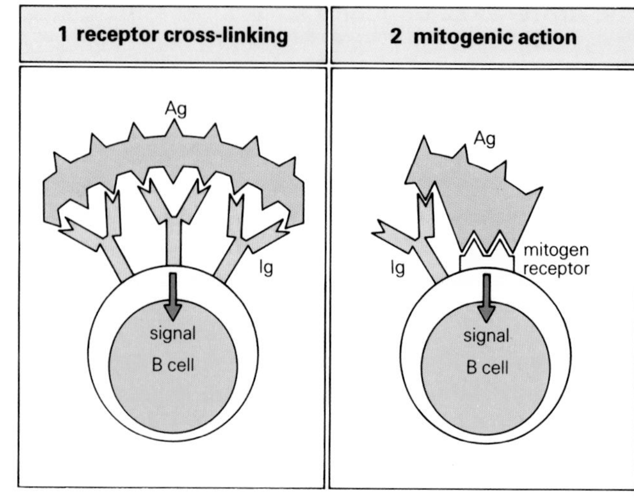

Fig. 8.23 Activation of B cells by T-independent antigens. Many T-independent (T-ind) antigens are polyvalent and appear to activate B cells without T cell help by cross-linking the antigen receptors (left); this emphasizes the importance of receptor cross-linking, which may also occur in T cell activation. Some T-ind antigens are mitogenic and these may be focused onto the B cell surface via the specific antigen receptor (right).

B CELL – T CELL INTERACTIONS

For B cells to be optimally activated to replicate *in vivo* or *in vitro* and produce immunoglobulin of all classes, it is essential that T cells are present. Although the mechanism of T cell and B cell interaction has been studied intensely for many years, it is only partly resolved. It is possible that an APC, for example a macrophage or a dendritic cell, which has taken up antigen, may attract T cells and B cells of the appropriate specificity; thus, T cells and B cells would be close enough for mediators released by T cells to have ready access to the B cells, at high concentration. This is the most likely scenario with unprimed T and B cells, which are present at low frequency. As discussed earlier, B cells after priming may present antigen directly to T-helper cells and such interactions have been visualized *in vitro*. The molecules IL-4, IL-5, IL-6, IL-2 and IFNγ, whose properties are listed in Fig. 8.24, mediate some of the effects of T cells on B cells, but this does not necessarily represent the full picture, particularly in the very early stages of B cell activation. There have been conflicting reports of antigen-specific T-helper factors in B cell activation which could be shed or secreted T cell receptors, but this remains controversial.

lymphokine	mol. wt	cell source(s)	main cell target(s)	main actions
IFNγ	40–50,000 (dimer)	T cells NK cells	lymphocytes monocytes tissue cells	immunoregulation B cell differentiation
IL-1α IL-1β	33,000 (precursor) 17,500	monocytes dendritic cells B cells fibroblasts epithelial cells endothelium astrocytes	thymocytes neutrophils T and B cells tissue cells	immunoregulation and inflammatory mediator
IL-2	15,000	T cells NK cells	T cells B cells monocytes	proliferation activation
IL-3	15,000	T cells	stem cells progenitors	pan-specific colony stimulating factor
IL-4	15,000	T cells	B cells	division and differentiation
IL-5	? 15,000 (153 amino acids)	T cells	B cells eosinophils	differentiation
IL-6	20,000	T cells fibroblasts macrophages	B cells thymocytes	differentiation

Fig. 8.24 Summary of the main features of interferon-γ and interleukins. In some cases the molecular weight data is derived from study of cDNA sequences. Only the most important targets and actions are shown.

FURTHER READING

Clevers, H., Alarcon, B., Wileman, T. & Terhorst, C. (1988) The T cell receptor/CD3 complex: A dynamic protein ensemble. *Annual Review of Immunology*, **6**, 629–662.

Durum, S.K., Schmidt, J.A. & Oppenheim, J.J. (1985) Interleukin-1: An immunological perspective. *Annual Review of Immunology*, **3**, 263–287.

Feldmann, M., Lamb, J.R. & Owen, M.J. (1989) *T Cells*. New York: J. Wiley & Sons.

Kishimoto, T. & Hirano, T. (1988) Molecular regulation of B lymphocyte response. *Annual Review of Immunology*, **6**, 485–512.

Kronenberg, M., Siu, G., Hood, L.E. & Shastri, N. (1986) The molecular genetics of the T-cell antigen receptor and T-cell antigen recognition. *Annual Review of Immunology*, **4**, 529–591.

Littman, D.R. (1987) The structure of the CD4 and CD8 genes. *Annual Review of Immunology*, **5**, 561–587.

Paul, W.E. & Ohara, J. (1987) B-cell stimulatory factor-1/Interleukin-4. *Annual Review of Immunology*, **5**, 429–459.

Schwartz, R.H. (1985) T-lymphocyte recognition of antigen in association with gene products of the major histocompatibility complex. *Annual Review of Immunology*, **3**, 237–261.

Taniguchi, T. (1988) Regulation of cytokine gene expression. *Annual Review of Immunology*, **6**, 439–464.

Unanue, E.R. (1984) Antigen-presenting function of the macrophage. *Annual Review of Immunology*, **2**, 395.

9 Cell-mediated Immune Responses

The term 'cell-mediated immunity' (CMI) was originally coined to describe localized reactions to organisms, usually intracellular pathogens, mediated by lymphocytes and phagocytes rather than by antibody (humoral immunity). However it is now often used in a more general sense for any response in which antibody plays a subordinate role.

It is not possible however to consider cell-mediated and antibody-mediated responses entirely separately. Cells are involved in the initiation of antibody responses, and antibody acts as an essential link in some cell-mediated reactions. Moreover no cell-mediated response is likely to occur in the total absence of antibody, which can modify cellular responses in numerous ways. For instance, antigen–antibody complexes may form during an immune response in which chemotactic molecules are released causing cellular aggregation and local inflammation. Antibody may block antigenic determinants which would otherwise be recognized by cells, or cause stripping or modulation of such determinants from target cell membranes. It may also be involved in linking antigens to T cells via their Fc receptors, thus modulating the cells' responses.

The various aspects of CMI are summarized in Fig. 9.1 which illustrates the most important functions of immunologically active cells (individual cells may perform more than one function). This figure does not include the secondary effects of the activities of these cell types, for example delayed hypersensitivity or granuloma formation.

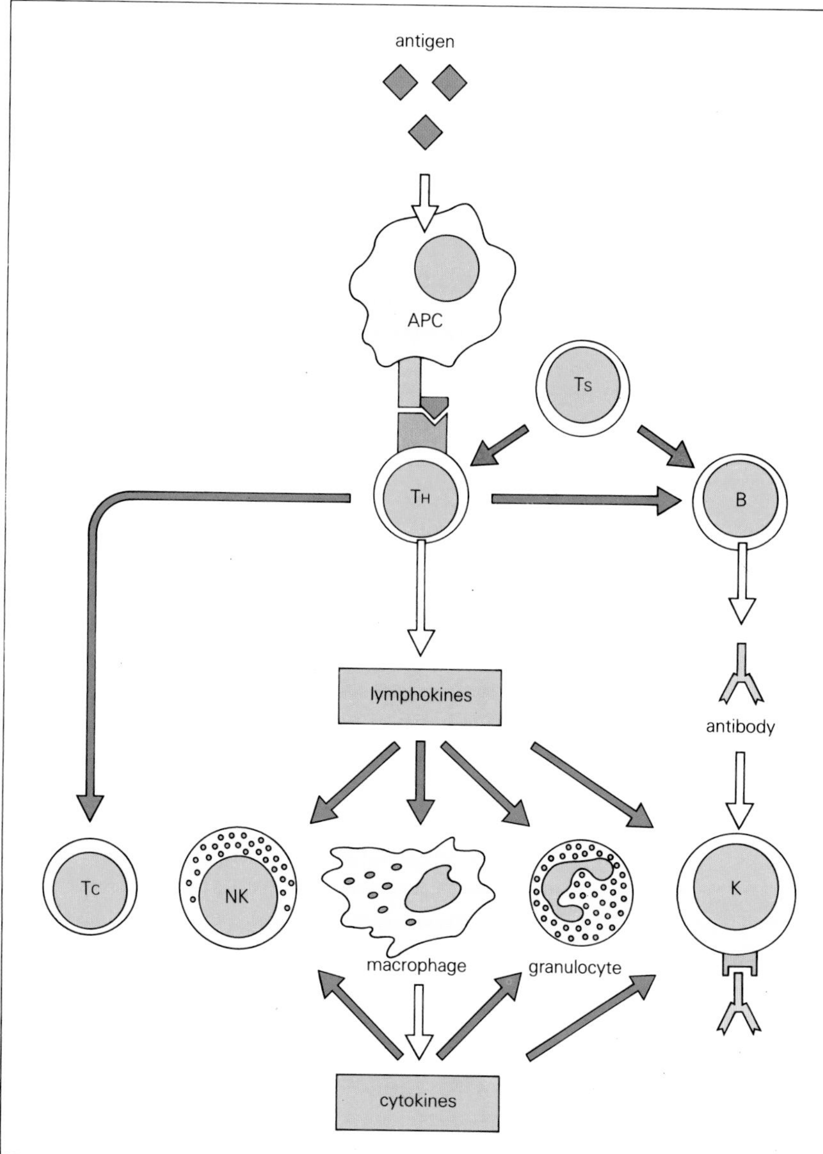

Fig. 9.1 Scope of cell-mediated immunity. Antigen-presenting cells (APC) present processed antigen to helper T cells (TH), which are central to the development of immune responses. They can help B cells to make antibody and modulate the actions of a variety of other effector cells, including cytotoxic T (Tc) cells, natural killer (NK) cells, macrophages, granulocytes and antibody-dependent cytotoxic (K) cells. Many of these effects are mediated by lymphokines, but cytokines from other cells, particularly macrophages are also important. Both T and B cells may in turn by influenced by suppressor T (Ts) cells.

T CELL FUNCTIONS

T cells are critical in the development of all cell-mediated immune reactions. It is important to distinguish the role of T-helper cells which control and modulate the development of immune responses from T-cytotoxic cells, which are effector cells with a particularly important role in the immune reactions against intracellular parasites and viruses. Cells which may be recognized by cytotoxic T cells, either because they are infected or because they are allogeneic, are often referred to as target cells. These different functional groups of T cells are described in Chapter 2, and the way in which T cells recognize antigen in association with Major Histocompatibility Complex (MHC) molecules is outlined in Chapter 7. Although most T cells recognize antigen in relation to MHC products on cell surfaces, not all T cells use the same MHC molecules. Broadly speaking the functional differences between T cell populations are mirrored in the different ways that they recognize antigen plus MHC. For instance, cytotoxic T cells usually recognize antigen in association with class I MHC products, which are expressed on all nucleated cells, while helper T cells and most of the T cells which proliferate in response to antigen *in vitro*, recognize antigen in association with class II products, which are expressed mostly on antigen-presenting cells, and also on some lymphocytes (Fig. 9.2).

There are several ways of demonstrating this MHC restriction experimentally. Cytotoxic T cells which kill virus-infected autologous cells, will not kill cells infected with the same virus, if the infected cells do not also express the same class I glycopeptides, even if the class II products are identical. Moreover, antibody to class I, but not to class II glycopeptides can block killing of infected autologous cells. The reverse results can be obtained in proliferative, or helper T cell assays. The relationship between function and the class of MHC glycopeptide to which T cells of that function are usually restricted 'makes sense' from an evolutionary point of view. Thus cytotoxic T cells may be required to kill virus-infected cells in any tissue, so they must 'see' antigen in relation to something expressed in all tissues. On the other hand, proliferation or help for antibody production, are regulatory 'decisions' within the lymphoid system, and are restricted by MHC products which are unique to that system and to specialized antigen-presenting cells (see Chapter 8 and below).

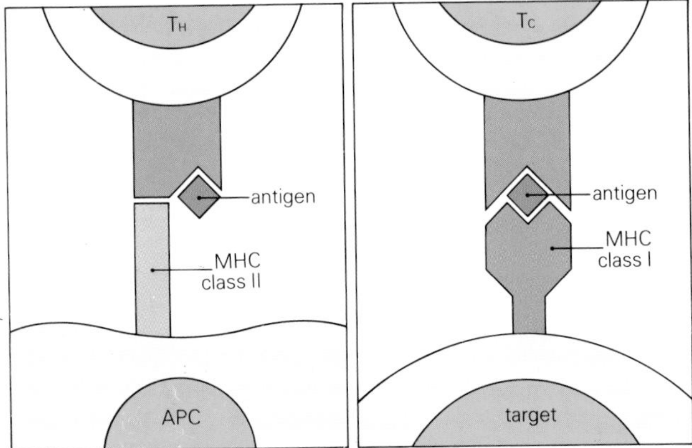

Fig. 9.2 MHC restriction in T cell responses. T-helper (TH) and T-cytotoxic (Tc) cells recognize antigen in association with different types of MHC molecule. Helper cells recognize processed antigen plus MHC class II on antigen-presenting cells, while most cytotoxic cells recognize antigen plus MHC class I on target cells.

T cells can be divided into two major subpopulations on the basis of their cell membrane glycoproteins, which can be defined with monoclonal antibodies. The $CD4^+$ subset expresses a 62 kD glycoprotein, while the $CD8^+$ subset expresses a 76 kD glycoprotein. There is a strong correlation between:

1. expression of CD4 and class II restriction
2. expression of CD8 and class I restriction.

This correlation has led to the suggestion that CD4 and CD8 are the receptors for class II and class I MHC glycopeptides respectively, which is supported by the observation that monoclonal antibodies against CD4 will block class II-restricted T cell activation while anti-CD8 will block killing by class I-restricted cells. Although CD4 and CD8 molecules appear to be involved in class II and class I restricted interactions, it is not certain that they are a mandatory part of the T cell antigen receptor complex in these interactions. It is possible that high affinity interactions between T cells and antigen–MHC do not require CD4 and CD8, while low affinity interactions are enhanced by the interaction of CD4 with class II or CD8 with class I.

The antigen-specific interactions mediated by T cells and antigen-presenting cells determine the antigen specificity of the cellular immune responses. However T cells also interact with other cells via lymphokines which they release following activation. Although the actions of lymphokines (detailed below) are antigen non-specific, they usually act with greatest effect on cells in the immediate vicinity of the active T cells. These will be cells expressing antigen–MHC. Thus lymphokines can act as mediators of antigen-specific immune reactions.

ANTIGEN-PRESENTING CELLS

T cells, particularly T-helper cells, cannot recognize free antigen; for recognition to occur, antigen must be presented together with MHC class II products. This presentation is performed by antigen-presenting cells.

Some cells of the monocyte/macrophage series express class II glycopeptides (Ia antigens) and can act as antigen-presenting cells for T cells or B cells. Other cell types, for instance vascular endothelial cells, may also act as antigen-presenting cells, and it has been recently shown that certain stimuli *in vitro* will cause class II glycopeptide expression on cells which do not normally do so, for example thyroid follicular cells. However it is not clear whether this automatically correlates with the antigen-presenting function.

Dendritic cells found in blood, lymph and other tissues are non-phagocytic Fc receptor negative cells which strongly express class II glycopeptides. Their relationship to the monocyte/macrophage series is doubtful. They are very efficient presenters of antigen to T cells in several *in vitro* and *in vivo* systems. They may be related to the strongly Ia positive Langerhans' cells found in the epidermis.

It should be remembered that other cell types, possibly variants of the macrophage lineage, may

antigen-presenting cell	characteristics			
	phago-cytosis	Fc/C3 receptors	class II MHC ex-pression	present to:
marginal zone macrophages	+	+	−	B
follicular dendritic cells	−	+	−	B
interdigitating dendritic cells	−	−	+	T
monocytes/ macrophages	+	+	+/−	T + B
Langerhans'cell	−	+	+	T

Fig. 9.3 The chief characteristics of different antigen-presenting cells (APCs). Those cells which present antigen to T cells have class II MHC molecules. B cells do not need to recognize antigen in association with MHC but can be stimulated by free antigen or complexed antigen which has bound to APCs with Fc and C3 receptors.

be involved in antigen presentation to B cells. These cell types probably do not express class II glycopeptides and therefore presumably do not present antigen to T cells. For example, some T-independent antigens localize in the marginal zone macrophages, which may be involved in the induction of T-independent antibody responses. Class II negative follicular dendritic cells (not to be confused with the Ia positive dendritic cells discussed above) express receptors for Fc and complement C3, and appear to pick up immune complexes via these receptors and induce B cell memory (T-dependently). The important characteristics of these antigen-presenting cells are tabulated in Fig. 9.3.

The initiation of T cell proliferation involves not only recognition of antigen and MHC determinants as already discussed, but also involves the passage of signals between the APC and lymphocytes via interleukins, including IL-1 and IFNγ (see Chapter 8). Macrophages release IL-1, but dendritic cells do not. Consequently it is thought that IL-1 is an accessory factor in T cell activation and not mandatory.

CELL-MEDIATED CYTOTOXICITY

Certain subpopulations of lymphoid cells, and under some circumstances, myeloid cells, can lyse target cells to which they are sufficiently closely bound. Much confusion has arisen because several receptors can be involved in this binding, and in the triggering of the killing pathways. Similarly there seem to be several killing mechanisms. The main types of receptor–ligand interaction involved are:

1. MHC-restricted T cell receptors (cytotoxic T cells)
2. determinants recognized by NK cells
3. antibody Fc receptors (K cells, antibody-dependent cell-mediated cytotoxicity).

These possible types of cell binding are illustrated in Fig. 9.4. However the situation is in reality rather more complex because other receptor–ligand interactions which are discussed later can also help to stabilize the bond between the cytotoxic cell and the target, and can even help to trigger the killing event. Similarly the mechanisms, which are shown in Fig. 9.4 are functional categories and more than one type of target cell interaction may be manifested by a particular morphological cell type.

The first three types of physiological cell-mediated cytotoxicity will now be described. Other mechanisms which involve the secretion of cytotoxic molecules, or activation of macrophages, will be considered in later sections.

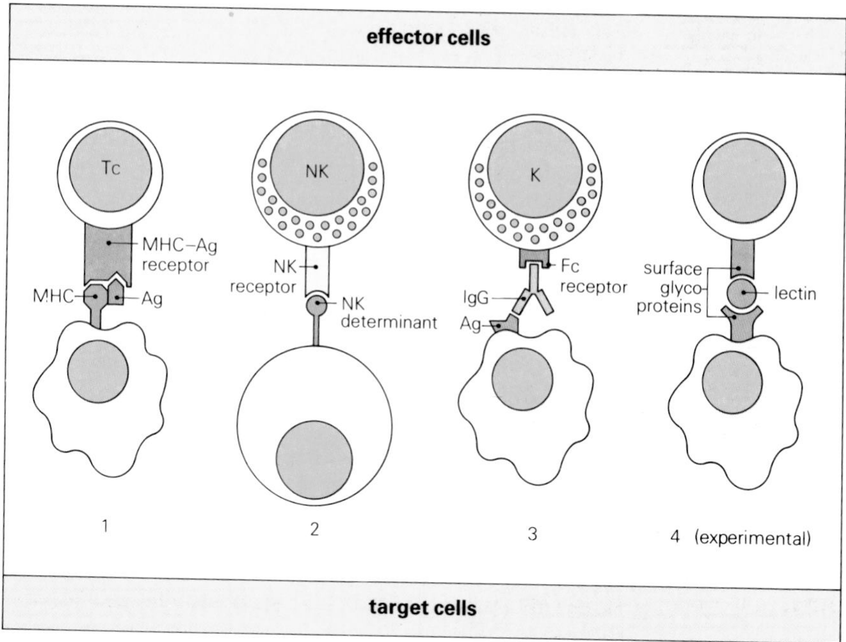

Fig. 9.4 Cell-mediated cytotoxicity. Four different types of cell binding in cell-mediated cytotoxicity.
1. Cytotoxic T cells (Tc) bind their target while recognizing antigen and MHC determinants.
2. NK cells recognize determinants expressed on neoplastic cells.
3. K cells recognize the Fc of IgG antibody bound to antigen on the target cell surface.
4. Experimentally, glycoproteins on the surface of effector and target can be cross-linked by lectins.

MHC-RESTRICTED CYTOTOXIC T CELLS

MHC-restricted cytotoxic T-cells are a subpopulation of small lymphocytes derived from non-lytic radiosensitive precursors. The majority are $CD8^+$ and recognize antigens in association with class I MHC molecules, or foreign class I alone on allogeneic/xenogeneic cells, since foreign class I may mimic syngeneic class I associated with antigens. About 10% of MHC-restricted cytotoxic T cells are $CD4^+$ and class II restricted. The interaction between CD4 or CD8 and the appropriate MHC molecule probably helps to stabilize the cell–cell recognition, and antibodies to any of these cell surface molecules can inhibit killing. The most important role of these cells may be elimination of virus-infected cells (see Chapter 16).

NON-SPECIFIC, MHC-UNRESTRICTED KILLER CELLS

Several, partly overlapping cell populations have been shown to possess the property of non-specific, MHC-unrestricted killing and include:

1. cells naturally present in spleen or peripheral blood populations, usually known as Natural Killer (NK) cells
2. cells activated by culture in relatively high concentrations of interleukin-2 (IL-2) – Lymphokine Activated Killer (LAK) cells
3. mixed populations with non-specific killing activity developing in mixed lymphocyte cultures, or cultures stimulated with the lectin phytohaemagglutinin (PHA)

NK Cells These cells are mostly derived from the 'large granular lymphocytes' (LGLs) which comprise about 5% of human peripheral blood lymphoid cells (Fig. 9.5). The majority of NK cells are $CD16^+$ (IgG Fc receptor), $NKH1^+$, $CD3^-$, and do not contain productive rearrangement of the T cell receptor genes. In rodents, NK cells express asialo GM_1 which is also found on macrophages and granulocytes, though the tissue distribution of NK cells is different from that of macrophages (Fig. 9.6). Cloned NK cells are heterogeneous in the range of targets which they will lyse. However, it is still not clear whether this is because NK cells are a distinct cell lineage with a clonally expressed diversity of receptors,

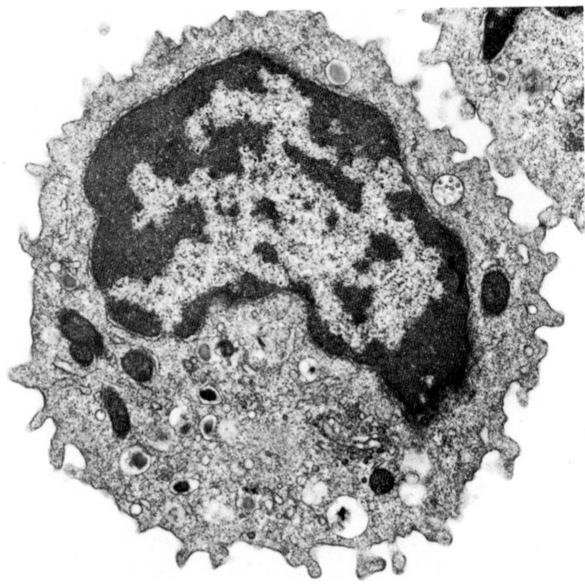

Fig. 9.5 A large granular lymphocyte. Large granular lymphocytes isolated by density gradient centrifugation contain the majority of serum NK effector activity.

	NK cells	macrophages
thymus	–	–
spleen	+++	+++
bone marrow	±	+++
peritoneal exudate	+++	+++
lymph node	±	++
thoracic lymph duct	–	–
blood	+++	+++

Fig. 9.6 Distribution of NK cells and cytolytic macrophages in lymphoid tissues. The distribution reveals that the two cell types are distinct, despite their common possession of Fc receptors.

or several distinct lineages. It is also possible that the apparent diversity is really due to variation in the degree of activation, and in the contribution of several other receptors to the NK–target cell binding, and to the triggering of killing, as outlined below.

LAK Cells There is increasing evidence that the enhanced cytotoxic activity of peripheral blood or spleen cell populations precultured with IL-2 is largely derived from precursors which are indistinguishable from NK cells. Thus LAK cells probably do not represent a separate lineage, but rather a consequence of activation. The differences in specificity may also be attributable to activation, and to the changing contribution of other receptors. This type of cell is undergoing trials for the treatment of cancer in man. The patients' own T cells are stimulated *in vitro* with IL-2, and then returned to the patient.

Mixed Populations with Non-specific Killing Activity Stimulation of peripheral blood cells by autologous tumour cells or mixed lymphocyte culture gives rise to many $CD3^+$, $CD8^+$ cells which show typical class I-restricted cytotoxicity. However, clonal analysis of these complex cultures, particularly when PHA has been used as a stimulus, reveals that some $CD3^+$ cells expressing the α and β, or the γ and δ chains of the T cell receptor, can exert cytotoxic effects which show little or no apparent MHC restriction. It is possible that such cells merely recognize determinants which are present on a wide range of target cells, or are recognizing an as yet undefined restriction element. The situation is further complicated by the fact that such cultures also contain LAK cells, presumably derived from NK cells in the presence of the IL-2 released in the culture.

OTHER RECEPTORS INVOLVED IN BINDING OR TRIGGERING EVENTS

Fig. 9.7 lists some of the other receptor–ligand interactions which may increase binding between the cytotoxic cell and its target, or even mediate the triggering of the killing event. Thus, experimentally, antibodies to CD3, CD2 (the sheep red cell receptor) and CD16 (the IgG Fc receptor) can all trigger killing of attached cells, and interaction with their natural ligands may also do so.

receptor	ligand	function
CD2(LFA-2)	LFA-3	binding and activation
LFA-1	ICAM-1	binding
CD16 (IgG Fc')	IgG, ? other members of Ig supergene family	binding and activation

Fig. 9.7 Antigen non-specific binding receptors on leucocytes.

THE RELATIONSHIP OF NK CELLS AND CYTOTOXIC T CELLS TO K CELLS

Cells with cytotoxic potential which also possess Fc receptors for IgG may bind to and lyse target cells coated with antibody of the relevant class (Fig. 9.8). Since some cytotoxic T lymphocytes (CTLs) and NK cells have such $Fc\gamma$ receptors, they can also perform this function. It is customary to refer to this as killer (K) cell activity but it is now clear that K cells represent a function rather than a separate cell type. Observations of single cells have proved that both K and NK activity can be properties of the same cell. The models most frequently studied involve antibodies to viruses expressed on the target cell membrane; tumour or MHC-associated determinants; haptens such as TNP conjugated onto the membrane; membranes of avian nucleated erythrocytes. Strictly speaking myeloid cells expressing Fc receptors can also express K cell activity, but it is not certain that the killing mechanisms are the same, and these cells are considered later.

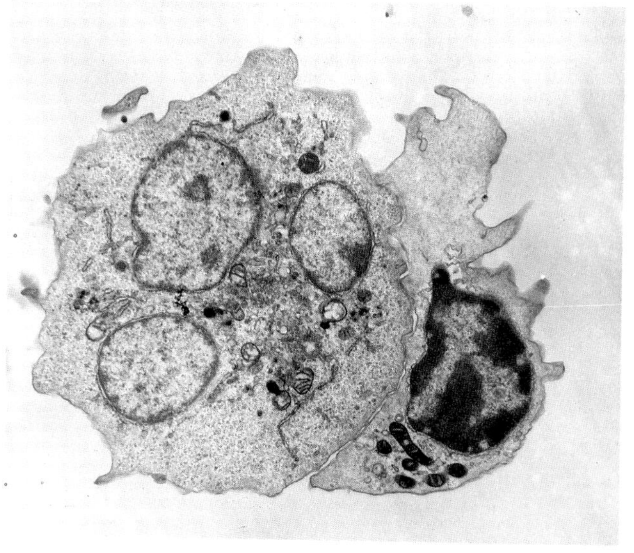

Fig. 9.8 Electronmicrograph of a K cell (right) engaging a target cell (left). x2500. (Courtesy of Mr P. Penfold.)

THE MECHANISM OF CELL-MEDIATED CYTOTOXICITY

It appears that the mechanisms involved in killing are similar whether CTL, NK or lymphoid K cells are involved, and whatever receptor–target interaction is responsible (Fig. 9.9). One view is that there are three distinct phases:

1. binding to the target
2. a Ca^{++}-dependent phase which involves secretion of vesicle contents which modify the target so that it is programmed for death
3. a late phase when the target undergoes apoptosis.

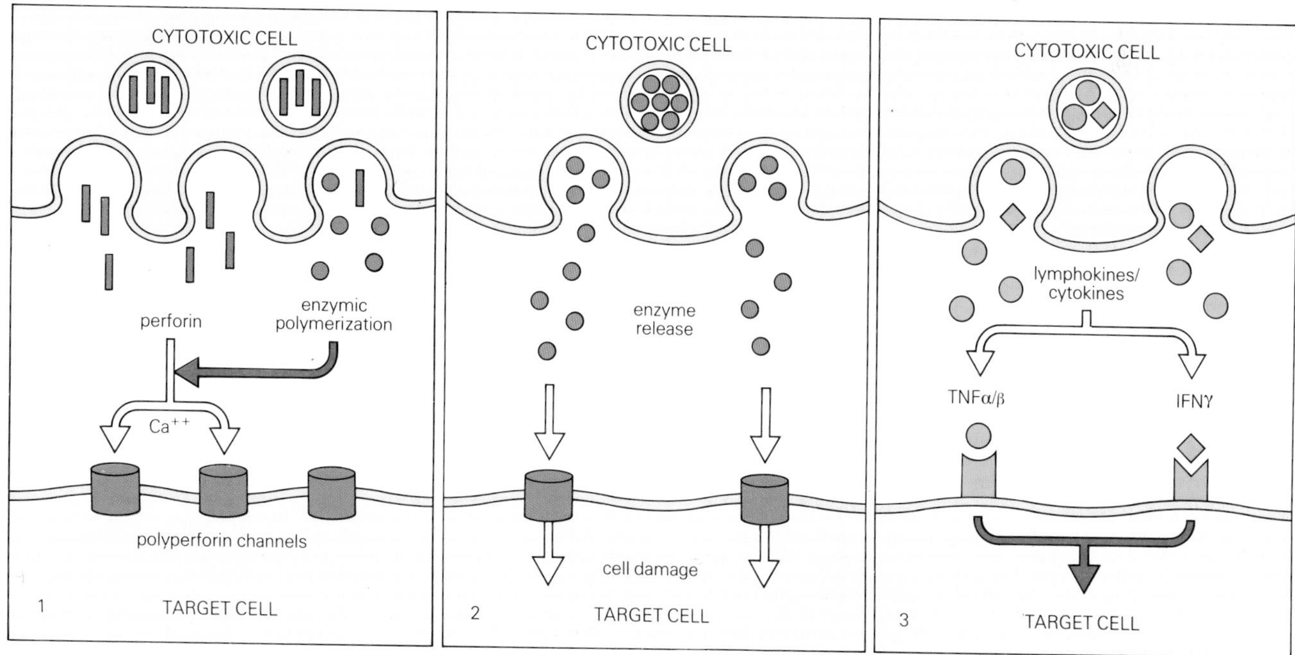

Fig. 9.9 Cytotoxicity. Three potential mechanisms for cytotoxic damage to target cells are presented.
1. The cytotoxic cell degranulates, releasing perforin and various enzymes into the immediate vicinity of the target cell membrane. In the presence of Ca^{++} there is enzymic polymerization of the perforin, to form polyperforin channels on the target cell. A mechanism specifically protects the cytotoxic cell from damage.
2. Degradative enzymes released from the cytotoxic cell pass through the channels on the target to cause cell damage.
3. Lymphokines and cytokines, including TNF and IFNγ from the cytotoxic cell, trigger the target cell via its receptors, modulating its protein synthesis and causing cytotoxic damage. This process takes longer than 1 or 2.

This model is based on the observation that the granules of LGLs, NK cells and some CTLs contain perforin, which is a monomeric pore-forming protein related to the lytic component (C9) of complement, and a serine esterase of unknown significance. In the presence of Ca^{++}, the perforin monomers bind to the target cell membrane and polymerize to form transmembrane channels. The cytotoxic cell survives, and can continue to kill further targets. It is suggested that it is protected from autodestruction by a proteoglycan (chondroitin sulphate A) which is also present in the granules, and may bind to the perforin.

The killing is in fact quite unlike the true lysis caused by complement. What is seen is apoptosis, with DNA fragmentation, blebbing, and disintegration into small membrane-bound fragments known as apoptotic bodies. Furthermore there are CTLs which do not seem to contain perforin, and can lyse targets in the absence of calcium. This is particularly striking with primary CTLs generated *in vivo.* It has been suggested that these cells must use some other mechanism, and that the perforin pathway is expressed only after exposure of the effector cells to high concentrations of IL-2.

The granules can also contain tumour necrosis factor-α (TNFα), lymphotoxin (LT or TNFß), and NK cytotoxic factor (NKCF) which is partially neutralized by antibody to TNF (discussed in greater detail below). The role of these cytokines is unclear because their known cytotoxic effects take much longer than the 3–4 hours required by cytotoxic lymphocytes. The various possible mechanisms of cytotoxicity are illustrated in Fig. 9.9.

ANTIBODY-DEPENDENT CELL-MEDIATED CYTOTOXICITY BY MYELOID CELLS

Monocytes, and according to some controversial reports, polymorphonuclear cells, may also be active against antibody-coated tumour targets. Myeloid cells (monocytes and eosinophils) are certainly important effectors of damage to antibody-coated schistosomulae (see Chapter 17). In this system (which may apply also to other parasites), the important antibody classes appear to be the anaphylactic ones (IgE in all species, IgG in mice, and IgG2a in rats). This raises the intriguing possibility that IgE acts by first triggering release of eosinophil chemotactic factor from mast cells, and then binding the arriving eosinophils onto the target (Fig. 9.10).

The mechanism of killing by these myeloid effectors of antibody-dependent cell-mediated cytotoxicity (ADCC) may differ from that of the NK/K cell group.

THE CENTRAL ROLE OF MACROPHAGES

Macrophages play a central role in cell-mediated immunity; they are involved both in the initiation of responses as antigen-presenting cells, and in the effector phase as inflammatory, tumoricidal and microbicidal cells, in addition to their regulatory functions (Fig. 9.11).

MACROPHAGE ACTIVATION BY T LYMPHOCYTE-DERIVED MEDIATORS

Many of the macrophage functions are enhanced by a process known as ‘activation’. The destruction of intracellular parasites and, *in vitro,* of some tumour cells at least requires activation of macrophages by signals derived from lymphocytes (Fig. 9.12). The classical experiment demonstrating this involved BCG (attenuated *Mycobacterium tuberculosis* used in vaccines against tuberculosis) and *Listeria monocytogenes* (Fig. 9.13). From these experiments it was concluded that the activation of macrophages involved antigen-specific triggering by a mechanism which subsequently led to an enhanced microbicidal activity but was not specific for that antigen. Antigen specificity was known to be a property of lymphocytes, and listericidal activity, a property of macrophages. The next step was to demonstrate *in vitro* that, when cultured with appropriate antigen (PPD), immune lymphocytes, for example, lymphocytes derived from a BCG-immunized mouse, would release mediators which non-specifically enhanced the ability of macrophages to kill or inhibit the immunizing organism, and often unrelated organisms as well. However, macrophage activation is a complex phenomenon and enhanced ability to kill one microorganism is not always accompanied by ability to kill all others.

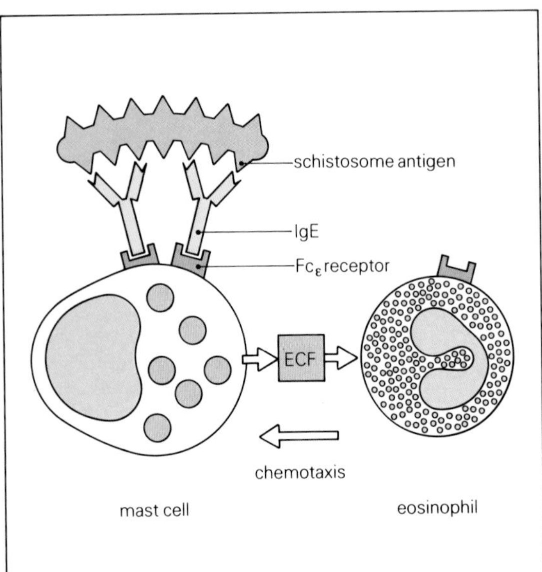

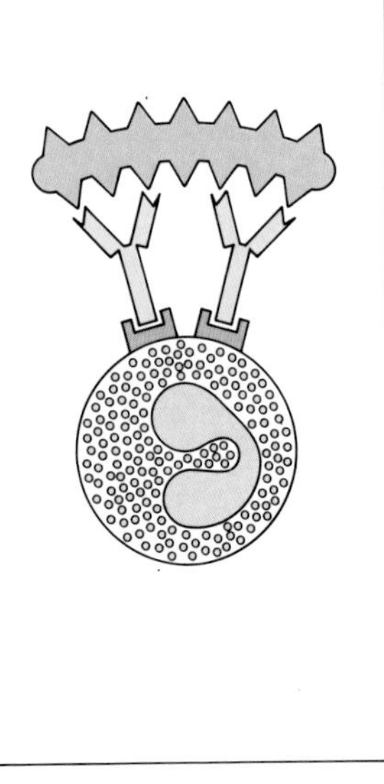

Fig. 9.10 Dual role for antibody in the immune reaction to schistosomes. Mast cells sensitized with IgE anti-schistosome release eosinophil chemotactic factor (ECF) following contact with antigen (left). The arriving eosinophils attach to the antibody-coated worm via their Fc receptors and are important effectors in damaging the parasites (right).

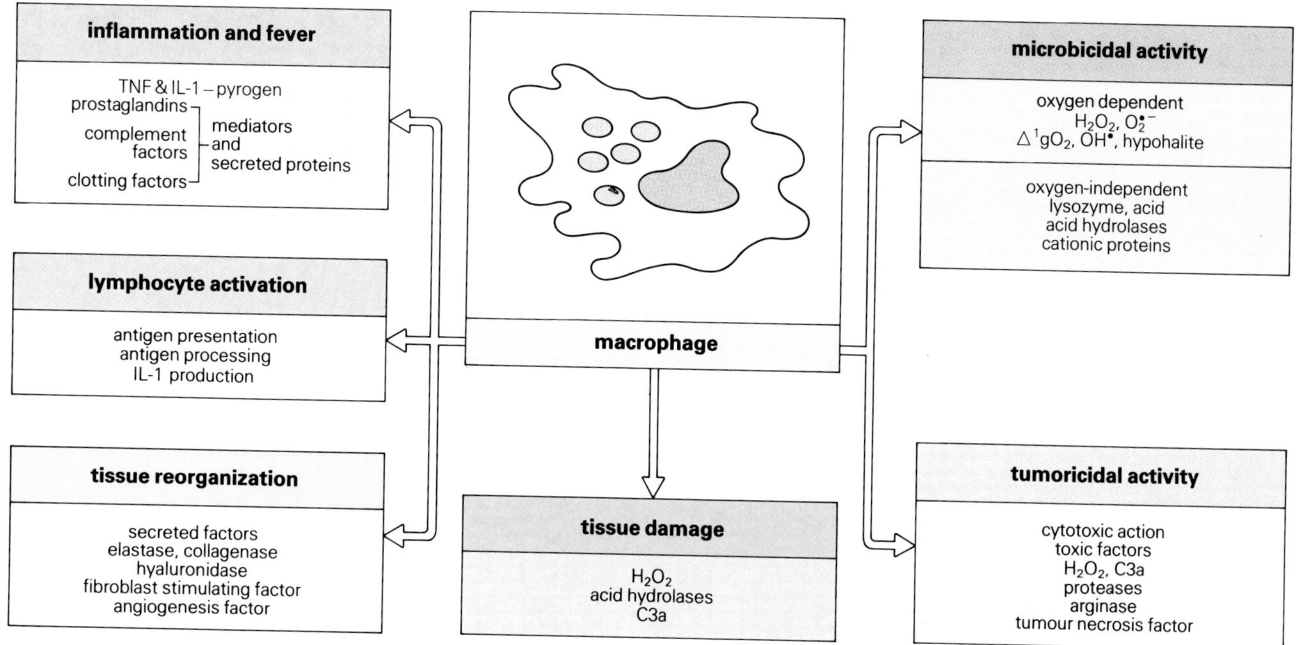

Fig. 9.11 The central role of macrophages. Macrophages and their products listed above are important in both the induction phases of inflammation and tissue reorganization and repair (left) and also perform their effector functions (right). The effector functions may cause tissue damage as in delayed hypersensitivity reactions.

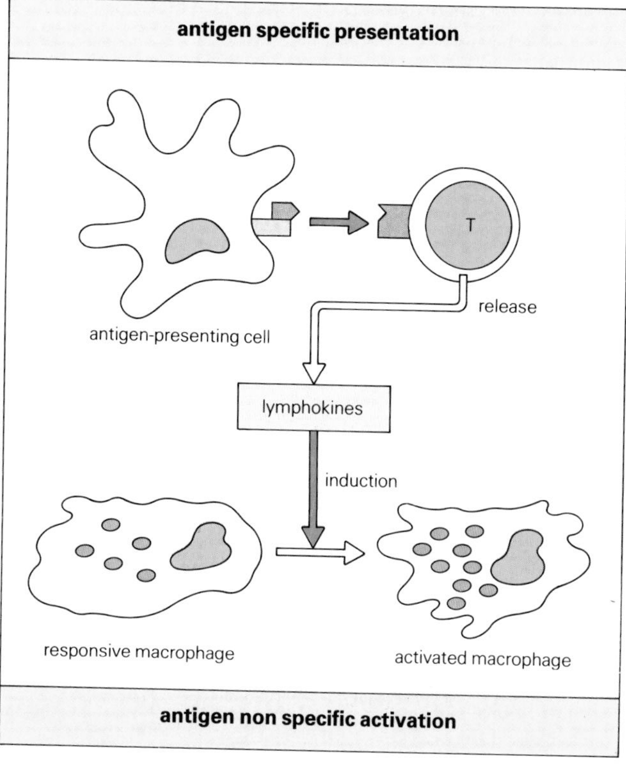

Fig. 9.12 Macrophage activation – I. When antigen is presented to T cells they are stimulated to release factors termed lymphokines, which act on macrophages, causing them in turn to become activated. Note that T cell activation is antigen-specific whereas subsequent macrophage activation is not antigen-specific. Thus, lymphokines released in response to one microorganism's antigens may bring about the destruction of a different microorganism residing in the activated macrophage. Note that macrophages themselves may present antigen to T cells, causing T cells to release cytokines into the immediate vicinity of the responding macrophages.

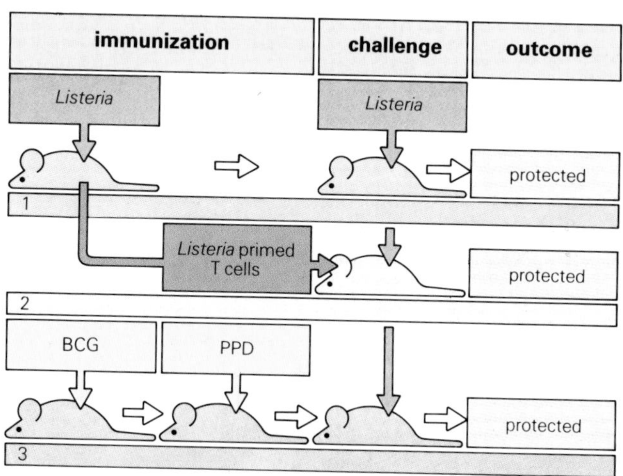

Fig. 9.13 Macrophage activation – II. Animals immunized with *Listeria monocytogenes* are protected against a subsequent challenge with viable bacteria (1). This effect is due to antigen-specific T cells since the immunity can be transferred with T cells from immunized animals (2). However, protection can also be induced by immunization with BCG followed by PPD (antigen of BCG) a few hours before challenge with *Listeria* (3). This implies that specific antigen triggering (T cells) can produce activation of antigen non-specific immune mechanisms (macrophages).

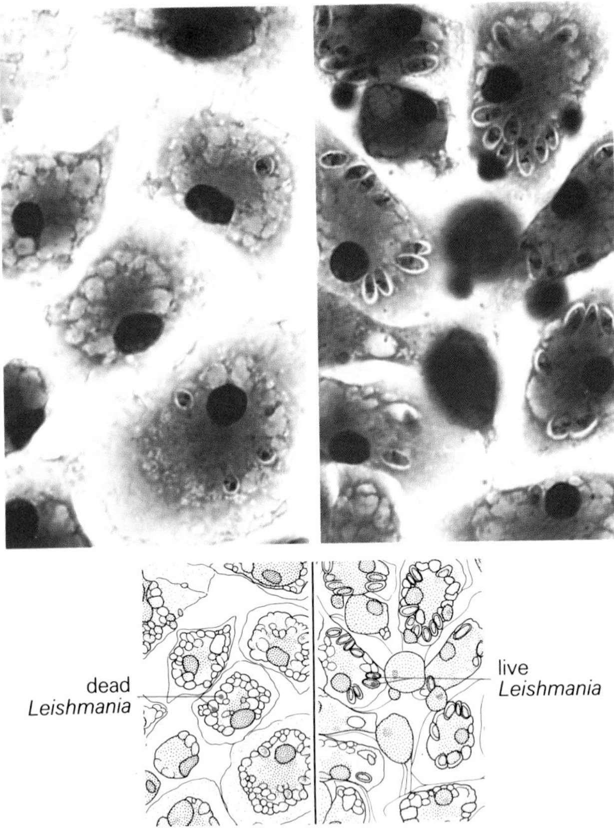

Fig. 9.14 Killing of *Leishmania* by activated macrophages. The destruction of *Leishmania enriettii* by C57 strain mouse macrophages is enhanced by lymphokines. Parasites within the macrophages are destroyed during 48-hour culture with a lymphokine (macrophage activating factor) (left) by comparison with control cultures containing no lymphokine (right). Giemsa stain, x800. (Courtesy of Dr J. Manuel.)

Fig. 9.14 shows macrophages that are infected with *Leishmania enriettii* and incubated with or without mediators derived from lymphocytes, illustrating the difference between activated and non-activated cells.

LYMPHOKINES

The experiments described above have led to the acceptance of the model whereby mediators released from antigen-activated T cells can then activate macrophages; these mediators are termed lymphokines. This raises a number of questions:

1. which lymphocytes can release lymphokines?
2. how many lymphokines are there?
3. does the effect of a lymphokine depend on the stage of maturation of the macrophage on which it acts?
4. can different functions of activated macrophages be dissociated from each other?
5. what is the relationship of this macrophage activation to immunopathological CMI (described in Chapter 22)?

Some of the answers to these questions are presented below and suggest that this macrophage-activation pathway should not be regarded as a single pathway, but as a family of related ones.

THE NATURE OF LYMPHOKINES AND THE CELLS OF ORIGIN

Lymphokines are glycosylated or non-glycosylated polypeptides. The lymphokines, and the macrophage-derived cytokines which may be produced in enhanced quantities under the influence of lymphokines, exert effects on most, perhaps all organ systems, and should be seen as part of a coordinated response to an immunological challenge. This is illustrated in Fig. 9.15. Lymphokines can be secreted by both T cells and B cells, though T cells are assumed to be the major source in cell-mediated responses. There is some evidence from work with T cell hybridomas and T cell clones that not all T cells secrete the same range of lymphokines. For instance it has been suggested that murine T cell clones can be divided into those secreting LT, IL-3, IL-2 and IFNϒ, and those secreting IL-3, IL-4 and IL-5. However not all laboratories find that their clones fit this classification. The major function of lymphokines in the context of this chapter is the activation of macrophages.

THE BIOLOGICAL ROLE OF THE LYMPHOKINES

The study of the biological role of lymphokines is extraordinarily difficult. The early work used crude supernatants of lymphocyte cultures, and was criticized as phenomenology because the active components were unknown. The genes for many of the lymphokines were then cloned, and large quantities of pure substances were made available, which resulted in a flood of publications containing data, often conflicting, on the effects of single mediators in specific experimental systems. This approach, while superficially more promising, can still be biologically misleading, since *in vivo* no lymphokine would ever operate in isolation.

It has recently been pointed out that three types of lymphokine-mediated effects can be recognized (Fig. 9.16):

1. effects mediated by a single lymphokine working alone
2. quantitative effects, increased or decreased according to the status of second signals
3. co-operative (synergistic) effects, where one mediator alone has no effect in the absence of a second one.

ACTIVATION OF MACROPHAGES TO RENDER THEM RESISTANT TO INFECTION

Exposure of murine macrophages to a crude lymphokine-rich spleen cell supernatant makes them resistant to infection by *Leishmania, Candida, Trypanosoma cruzi, Rickettsia,* and *Legionella.* This is an example of the synergistic interactions of lymphokines, since pure recombinant IL-2, IL-4, GM-CSF, or IFNϒ are all unable to cause this effect. However, a combination of IFNϒ and any of the others is active. The only mediator which was shown to be active by itself was TNF.

It is possible that the apparent resistance to infection in this model is in reality due to killing of the organisms on contact with the appropriately activated cells.

ACTIVATION OF MACROPHAGES TO KILL INGESTED ORGANISMS

Circulating monocytes possess the ability to kill some organisms (see Chapter 16). Much of this ability is lost if they are cultured *in vitro,* but exposure to lymphokines, particularly IFNϒ, restores it, and also activates additional killing pathways.

cytokine	immune system source	other cells	principal targets	principal effects
IL-1α IL-1β	macrophages, LGLs, B cells	endothelium, fibroblasts, astrocytes, etc.	T cells, B cells, macrophages, endothelium, tissue cells	lymphocyte activation, macrophage stimulation, ↑ leucocyte/endothelial adhesion, pyrexia, acute phase proteins
IL-2	T cells		T cells	T cell growth factor
IL-3	T cells		stem cells	multilineage colony stimulating factor
IL-4	T cells		B cells, T cells	B cell growth factor
IL-5	T cells		B cells	B cell growth/differentiation
IL-6	T cells, B cells macrophages	fibroblasts	B cells, hepatocytes	B cell growth/differentiation, 'acute phase' response
TNFα	macrophages, lymphocytes		macrophages, granulocytes, tissue cells	activation of macrophages, granulocytes and cytotoxic cells, ↑ leucocyte/endothelial cell adhesion, cachexia, etc.
TNFβ (LT)	T cells			
IFNα	leucocytes	epithelia, fibroblasts	tissue cells	MHC class I induction, antiviral effect
IFNβ	—			
IFNγ	T cells, NK cells	epithelia, fibroblasts	leucocytes and tissue cells	MHC induction, macrophage activation ↑ endothelial cell/lymphocyte adhesion
M-CSF	monocytes	endothelium, fibroblasts		
G-CSF	macrophages	fibroblasts	stem cells	stimulate division and differentiation
GM-CSF	T cells, macrophages	endothelium, fibroblasts		
MIF	T cells		macrophages	migration inhibition

Fig. 9.15 List of the major cytokines. The cytokines in the list above have all been identified as distinct by genomic cloning with the exception of MIF. Note that only the principle sources, targets and effects have been included in this table. Most cytokines act in concert with others to produce their biological effects *in vivo*.

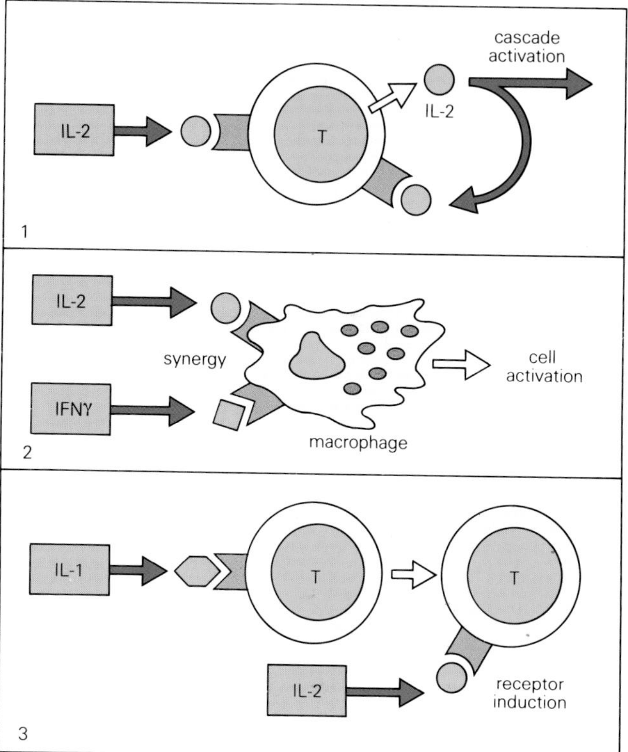

Fig. 9.16 Lymphokine synergy. Many lymphokine actions are synergistic. This diagram illustrates three kinds of synergy, with particular examples.
1. Cascade activation. A T cell is triggered to divide by a signal which includes IL-2. The activated cell releases more IL-2 which can act both on the original cell and on other responsive T cells.
2. Synergy by dual activation. Some cells such as macrophages require triggers from two different cytokines together, before developing their full range of functions.
3. Receptor induction. In the presence of IL-1, expression of IL-2 receptors is up-regulated on T cells, thereby making the cell more responsive to IL-2.

MACROPHAGE ACTIVATION AND TUMOUR CELL KILLING

Macrophage activation is a complex phenomenon and the various effector functions can be dissociated from one another. Thus it is possible to activate murine macrophages so that they have an increased ability to kill *Listeria monocytogenes* without increasing their ability to kill tumour cells, or mycobacteria. There are two reasons for this complexity.

1. The monocyte/macrophage series is very heterogeneous and cells taken from different sites differ in such relevant characteristics as expression of class II MHC glycopeptides, Fc receptors, lymphokine responsiveness and production of peroxidase. Most authors nevertheless believe that there is only one lineage of macrophages and that these differences are due to environmental and maturational effects.
2. As hinted in the previous section, the functions activated may depend not only on the pre-existing functional and maturational stage of the macrophage, but also on the precise 'blend' of lymphokines and inflammatory stimuli to which it is exposed. Fig. 9.17 shows some of the changes which can be induced by inflammation alone as well as by lymphokine treatment *in vitro*.

It is suggested that activation occurs in stages, and requires sequential stimuli, which include lymphokines, endotoxin, various mediators and regulators of inflammation (*in vitro*, plastic or glass surfaces and tissue culture media are important). Different effector functions may be expressed at each stage. There is also evidence that activated macrophages can be de-activated. It has been suggested that prostaglandin E may have this effect.

characteristic		inflammatory macrophage	lymphokine-treated *in vitro*
cell volume		↑	↑
spreading		↑	↑
pinocytosis		↑	?
phagocytosis	via Fc receptor	↑	?
	via C3 receptor	↑	?
secretion of O_2-reduction products (O_2 and H_2O_2)		↑	↑
secretion of neutral proteases	plasminogen activation	↑	↑
	collagenase	↑	↑
hydrolase content of lysosomes		↑	↓?
plasma membrane 5'-nucleotidase		↓	↓

Fig. 9.17 Changes occurring in inflammatory, or lymphokine-activated macrophages. Some of the changes may be due to recruitment of monocytes. It is difficult to study purely lymphokine-mediated effects without any contribution from inflammatory or environmental factors, such as culture plates, or synthetic media. These findings are based on mouse peritoneal macrophages. The common decrease in plasma membrane 5'-nucleotidase is shown to indicate that the activation has some specificity and that not all properties and enzyme activities increase in parallel.

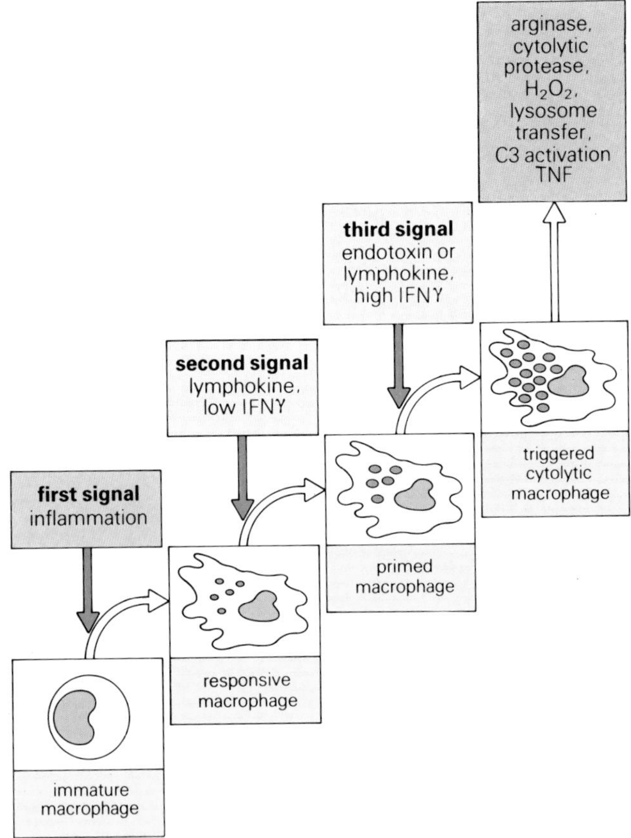

Fig. 9.18 A hypothetical scheme for the activation of murine peritoneal macrophages to destroy tumour cells. It is thought that macrophage activation occurs in a series of steps.

Fig. 9.18 shows a scheme for the activation of the tumoricidal function of murine peritoneal macrophages. Binding to the tumour cells occurs via a receptor for an unknown feature of tumour membranes, or via Fc-receptors and antibody. There may be distinct slow, and rapid mechanisms for tumour cell damage.

MACROPHAGE-DERIVED CYTOKINES

As shown in Fig. 9.15, monocytes and macrophages release a number of regulatory mediators or cytokines. Macrophages which have been activated by lymphokines have an enhanced potential for release of these mediators, though this may require a further triggering signal. Killing of tumour cells by tumour necrosis factor (TNF) requires such a second signal (Fig. 9.18) which can be provided by lipopolysaccharide, a number of other bacterial products, or sometimes by the tumour cells themselves.

TNF, acting in synergy with IL-1 and perhaps IL-6 is particularly important to an understanding of the consequences of infection and the immunopathology which can accompany cell-mediated responses.

TUMOUR NECROSIS FACTOR (TNF-α)

Two experimental systems led independently to the discovery of tumour necrosis factor (TNF-α). The first was the induction of necrosis in tumours by injection of factor-containing sera into the tumour-bearing animal. This phenomenon occurred if the donor animal was prepared by an injection of BCG, *Corynebacterium parvum*, or schistosome ova, about 2 weeks before an injection of LPS. The activated macrophages associated with the T cell-dependent granulomata are probably the source of the TNF. The second system was the weight loss and hypertriglyceridaemia which accompanies some parasitic infections such as trypanosomiasis in cattle and rabbits. This was found to be due in part to down-regulation of lipoprotein lipase by a factor released mainly from macrophages. Release could be provoked by endotoxin (LPS).

The TNF gene is situated close to the gene for lymphotoxin, to which it shows a 28% sequence homology. Interestingly it is also 70 kilobases from the D locus of the MHC. The major sources are monocytes and activated macrophages, though other cells such as cytotoxic lymphoid cells also express the gene. It is present on the membrane of macrophages, and may be released from them by cleavage of the membrane-bound form. Numerous stimuli will cause its release, including components of bacteria and protozoa, and some tumour cells.

Fig. 9.19 shows some of the effects of TNF. *In vivo* TNF acts in synergy with numerous other cytokines, particularly IL-1, with which it shares some properties and also IFNγ. Some of the effects shown are clearly beneficial components of cell-mediated immunity. However, under other circumstances, TNF is responsible for important immunopathology.

Harmful Effects of TNF Of particular importance in this context are the harmful effects of TNF on endothelial cells and neutrophils. Endothelial cells lose their usual anticoagulant properties, and enhance fibrin deposition. This may result in diffuse intravascular coagulation, and eventually the plasma becomes depleted of clotting factors, and will not clot. TNF also promotes adherence of polymorphonuclear cells to the endothelium, and causes them to degranulate and form reactive oxygen intermediates such as the superoxide anion and hydrogen peroxide. As a consequence of these and other properties, TNF is now thought to be a major mediator of the circulatory collapse and widespread tissue necrosis which can accompany bacterial septicaemia (Fig. 9.20). Neutralizing antibodies will prevent death in appropriate models, and injections of pure recombinant TNF will mimic many of the effects. TNF was readily detected in the serum of children dying from *Neisseria meningitidis* septicaemia. Moreover antisera to TNF will also modulate acute graft versus host reactions implying its importance in local as well as systemic immune reactions. These phenomena are discussed further in relation to bacterial infections in Chapter 16.

Protective Effects of TNF

1. Tumours. TNF appears to be responsible for most of the tumoricidal activity of human monocytes, and as mentioned earlier, it may play a role in the action of cytotoxic lymphoid cells. However, not all tumour lines are sensitive to it. The standard bioassay *in vitro* makes use of the fact that certain tumour lines are exquisitely sensitive to TNF in the presence of metabolic inhibitors such as emetine or actinomycin D. The necrosis evoked in tumours *in vivo* is probably due more to damage to the

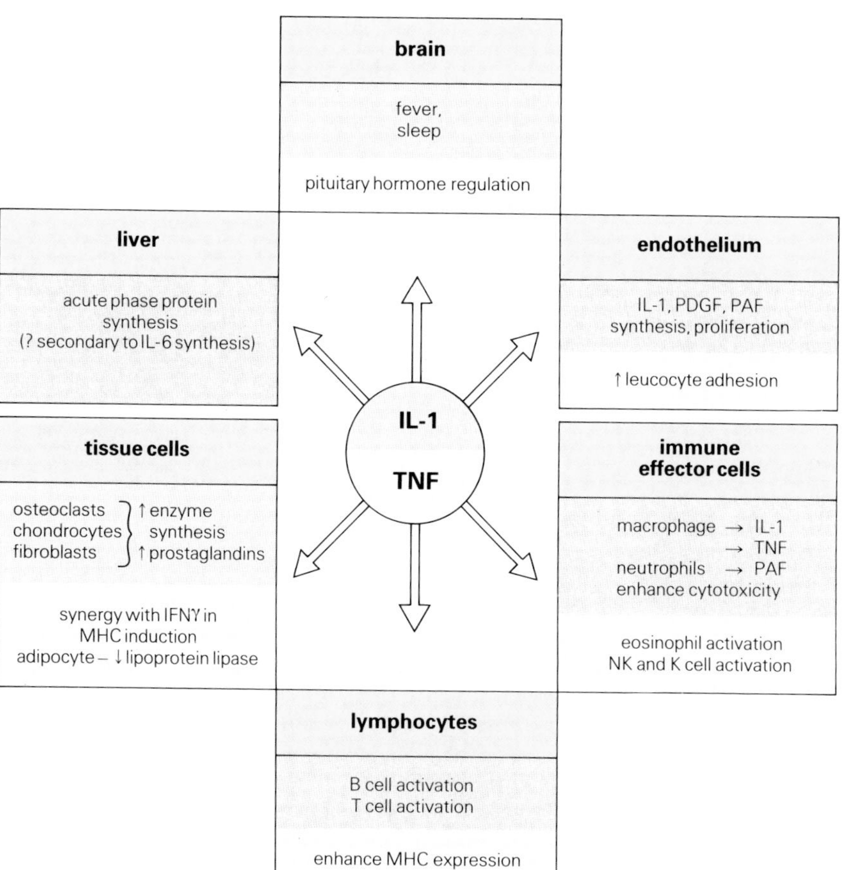

Fig. 9.19 Actions of IL-1 and TNF. IL-1 and TNF have many effects in common, both on leucocytes and on other tissues of the body. In this diagram those effects primarily mediated by IL-1 are pink, those by TNF are blue, and those mediated by both are purple. There is however considerable overlap of all these functions, particularly across different species.

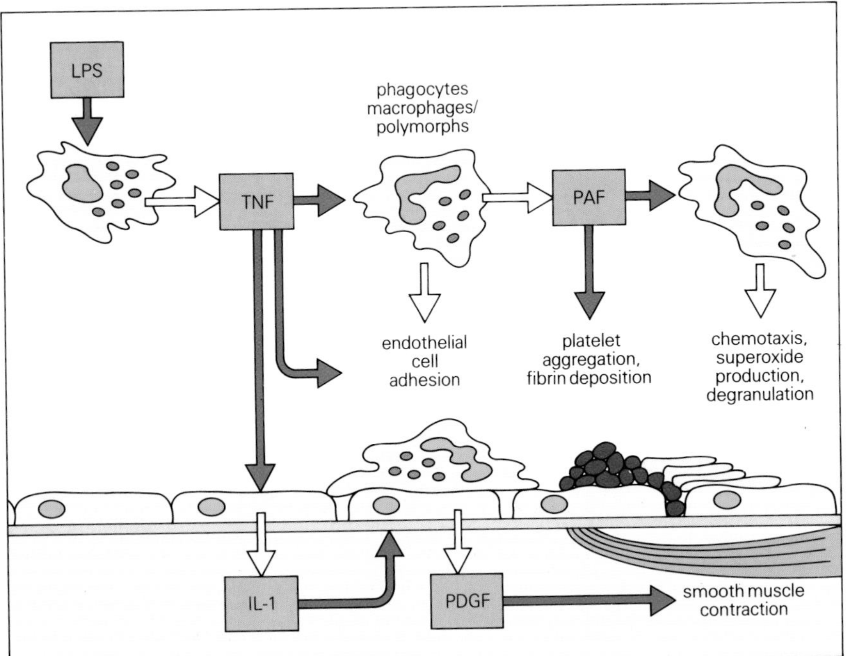

Fig. 9.20 Role of TNF in endotoxic shock. LPS activation of primed macrophages causes the release of TNF which generates a cascade of reactions including endothelial cell, macrophage and neutrophil activation. These reactions lead to diffuse intravascular coagulation and tissue damage mediated by platelet activating factor (PAF), smooth muscle contraction, and alterations in the endothelium causing leucocyte adhesion and fibrin deposition.

vasculature of the tumour by mechanisms discussed in the previous section, than to direct effects on tumour cells. This implies that for some reason the vasculature of some tumours is more sensitive to TNF than the vasculature in normal tissues. Trials of TNF for the treatment of human neoplasia have had variable success.

2. Microorganisms. As shown in Fig. 9.19, TNF can activate some functions of eosinophils, neutrophils, and macrophages, and this may be relevant to protection against pathogens. *In vivo* TNF can protect mice from malaria, and some *Legionella*. Moreover TNF can induce resistance to both RNA and DNA virus infection in some cell types, and selectively kills virus-infected cells. These effects are synergistic with those of IFNγ (see Chapter 16).

CHRONIC CELL-MEDIATED RESPONSES

When foreign antigenic material cannot be degraded, T cells accumulate and release lymphokines. This leads to the aggregation and proliferation of macrophages and the characteristic appearance of a nodular mass called a granuloma which consists of multinucleate giant cells, epithelioid cells and activated macrophages. The granuloma isolates the focus of the infection (Fig. 9.21).

A granuloma can be produced experimentally using soluble antigen conjugated covalently onto an insoluble particle, such as a sepharose bead. Antigen-coated beads will evoke T cell-dependent granulomata in appropriately immunized mice, whereas control beads will not (Fig. 9.22). If such granulomata are explanted *in vitro* they can be shown to release mediators, presumably lymphokines, with macrophage-activating and chemotactic properties. Thus the T cell plays a dual role in granuloma formation by causing both accumulation and activation of phagocytes. Such granulomata are characteristic of infections with either organisms which live at least partly intracellularly (for example, *Mycobacterium tuberculosis, M. leprae, Leishmania, Listeria*

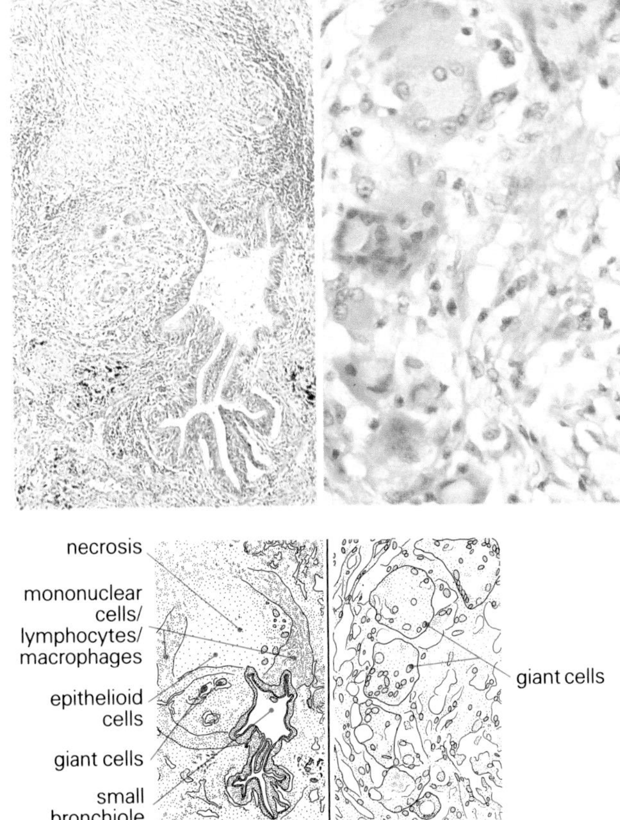

Fig. 9.21 A granulomatous reaction in pulmonary tuberculosis. The central area of caseous necrosis in which much of the cellular structure is destroyed is characteristic of tuberculosis in the lung. This is surrounded by a ring of epithelioid cells and mononuclear cells. Multinucleate giant cells, thought to be derived from the fusion of epithelioid cells, are also present (left, x170). Giant cells are illustrated at a higher magnification (right, x 270). H&E stain. (Courtesy of Dr G. Boyd.)

monocytogenes), or organisms which are large and persistent (for example, schistosome ova). Granulomata are a site of localization and destruction of organisms by activated macrophages, and a component of the immunopathology of the diseases. Analysis of the T cells in granulomatous foci indicate that CD4$^+$ cells are located at the centre and CD8$^+$ cells around the periphery, suggesting that CD4$^+$ cells are of prime importance in antigen recognition and accumulation of other lymphocytes and macrophages (Fig. 9.23). In mice, the activity of T cell dependent granulomata eventually wanes under the influence of suppressor T cells.

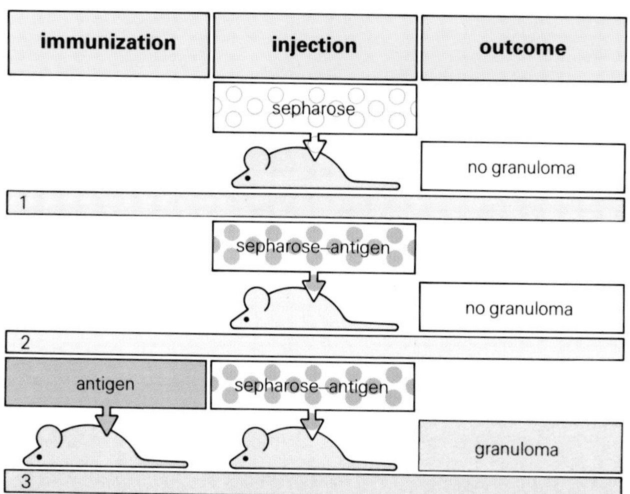

Fig. 9.22 Artificial production of a granuloma. Mice injected with either normal sepharose beads (1) or sepharose beads coupled to antigen (2) do not develop any local granulomatous reaction, but if the animal is previously immunized to the antigen (3) it does. If the granulomatous tissue and beads are recovered from animal 3 they release, into culture, factors with macrophage-chemotactic and activating properties.

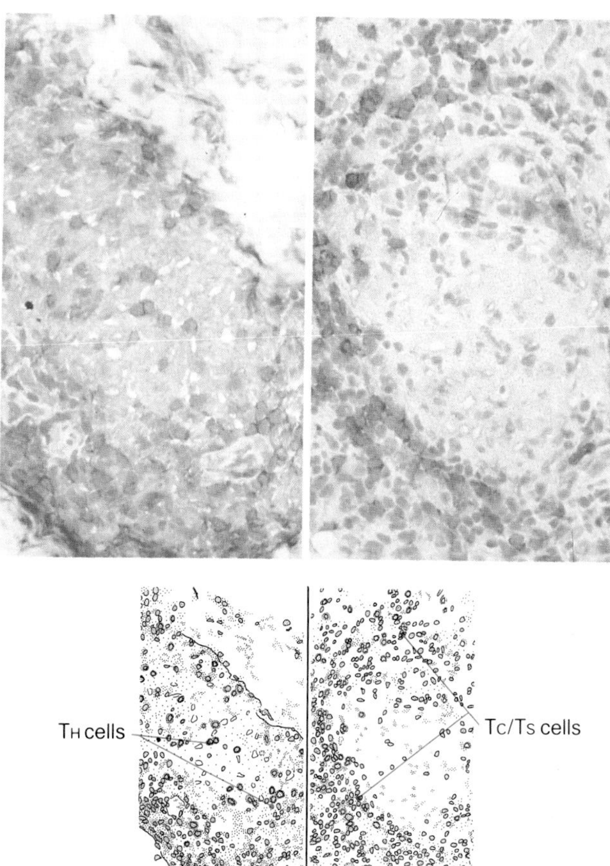

Fig. 9.23 CD4 and CD8 staining of a granuloma. Shown here is a dermal granuloma from a patient with borderline tuberculoid leprosy stained red with peroxidase-coupled antibodies to Leu 3 (equivalent to CD4) (left) and Leu 2 (equivalent to CD8) (right). Leu 3 T-helper cells are present in and around the lesion while Leu 2 cytotoxic/suppressor T cells occur mainly on the periphery. (Courtesy of Dr R. L. Modlin and Dr T. H. Rea.)

FURTHER READING

Adams, D. (1982) Molecules, membranes, and macrophage activation. *Immunology Today*, **3**, 285.

Carrick, L. & Boros, D.L. (1980) The artificial granuloma 1. *In vitro* lymphokine production by pulmonary artificial hypersensitivity granulomas. *Clinical Immunology and Immunopathology*, **17**, 415.

Cerami, A. & Beutler, B. (1988) The role of cachectin/TNF in endotoxin shock and cachexia. *Immunology Today*, **9**, 28.

Eckels, D.D., Lamb, P., Lake, P., Woody, J.N., Johnson, A.H. & Hartzman, R. (1982) Antigen-specific human T lymphocyte clones. Genetic restriction of influenza virus-specific responses to HLA–D region genes. *Human Immunology*, **4**, 313.

Kohl, S. & Loo, L.S. (1982) Protection of neonatal mice against herpes simplex virus infections: probable *in vivo* antibody-dependent cellular cytotoxicity. *Journal of Immunology*, **129**, 370.

McMichael, A.J., Gotch, F. & Noble, G.R. (1983) Cytotoxic T cell immunity to influenza. *New England Journal of Medicine*, **309**, 13.

Nathan, C.F., Murray, H.W., Wiebe, M.E. & Rubin, B.Y. (1983) Identification of interferon-γ as the lymphokine that activates human macrophage oxidative metabolism and antimicrobial activity. *Journal of Experimental Medicine*, **158**, 670.

Oppenheim, J.J. & Geryl, I. (1982) Interleukin-1 is more than an interleukin. *Immunology Today*, **3**, 113.

Ritz, J., Schmidt, R.E., Michon, J., Hercend, T. & Schlossman, S.F. (1988) Characterisation of functional surface structures on human natural killer cells. *Advances in Immunology*, **42**, 181.

Rook, G.A.W. (1988) The role of activated macrophages in the immunopathology of tuberculosis. *British Medical Bulletin*, **44(3)**, 624.

Rosenstein, M., Eberlein, F.J. & Rosenberg, S.A. (1984) Adoptive immunotherapy of established syngeneic solid tumours: role of T lymphoid subpopulations. *Journal of Immunology*, **132**, 2117.

Steinman, R.M. & Nussenzweig, M.C. (1980) Dendritic cells: features and functions. *Immunological Reviews*, **53**, 127.

Unanue, E.R. (1984) Antigen-presenting function of the macrophage. *Annual Review of Immunology*, **2**, 395.

Warner, J.F. & Dennert, G. (1982) Effects of a cloned cell line with NK activity on bone marrow transplants, tumour development, and metastasis *in vivo*. *Nature*, **300**, 31.

Young, J.D. & Liu, C. (1988) Multiple mechanisms of lymphocyte-mediated killing. *Immunology Today*, **9**, 140–144.

Zinkernage, R.M. & Doherty, P.C. (1979) MHC-restricted cytotoxic T cells. Studies on the biological role of polymorphic major transplantation antigens determining T cell restriction specificity, function and responsiveness. *Advances in Immunology*, **27**, 51.

10 Regulation of the Immune Response

Once an immune response is initiated the components of that response, for example B cells, are capable of immense replication as seen in the classical secondary response, and in experiments involving the transfer of lymphocytes into X-irradiated recipients (Fig. 10.1). Thus immune responses must normally be subject to strict and specific controls affecting not only the magnitude of the response but also a host of other parameters governing the type of reaction elicited, referred to as the modality of the response. For example, the immune system determines what type of cell-mediated or antibody response is produced to any particular antigen, and also the spectrum of antibody isotypes generated.

The primary regulator of the immune response is of course the antigen itself, which can either produce an immune reaction as described in Chapters 8 and 9, or induce a state of tolerance (see Chapter 12). The pivotal role of antigen is so important that the immune system can be considered as a tissue with the principal homeostatic function of eliminating antigen. The complexity of the system arises from the wide variety of antigens in the environment, their various points of entry into the body and the necessity of mounting an appropriate reaction to each. Although antigen is crucial, there are also a number of other regulatory mechanisms which are intrinsic to the immune system. Although these other immunoregulatory controls may interact with antigen at some points, many involve only internal components of the immune system.

THE REGULATORY EFFECT OF ANTIBODY

The simplest and longest-known mechanism for regulating humoral immunity is that by which circulating antibody regulates the production of antibody. Fig. 10.2

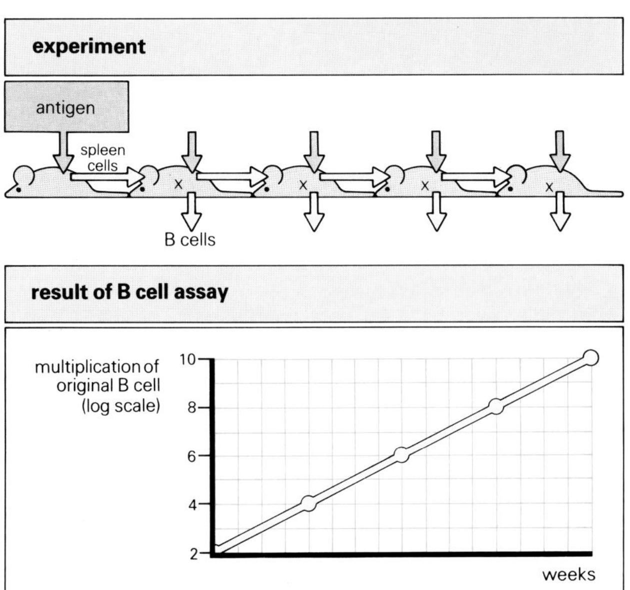

Fig. 10.1 Replicative potential of a B cell clone. A mouse was immunized with antigen and the antigen-primed spleen cells (5×10^6) were transferred into X-irradiated recipient mice, which were then injected with the same antigen. Some recipients produced homogeneous antibody indicating that a single clone had been transferred. Assay of these B cells after each transfer revealed that the clone continued to multiply through three further transfers as shown in the graph. The transferred cells of such a clone increased 100-fold between each transfer, therefore a B cell must have the potential to produce at least 10^{10} cells.

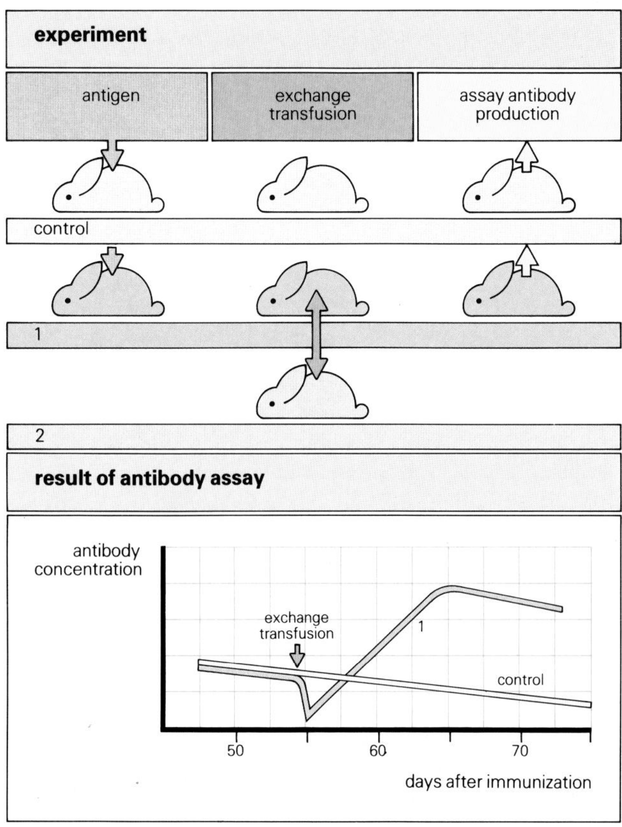

Fig. 10.2 Demonstration of the role of antibody in regulating its own production. Two rabbits (control, 1) are injected with antigen. Rabbit 1 has its serum exchanged with that of a non-immunized rabbit (2) in order to reduce its serum antibody concentration. The production of antibody by both the control rabbit and the exchange-transfused rabbit is then assayed. If the antibody is artificially reduced (1), the rate of specific antibody production is increased causing the concentration to overshoot that expected without exchange transfusion. Exchange transfusion does not remove the antigen because it is fixed in the lymphoid tissues.

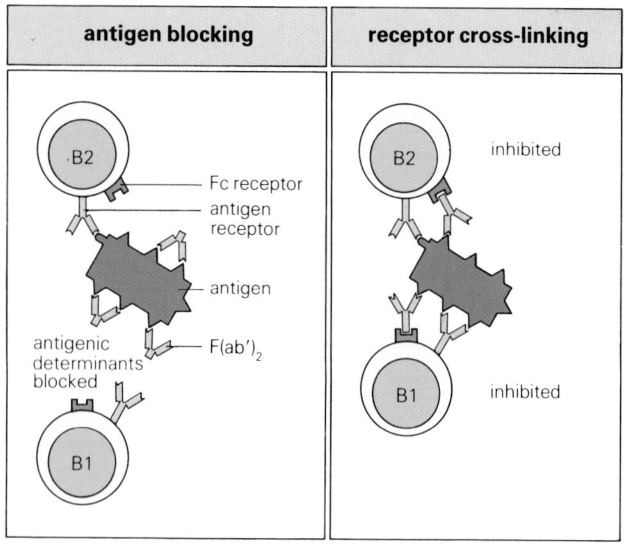

Fig. 10.3 Antibody-dependent B cell regulation – two ways in which antibody feedback can suppress the antibody response.
Antigen blocking. High doses of antibody (or its $F(ab')_2$ fragment) block the interaction between an antigenic determinant (epitope) and B cell receptors for that determinant, which are then effectively unable to recognize the antigen (B1). This receptor blocking mechanism also prevents B cell priming. B cells with receptors for different epitopes are unaffected (B2).
Receptor cross-linking. Low doses of antibody – but not $F(ab')_2$ – allow cross-linking between a B cell's Fc receptors and its antigen receptors. This inhibits the B cell from entering the phase of antibody synthesis but does not inhibit B cell priming. The effect is not epitope-specific.

illustrates a direct demonstration of this; there is a prompt increase in the rate of antibody synthesis in a long-term immunized rabbit when its antibody is removed by replacing its serum with normal serum.

There are two ways in which antibody is known to suppress the production of further antibody: antigen blocking and receptor cross-linking (Fig. 10.3).

Antigen blocking occurs when antibody combines with the antigen and thus competes with the antigen receptors of responding B cells. As might be expected this mechanism depends strictly on the concentration of the antibody and its affinity compared to that of the cellular receptors, and is independent of the Fc portion of the antibody.

In many situations, however, antibody can be shown to have a suppressive effect which is Fc-dependent. As a result of experiments *in vitro* (which overcome the problem that $F(ab')_2$ fragments are so rapidly cleared *in vivo*), the Fc-dependent effect has been shown to interfere with the productive response of T dependent B cells, but to leave the priming of both T and B cells unimpaired. It is postulated that the whole antibody molecule inhibits B cell differentiation by cross-linking the antigen receptor with the Fc receptor (Fig. 10.3). The $F(ab')_2$ fragment, on the other hand, has no effect at the low concentrations at which whole antibody works, but by its blocking activity at higher concentrations it is able to inhibit both T and B priming and the productive response.

Doses of antibody which are insufficient to completely inhibit the production of antibody have the effect of increasing its average affinity (Fig. 10.4). For this reason antibody feedback is thought to be an important factor driving the process of affinity maturation. It is thought that this process involves competition between the free antibody and the B cell antigen receptors. Antibody binds to the stimulating antigen, thus reducing the free antigen concentration; consequently only those B cells with high affinity receptors bind to the antigen and are stimulated into division and maturation.

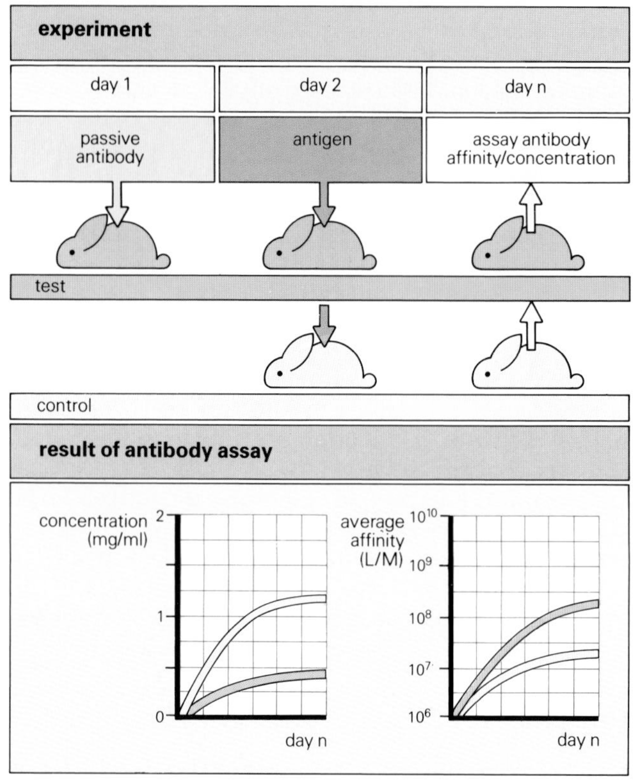

Fig. 10.4 Effect of passive antibody on the affinity and concentration of secreted antibody. One of two rabbits was injected with antibody (passive antibody) on day 1. Both rabbits were immunized with antigen on day 2 and the affinity and concentration of antibody raised to this antigen were assayed at a later time (day n). The results of the antibody assay show that passive antibody reduces the concentration but increases the affinity of antibody produced.

THE REGULATORY EFFECT OF IMMUNE COMPLEXES

It was seen in the preceding section that antibody, in its Fc-dependent mechanism, only regulates the B cell after first forming an immune complex with the antigen. Thus it is not surprising that preformed immune complexes often suppress B cell activation. Sometimes, however, they may augment the immune response, particularly when the ratio of antigen to antibody is high. This enhancing effect is also Fc-dependent, and may operate by encouraging fixation of the antigen on certain antigen-presenting cells, which is consistent with the greatly enhanced localization of antigen in germinal centres (where some antigen-presenting cells occur)

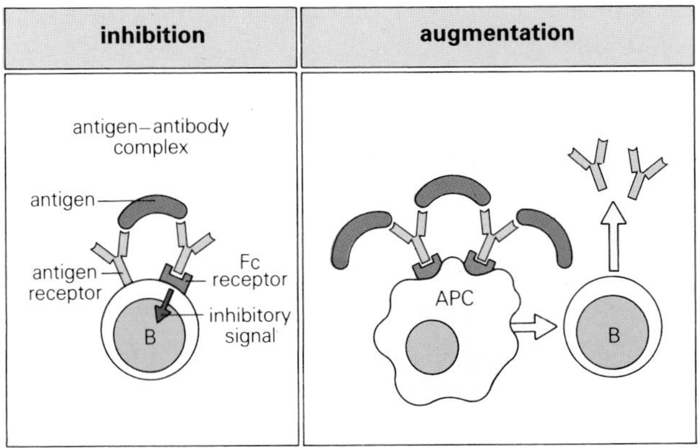

Fig. 10.5 Regulatory effects of immune complexes – inhibition and augmentation.
Inhibition. When the B cell's Fc receptor is cross-linked to its antigen receptor by an antigen–antibody complex, a signal is delivered to the B cell inhibiting it from entering the antibody production phase.
Augmentation. Antibody encourages presentation of antigen to B cells when it is present on an antigen-presenting cell (APC), bound via Fc receptors. (Complexes can also activate complement and bind to APCs via their C3b receptors in an analagous way.)

when complexed to antibody. The postulated mechanisms for the action of immune complexes are illustrated in Fig. 10.5.

In a general sense it could clearly be useful for early appearing antibody to augment the response, and for later appearing antibody to inhibit it when the antibody concentration exceeds that required to neutralize the antigen. The effect of antibody and of complexes is greatly influenced by the antibody's isotype. In general, IgM antibodies have the strongest tendency to enhance the response, while IgG is more often suppressive. There are interesting differences among the IgG isotypes, but it is not profitable to particularize in the present context.

IDIOTYPIC REGULATION

An antibody's variable (V) and hypervariable regions may act as antigenic determinants. The experimental induction of anti-idiotype antibodies shows that lymphocytes exist which are capable of recognizing and responding to the combining sites of antibodies and receptors on other lymphocytes. Thus there may be regulatory interactions between the lymphocytes and antibodies of the immune system via their antigen combining sites.

To facilitate discussion of this field, it is first necessary to define the structures which may be involved in these regulatory interactions (Fig. 10.6). The antigenic constitution of the V region of an immunoglobulin is known as its idiotype. The antigenic determinants of which the idiotype is made up are referred to as idiotopes. Finally, that part of the V region which forms its specific binding site is called its paratope. Some idiotopes will be found within the paratope, but others will be outside it.

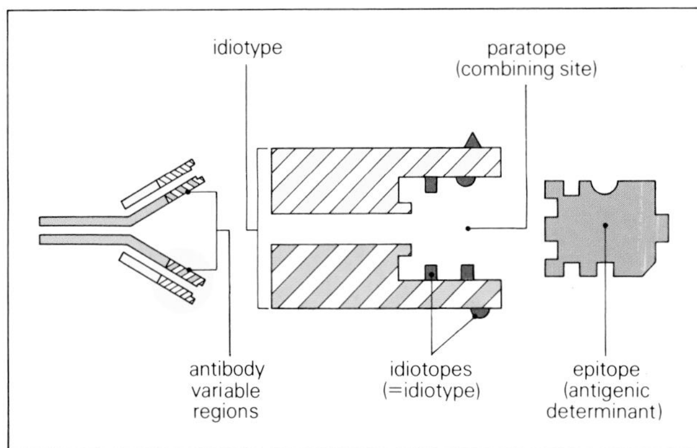

Fig. 10.6 Nomenclature in relation to the antibody variable domain. The determinants making up the antibody V region are termed idiotopes. Some idiotopes are located in the combining site (also referred to as the paratope), whilst others occur outside the paratope. The full set of V region determinants is termed the idiotype of the antibody molecule. Determinants on the antigen molecule are called epitopes.

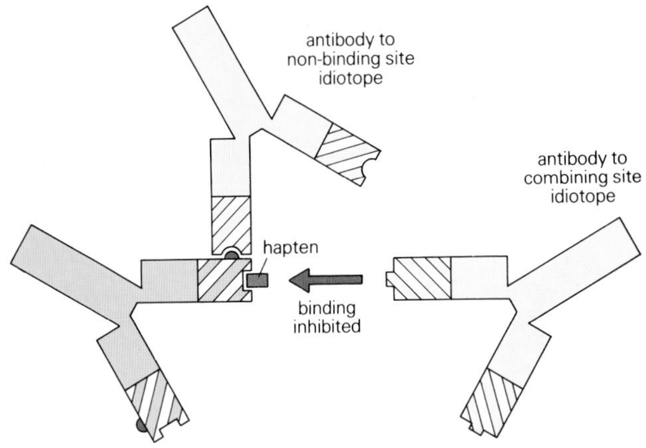

Fig. 10.7 Distinction between idiotopes inside and outside the antibody combining site. An anti-idiotype serum may contain some antibodies directed to idiotopes associated with the combining site (site associated). The binding to these can be inhibited by hapten. Antibodies to non-binding site idiotopes (non-site associated) will not be inhibited by hapten.

Anti-immunoglobulin sera do not normally contain a high concentration of antibody directed against a particular idiotype (anti-idiotype). This is because the normal immunoglobulin used for immunization is too heterogeneous in its V region to induce a particular anti-idiotype. Using a myeloma protein however, or homogeneous antibody, it is possible to produce an anti-idiotype serum which reacts with one or more idiotopes in the V region of the immunizing antibody.

Anti-idiotypes, directed against idiotopes within the combining site and anti-idiotypes directed against idiotopes outside the combining site can be distinguished: only those binding to the antigen combining site inhibit the interaction between that combining site and a hapten (Fig. 10.7). Thus, it is clearly possible for anti-idiotype to substitute for the original antigen (Fig. 10.8). Like antigen it may either stimulate or depress the immune response. Anti-idiotype, unlike

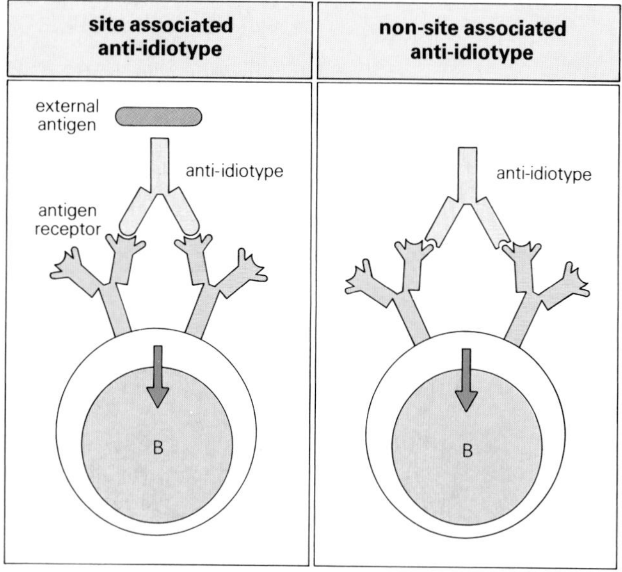

Fig. 10.8 Regulation by site associated and non-site associated anti-idiotype. Site associated anti-idiotype mimics the external (original) antigen and cross-links the B cell's antigen receptors. This delivers a signal to the B cell. Since non-site associated anti-idiotype also cross-links the B cell's antigen receptors, it can also deliver a signal. The direction of its effect depends on many factors, most of which are unknown.

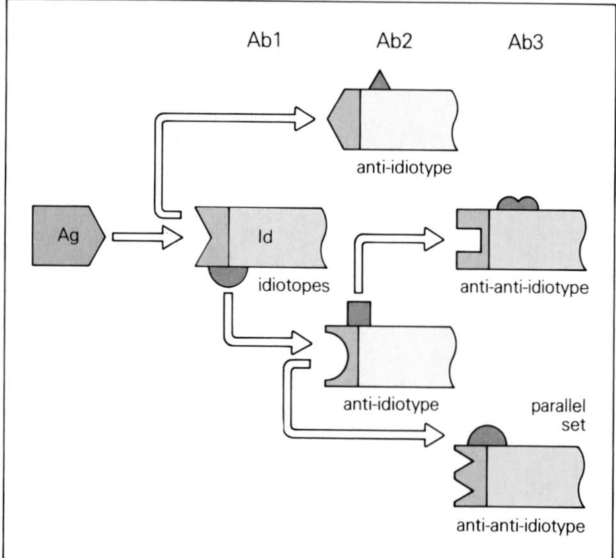

Fig. 10.9 Jerne's Network Hypothesis. In this conceptual framework, antigen stimulates the production of an antibody bearing the original idiotype (Id) comprising a number of idiotopes (pink and red). The Id stimulates anti-idiotypes which regulate production of the Id. The anti-idiotypes are in turn regulated by anti-anti-idiotypes. The sets of antibodies comprising these chains of recognition are sometimes referred to as Ab1, Ab2, Ab3, etc. Note that the upper anti-Id has an idiotope resembling the external antigen and is known as the internal image of the antigen. Some antibodies share idiotopes with the original Id but do not share paratopes; these parallel sets of antibodies will be regulated in tandem. The hypothesis does not make specific predictions on the degree of regulation or even its direction (stimulation or inhibition).

antigen bears an Fc region and can therefore interact with Fc receptors (Fig. 10.5).

Knowing that such interactions between idiotypes and anti-idiotypes are possible, Jerne has built up a conceptual framework indicating how they may function in the maintenance of immunological homeostasis by forming a network with widespread connections (Fig. 10.9). This very general concept is currently undergoing more detailed investigation. The evidence that such a network may exist is mainly indirect, and is discussed in the next section.

EVIDENCE THAT IDIOTYPIC INTERACTIONS ARE IMPORTANT IN IMMUNOREGULATION

Striking evidence has been obtained that anti-idiotypes can affect the representation of recognized idiotypes in immune responses. Depending on the experimental conditions, either enhancement or suppression may occur. When mice of the C57BL/6 strain are challenged with the hapten, NP, they produce antibodies of which a high proportion are restricted to a few defined idiotypes, for example, idiotype 146. Anti-idiotype to this antibody can enhance or suppress the production of idiotype 146, depending on the amount of anti-idiotype given (Fig. 10.10), when these mice are subsequently challenged

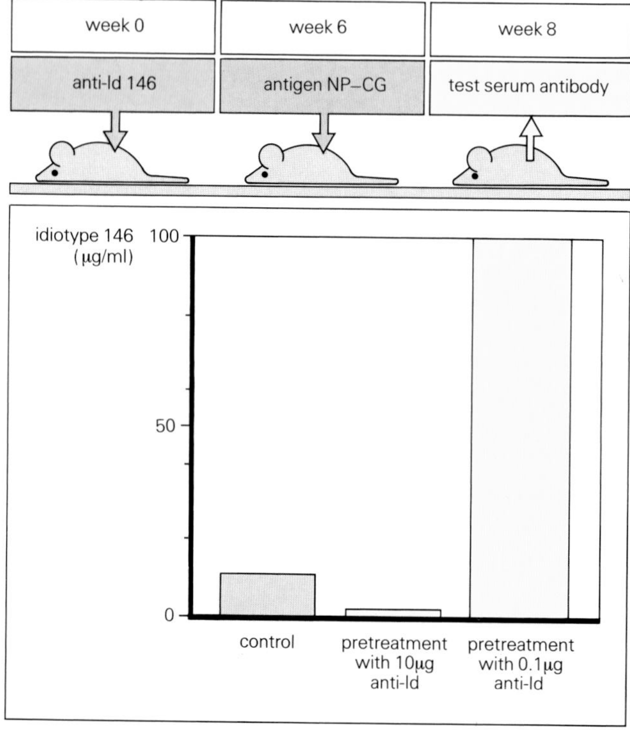

Fig. 10.10 Modulation of idiotype by anti-idiotype. Mice were injected at time O with either 10μg or 0.1μg of anti-idiotype (anti-Id) to the nitrophenyl (NP) binding antibody 146. The animals were then challenged 6 weeks later with NP on the carrier chicken globulin (CG). Two weeks later the serum titres of idiotype 146 (bar diagram), and total anti-NP (not shown) were assayed. Mice pretreated with 10μg anti-Id showed suppression of idiotype 146 while mice treated with 0.1μg showed enhanced production of idiotype 146, although the overall levels of anti-NP were similar in both groups.

with NP on a carrier protein. The suppression is idiotype specific as the level of anti-NP is hardly affected. Most importantly, the amounts of anti-idiotype causing these effects are in the physiological range for particular idiotype bearing antibodies, which suggests that idiotypic regulation may occur *in vivo*. Similar effects have been seen in a number of other systems using different antigens.

Some of the most dramatic effects are seen in neonatal animals where the effect of neonatally administered anti-idiotype can be lifelong. For example, the ability of neonatal mice to mount an anti-phosphorylcholine response after being injected with anti-idiotype to T15 (T15 is a major idiotype in the response to phosphorylcholine), is greatly reduced for many months. It has also been found that maternal anti-idiotype antibodies which are transmitted to offspring across the placenta, can greatly alter the representation of those idiotypes in the offspring. This means that immunological events within the mother can have long-lasting effects on the immune response of the offspring. Cell transfer experiments have shown that idiotype specific priming and suppression are maintained by specific T cell populations.

When a response is made to an antigen for the first time, the sharp rise in concentration of the complementary antibodies is itself a potential antigenic stimulus. Idiotype suppression may therefore be a mechanism by which tolerance is induced towards these V regions, and a positive feedback crisis averted. Conversely, the low dose priming mechanism ensures that antibodies do not suppress each other out of existence. These processes may be particularly important for the generation and stabilization of the antibody repertoire during ontogeny, before the cells encounter antigen.

Although the anti-idiotype in the foregoing experiments was produced by artificial means, there is increasing evidence that anti-idiotypes may be produced during natural immune responses. Anti-idiotypes can be found in plasma cells in lympoid tissue, or even in the serum, coexisting with their specific idiotype, presumably in the form of immune complexes (Fig. 10.11).

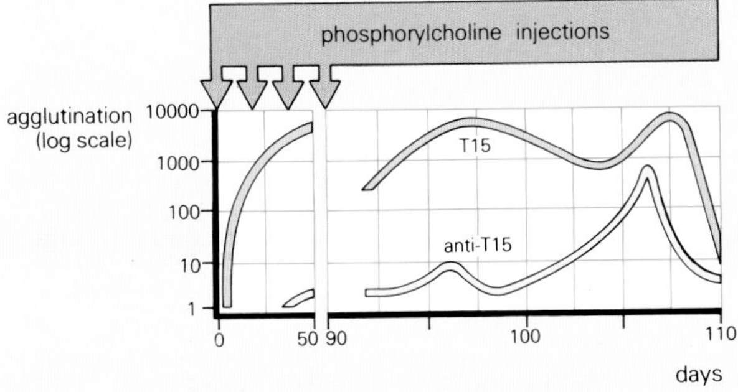

Fig. 10.11 Anti-idiotype production during the response to an antigen. Mice were repeatedly immunized with pneumococcal vaccine bearing the phosphorylcholine (PC) determinant for 90 days. The resulting antiserum was assayed for both the idiotype T15 (anti-PC) and anti-T15 antibodies. As shown, anti-idiotype is produced during the course of the anti-PC response. T15 and anti-T15 production occur in synchronous waves, suggesting that anti-T15 acts as a feedback control on T15 production.

T CELL IDIOTYPES

T cells, like B cells bear receptors with V regions. Although T cell V regions are the product of a different set of genes to those encoding B cell V regions, there is

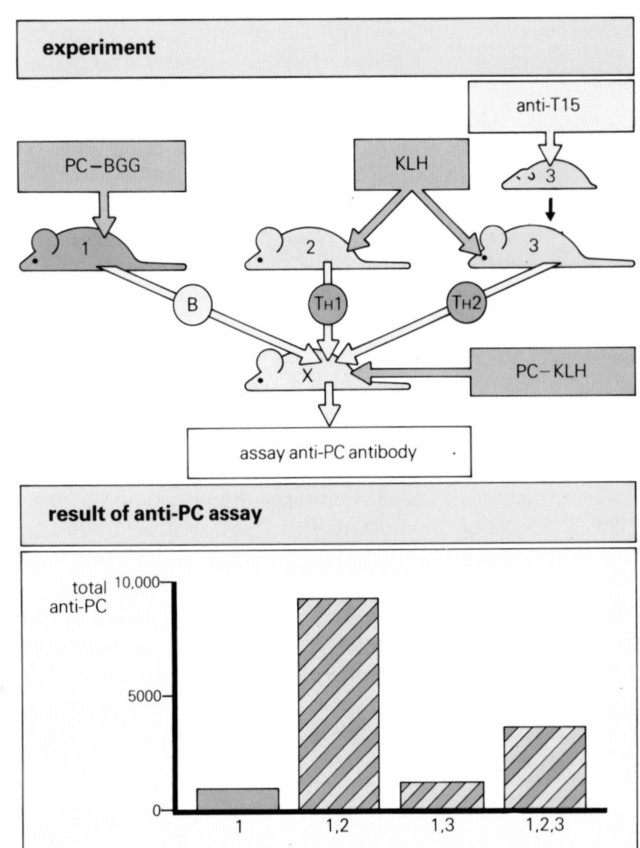

Fig. 10.12 Requirements for antigen-specific and idiotype-specific T-helper cells for a normal antibody response. X-irradiated mice were reconstituted (spleen cell transfer) with B cells primed to phosphorylcholine (PC) from a mouse immunized with PC – bovine gammaglobulin (PC–BGG).

Some of these mice were then given either TH cells from a mouse immunized with keyhole limpet haemocyanin (KLH) (these mice normally have TH cells capable of expanding the B cell population carrying the T15 idiotype), or TH cells from a mouse primed with KLH but whose T15-bearing lymphocytes were suppressed with anti-T15 antibody soon after birth. Other mice were given both types of TH cells. All of the mice were then challenged with PC–KLH, and the anti-PC response was assayed (represented by the plaque forming cells/spleen).

When the recipient mouse is reconstituted with B cells specific to PC (1) in the absence of T cell help, very little anti-PC antibody is raised. When TH cells primed to KLH (2) are introduced, the B cells generate a normal antibody response – most of this antibody carries the T15 idiotype. If, however, the mouse donating the TH cells is suppressed for T15 (3), the T15 response is suppressed, but is partly restored when spleen cells from mouse 2 are added, presumably by the activity of T15-specific TH cells. In this system, T15 forms over 80% of the total anti-PC antibody and there is little tendency for compensation by other idiotypes when it is suppressed, for example, in mouse 3.

now much evidence that anti-idiotypes prepared against antibodies can both bind to T cell receptors and exert functional influences on T cells. Indeed the stimulatory and suppressive effects of anti-idiotypes are often mediated as much, if not more, by their effect on T cells, either T-helper (TH) or T-suppressor (Ts) cells, than by their effect on B cells. One line of evidence comes from the fact that idiotype priming or suppression can be transferred to naïve animals with T cells alone. Furthermore, idiotypic clones of T cells have been isolated, and can be stimulated by anti-idiotypes to proliferate and release interleukin-2 *in vitro*.

There is also evidence that regulatory cells may be idiotype-specific rather than antigen-specific and thus control expression of different idiotypes in an immune response. For example, it may be demonstrated that the development of a normal immune response requires both antigen-specific and idiotype-specific TH cells (Fig. 10.12). The antigen-specific 'TH1' cells amplify the responses of B cells to different epitopes on the antigen, while the idiotype-specific 'TH2' cells amplify certain of the idiotype bearing B cell clones. In this scheme the antigen-specific TH1 cells are MHC restricted, while the idiotype-specific TH2 cells are not (Fig. 10.13).

To summarize, the network hypothesis is still the subject of considerable debate, but there is good evidence that idiotypic interactions can modulate the immune response, although the relative importance of these interactions in the resting state and the immune state has not been determined finally. On balance it appears that antigen is of prime importance in regulating the active immune state, but that idiotypic regulation may direct the antibody response towards a particular spectrum of idiotypes. In the resting state where antigen has not yet impinged on the immune system, idiotype/anti-idiotype regulation may be important in determining the initial state of the immune system in which it encounters antigen.

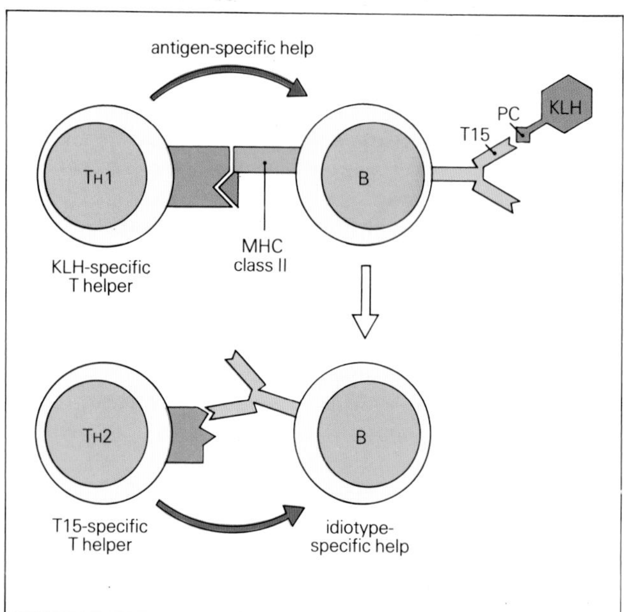

Fig. 10.13 Antigen-specific and idiotype-specific help. Two types of T-helper (TH) cell may be distinguished. TH1 is the classical T helper cell which recognizes processed antigen (KLH–PC in this example) in association with class II molecules on the B cell surface. The B cells are specific for the phosphorylcholine (PC) hapten. TH2 is an idiotype-specific helper cell which selectively expands only those B cell clones carrying the T15 idiotype. This interaction is not MHC restricted.

REGULATION BY CELLULAR MECHANISMS – SUPPRESSOR AND CONTRASUPPRESSOR CELLS

While some lymphocytes either possess their own effector function, for example cytotoxic T cells, or instruct non-specific cells to exert an effector function in the way that B cells instruct polymorphs and macrophages via antibody, and T cells activate macrophages, others function purely as regulators of other lymphocytes. The best known of these is the helper T cell. Besides helpers, however, there are T cells which specifically suppress immune responses; these are T-suppressor (Ts) cells. Ts cells can become activated after certain procedures designed to induce immunological tolerance and can be demonstrated in cell transfer experiments by their suppression of the response of normal cells (Fig. 10.14). Ts

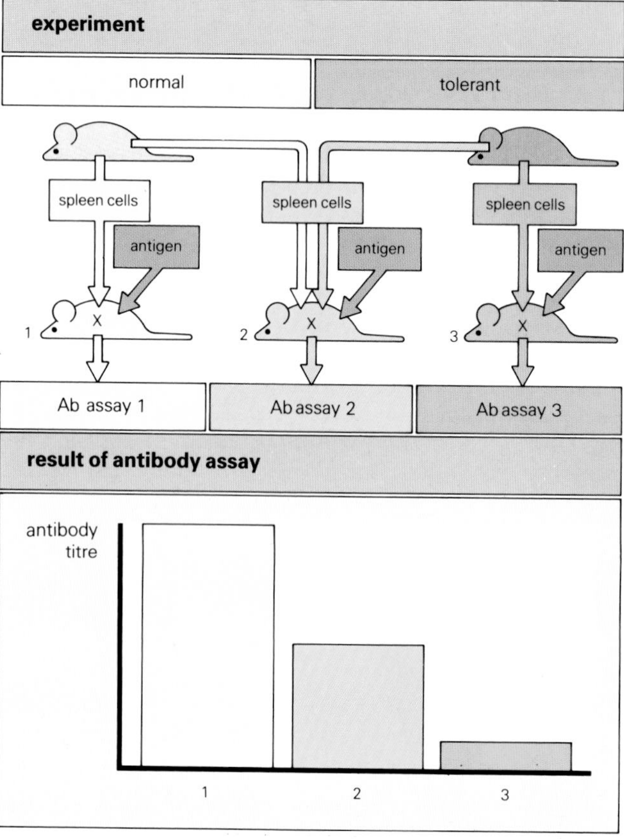

Fig. 10.14 Demonstration of T-suppressor cells. Three X-irradiated mice (1, 2, 3) are reconstituted with:
1. spleen cells from a normal mouse
2. spleen cells from both a normal mouse and a mouse rendered tolerant to the antigen; sheep red blood cells
3. spleen cells from the tolerant mouse only.
All three mice are then immunized with the antigen, and the antibody produced to the antigen is assayed. Mouse 1 produces a normal response, mouse 3 produces a weak response and the response of mouse 2 is intermediate, demonstrating that cells from the tolerant mouse can suppress the response of normal cells.

cells can act on either T cells or B cells in different experiments. Ts cell activity can also be demonstrated during normal immune responses, suggesting that they play a continuous role in regulation.

In addition to Ts cells, a further level of control has now been established, both in man and in mice, in the form of T-contrasuppressor (Tcs) cells, which interfere with suppression in a manner distinct from that of TH cells. Tcs cells make TH cells impervious to the actions of Ts cells and so allow TH cells to exert their helper activity, but are inactive in the absence of TH or Ts cells. Animals in which contrasuppression (but not help) has been induced do not become immune, but become refractory to the induction of tolerance.

With Tcs cells, the immune system gains another level of control, which doubtless enables it to make more complex patterns of response. One of these is the localization of immune responses, as occurs for example, after oral immunization, which induces a local response in the gut (and other mucosae), and at the same time induces a state of partial tolerance towards systemic administration of the same antigen. This so-called oral tolerance probably serves to prevent systemic (allergic) responses to food antigens while promoting the local defence of the gut.

THE ROLE OF THE I–J REGION

During the study of Ts cells it was often found that functional interactions between Ts cells and their targets only occurred when both the Ts cell and its target cell were genetically homologous in the H-2I region, that is, Ts activity was usually MHC restricted. This provided the first clue to a story which, though still confusing and incomplete, indicates the existence of a molecular system important for communication between T cells.

Initially, genetic mapping of MHC restricted Ts activity indicated that a locus between I–A and I–E controlled T cell suppression, and this was termed the I–J region. The Ts cells were said to be I–J restricted. However, when gene maps were made of the mouse class II region, it was found that there were no genes coding for proteins other than the I–A and I–E encoded class II molecules described in Chapter 4. Nevertheless, when class II I–Eα genes from a mouse of one I–J phenotype were transfected into the embryo of a mouse of a different phenotype, it altered the I–J phenotype in the recipient. This experiment shows that the I–Eα gene can control the I–J phenotype.

Antisera raised by cross-immunization between mouse strains of different I–J types will inhibit Ts activity. These antisera (anti-I–J) define at least two serological determinants which are expressed on the surface of some T cells (less than 10%), antigen-presenting cells (including some macrophages), and some antigen-specific T cell factors. The determinants are not, however, present on conventional class I restricted cytotoxic T(Tc) cells or class II restricted TH cells. The current view is that MHC class II influences the I–J phenotype of an animal, but does not encode the I–J gene products.

Additional evidence suggests that at least two genes, in addition to MHC class II, control I–J restricted interactions. One of these affects cell surface expression of the I–J gene product, while another gene(s) determines the gene product itself. One way to resolve these data is to postulate that the I–J gene product acts on the class II molecules, for example by a post-transcriptional modification of I–E. An alternative hypothesis is that the I–J gene product is a receptor molecule which recognizes class II molecules and is thus influenced by the class II haplotype.

Thus, in conclusion, anti-I–J antisera recognize one or more types of molecule involved in Ts cell interactions, but the molecular nature of the proteins expressing I–J determinants has yet to be elucidated.

T CELL FACTORS

It is important to realize that two cells can communicate either by recognizing the idiotypes of each others' receptors, or by both recognizing separate epitopes on an antigen particle when the antigen acts to link the cells, apparently through an antigen bridge (Fig. 10.13). Originally it was thought that the whole antigen could physically cross-link the two cells, but present understanding of MHC restricted interactions now leads us to think that the antigen bridge effect is mediated by the recognition of processed antigen on the surface of one cell by another.

There is increasing evidence that physical contact between lymphocytes is not necessary for communication, since antigen-specific factors can convey messages. Since these factors have been found *in vitro*, but not *in vivo*, it is probable that they act only over a short range within a limited area of lymphoid tissue.

A number of factors have been described, for the actions of both Ts and Tcs cells. These factors are protein molecules which, in many cases, consist of two polypeptide chains of approximately 45 kD and 28 kD, linked either non-covalently or by a disulphide bond(s). The two chains are not necessarily produced by the same cell. The larger chain is antigen-specific while the smaller chain expresses I–J determinants (Fig. 10.15). This description applies to just one group of antigen-specific

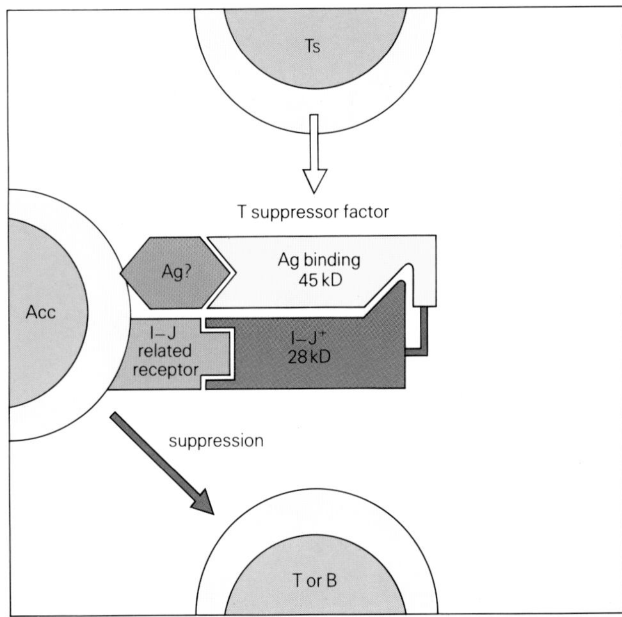

Fig. 10.15 T suppressor factor. This illustrates the structure of one class of T suppressor factors, which consists of an antigen-binding portion and an I–J-bearing portion which may be linked by disulphide bonds. The factor is released by suppressor T (Ts) cells and binds to an acceptor cell (Acc) via I–J related structures and possibly also via recognition of antigen on the Acc. The Acc in turn suppresses T or B cells.

factors. Another group of suppressor factors appears to bind to antibody and may be important in regulating the isotype profile of immune responses. These also express I–J determinants.

T CELL CIRCUITS

The way in which TH, Ts, Tcs and B cells interact to produce fine levels of regulation is only partly understood. Many of the experiments are based on studies *in vitro* and the relevance of the findings to physiological regulation *in vivo* is difficult to determine. What is clear is that a number of cells act in sequence before the final suppression or contrasuppression is exerted on T or B cells. Each cell acts on the next by a direct interaction or by factors. The last link in the sequence is the activation of an acceptor cell which then releases a non-specific immunosuppressive factor to modulate the action of T or B cells. Acceptor cells may express surface markers of T cells or macrophages.

Although a coherent picture of immunosuppression cannot be drawn from all the experiments performed so far, several studies have suggested the sequence of events shown in Fig. 10.16. To extrapolate the findings to the immune system as a whole, it might be postulated that suppressive factors released by Ts cells bind to antigen-presenting cells and other cells in secondary lymphoid tissue, and that these cells subsequently suppress effector cells which arrive in that tissue.

Most of the interactions of the factors with cells show some kind of genetic restriction, suggesting that another

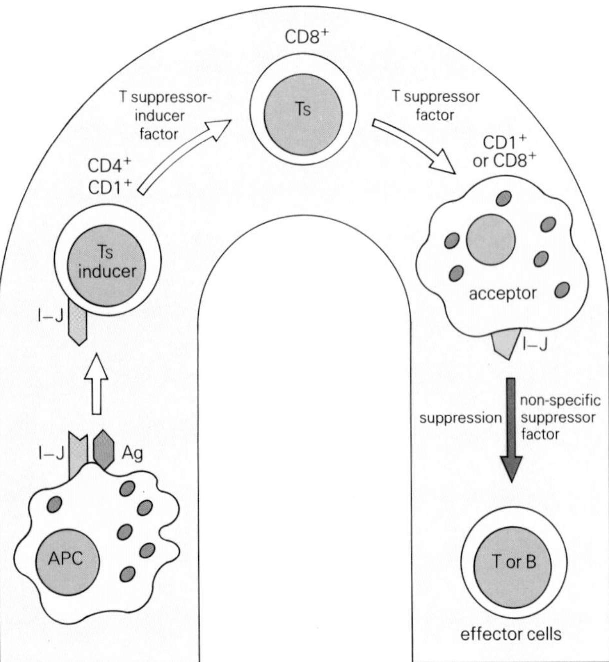

Fig. 10.16 Suppressor T cell circuit. Antigen-presenting cells (APCs) stimulate a T-suppressor (Ts) inducer cell to release a factor which activates the classical CD8$^+$ Ts cell. This cell then releases an I–J-bearing factor which is taken up by an acceptor cell to suppress effector cells. Some evidence suggests that the cells have the surface phenotypes indicated. A similar pathway for the development of contrasuppression has been proposed.

specific interaction must accompany the recognition of antigen and guide the factor to its allotted target cell (as in class II restriction of TH cells). In some cases the interactions are IgH restricted, which suggests a recognition of idiotype related structures, whereas in other cases the interactions are I–J restricted. In each case the structures involved in recognition are probably not coded by IgH or I–J genes themselves, but only appear to be restricted to these elements due to the selection of cells recognizing these structures during ontogeny. The genes which actually recognize the IgH or I–J are not known, but may belong to the T cell receptor complex.

REGULATION OF THE MODE OF RESPONSE

There are good reasons why different modes of response should be appropriate to cope with different infections. For example, cytotoxic cells may be appropriate for many virus infections, complement-fixing antibody for acute bacterial infections, and macrophage activation for those organisms which would normally resist the microbicidal powers of macrophages. Just how the response is directed into these different modes is not clear. The discovery that different types of antigen-presenting cells exist in different parts of the body offers a partial answer. For example, the Langerhans' cells in skin seem to be particularly adapted for the mediation of delayed hypersensitivity and thus account for the tendency of antigens to cause this type of response on cutaneous application. On the other hand the dendritic cells of lymphoid follicles probably mediate the priming of B cells for antibody production.

How does an antigen-presenting cell engage with the correct type of lymphocyte to bring about a particular type of response? It is suggested that this is a function of MHC products or other cellular interaction molecules, which force a lymphocyte to notice antigen only in the context of messages from antigen-presenting cells or other lymphocytes via their factors. Examples are the association of class I/CD8 with the cytotoxic response, class II/CD4 with help, and I–J with suppression and contrasuppression (Fig. 10.17). More associations such as these probably exist.

Information relevant to the mode of response is also processed by the regulatory T cell circuits. Thus there can be helper and suppressor cells specific for immunoglobulin isotype. These are responsible in part for the maintenance of situations in which particular isotypes predominate, for example, IgE in worm infestation, IgA in responses at mucous membranes, and particular IgG isotypes depending on the antigen and the organ in which they are produced.

It is also likely that the mode of response depends to a large extent on certain physical or chemical properties of the antigen or infective organism, which are perceived in a way which is not immunologically specific. Although these properties of the antigen can be either suppressive or stimulatory, it is convenient to lump them together as the 'adjuvanticity' of the antigen. It is well-known that different adjuvants injected with the same antigen tend to favour different modalities of response, and the available evidence often points to antigen-presenting cells as the immediate site of action of these adjuvant effects. It has been found, for example, that when lipids

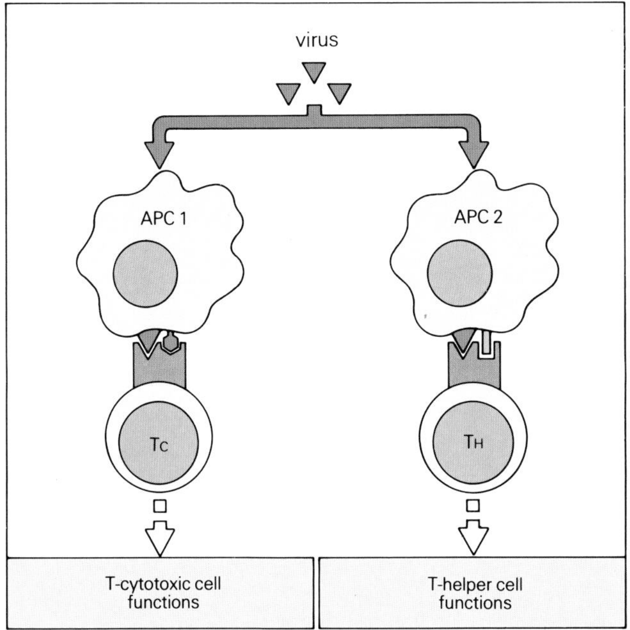

Fig. 10.17 Mode of response regulated by antigen presentation. This scheme shows how an antigenic stimulus, in this case a virus, may activate two different cell classes. The virus will activate cytotoxic T cells (Tc) if seen on the antigen-presenting cell 1 (APC 1) in association with the class I K or D MHC antigen (mice), or will activate helper T cells (TH) if seen on the APC (APC 2) in association with Class II Ia antigens. Some TH cells will subsequently help cytotoxic reactions while others will help antibody production.

are coupled to protein antigens they tend to induce delayed hypersensitivity rather than antibody production and to localize in T-dependent rather than B-dependent areas of lymphoid tissues. This suggests that lipophilic properties direct the antigen to a different set of antigen-presenting cells, programmed to trigger a different modality of response.

REGULATION VIA THE ENDOCRINE AND NERVOUS SYSTEMS

The immune system is by no means isolated from other control systems of the body; indeed, there are many possibilities for communication between the nervous, endocrine and immune systems. This can be deduced from morphological evidence of the innervation of lymphoid tissues. The fibres connect not only to blood vessels, which modulate cellular traffic, but also to neuroendocrine cells which release hormones that can influence lymphocytes. Lymphocytes themselves have receptors for a wide variety of hormones, including corticosteroids, insulin, catecholamines, growth hormone and met-enkephalin. Moreover, virtually every hormone investigated has some effect on the immune system, although not all of the effects are very direct. There is evidence that the thymus may play a central role, both receiving nervous and hormonal signals and relaying them to the immune system via its own hormones (see Chapter 14). Some pathways of neuroendocrine action on the immune system are shown in Fig. 10.18.

The physiological reality of neuroendocrine control of the immune system can be seen in the effects of stress on immune responses. An immunosuppressive effect has usually been noted, mediated principally by corticosteroids, endorphin and met-enkephalin. This may be seen as a general effect resulting from degradation of the integrity of the body's control systems by stress. Interestingly however, when the challenge of the stressing agent is met by an adequate coping response, the immune system may be unaffected or even stimulated to respond more strongly than usual. This coping response may also be mediated by the nervous system, since the pineal hormone, melatonin, can reverse the immunosuppressive effect of stress on the immune response of animals responding to a virus infection.

It is unlikely that the nervous or endocrine systems can process information directly related to immunological specificity. Nevertheless there are many opportunities for them to control not only the intensity, but also the modality, kinetics and localization of immune responses. With this in mind, the increasing use of psychotherapy in immune-related diseases and cancer

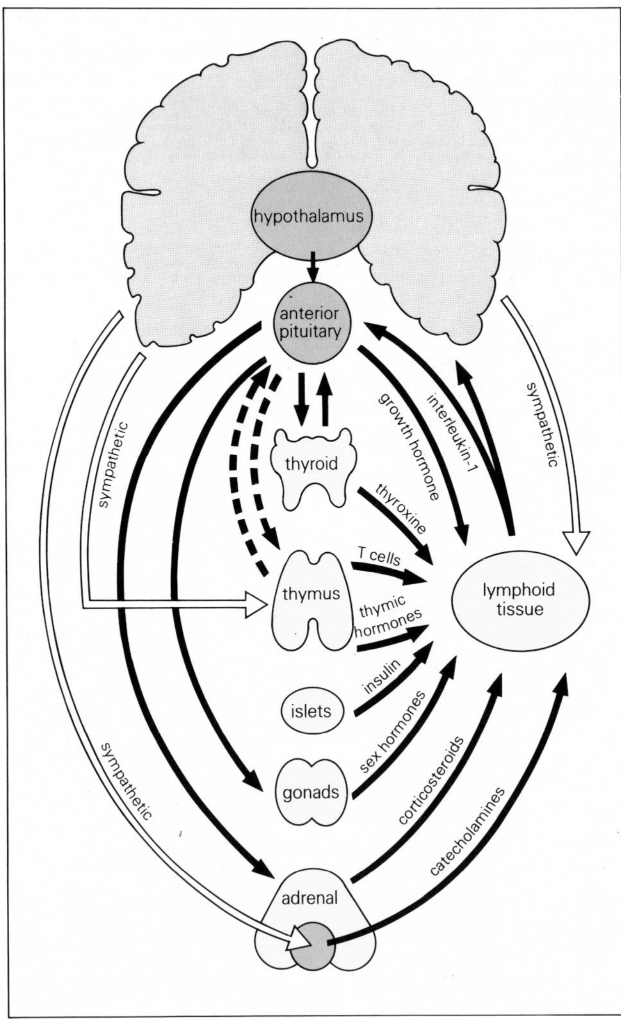

Fig. 10.18 Neuroendocrine interactions with the immune system. The diagram indicates some of the potential connections between the endocrine, nervous and immune systems. Open lines indicate nervous connections, black lines indicate hormonal interactions, and dotted lines indicate postulated connections for which the effector molecules have not been established.

does not seem to be totally unreasonable. It should also be remembered that lymphoid cells themselves can produce immunoreactive hormones such as ACTH, FSH and TSH, which may have further modulating effects on the immune response.

IMMUNOREGULATION IN SELF/NON-SELF DISCRIMINATION

Certain elements of tolerance induction impinge on the role of Ts cells. Under some conditions both T and B cells may be functionally deleted, but there is increasing evidence, such as finding lymphocytes with specificity for self molecules in normal individuals, that such deletion is neither necessary nor sufficient to account for self tolerance. This includes not just Tc and B cells, but also the TH cells which could stimulate them. Thus, there are grounds for considering self/non-self discrimination as a regulatory phenomenon. As such it would not depend entirely on the presence or absence, or even relative abundance of particular clones but could, to some extent, be a function of the dynamics of the whole system. Such a functional pattern, which might be seen as the operational balance of the immune system, will not reveal itself to study by techniques which disturb it too greatly. The major elements discussed in this chapter are summarized in Fig. 10.19.

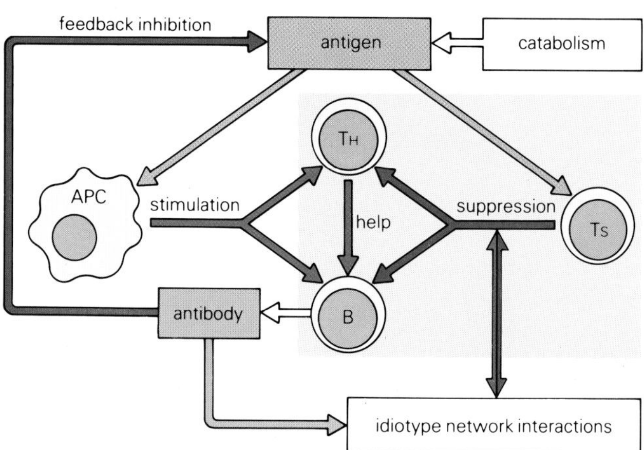

Fig. 10.19 Regulation of the immune response: a summary. This diagram outlines a minimum model for immunoregulation involving the feedback inhibition by antibody on antigen and through the idiotype network. Antigen is presented to T-helper (TH) and B cells by an antigen-presenting cell (APC) which stimulates them. Once activated, TH cells help their specific B cells to produce antibody. T-suppressor (Ts) cells are also stimulated by antigen and regulate both TH cells and B cells. Antibody and idiotype-specific T cells interact with the antigen-specific cells (blue box) to regulate the response. The stimulating effect of antigen on the immune system is diminished by complexing with antibody and by its catabolism.

FURTHER READING

Ader, R. & Hadden, J.W. (1987) Neuroimmunologic interactions: Proceedings of the 2nd international workshop on neuroimmunoregulation. *Annals of the New York Academy of Sciences*, **496**.

Asherson, G.L., Collizzi, V. & Zembala, M. (1986) An overview of T-suppressor cell circuits. *Annual Review of Immunology*, **4**, 37.

Besedovsky, H.O., Del Ray, A.E. & Sorkin, E. (1983) What do the immune system and the brain know about each other? *Immunology Today*, **4**, 342.

Bona, C.A. (1987) *Regulatory Idiotypes* (*Modern Concepts in Immunology* Vol II) New York: Wiley.

Borysenko, M. (1987) Area review: psychoneuroimmunology. *Annals of Behavioural Medicine*, **9**, 3.

Dorf, M.E. & Benacerraf, B. (1984) Suppressor cells and immunoregulation. *Annual Review of Immunology*, **2**, 127.

Green, D.R., Flood, P.M. & Gershon, R.K. (1983) Immunoregulatory T cell pathways. *Annual Review of Immunology*, **1**, 439.

Green, D.R., & Ptak, W. (1986) Contrasuppression in the mouse. *Immunology Today*, **7**, 81.

Jerne, N.K. (1974) Towards a network theory of the immune system. *Annals of Immunology* (Paris), **125C**, 373.

Kelsoe, G., Reth, M. & Rajewsky, K. (1981) Control of idiotype expression by monoclonal anti-idiotype and idiotype-bearing antibodies. *European Journal of Immunology*, **11**, 418.

Lehner, T. (1986) Antigen-presenting, contrasuppressor human T-cells. *Immunology Today*, **7**, 87.

Moller, G. (ed.) (1980) Regulation of the immune response by antibodies against the immunogen. *Immunological Reviews*, **49**.

Moller, G. (ed.) (1984) Idiotype networks. *Immunological Reviews*, **79**.

Moller, G. (ed.) (1985) I–J. *Immunological Reviews*, **89**.

Taylor, R.B. (1982) Regulation of antibody responses by antibody towards the immunogen. *Immunology Today*, **3**, 47.

Teale, J.M. & Abraham K.M. (1987) The regulation of antibody class expression. *Immunology Today*, **8**, 122.

11 Genetic Control of Immunity

There are many potential sites at which genetic factors could play a role in the generation of an immune response. It was in the latter half of the nineteenth century that Jacobi noted that genetic factors influenced susceptibility to disease. The observation that diphtheria tended to occur in families prompted the tentative proposal that resistance or susceptibility of an individual to *Corynebacterium diphtheriae* might be an inherited trait. This proposal was supported by the finding that different strains of guinea-pig displayed different resistance patterns to diphtheria and that the characteristic was inherited. Fjord-Scheibel demonstrated in 1943 that the production of diphtheria antitoxin was controlled by a gene inherited in a Mendelian dominant fashion, by selective breeding of high and low responder guinea-pig strains. This study was the first demonstration of the dominance of high responsiveness since 90% of the offspring of the two high responder strains were antitoxin producers in the first generation whereas it took five generations of inbreeding non-producers to achieve 90% of the offspring as non-producers.

In the 1920s and 30s Webster noted that in a stock of outbred Swiss mice, susceptibility to infection by *Bacillus enteritidis* varied. By selective in-breeding, Webster obtained two lines of mice; one resistant to *B. enteritidis* (BR) and the other susceptible (BS). Studies on the susceptibility of these lines to virus infection allowed development of further lines which were either susceptible (BSVS and BRVS) or resistant (BSVR and BRVR) to these viral infections. The BSVS line was therefore highly susceptible to both bacterial and viral infections. Once again, breeding studies demonstrated that responsiveness was a dominant trait since F1 hybrid mice derived from parental lines BSVR and BRVS were resistant to both bacterial and viral infections. These experiments laid the groundwork for further studies on the role of immune response genes.

GENES CONTROLLING THE IMMUNE RESPONSE

By using inbred strains of animals and employing antigens of a more defined composition it became possible to subject the genetic regulation of immune responsiveness to a finer analysis. Therefore, instead of using complex antigens like bacteria or red blood cells, researchers used small proteins such as insulin, or synthetic polypeptides like poly-L-lysine (PLL) or (T,G)-A--L, (H,G)-A--L and (P,G)-A--L. These have an alanine-lysine copolymer backbone substituted with glutamic acid and tyrosine, histidine, or phenylalanine branches.

Benacerraf and his colleagues found that outbred guinea-pigs either made a delayed hypersensitivity response and antibodies to the antigen DNP–PLL, or failed to make a delayed hypersensitivity response or antibodies. By selective inbreeding it was possible to show that such responses were inherited, the dominant trait being attributable to a single gene. If DNP–PLL was coupled to another antigen, for example ovalbumin, the resulting immunogen was found to induce antibodies to DNP–PLL in the non-responder strain, but it did not induce delayed hypersensitivity.

MHC LINKED IMMUNE RESPONSE GENES

In the 1960s, McDevitt and Chinitz followed the observation of John Humphrey that sandy lop rabbits differed from the Himalayan strain in their responses to synthetic branched amino acid copolymers. Using inbred strains of mice and the antigen (T,G)-A--L, McDevitt and colleagues demonstrated that the response to (T,G)-A--L was under the control of a single autosomal dominant gene or gene cluster, termed the immune response 1 (Ir-1) gene and found to be linked to the mouse major histocompatibility complex (MHC) – H-2 (Fig. 11.1).

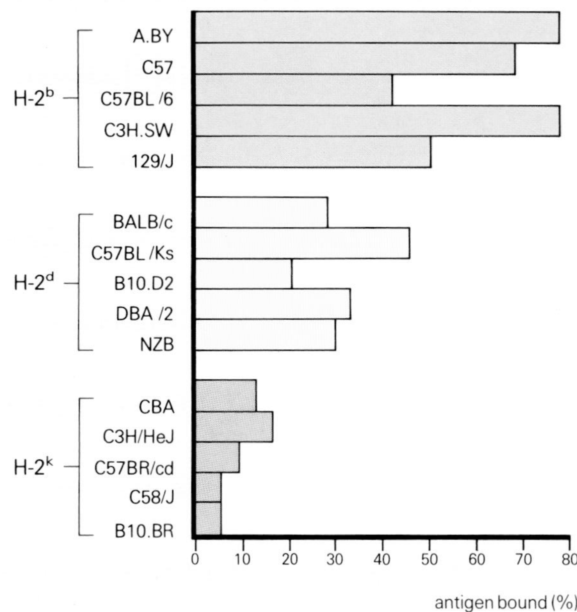

Fig.11.1 Strain differences in the antibody response to (T,G)-A--L. Fifteen strains of mice were given a standard dose of the synthetic antigen (T,G)-A--L. Antibody responses are expressed as the antigen-binding capacity of the antisera. Animals with the H-2^b haplotype are high responders, H-2^d are intermediate and H-2^k are low responders. Note that there is some overlap between the level of response in the different haplotypes indicating that the H-2 linked genes are not the only ones to control the response.

Using another synthetic antigen, (H,G)-A--L, genetic mapping localized the Ir-1 gene to the I–A subregion of the mouse MHC (Fig. 11.2). After this first demonstration of an MHC-linked immune response gene the responses to a large number of T-dependent antigens have been found to be under the control of genes located in this part of the MHC. These antigens include linear and branched chain synthetic amino acid copolymers, other antigens, for example alloantigens, the male antigen H-Y, and protein antigens including insulin, hen egg lysozyme, cytochrome C and myoglobin. It is notable, however, that a high responder strain for one antigen is a low responder for other antigens, while other strains have the opposite high and low response patterns, as tabulated in Fig. 11.3. Thus the MHC-linked Ir genes act in an antigen-specific fashion, but not all the immune response genes are linked to the MHC. Most of these non-MHC immune response genes do not seem to have the degree of antigen specificity which MHC-linked Ir genes have. It is likely that Ir genes play a role in determining the level of a response to any T-dependent antigen. Since an Ir gene may control the recognition of a given epitope on an antigen, antigens which are antigenically complex will provide many determinants subject to Ir gene control. This was demonstrated by Berzofsky's studies on sperm whale myoglobin in which separate determinants on the molecule are shown to be under the control of distinct Ir genes (Fig. 11.4).

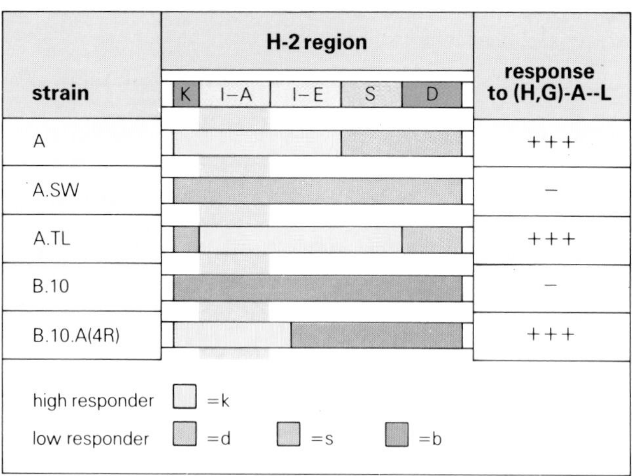

Fig.11.2 Mapping of the immune response (Ir) gene controlling responses to (H,G)-A--L. The H-2 regions of five strains of mice are illustrated; three strains are high responders to (H,G)-A--L and two are low responders. All three high responder strains have only the H-2[k] I–A region in common, indicating that the gene present in H-2[k] mice controlling the immune response to (H,G)-A--L is in the I–A region. Colours represent haplotypes.

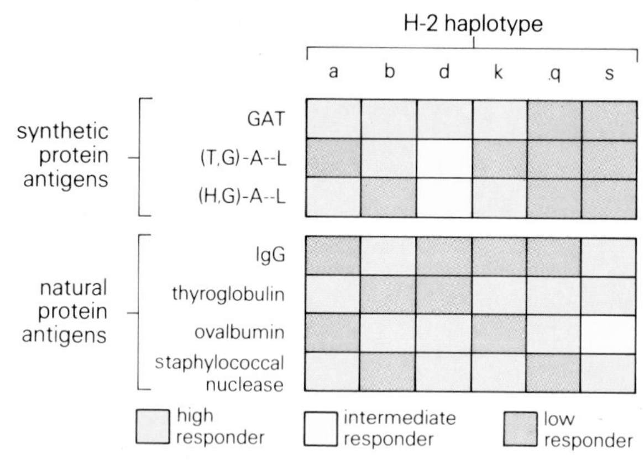

Fig.11.3 High and low responder haplotypes. This table shows the response of six inbred strains of mice, with different H-2 haplotypes, to seven different antigens. High responders to some antigens produce low responses to others, and the pattern of response is quite unsystematic. Even with very closely related antigens, for example, (T,G)-A--L and (H,G)-A--L, the response is different in H-2[a] and H-2[b] strains.

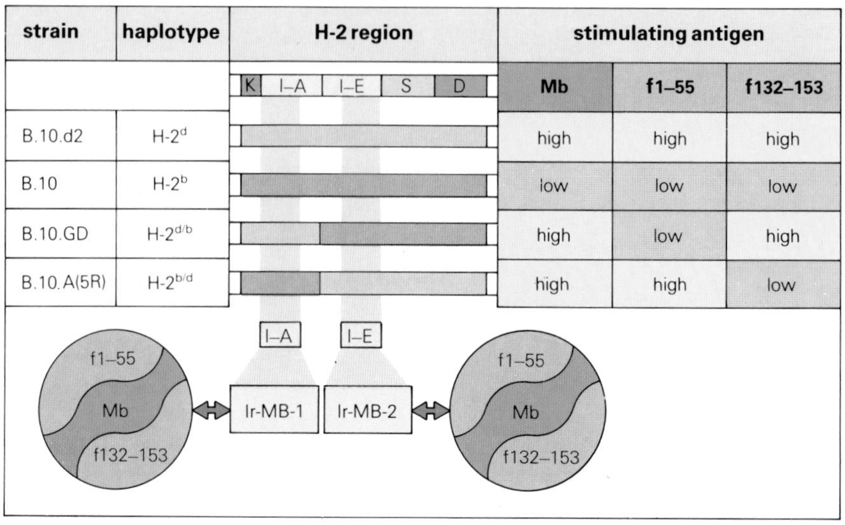

strain	haplotype	H-2 region (K, I–A, I–E, S, D)	stimulating antigen: Mb	f1–55	f132–153
B.10.d2	H-2[d]		high	high	high
B.10	H-2[b]		low	low	low
B.10.GD	H-2[d/b]		high	low	high
B.10.A(5R)	H-2[b/d]		high	high	low

I–A   I–E

f1–55   Mb   f132–153 ↔ Ir-MB-1   Ir-MB-2 ↔ f1–55   Mb   f132–153

Fig.11.4 Genetic control of the responses to myoglobin. Mice of four different strains were immunized with myoglobin (Mb). The different strains were genetically identical except at the H-2 locus, where they were either H-2[d] (purple), H-2[b] (pink) or recombinants containing part b and part d (pink and purple). The spleen cells from the immunized animals were set up in cultures containing either whole Mb antigen or fragments of the antigen, consisting of amino acids 1–55 (f1–55) or amino acids 132–153 (f132–153). Proliferation of T cells in response to the antigen or fragments was measured and the strains showed either high responses or low responses. H-2[d] mice showed high responses to the whole antigen and fragments whereas H-2[b] mice showed low responses. B.10.GD mice which have a high responder I–A region make a high response to the whole antigen and to f132–153 while B.10. A(5R) mice, which have a high responder I–E region respond to f1–55 but not f132–153. Thus a gene in I–A (Ir-MB-1) controls the response to f132–153 while a gene in I–E (Ir-MB-2) controls the response to f1–55 in H-2[d] mice. H-2[b] mice lack these genes. These conclusions are summarized in the lower part of the diagram.

LEVEL OF ACTION OF IMMUNE RESPONSE GENES

MHC-linked immune response (Ir) gene control is very specific; in many cases a single amino acid substitution will affect responsiveness. For example in Fig. 11.3 it was shown that whereas H-2^b mice are high responders to (T,G)-A--L but not to (H,G)-A--L, H-2^k mice are the opposite, being high responders to (H,G)-A--L but not to (T,G)-A--L. However, both H-2^k and H-2^b mice respond to (P,G)-A--L. This pattern of responsiveness would not be predicted in terms of antibody specificity since substantial cross-reactivity is observed between the antibodies to (H,G)-A--L, (T,G)-A--L and (P,G)-A--L. This led to the proposal that MHC-linked Ir genes exert their control at the level of T cell recognition of antigen and not at the level of B cells (Fig. 11.5).

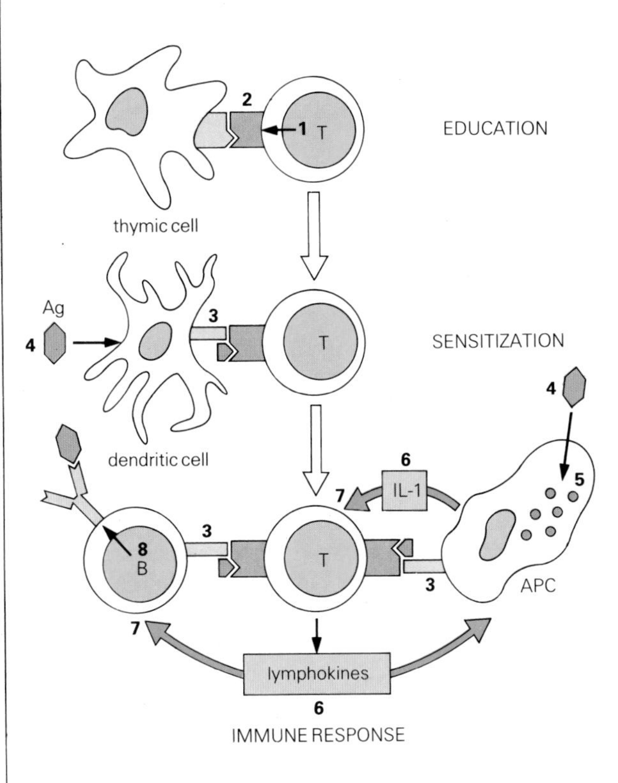

Fig. 11.5 Levels of action of immune response genes. Many genes affect immune responsiveness. This diagram illustrates possible points of action. T cells generate their antigen receptors from germ line genes (1) and are then selected by education in the thymus (2). T cells become sensitized by contact with antigen on antigen-presenting cells, including dendritic cells, a process which involves presentation of the antigen in association with class II MHC molecules (3) and which may also be influenced by genes which control antigen uptake and processing. During the development of the immune response, cellular cooperation again requires recognition, antigen processing, and presentation (3, 4, 5) and is mediated by the generation of cytokines and lymphokines (6). The response to these signals depends on cellular receptors for the cytokines and signal transduction (7). Antibody responses depend on cellular cooperation but the specificity of the antibodies available depends to some extent on the antibody genes (8). Since cytokine-mediated signalling is a short range event, the cooperation between B cells and macrophages with T cells is most effective when the T cells recognize antigen–MHC on their surface.

ANTIGEN PRESENTATION AND T–B COOPERATION

Analysis of the levels at which Ir genes exert their control on cellular interactions has focused on Ir genes controlling antigen presentation between macrophages and T cells, and Ir genes regulating T cell–B cell cooperation.

Rosenthal and Shevach clearly demonstrated that a T cell proliferative response to antigen only occurred if the T cells and antigen-presenting cells (APCs) were derived from guinea-pigs of the same strain (Fig. 11.6). A similar requirement for MHC I region compatibility was demonstrated for T–B collaboration in the immune response of mice to hapten–carrier conjugates. T cells recognizing carrier cooperate with B cells recognizing hapten if they are the same H-2 type, as demonstrated *in vivo* (Fig. 11.7). This has also been demonstrated *in vitro* in a T-dependent antibody response, in which responsiveness was only restored to a macrophage-depleted population by the addition of macrophages of a responder genotype (isolated by adherence to a plastic plate). In the response to TNP–(T,G)-A--L this ability to restore the response was mapped to the I–A subregion of the mouse MHC.

In F1 animals it can be shown that T cells are genetically restricted to one or other of the two parental strains. An elegant *in vitro* demonstration of this is illustrated in

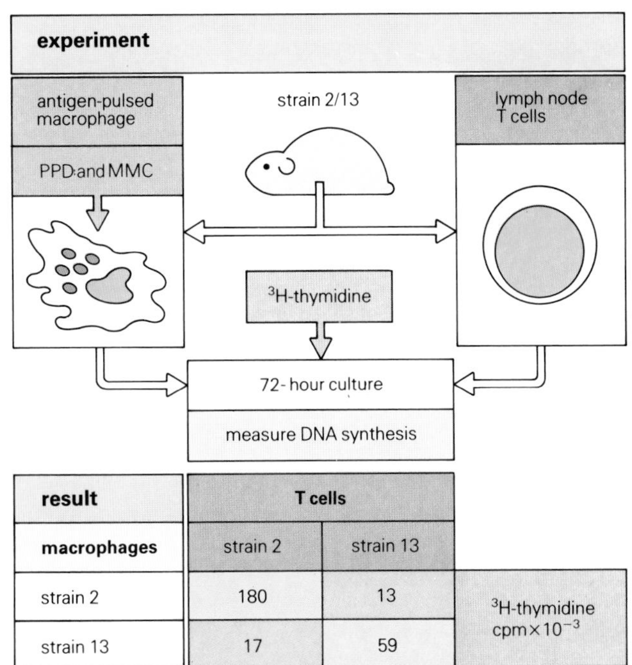

result	T cells		
macrophages	strain 2	strain 13	
strain 2	180	13	^{3}H-thymidine cpm$\times 10^{-3}$
strain 13	17	59	

Fig. 11.6 Genetic restriction in macrophage–T cell cooperation. Peritoneal macrophages and T cells were isolated from antigen-primed strain 2 and strain 13 guinea-pigs. The macrophages were pulsed with antigen (PPD), and mitomycin C (MMC) to prevent the macrophages proliferating. The T cells and antigen-pulsed macrophages were co-cultured and DNA synthesis by the T cells measured by incorporation of tritiated thymidine (^{3}H-thymidine). The incorporation is given in the table. Lymphocytes of both strains respond well when the antigen is presented on syngeneic macrophages, but poorly when presented on allogeneic macrophages.

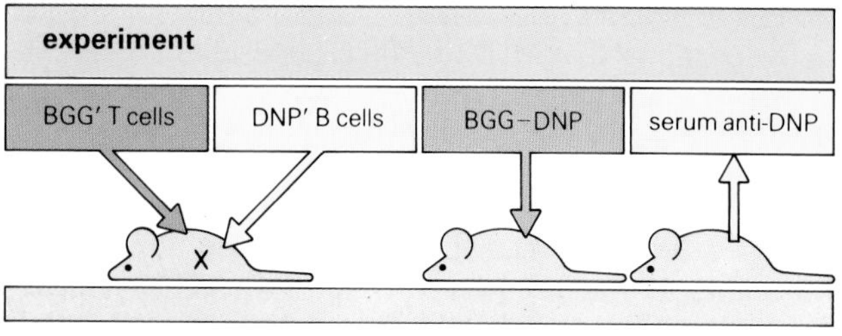

result				
experiment	T cells	B cells	recipient	response
1	C	C	CxD	+
2	D	D	CxD	+
3	C	D	CxD	–
4	D	C	CxD	–
5	CxD	D	CxD	+

Fig.11.7 Genetic restriction in T–B cooperation. Mice were X-irradiated and reconstituted with T cells primed to bovine gammaglobulin (BGG') and B cells primed to the hapten dinitrophenol (DNP'). The animals were challenged with BGG–DNP and the anti-DNP response measured. This experiment was performed using different combinations of strain C and D, B cells and T cells, with hybrid mice (CxD) as the recipients. The responses obtained with different combinations of T and B cells are shown. Strain C T cells cooperate with strain C B cells (1) and strain D T cells also cooperate with strain D B cells (2). However, strain C T cells cannot cooperate with strain D B cells and vice versa (3 and 4). Sharing of one haplotype between T cells and B cells is sufficient to produce a response, as demonstrated by using T cells from hybrid (CxD) mice (5).

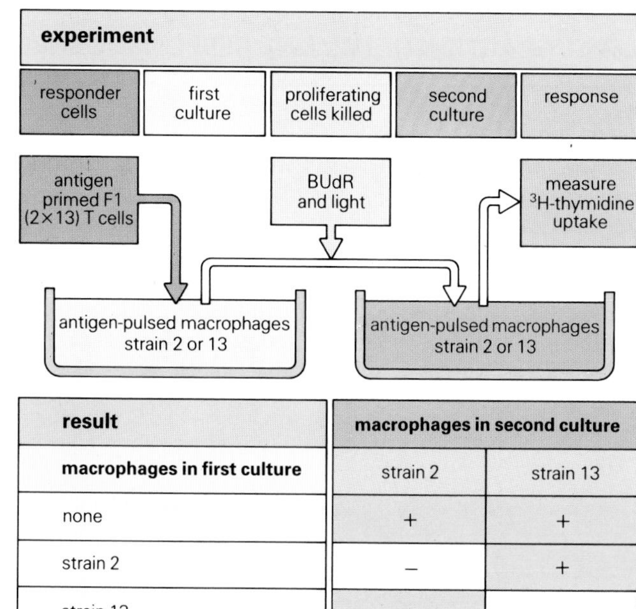

result	macrophages in second culture	
macrophages in first culture	strain 2	strain 13
none	+	+
strain 2	–	+
strain 13	+	–

Fig.11.8 Demonstration of two types of genetically restricted T cells in F1 animals. T cells (responder cells) from an F1 (strain 2 × strain 13) guinea-pig were cultured on an antigen-pulsed layer of macrophages (antigen-presenting cells from a strain 2 or strain 13 animal). The T cells were harvested and exposed to bromodeoxyuridine (BUdR) and light which killed the responding, proliferating cells. The surviving, non-responding cells were then cultured with a second layer of antigen-pulsed macrophages and their response was measured by the uptake of ^{3}H-thymidine. The table shows that F1 cells with no first culture respond to antigen presented on macrophages of either parental strain in the second culture. If the T cells are first cultured on strain 2 macrophages and the proliferating cells killed, there are no cells to proliferate in a second culture containing strain 2 antigen-presenting cells, but there are cells which can respond to antigen on strain 13 cells. The converse occurs with preculture on strain 13 macrophages. Thus, there are two sets of T cells in the F1 animal; one responds to antigen presented by cells of one parental haplotype, the other responds to antigens presented by cells of the other haplotype.

Fig. 11.8. This phenomenon can also be demonstrated *in vivo*. Cells from F1 hybrid mice can transfer delayed hypersensitivity to only one of the two parental strains if the F1 mouse is primed only with antigen-pulsed APCs of that parental strain. Using T cell lines or clones this restriction of recognition between APCs and T cells has been fully substantiated. Interestingly the use of such T cell clones has allowed Sredni and Schwarz to demonstrate that T cells also exist in F1 animals which are restricted to unique elements on F1 APCs and arise through mixed (heterologous) pairing of parental α and β class II chains, as well as T cells restricted to parental MHC molecules. In some situations, however, preferential pairing of chains can occur resulting in the virtual absence of expression of one parental haplotype class II molecule on the surface of the F1 APC.

CYTOTOXIC T CELLS

The need for MHC compatibility is also noted in the activity of specific cytotoxic T cells which are directed against virally-modified targets, chemically-modified self-antigens or a variety of minor histocompatibility antigens, including the male antigen H-Y, for which expression is determined by genes on the Y chromosome. The requirement for compatibility is primarily restricted to the H-2K or H-2D regions of the mouse MHC (that is, class I antigens). Thus specific cytotoxic T cells can only lyse virally-infected cells or TNP-modified target cells if they are matched with the targets at the H-2K or H-2D regions (Fig. 11.9). The way in which viral proteins are associated with the MHC class I products has been examined by precipitating the surface proteins of virally-infected cells with specific antisera. It is found in some cases that precipitation of the surface MHC antigens with antibody specific for class I products co-precipitates viral proteins and vice versa, implying that the class I antigens are physically associated with viral antigens on the membrane. It is notable that the presence of virus in these cells modifies the β_2-microglobulin-dependent transport of the class I MHC antigens to the Golgi apparatus. The mechanism by which MHC restriction of cytotoxic cell activity occurs has been broadly established by using radiation-induced bone marrow chimaeras (Fig. 11.10). It can be seen that an irradiated parental type A mouse reconstituted with F1(A × B) bone marrow develops T cells which can only

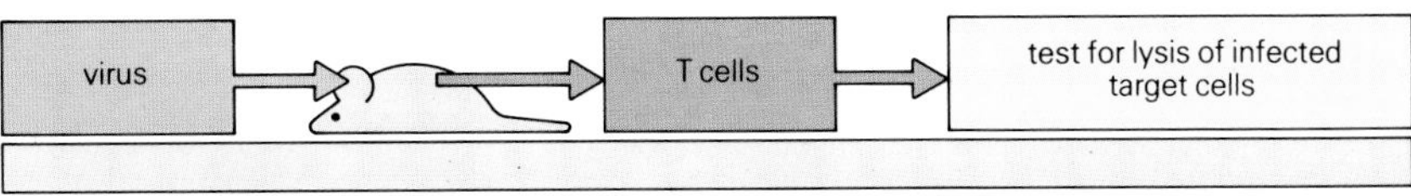

virus	mouse strain	H-2 region	lysis of infected targets of haplotype (%)		
		K I S D	$H-2^s$	$H-2^k$	$H-2^d$
LCM	A.TL		25	1	64
Sendai	A.TL		63	4	24
LCM	CBA		2	34	1
LCM	A/J		0	30	64

Fig.11.9 Genetic restriction of cytotoxic cells. The cytotoxic cells of virus-infected adult mice of different strains were tested for their ability to kill virus-infected target cells of different H-2 haplotypes (k, s and d). The strain A.TL is $H\text{-}2K^s$, $H\text{-}2I^k$ and $H\text{-}2D^d$ and its cells kill target cells infected with lymphocytic choriomeningitis virus (LCM) only if the targets share the $H\text{-}2K^s$ or the $H\text{-}2D^d$ haplotypes. Haplotype identity between the cells and targets at the H-2I locus does not produce cytotoxicity. Note that the cytotoxicity is determined mostly by the H-2D locus. By comparison, in A.TL mice infected with Sendai virus the cytotoxicity is principally determined by the H-2K locus. Infection of CBA mice with LCM confirms the importance of genetic restriction in these responses, while the infection of A/J mice with LCM confirms the finding that cytotoxicity to LCM is strongest to the H-2D-matched infected targets. It is thought that different viruses may associate preferentially with particular H-2K or H-2D MHC molecules in order to present a target for cytotoxic cells.

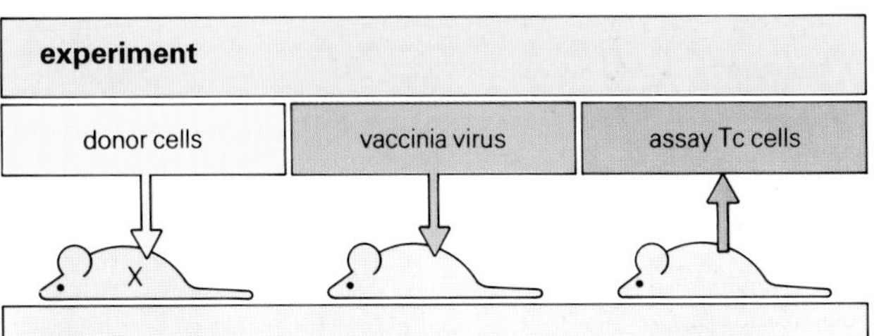

results			cytotoxicity to:	
experiment	donor cells	recipient	A-vaccinia	B-vaccinia
1	AxB(BM)	A	+	–
2	AxB(BM)	B	–	+
3	AxB(spleen)	A	+	+
4	AxB(spleen)	B	+	+

Fig.11.10 Education of cytotoxic T cells. Recipient mice (type A and B) were X-irradiated and reconstituted with donor lymphocytes (bone marrow or spleen cells). This produced chimaeric animals, in which the lymphocytes were of the donor type and other tissues were of the recipient type. The chimaeras were then challenged with vaccinia virus and the spleen cells removed and assayed for cytotoxicity against either type A or type B cells infected with vaccinia (A-vaccinia and B-vaccinia). Four experiments using different combinations of donor cells and recipient mice were conducted. Experiments 1 and 2 demonstrate that mice reconstituted with A × B bone marrow (BM) cells can only kill infected targets of the same type as the recipient. Experiments 3 and 4 show that mature adult A × B spleen cells can kill both A and B infected targets. The interpretation is that immature stem cells (BM) are educated to recognize antigen only in association with the recipient's MHC haplotype, whereas mature cells (spleen) have already been educated.

respond cytolytically to virally-infected parental type A cells but not to B cells infected with this virus. This experiment demonstrates the critical role played by the environment in which the T cell matures. The educative function performed by the thymus has also been demonstrated by placing parental type B or A thymus grafts in a thymectomized and lethally-irradiated F1 mouse reconstituted with T cell-depleted bone marrow; T cells from such mice are restricted to the parental thymus MHC type. These experiments illustrate the principle that MHC restriction manifesting itself in mature T cells may be an outcome of T cell education.

MOLECULAR CONTROL OF IMMUNE RESPONSES

ANTIGEN RECEPTOR GENES

It is clear that MHC class II molecules have a major effect in determining an individual's immune response to particular antigens. This is due to their central role in antigen presentation to T-helper cells, and ultimately is also seen in the way particular MHC haplotypes confer susceptibility to different diseases.

It might be anticipated that genes for the T cell antigen receptor and antibody would also determine the ability to make immune responses. However the haplotype of an individual's antigen receptor genes has much less influence on their immune responsiveness than their MHC haplotype. The reason for this is that the antibody genes and T cell receptor genes undergo rearrangement and diversification during ontogeny, so that each individual can make an enormous number of receptor types, regardless of the genetic variation in their germ line receptor genes. In contrast, the MHC molecules are fixed within an individual, although they are extremely polymorphic within the population as a whole. Consequently MHC molecules are highly variable between individuals but receptor genes produce populations of receptor molecules which are functionally equivalent, in

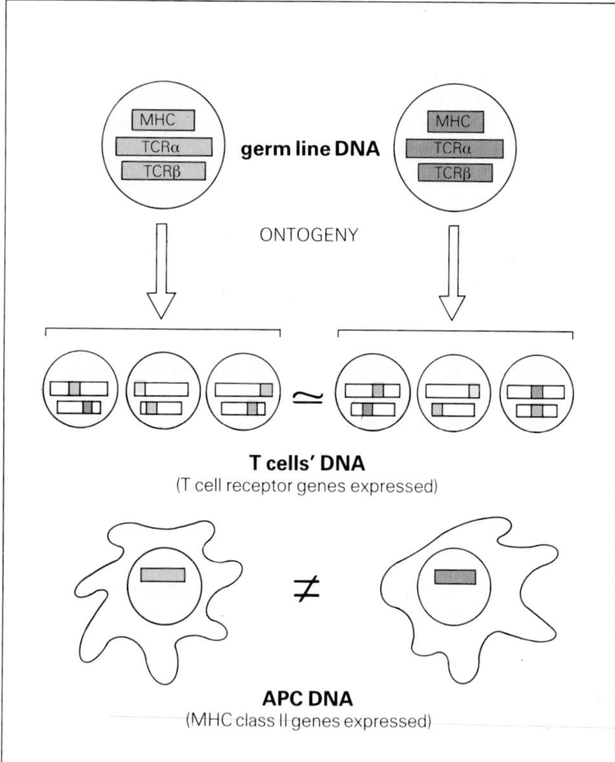

Fig. 11.11 Polymorphism of MHC and T cell receptor genes. The germ line DNA of different individuals, A and B, (red and purple) contain distinct haplotypes of T cell receptor and MHC genes. During ontogeny, rearrangement of the T cell receptor genes in different cells generates a population of T cells which can recognize an enormous range of antigens and is functionally similar between individuals with respect to what the T cells can recognize. The MHC however has a smaller number of genes and does not diversify during ontogeny, so that the class II genes expressed on the antigen-presenting cells (APCs) of different individuals are functionally different with regard to the antigens they can present. Consequently MHC haplotype has a major effect on variations in antigen-specific immune responsiveness between individuals.

	antigen	recipient	delayed hypersensitivity to: PLL		antibody to: DNP	
			strain 2	strain 13	strain 2	strain 13
1	PLL–DNP	normal	+	–	+	–
2	BSA–PLL–DNP	normal	+	–	+	+
3	BSA–PLL–DNP	BSA-tolerant	+	–	+	–

Fig.11.12 Holes in the repertoire of T cell responses. Strain 2 and strain 13 guinea-pigs were immunized with the antigens shown, the T cell response was measured by delayed hypersensitivity to poly-L-lysine (PLL) and the TH cell response was measured by the ability to cooperate with B cells in the production of antibody to DNP. (1). Strain 13 animals do not respond to PLL or DNP whereas strain 2 do, suggesting a hole in the functional T cell repertoire. (2). The lack of antibody response can be bypassed for the TH cells by adding a BSA carrier to the PLL–DNP. (3). If the animal is tolerant to BSA the BSA–PLL–DNP no longer stimulates the TH cells, confirming that bypass is via the new BSA carrier. It is not certain whether the hole in the T cell repertoire is at the point of education, presentation or in the antigen receptor.

different individuals. This idea is illustrated in Fig. 11.11. There has been some debate as to whether the lack of response in low responder strains is due to the failure of the MHC molecules to present antigen, or the failure of the T cell population to recognize it – referred to as a hole in the T cell receptor repertoire. Experimentally it is difficult to distinguish these possibilities (Fig.11.12). On balance, failure of presentation appears more important, although there are some cases where holes in the T cell repertoire are implicated. Thus, although the antigen receptor genes do have a profound influence on the initial repertoire of T cell receptors, the repertoire becomes modified considerably during ontogeny. This effect is seen in the skewing of the spectrum of expressed T cell receptor V genes which occurs following selection of T cells in the thymus. Recent experiments of Kappler and Marrack have indicated that the expressed T cell repertoire may be affected by the Mls gene locus. It is known that a large proportion of T cells in a mouse with the b allele of Mls recognize Mls^a. Close linkage was found between reactivity to Mls^a and the use of the $V\beta8$ T cell receptor gene. Studies of animals expressing Mls^a revealed that T cells using $V\beta8$ were deleted during development in the thymus. Thus tolerance to this particular self-antigen results in elimination of T cells using $V\beta8$. Similarly, mice expressing the I–E molecule undergo a deletion of T cells bearing $V\beta17$ (see Chapter 12).

CROSS-REACTIVE IDIOTYPES

The antibody genes partly determine which idiotypes are seen on the antibodies in animals of different strains. Particular idiotypes occur at high levels in all animals of a strain in the antibody response to particular antigens. This form of dominant idiotype expression has been noted in the response to many antigens and they are called cross-reactive idiotypes. Fig. 11.13 shows the distribution patterns of responsiveness to simple antigens which suggests that idiotype expression is linked to the Ig heavy chain haplotype. However it is clear that the association between haplotype and idiotype is not complete. This is explained by the gene rearrangements and mutation occurring during B cell development. Thus some animals will acquire a dominant idiotype from their germ line genes, while others may develop it during ontogeny. This occurs in the antibody response of different mouse strains to the arsonate hapten where strains of different Ig haplotype have developed a similar heavy chain DJ region and consequently share an idiotype.

It seems then that the occurrence of particular cross-reactive idiotypes in different strains represents a genetic predisposition to make particular antibodies, and as such it is the opposite of a hole in the repertoire. It is likely that cross-reactive idiotypes play a role in the regulation of the immune response, since they provide a target for idiotype-specific T-helper or T-suppressor cells.

MHC MOLECULES

The central role of MHC haplotype in immune responses cannot be overemphasized. Even small changes in the structure of MHC molecules have profound effects on immune recognition. The use of mice with mutant alleles coding for the H-2K antigens has greatly facilitated the studies on the fine specificity of cytotoxic T cells. For example, mutant animals spontaneously arising in the wild type C57BL/6 mouse strain (H-$2K^b$) have been studied extensively at the functional and structural levels. These mice are referred to as the bm series and have haplotypes designated H-2^{bm} (Fig. 11.14). The H-2K glycoproteins of the mutant mouse H-$2K^{bm1}$ are serologically almost indistinguishable from the wild type. However cytotoxic T cells can discriminate between H-$2K^b$ and H-$2k^{bm1}$ virally infected targets. The effects caused by haplotype differences in class II molecules were studied by Buus who showed how different antigenic peptides would associate with class II molecules of different haplotype (Fig. 11.15). In general, MHC restriction of the immune response to a particular antigen in a strain is reflected in how well antigenic peptides bind to the different MHC molecules. For example, the peptide OVA (323–339) is recognized in H-2^d animals but not H-2^k animals. This peptide binds to the I–A^d class II molecule, but not to I–A^k or I–E^k molecules.

The MHC haplotype of an animal may also affect the balance between T cell help and suppression as shown by studies on hen egg-white lysozyme (HEL) and its peptides, N–C, L II and L III. The response to HEL is under immune response (Ir) gene control and it is possible to demonstrate T cell proliferation and generation of T-helper cells to HEL in responding strains following priming by the N–C peptide or the L II peptide. When intact HEL is used for priming, T-helper activity is triggered predominantly by epitopes of the L II peptide (Fig. 11.16). Mice of the H-2^b haplotype do not develop this pattern of reactivity, and Sercarz and colleagues have shown that non-responsiveness of certain mouse strains to HEL is due to the development of T-suppressor cells generated by the N–C peptide. Responder strains primed by N–C develop some T cell help specific for HEL while non-responder strains subjected to the same immunization develop T-suppressor cells. The pattern of response is therefore determined by the balance of help to suppression which is in turn affected by the animal's MHC haplotype.

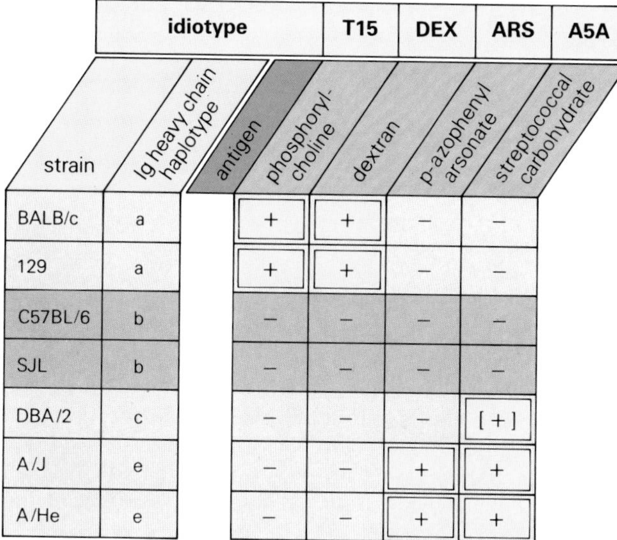

strain	Ig heavy chain haplotype	idiotype: T15 (antigen: phosphoryl-choline)	DEX (dextran)	ARS (p-azophenyl arsonate)	A5A (streptococcal carbohydrate)
BALB/c	a	+	+	–	–
129	a	+	+	–	–
C57BL/6	b	–	–	–	–
SJL	b	–	–	–	–
DBA/2	c	–	–	–	[+]
A/J	e	–	–	+	+
A/He	e	–	–	+	+

Fig.11.13 Cross-reactive idiotypes. The four main idiotypes to four different antigens in different strains of mice are shown. These idiotypes appear to be linked to the Ig heavy chain locus. In general, each idiotype is present in mice of only one heavy chain haplotype. Sometimes however, the idiotype may be found in a different haplotype strain also, such as the A5A idiotype detectable in DBA/2. The A5A idiotype is present in lower amounts than in Ig^e strains and it is thought that either (a) the shape of the A5A idiotype has been generated on a protein with a different sequence to that of the A/J strain or (b) mutation and recombination generated the A5A amino acid sequence from a different germ line gene than in the Ig^e haplotype strains.

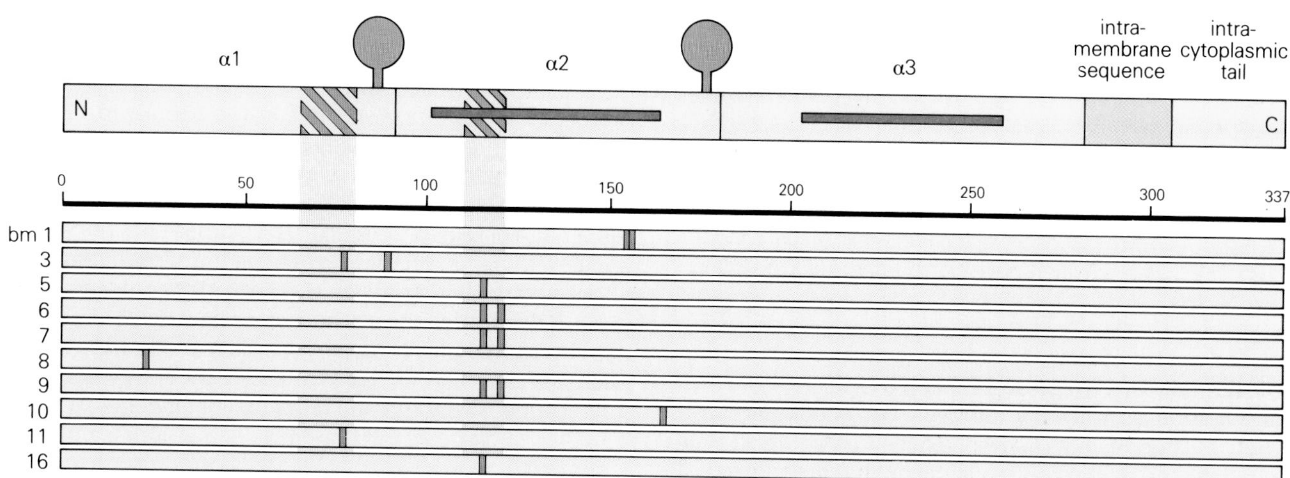

Fig.11.14 Mutation in the MHC. In this representation of an H-2K molecule, blue = carbohydrate, red = intradomain disulphide bonds, and hatching = proposed allotypic sites. Mutations in the H-2K locus of mice in the bm series were identified by skin grafting between a very large number of mice of a single strain (H-2^b). The mutations in the H-2K locus of ten animals are clustered in the α1 and α2 domains with particular sites being especially mutable. These findings indicate that MHC genes have the highest mutation rate of any germ line genes yet studied.

peptide	H-2d I-A	H-2d I-E	H-2k I-A	H-2k I-E
OVA (323–339)	++			
HEL (46–61)			+++	
MYO (132–153)		++		
p.CYT (88–104)			(+)	++
λ repr (12–26)	(+)	++		(+)

Fig 11.15 Antigen binding to MHC class II molecules. The binding of peptides to I–A and I–E encoded molecules of H-2^d and H-2^k haplotypes is indicated. (+++ = strong, (+) = very weak). Pink shaded blocks indicate known MHC restrictions *in vivo*. This usually corresponds with the MHC molecule to which the antigenic peptide binds best. (OVA = ovalbumin ; HEL = hen egg-white lysozyme ; MYO = myoglobin ; p.CYT = pigeon cytochrome C; λ repr = λ repressor.)

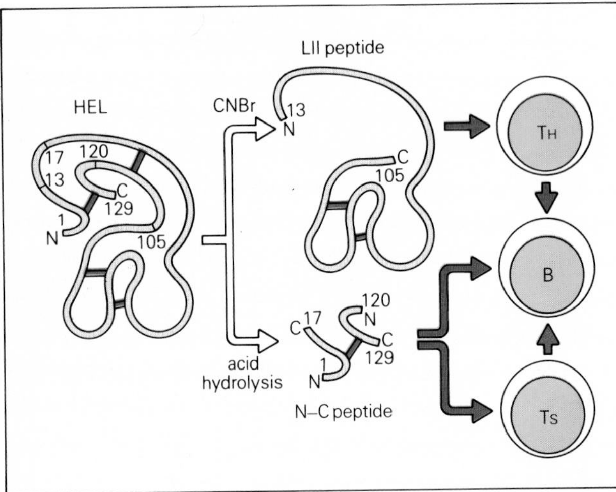

Fig.11.16 Immune response to hen egg-white lysozyme (HEL). The structure of HEL is shown with disulphide bonds in red. Certain amino acids are marked. The molecule can be cleaved by acid hydrolysis to yield an N–C peptide or by CNBr to yield a large peptide, LII. The LII peptide is recognized by T-helper (TH) cells. B cells recognize a determinant on the N–C peptide, and T-suppressor (Ts) cells also recognize the N–C peptide; thus the antibody response results from the balance between help and suppression. H-2^a high responder animals have T cells which recognize LII but no Ts cells recognizing N–C; H-2^b low responders have high numbers of Ts cells and few TH cells.

OTHER IMMUNE RESPONSE GENES

The responses to many antigens are under polygenic control. High or low responsiveness to a complex antigen could arise in many ways; through macrophages, T cells or B cells. Biozzi noted that within an outbred mouse colony some mice were high responders (in terms of antibody production) to erythrocyte antigens whereas other mice were low responders. Following selective inbreeding of high responder mice and separate inbreeding of low responder mice Biozzi had, after

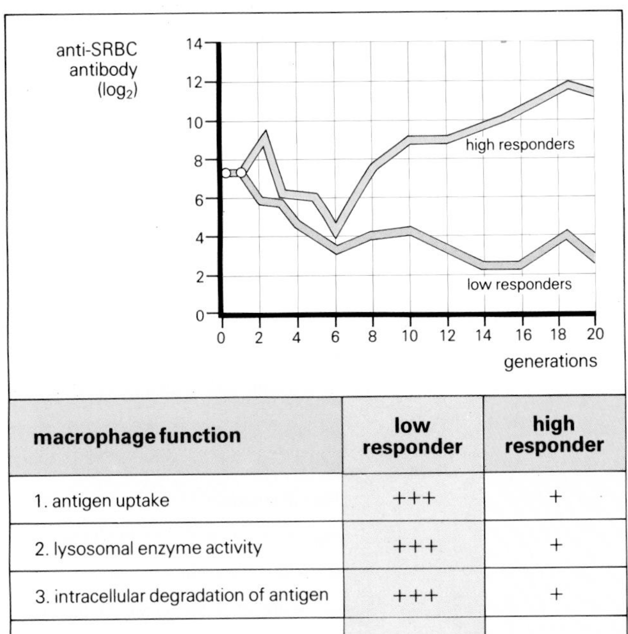

macrophage function	low responder	high responder
1. antigen uptake	+++	+
2. lysosomal enzyme activity	+++	+
3. intracellular degradation of antigen	+++	+
4. surface persistence of antigen	+	+++

Fig.11.17 Macrophage functions in high and low responder mice. Mice giving high responses and low responses to sheep red blood cells (SRBC, a complex multideterminate antigen) were inbred over 20 successive generations to produce separate high and low responder strains – Biozzi mice. As shown in the table, the low responder strain processes antigen in the macrophages faster than the high responder strain.

20 generations, established two strains of mice; one producing a high response to erythrocyte antigens the other producing a low response. The differences between the two strains is attributed to at least 10 genes, some of which affect macrophage functions. The high responder Biozzi mice present the antigen on the surface of the presenting cell for a longer time than the low responder strain. The macrophages of the low responders appear to be highly efficient at taking up the antigen and degrading it within the lysosomes (Fig. 11.17). This high lysosomal activity in the low responder mice also renders them less susceptible to intracellular parasites.

Resistance or susceptibility to *Leishmania donovani, Salmonella typhimurium* and *Mycobacterium bovis* appears to map to a gene locus on chromosome 1 of the mouse. Thus the genes Lsh, Ity and Bcg, which determine innate responsiveness to these infectious agents respectively, may be identical. Resistance to *L. donovani* appears to be linked to macrophage function. Therefore although the MHC has been shown to play a role in determining the course of viral and some bacterial infections it is apparent that resistance to some parasites and some bacteria is either wholly controlled by some non-H-2 linked genes or by H-2 and non-H-2 linked genes.

GENETICALLY IMMUNODEFICIENT MOUSE STRAINS

CBA/N mice carry an X-linked B cell defect (xid) which is manifest in the inability to respond to certain

		CBA/N	normal
antibody response	poly I:C 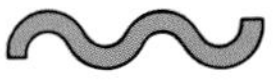	–	+
	poly I:C–BSA 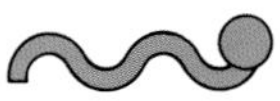	+	+
spleen (B) cell colony formation from 5×10^4 cells	spontaneous	0	49
	LPS	0	248
$CD5^+$ spleen cells (%)		0%	30%

Fig.11.18 Genetic defects of CBA/N mice. Antibody response: CBA/N mice are unable to respond to the T-independent antigen, poly I:C, but can recognize the antigen when it is coupled to a T-dependent carrier, BSA. Spleen cell colony formation: CBA/N spleen cells (5×10^4) fail to produce colonies spontaneously, or when stimulated with LPS. They appear to lack a subset of $CD5^+$ B cells.

	♂ response			♀ response		
BALB/c	X	Y	+	X	X	+
DBA/2Ha	X	Y	–	X	X	–
BALB/c(♀)×DBA/2Ha(♂)	X	Y	+	X	X	+
DBA/2Ha(♀)×BALB/c(♂)	X	Y	–	X	X	+

Fig.11.19 TRF receptor defect in DBA/2Ha mice. Male and female mice were assayed for their response to T cell replacing factor (TRF). Male (XY) and female (XX) BALB/c mice respond to the factor, whereas neither male nor female DBA/2Ha mice do. Offspring of crosses between these responder and non-responder strains were tested. If BALB/c females are crossed with DBA/2Ha males both male and female offspring respond, whereas in the reciprocal cross only the females respond. This implies that a gene on the DBA/2Ha X chromosome is defective. In the F1 mice those animals which have at least one normal BALB/c X chromosome can respond.

T-independent antigens such as TNP–Ficoll, and to have decreased IgM and IgG3. These mice may have a B cell maturational defect and lack a subset of B cells bearing CD5. CBA/N mice have also been shown to lack a clonable B cell population (Fig. 11.18). Interestingly, patients with Wiskott-Aldrich syndrome (an X-linked condition) are also incapable of responding to some polysaccharide antigens and they may also lack a B cell subset. Therefore, non-responsiveness to a given antigen could in some cases be attributed not only to overriding T-suppressors, or lack of T-helpers, but also to a lack of a relevant B cell subset.

Mutant mice have been described with severe combined immunodeficiency (SCID) attributed to an autosomal recessive gene, scid. Homozygous mice (scid/scid) have depressed T and B cell numbers, impaired immune responses and hypogammaglobulinaemia. The scid defect appears to be due to the impaired development of the lymphopoietic stem cells since SCID bone marrow cannot fully reconstitute the lymphoid system of normal irradiated MHC compatible recipients. The strain appears to be a good model of human severe combined immunodeficiency.

There is some evidence which suggests that B cells are sensitive to some non-specific T cell factors. A T cell replacing factor (TRF) has been found in the supernatants of suitably stimulated murine spleen cell cultures. TRF can be shown to overcome the usual MHC-restricted interaction of T and B cells. Recently a mouse strain DBA/2Ha has been described which is unable to respond to TRF since its B cells lack a receptor for it. This has been shown to be an X-linked disorder (Fig. 11.19). Another mouse strain which expresses a B cell function abnormality is the C3H/Hej mouse. These mice do not respond to the lipid A extract of LPS but do respond to the lipoproteins. Functionally this defect results in a greater than 1000-fold reduction in the number of B cell precursors which respond to LPS. The lack of responsiveness to LPS has been attributed to the lack of a relevant receptor for LPS on the surface of the C3H/Hej B cell.

MODELS OF AUTOIMMUNE DISEASE

Several animal models of autoimmunity exist which partly mimic the human diseases. These models exist for both organ specific and non-organ specific autoimmune disease (Fig. 11.20).

Perhaps the best studied models of non-organ specific autoimmunity have been those spontaneously arising in mice. The NZB, NZB×NZW F1 and MRL/1pr mice are animal models of Coombs' positive haemolytic anaemia, systemic lupus erythematosus (SLE) and rheumatoid arthritis respectively. These animals have a variety of disorders and regulatory disturbances associated with the spontaneous occurrence of autoimmunity. In an attempt to analyse whether some of these disorders were of primary importance in the development of autoimmunity in the NZB mouse, Wiegert and Riblet constructed recombinant inbred lines of mice using the non-autoimmune C58 and the autoimmune NZB mouse as the two parental strains. These studies allowed them to confirm and extend previous observations and thus to

abnormal function	strain(s) affected
thymic epithelium	NZB × NZW (F1)
thymic hormone levels	NZB
pre-T cells	NZB
T cell immunoregulation	NZB, MRL /lpr
IL-2 levels	MRL /lpr
generation of non-specific suppression	NZB × NZW (F1)
tolerance induction	NZB, NZB × NZW (F1)
B cell hyperactivity	NZB, Me^v
DNA repair	NZB

Fig.11.20 Defects in genetically autoimmune mice.

conclude that the development of autoimmunity in NZB mice was:

1. under polygenic control involving at least 7 genes
2. not linked to MHC haplotype
3. not related to B cell hyperactivity
4. not linked to defective autologous mixed lymphocyte reactivity
5. not linked to inherited V region genes.

The NZB×NZW F1 hybrid mouse develops an SLE-like disease and dies of glomerulonephritis, whereas the NZB parent develops haemolytic anaemia with mild kidney disease and the NZW is non-autoimmune. Breeding studies have shown that the genetic contribution of the NZW to the development of kidney disease in the F1 is linked to the MHC. While it is always tempting to attribute any MHC-linked gene effect to an MHC molecule, recent studies by McDevitt and colleagues have clearly shown that a polymorphism in the TNFα gene (located within the MHC) of the NZW mouse results in reduced levels of production of TNFα. Treatment of NZB×NZW F1 mice with TNFα significantly delays the development of glomerulonephritis in these animals and prolongs their lifespan.

Another autosomal recessive mutation, motheaten viable (me^v) causes immunodeficiency and autoimmune disease. Homozygous me^v/me^v mice produce high levels of serum immunoglobulins and develop multiple autoantibodies and immune complex depositions in skin, kidney and lungs. The elevated B cell responses of these animals has been attributed to hyperinduction of B cell growth and maturation factors. An interesting feature of these animals is the almost complete usage of $CD5^+$ B cells. Taken together with the spontaneous production of IgM autoantibodies by this subpopulation of B cells and the non-development of autoimmunity in NZB mice into which x-linked immunodeficiency (xid) gene (the defective gene of the CBA / N strain) has been introduced, this has lead Herzenberg and others to propose that the $CD5^+$ B cell is involved in the development of autoimmune disease.

With regard to models of organ specific autoimmune disease, the obese strain chicken is perhaps the best animal model of Hashimoto's thyroiditis in man (see Chapter 23). Two good spontaneous models of insulin-dependent diabetes mellitus (IDDM) exist. These are the BB rat and the NOD mouse. The development of disease in these two animal models has been shown, as in the human, to be under polygenic control. In the mouse, genetic studies have implicated three recessive genes in the development of IDDM. One of these, as in man, is linked to the MHC, a second gene has been shown to be located on chromosome 9 close to Thy-1 while the third gene remains to be identified. McDevitt and his colleagues have recently carried out sequence analysis of the Aβ chain of the NOD mouse which does not express I–E and uses $A\alpha^d$, and have shown that the first external domain of this class II I–Aβ chain is unique, leading to the suggestion that this sequence directly contributes to disease susceptibility. This proposal has been strengthened by comparative analysis of sequence data for DQβ of diabetic and non-diabetic individuals which suggests that the amino acid at position 57 of the β chain determines whether an autoimmune response against the pancreatic β cell will occur.

FURTHER READING

Acha-Orbea, H. & McDevitt, H.O. (1987) The first external domain of the non obese diabetic mouse class II I–Aβ chain is unique. *Proceedings of the National Academy of Sciences (USA)*, **84**, 2435.

Benjamin, D.C. & Berzofsky, J.A. *et al.* (1984) The antigenic structure of proteins: a reappraisal. *Annual Review of Immunology*, **2**, 67.

Bocchieri, M., Cooke, A., Smith, B., Weigert, M. & Riblet, R. (1982) Independent aggregation of NZB: immune abnormalities in NZB × C58 recombinant inbred mice. *European Journal of Immunology*, **4**, 349.

Green, M.C. & Schultz, L.D. (1975) Motheaten, an immunodeficient mutant of the mouse. I. Genetics and pathology. *Journal of Heredity*, **66**, 250.

Heber-Katz, E., Hansburg, D. & Schwartz, R.H. (1983) The Ia molecule of the antigen-presenting cell plays a critical role in immune response gene regulation of T cell activation. *Journal of Molecular and Cellular Immunology*, **1**, 3.

Jacob, C.O. & McDevitt, H.O. (1988) Tumour necrosis factor-α in murine autoimmune 'lupus' nephritis. *Nature*, **331**, 356.

Jareway, C.A. (1983) Immune response genes, the problem of the non-responder. *Journal of Molecular and Cellular Immunology*, **1**, 15.

Kappler, J.W., Staerz, U., White, J. & Marrack, P.C. (1988) Self-tolerance eliminates T cells specific for M1s-modified products of the major histocompatibility complex. *Nature*, **332**, 35.

Krco, C.J. & David, C.S. (1981) Genetics of the immune response: a survey. *C.R.C. Critical Reviews in Immunology*, **1**, 211.

Longo, D.L., Matis, L.A. & Schwartz, R.H. (1981) Insights into immune response gene function from experiments with chimeric animals. *C.R.C. Critical Reviews in Immunology*, **2**, 83.

Marchalonis, J.J., Vasta, G.R., Warr, G. & Barker, W.C. (1984) Probing the boundaries of the extended immunoglobulin family of recognition molecules: jumping domains, convergence and minigenes. *Immunology Today*, **5**, 133.

Robson Macdonald, H., Schneider, R., Lees, R.K., Ho, R.C., Acha-Orbea, H., Festenstein, H., Zinkernagel, R.M. & Hengartner, H. (1988) T cell receptor Vβ use predicts reactivity and tolerance to $M1s^a$ encoded antigens. *Nature*, **332**, 40.

Scher, I. (1982) CBA/N immune defective mice; evidence for a failure of a B cell subpopulation to be expressed. *Immunological Reviews*, **64**, 117.

Schultz, L.D., Colman, D.R., Bailey, C.L., Beamer, W.G. & Sidman, C.L. (1984) 'Viable motheaten' a new allele at the motheaten locus. I. Pathology. *American Journal of Pathology*, **116**, 179.

Todd, J.A., Bell, J.I. & McDevitt, H.O. (1987) HLA–DQβ gene contribution to susceptibility and resistance to insulin dependent diabetes mellitus. *Nature*, **329**, 599.

12 Immunological Tolerance

Immunological tolerance is the acquisition of non-reactivity towards particular antigens (referred to in this context as tolerogens), and as such it is the converse of immunity. The importance of tolerance to self-antigens was appreciated early in the development of immunology by Ehrlich and is fundamental to the normal functioning of the immune system. However, in the 1920s, it was discovered that tolerance could also be induced in animals to non-self antigens. For example, it was noted that sufficiently large doses of diphtheria toxoid would suppress the immune response normally elicited by smaller antigen doses.

A major breakthrough in understanding the mechanisms by which tolerance can be induced was made in 1945 when it was discovered that dizygotic cattle twins (developed from two fertilized ova and therefore, non-identical) became tolerant to each other's tissue antigens if they had exchanged embryonic blood following placental fusion (Fig. 12.1). These non-identical animals would normally be expected to reject tissue grafts from the other twin, but having exchanged embryonic blood it was found that the animals were stable chimaeras (composed of cells of two genetically different tissue types) with respect to their haemopoietic tissue and could mutually exchange skin grafts. This phenomenon was examined experimentally by Billingham, Brent and Medawar who injected spleen cells of adult mice into newborn mice of a different strain. Upon maturation the recipient mice were tolerant to skin grafts of the donor strain but rejected grafts of unrelated strains (Figs 12.2 and 12.3).

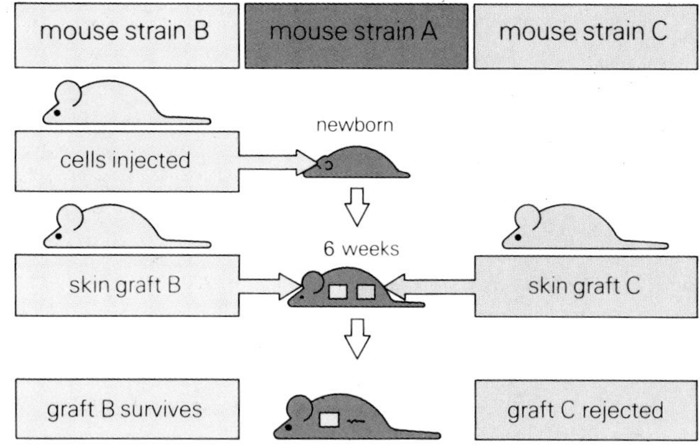

Fig. 12.2 Billingham, Brent and Medawar's neonatal grafting experiment. This demonstrates the induction of specific tolerance to grafted skin in mice by neonatal injection of spleen cells from a different strain. Mice of strain A normally reject grafts from strain B. However, if newborn mice of strain A receive cells from strain B mice and 6 weeks later are grafted with skin from mice of strains B and C, the mice show tolerance towards skin grafts from the donor strain B, but reject grafts from other strains (C).

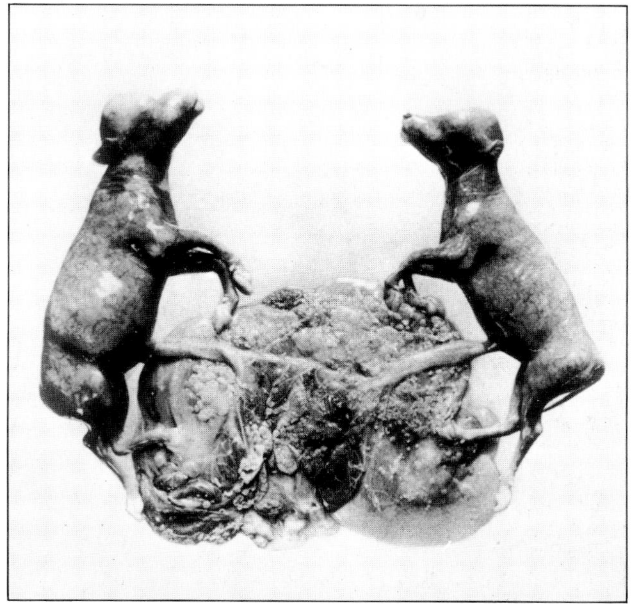

Fig. 12.1 Dizygotic cattle twins fused at the placentae (Dr Ray Owen's observation). Fusion of the placentae leads to exchange of blood cells in fetal life. Following separation the animals permanently retain the cells of the other twin, and are permanently tolerant to grafts of that twin's tissue type.

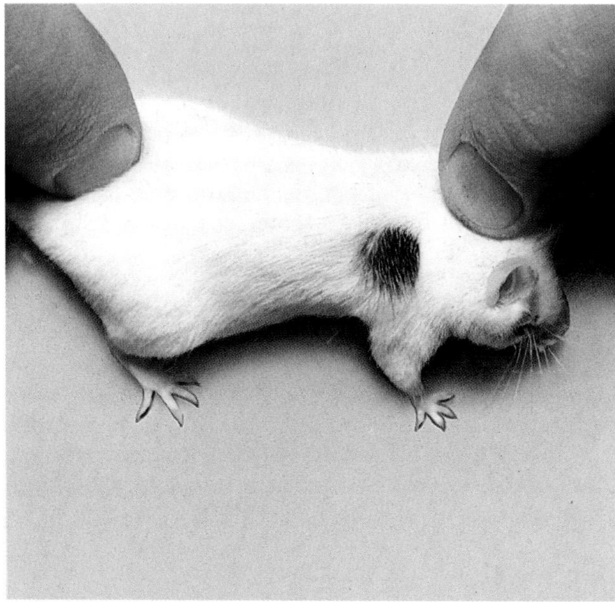

Fig. 12.3 A healthy brown hair graft growing on a tolerant white mouse 45 days after grafting.

The historical development of the concept of tolerance may be summarized as follows.

1. High doses of antigen in adult life lead to specific unresponsiveness. Antigens observed include:
   - 1924 protein (diphtheria toxoid)
   - 1927 polysaccharide (pneumococcal)
   - 1929 simple chemical (neoarsphenamine).
2. Exposure of antigen in embryonic life leads to specific unresponsiveness.
   - 1945 stable haemopoietic chimaerism in dizygotic cattle twins (see Fig. 12.1).
   - 1949 natural or artificial exposure to antigen (non-self) in embryonic life created tolerance (as for self)
   - 1951 skin grafts exchanged reciprocally in chimaeric cattle twins found to survive
   - 1953 chimaerism induced in neonatal mice which accepted skin grafts from each other in adult life
   - 1959 maturation of lymphocytes involved a stage where exposure to an antigen led to an alteration in the lymphocyte's development involving the loss of its immune function – that is, the lymphocytes become tolerant to that antigen.
3. In the early 1960s it was appreciated that tolerance and immunity could be induced with all classes of antigens in neonatal and adult animals – whether immunity or tolerance is produced depends upon the dose.

Although a single mechanism accounting for the generation and maintenance of the tolerant state has not been discovered, many studies have defined important characteristics of the phenomenon.

PATHWAYS TO TOLERANCE

By 1960 it had become evident that there were several pathways to immunological tolerance, and recent data suggests that both B cells and T cells may become tolerized under particular circumstances and that they are affected independently and differently. Not only do these cells differ in the ways in which they can be tolerized, they also vary in their susceptibility to tolerance throughout their clonal ontogeny. Immature B cells are particularly susceptible to tolerization by contact with antigen, but following development into mature B cells and subsequently into antibody-forming cells (AFCs) they become increasingly resistant. In effect, the further the B cell has progressed along its maturation pathway, the higher the dose of antigen required to tolerize the cell. T cells, by contrast do not vary in their susceptibility during ontogeny to such a marked extent. During fetal development of the immune system, and in the first weeks of neonatal life, none of the cells of the immune system have reached maturity, and so the entire immune system of an animal is particularly susceptible to tolerance induction at this stage.

It is now recognized that fundamentally different mechanisms for establishing tolerance may lead to similar effects on the overall action of the immune system; indeed several mechanisms may operate simultaneously in a single animal.

PATHWAYS TO B CELL TOLERANCE

Four pathways leading to the tolerization of B cell function are described, and summarized in Fig. 12.4.

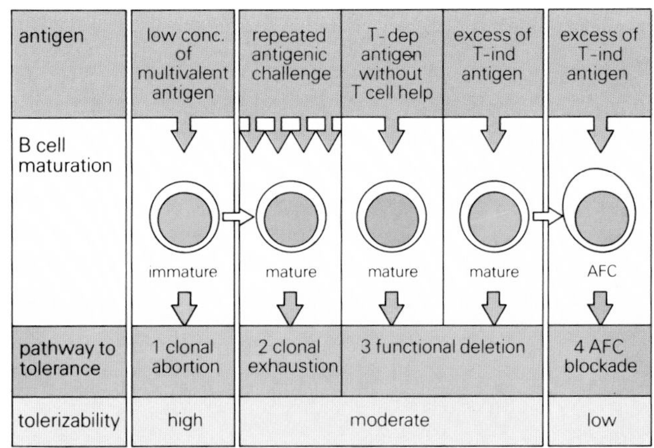

Fig. 12.4 Pathways to B cell tolerance. As an immature B cell matures into an antibody-forming cell (AFC) it becomes increasingly resistant to tolerization, and tolerizability, the susceptibility to tolerization, decreases. At the same time, the form of antigen presentation which will produce tolerance also varies. The type of tolerance induced is therefore dependent on the maturity of the cell, the antigen, and the manner in which the antigen is presented to the immune system.
1. Clonal Abortion. Low concentrations of multivalent antigen may cause the immature clone to abort. Tolerizability of immature B cells is high.
2. Clonal Exhaustion. Repeated antigenic challenge with a T-independent (T-ind) antigen may remove all mature functional B cell clones. Tolerizability of mature B cells is moderate.
3. Functional Deletion. Absence of T cell help, concurrent with the presence of T-dependent (T-dep) antigen (or with T-suppressor cells) or an excess of T-ind antigen prevents mature B cells from functioning normally.
4. AFC Blockade. Excess of T-ind antigen interferes with the secretion of antibody by the AFC. Tolerizability of AFCs is low.

Clonal Abortion Immature B cells encountering antigen for the first time are particularly susceptible to tolerization in the presence of low concentrations of antigen. In these circumstances the normal maturation of the B cell is aborted so that subsequently it is unable to respond normally to antigenic challenge.

Clonal Exhaustion Repeated antigenic challenge with immunizing doses of a particular T-independent (T-ind) antigen may cause clonal exhaustion. In this form of tolerance, all the mature B cells capable of responding to the antigen are stimulated to differentiate into short-lived AFCs (the terminal stage for B cell differentiation). If all mature responding B cells undergo this exhaustive terminal differentiation, there are no cells left capable of responding to a subsequent challenge with the antigen.

Functional Deletion The presence of T-dependent (T-dep) or T-ind antigens may lead to functional deletion of the B cells as follows.

1. Normal B cell responses to T-dep antigens require the help of specific T cells; the B cell binds to one determinant on an antigen and receives T specific help directed to another determinant. If the T help is not available the B cell may be unable to respond normally and is therefore functionally deleted.

2. T-ind antigens are high molecular weight polymers with repeating antigenic determinants capable of forming multiple bonds to the B cells, thus circumventing the requirement for T cell help. If, however, a T-ind antigen is presented to a B cell in excess or in a non-immunogenic form, the B cell will not respond normally and will therefore be functionally deleted.

Antibody-Forming Cell Blockade Although it is very difficult to tolerize AFCs, it is noted that very large doses of T-ind antigens can sometimes lead to an effective tolerization. In these circumstances it appears that the high concentrations of antigen are blockading the surface receptors of the cell and thereby interfering with antibody secretion.

PATHWAYS TO T CELL TOLERANCE

The pathways to T cell tolerance are superficially similar to those for B cell tolerance, for example, there is some evidence that immature T cells may be clonally aborted in a manner similar to that noted above. However, whereas all B cell clones have identical cellular functions ultimately leading to antibody synthesis, there are several subsets of T cells performing very different functions. The T-helper (TH) and T-cytotoxic (TC) subsets may be deleted under different circumstances leading to tolerization with respect to only one of the T cell functions. For example, precursors of mouse TC cells may be tolerized by exposure to mouse H-2 K and D antigens, whereas TH cells are tolerized only by I region antigens. Evidently, T cell subsets may only be tolerized to those antigenic determinants which they normally recognize. One other T cell subset is considered to be involved in the development and maintenance of certain states of tolerance – the T-suppressor (TS) cells.

T-SUPPRESSORS

The TS cell subset possesses the ability to suppress the function of B cells or other T cell subsets. Although it has been suggested that they act by bringing about deletion of either T or B cell clones, they probably directly suppress T and B cells. TS cells are antigen-specific and can be generated experimentally under certain injection schedules. The action of TS cells in these experimental systems can be demonstrated by transferring tolerance to a recipient by T cells. In this case the tolerance is temporary and is only maintained by the continued presence of TS cells. Experimental systems of this type in which tolerance may be transferred display 'infectious tolerance'. A shift of emphasis has arisen from more recent studies. It is argued that long-lived TS cells, which are functionally silent, rather than short-lived effector TS cells, could play a major role in the maintenance of tolerance. The pathways to T cell tolerance are summarized in Fig. 12.5.

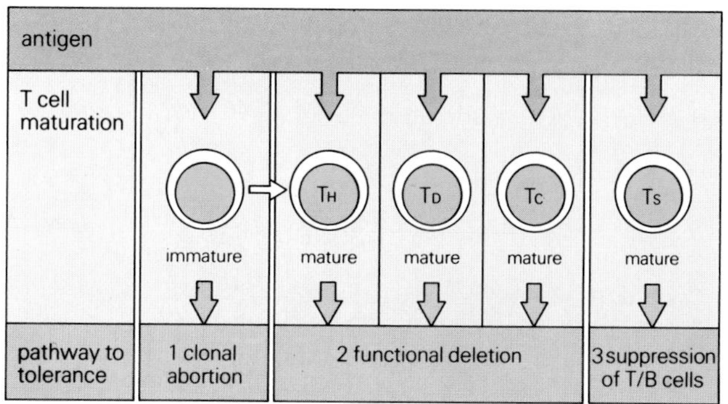

Fig. 12.5 Pathways to T cell tolerance. T cells do not show marked differences in their tolerizability at different stages of maturation. The antigen required to produce tolerance (not specified here) and the circumstances of its presentation, is particular to each individual T cell subset.
1. Clonal Abortion. Immature T cell clones may be aborted in a similar manner to B cells.
2. Functional Deletion. The subsets of mature T cells (TH, TD and TC) may be individually deleted leading to the loss of only one of the functions of the T cell group.
3. T Suppression. TS cells actively suppress the actions of other T cell subsets or B cells.

GENERAL CHARACTERISTICS OF T CELL AND B CELL TOLERIZATION

B and T cells differ in their susceptibility to tolerization *in vivo* with respect to the time course of tolerance induction, its duration and also the levels of antigen required to tolerize the cells (Fig. 12.6).

INDUCTION TIME

T cells from the spleen and thymus are tolerized rapidly with T-dep antigens – within hours of challenge. Such antigens tolerize adult splenic B cells within 4 days, but tolerization of bone marrow B cells may require up to 15 days. On the other hand T-ind antigens tend to tolerize B cells more quickly. This may be related to the higher avidity of these multivalent antigens for the B cells, or to the preferential handling of these antigens by different B cell classes.

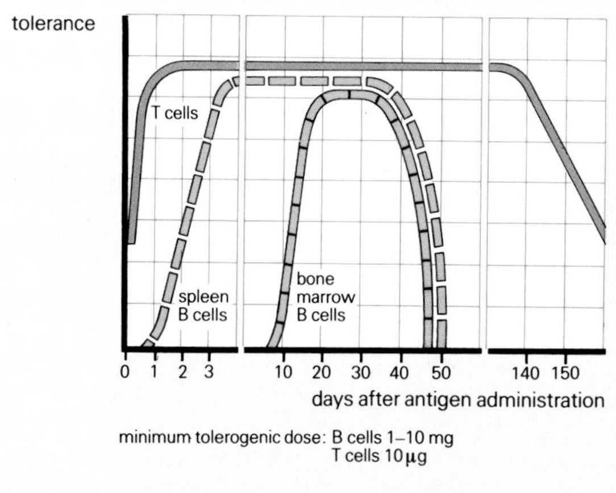

Fig. 12.6 The relative susceptibilities of T cells and B cells to tolerization *in vivo*. A mouse is administered antigen (human gammaglobulin – a T-dependent antigen) at a dose which produces tolerance (a tolerogenic dose), and the duration of tolerance is measured. T cell tolerance is more rapidly induced and more persistent than B cell tolerance. This is true whether the B cells are derived from the spleen or bone marrow, although bone marrow B cells may take considerably longer than splenic B cells to tolerize. Typically, much lower antigen doses are sufficient for T cell tolerization: 10 μg as opposed to 1–10 mg (i.e. a 1000-fold difference).

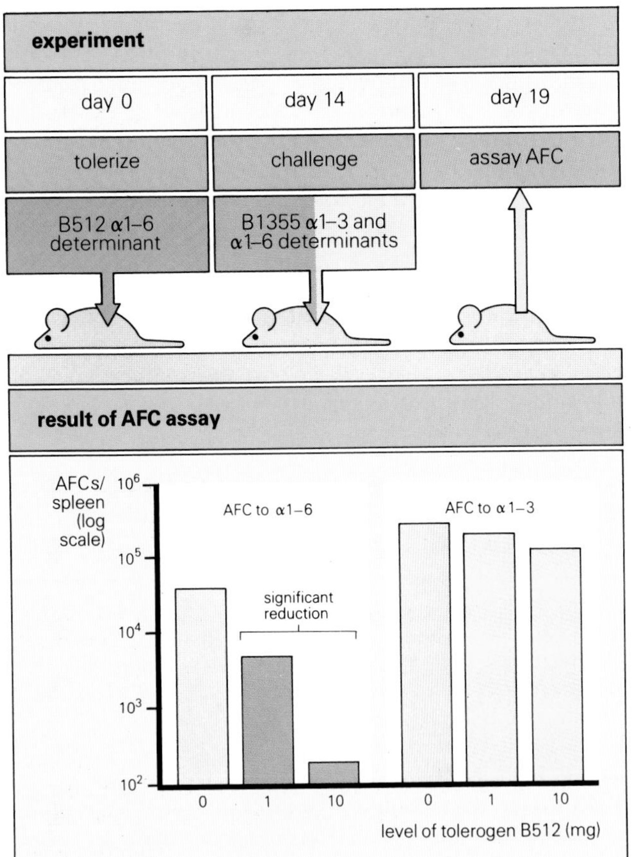

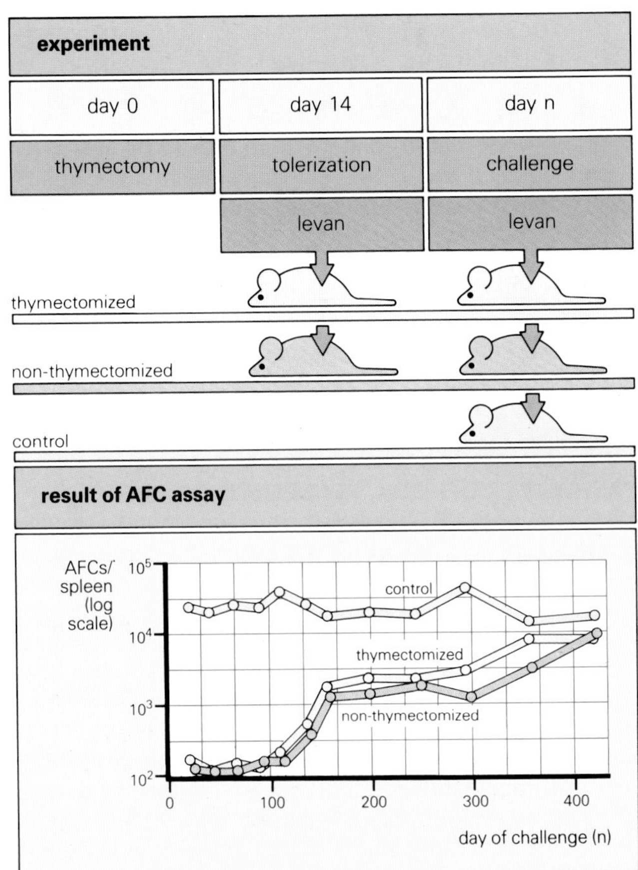

Fig. 12.7 Specificity of tolerance to one determinant, but not to another on the same antigen. The tolerogen used in this experiment was dextran B512 polysaccharide which possesses the α 1–6 glucosyl determinant. Three groups of mice were used: the first group received no tolerogen (control), the second group received 1 mg, and the third group received 10 mg. On day 14 all mice were challenged with an immunogenic dose of another polysaccharide, dextran B1355, possessing both the α 1–6 and the α 1–3 determinants. The antibody produced to these determinants was estimated on day 19 by assaying AFCs/spleen. The results of the assay are shown in the bar charts. The left hand chart shows the antibody response to the α 1–6 determinant: the response is significantly reduced and, moreover, the tolerance produced increases as the tolerogenic dose rises. The right hand chart representing the response to the α 1–3 determinant shows no significant reduction.

Fig. 12.8 Duration of tolerance – recovery from levan tolerance is similar in both thymectomized and non-thymectomized animals. On day 0, one of three groups of mice was thymectomized. On day 14 both the thymectomized group and a non-thymectomized group were tolerized with levan. At a later day (day n) both groups and a control group were challenged with an immunogenic dose of levan. The antibody response (AFCs/spleen) was then assayed and plotted against the day of levan challenge. The antibody response increases with the time interval between tolerization and antigen challenge. This recovery from tolerance shows a similar pattern for both thymectomized and non-thymectomized groups indicating that T cells are not responsible for the tolerance to this antigen.

ANTIGEN DOSE

Although B cells vary in their susceptibility to tolerance induction as they mature, the levels of antigen required to tolerize B cells are usually 100–1000-fold larger than those needed to tolerize T cells. The B cell requirement for high doses of antigen is reduced when high avidity binding between the B cell and tolerogen occurs as in reactions involving high affinity B cell receptors or multivalent antigens. Although it was initially observed that tolerance was best induced with high doses of antigen (referred to as high zone tolerance), subsequent research has shown that some weakly immunogenic antigens also induce tolerance if administered in minute quantities, typically several orders of magnitude less than would produce high zone tolerance. It has been determined that this form of tolerance is maintained by the action of Ts cells, which are triggered at much lower antigen doses than the TH cells. This form of tolerance (termed low zone tolerance) is partial however, and only affects some of the immunocytes.

ANTIGEN PERSISTENCE

Generally speaking it seems that antigen must be continually present to maintain the state of tolerance; therefore tolerance to slowly catabolized antigens, such as a D-amino acid polymer, is more persistent following a single injection (up to 1 year in mice) than tolerance to rapidly catabolized antigens. The ways in which antigens are handled *in vivo* is a major cause of discrepancy between *in vivo* and *in vitro* studies in this field.

SPECIFICITY

Experiments have shown that tolerance is developed for particular antigenic determinants, and not for particular antigens (Fig. 12.7). This can lead to tolerance to a variety of different antigens when T cells become tolerized to a single antigenic determinant which is shared by all the antigens. This tolerance can be maintained by just one of the mechanisms described above.

DURATION

Since the persistence of antigen plays a major role in maintaining tolerance, the duration of tolerance is best studied by transferring cells from tolerant animals into recipients whose immune system has been rendered non-functional by X-irradiation. It is then found that T cell tolerance is more persistent than B cell tolerance.

When tolerance is due to clonal deletion, recovery is related to the time required to regenerate mature lymphocytes from the stem cell population. If on the other hand tolerance is due to blockade of AFCs (for example, the tolerance produced by high doses of lipopolysaccharide), transfer of the tolerant cells to an environment free of antigen leads to a rapid loss of tolerance.

The duration of tolerance may also be studied experimentally by thymectomizing an animal, tolerizing it to a particular antigen and then comparing its recovery from tolerance with that of a similarly treated non-thymectomized individual. It is found that when a T-ind antigen, such as levan, is used, the profile of the thymectomized individual's recovery is identical to that of the non-thymectomized animal (Fig. 12.8). Both immunity and tolerance to T-ind antigens are B cell functions, therefore the lack of a thymus does not affect the development of tolerance or recovery from it.

INCOMPLETE TOLERANCE

Tolerance to an antigen need not necessarily be complete, but rather involve the deletion of some aspects only of the immune response.

Under normal circumstances the antibody response to a second challenge with an antigen leads to a shift in the isotype of antibody produced from IgM to IgG, with an associated increase in the overall affinity. The antibody response may however fail to mature in the normal way following tolerance induction with the result that second challenge with an antigen leads to a response marked by either an altered spectrum of immunoglobulin isotypes or antibodies of lower affinity than normal. This may be due to the preferential tolerization of high affinity B cells, blockade of AFCs of a particular isotype and/or the selective action of Ts cells. The order of susceptibility of B cell isotypes to tolerization is $B_\varepsilon > B_\gamma > B_\mu$ with T-ind antigens, and $B_{\gamma 1} > B_{\gamma 2}$ with some T-dep antigens.

Antigens in particular forms or doses may preferentially tolerize particular populations of lymphocytes (B cells or T cell subsets). Thus it is possible for an antigen to produce an antibody (humoral) response to an antigen but fail to produce sensitization when applied to the skin (T cell-mediated response). This difference in response may be due to the effects of cells regulating the immune response according to the antigen's dose, chemical modification or manner of presentation.

The phenomenon in which tolerance to one determinant on an antigen may be induced independently of any other determinants on that antigen has been discussed (see Fig. 12.7). In this case the determinant's size and density or differences in B cell receptor affinity may provide the basis for the discrimination observed.

It may occur that an animal (strain A) tolerized to tissue antigens of another strain (B) by neonatal injection of haemopoietic cells is not tolerant to skin cells of strain B. This is due to the host (A) recognizing foreign alloantigens on the strain B skin cells which are not expressed on the strain B haemopoietic cells to which the strain A animal has become tolerant. These different types of incomplete tolerance are summarized in Fig. 12.9.

level	phenomenon	basis
affinity and isotypes	antibody secretion impaired in quantity and affinity maturation, selective tolerization of isotype precursor B cells	preferential tolerance in high affinity B cells, AFC blockade, Ts cells, order of susceptibility $B_\varepsilon > B_\gamma > B_\mu$ (T-ind Ags) $B_\mu > B_{\gamma 2} > B_{\gamma 1}$ (some T-dep Ags)
humoral/CMI responses	suppression of one response independently of the other	regulatory cell interactions involving critical dosage or chemically modified antigen
determinants	different determinants on an antigen may be tolerized independently of one another	determinant size and density B cell receptor affinity
tissue specificity	animal tolerized to haemopoietic cells may not be tolerant to skin from donor strain	epidermal alloantigens not expressed by haemopoietic cells

Fig. 12.9 Incomplete tolerance. This table summarizes the types of incomplete tolerance which may be independently established and suggests the bases for the resulting phenomena observed.

MECHANISMS OF TOLERANCE INDUCTION

B CELL TOLERANCE

B cells may be tolerized to a variety of T-ind antigens. Generally speaking these antigens are slowly metabolized *in vivo* and therefore tend to promote relatively long lasting tolerance. The response of B cells to T-ind antigens is dependent on the dose of antigen injected (Fig. 12.10).

Despite their higher avidity for the B cells, T-ind antigens are required in higher doses than T-dep antigens, to act as effective tolerogens. T cells play no role in the tolerance to T-ind antigens, hence tolerization to these antigens is still seen in nude (athymic) mice. It can also be shown that humoral factors are not involved in the development of this form of tolerance since serum transfer from suppressed to normal mice does not transfer the tolerance. Studies demonstrating the lack of any humoral factor in the induction of tolerance in mature B cell clones suggests that clonal deletion or AFC blockade are the mechanisms responsible. The requirement for a large antigen dose supports this conclusion. Indeed it might be expected that the large doses of antigen used in some experiments, for example that shown in Fig. 12.10, would be capable of producing AFC blockade. However, the phenomenon of tolerance

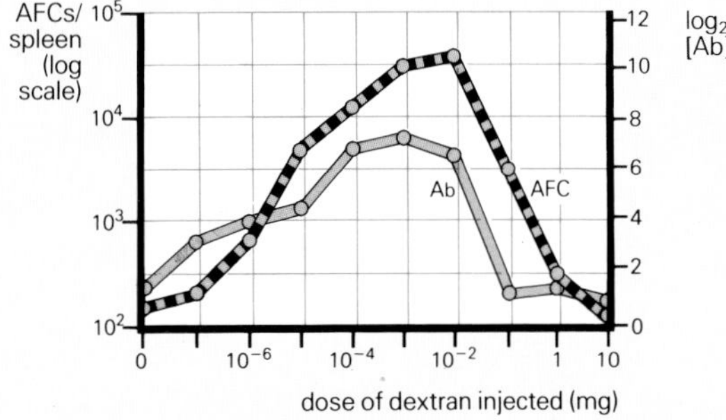

Fig. 12.10 The immune response to a T-independent antigen, dextran B512, depends upon the dose. Different groups of mice were injected with different doses of dextran and the resulting levels of antibody and AFCs/spleen were assessed and plotted against the different antigen doses. The dose of dextran required for tolerance induction appears to be lower with the antibody assay than with the AFC counts. This is attributable to peripheral neutralization of antibody by higher antigen doses. The AFC curve thus represents tolerance at the B cell level.

		B cell functional deletion	**AFC blockade**
		deletion	inhibits Ab secretion
minimum effective tolerogenic doses (mg)	dextran (500 kD)	1	0.01
	levan (6 kD)	10	inactive
isotype susceptibility		IgG >IgM	IgM >IgG
tolerance attainable		complete	partial

Fig. 12.11 Different characteristics of B cell clonal deletion and AFC blockade. Binding of the T-independent antigen to the B cell's receptors may cause functional deletion of the B cell clone. Alternatively, antigen binding to the AFC reduces antibody production by interfering with processes involved in antibody secretion. These two mechanisms of tolerance induction may be distinguished by the minimum effective dose of tolerogens and their molecular weight, the relative susceptibility of different classes of antibody affected and the level of tolerance attainable.

by B cell deletion or AFC blockade displays different characteristics in respect of the doses required to produce tolerance and in the degree of antibody suppression produced, which in turn is related to the difficulty encountered in trying to suppress the fully differentiated AFCs. AFC blockade and B cell clonal deletion are dissociable phenomena (Fig. 12.11).

In contrast with mature B cells, neonatal B cells are much more susceptible to tolerance induction. It is found that the levels of antigen which will produce B cell tolerance in neonates are approximately 100-fold smaller than those in adults (Fig. 12.12).

There appear to be two elements involved in the failure of pre-B cell maturation in the presence of

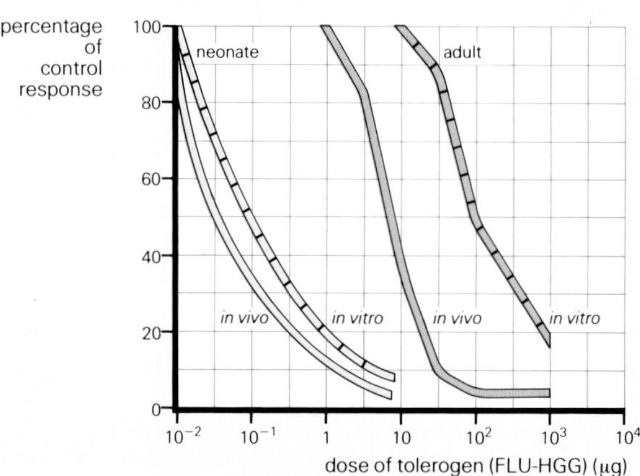

Fig. 12.12 Tolerance susceptibility of neonatal B cells to a T-independent antigen (FLU-HGG) *in vivo* and *in vitro*. The antibody response is represented as a percentage of the normal response. The dose required to achieve a tolerant state in the neonate is about 100-fold smaller than that required in the adult, since in the neonatal period all B cells are at an early stage of their clonal ontogeny and are relatively easily tolerized. It is easier to tolerize B cells *in vivo* than *in vitro*, a phenomenon probably related to the different methods of antigen presentation in the lymphoid tissue *in vivo*.

antigen. These were examined by Pike and colleagues who used anti-IgM to mimic the effect of antigen cross-linking the B cell antigen receptor. They found that 10 μg/ml of anti-IgM prevented the development of IgM^+ B cells from a pool of lymphocytes containing pre-B cells. However they also found that at lower concentrations (0.1 μg/ml), the capacity of B cells to respond to the mitogen LPS was markedly impaired, even though normal numbers of B cells were appearing. This implies that both cell numbers and cell function can be modulated via their membrane immunoglobulin at an early stage of development.

The production of B cell tolerance to T-dep antigens in the adult is a more difficult procedure to study since TH cells will normally supply help directed to determinants on the antigen (carrier determinants) enabling them to trigger B cells into a response. Thus, tolerance to these antigens can only be produced where this mechanism is circumvented such as when the animals lack T cells (nude mice) or where the T cells are effectively tolerant to the carrier determinants (Fig. 12.13).

T CELL TOLERANCE

Mature T cell tolerance may either be due to functional deletion of T cells or be related to the induction of Ts cells. Some of the ways of distinguishing the two types of tolerance were briefly mentioned earlier. It is found that:

1. TH cell deletion occurs more rapidly than Ts cell generation
2. TH cell deletion can be induced by stimuli that do not induce Ts cell generation (for example by the drug cyclophosphamide, whose action is discussed later)
3. tolerance due to TH deletion may not be transferred to recipient animals by cells of a tolerized animal
4. tolerance due to deletion of TH cells persists even after the loss of Ts cells.

These points are summarized in Fig. 12.14

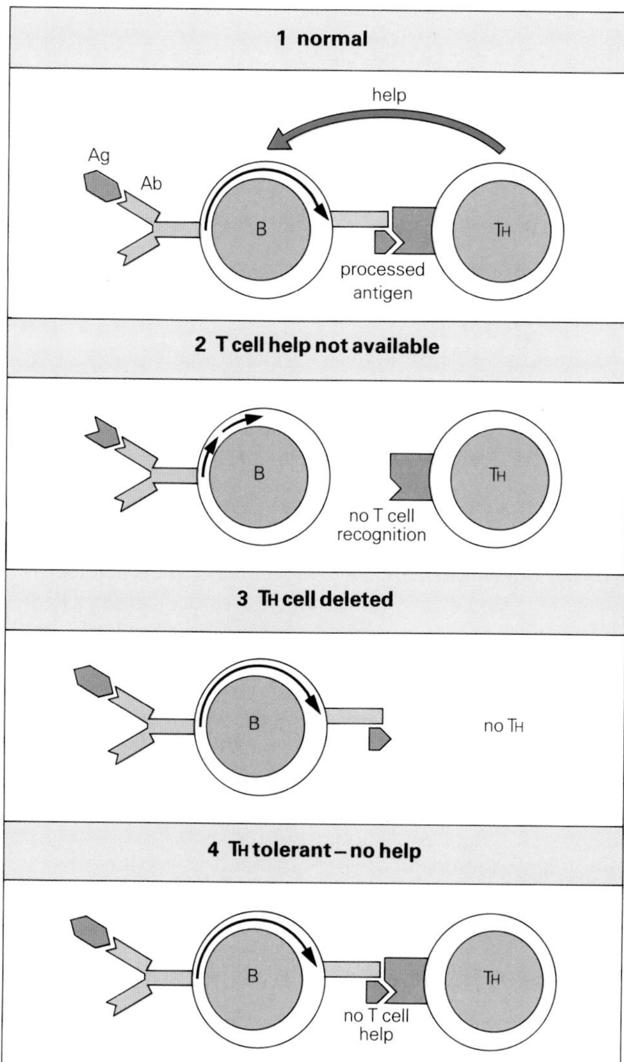

Fig. 12.13 Induction of B cell tolerance in adults to T-dependent antigens. Normally TH cells deliver help to responding B cells via recognition of processed antigen and class II MHC molecules expressed on the B cell surface (1). The scheme of tolerance is based on the failure of TH cells to deliver help to antigen-specific B cells. If the B cell fails to present a recognizable signal to the T cell (e.g. with univalent deaggregated gammaglobulin), no help will be delivered (2). The T cells may be deleted as in nude mice (3) or they may be functionally tolerized so that they do not deliver help, even if they recognize the antigen on the B cell (4).

evidence for clonal deletion in antigen-induced T cell tolerance

- rapid onset of TH cell deletion precedes Ts cell generation
- induced when Ts cell generation is suppressed (e.g. cyclophosphamide)
- tolerance broken *in vivo* by normal lymphocytes (parabiosis)
- tolerance persists after loss of Ts cells

Fig. 12.14 Evidence for clonal deletion in antigen-induced T cell tolerance: dissociability from Ts cell generation. These experimental findings favour the view that the tolerance produced in the experiments performed is due to Ts cell deletion rather than the induction of Ts cells.

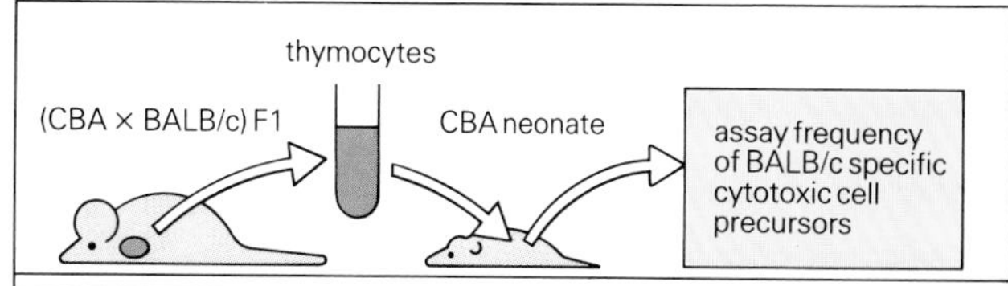

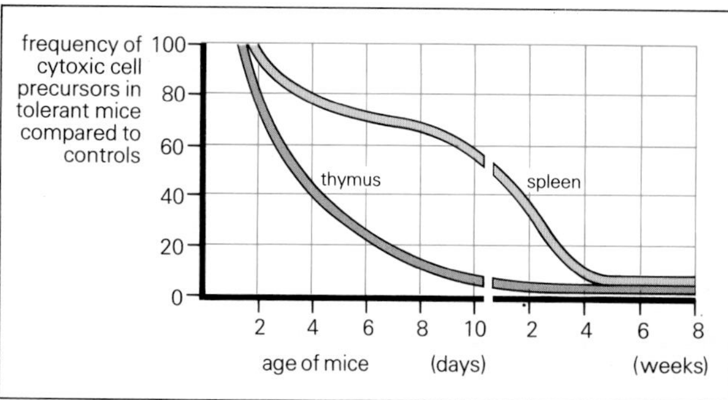

Fig. 12.15 T cell tolerance induced by clonal deletion. Neonatal CBA mice were tolerized to BALB/c by injection of 5×10^7 adult (CBA × BALB/c)F1 thymocytes. The frequency of cytotoxic cells specific for BALB/c in the spleen and thymus of these animals was measured over the following 8 weeks, using a limiting dilution assay. The frequency is shown in comparison with the frequency of cytotoxic cells in control animals of the same age which did not receive the tolerizing injection (=100%). The levels of cells fall rapidly in the tolerized animals to about 3% of that seen in controls. The fall in the thymus precedes the fall in the spleen, suggesting that the effects of clonal deletion occur first in the thymus. (Based on data of Nossal and Pike (1981).)

In practice, the evidence for the deletion of T cell classes is strongest in some transplantation systems, which cannot be explained by the presence of Ts cells.

1. In neonatally produced chimaeras fully tolerant to a foreign donor H-2 haplotype, the number of T cells capable of recognizing the foreign tissue type is drastically reduced and Ts cells are not found, in spite of the chimaera being permanently in contact with potentially antigenic cells (Fig. 12.15).
2. When X-irradiated F1 mice are repopulated with donor cells of both parental strains (the mice becoming radiation chimaeras), the donor cells do not react against one another as would be normal, and a stable chimaera is produced. Since no Ts cells are found it is concluded that the tolerance is due to deletion of the donor Tc cells, which recognize and destroy cells carrying allotypic markers of the other parental strain.
3. Although neonatally induced tolerance can be broken by the immunological termination of chimaerism, this breaking of tolerance does not occur in thymectomized animals, since they are unable to produce new mature T cells capable of reacting with the foreign tissue type. Such thymectomized animals will still accept tissue grafts of donor type despite procedures which would normally break their neonatally induced tolerance.
4. Although T and B cell receptors for self-antigens are encoded in the germ line, functional cells expressing them are absent from mature lymphocyte populations. The murine T cell receptor Vβ17a reacts with the I–E encoded molecules of the MHC and is only present on mature lymphocytes of mouse strains which are I–E

negative. Nevertheless, this receptor is present on immature thymocytes of I–E positive strains and disappears during ontogeny. This provides direct evidence for clonal elimination.

The evidence for T cell deletion derived from transplantation systems is summarized in Fig. 12.16.

T cells are much more susceptible to tolerization than B cells, particularly in adult life. Additionally, it appears that tolerance due to T cell deletion differs from B cell deletion in its initial stages, particularly in respect of the dose and form of the antigen needed. For example, T cells may be tolerized by the monomeric form of the protein, flagellin, whereas B cells require polymerized flagellin. Thus, it seems that it is not necessary to cross-link the T cells' receptors with high doses of multivalent antigens to induce tolerance, implying that T cell tolerance can be induced by a single signal to the T cell.

Until recently, it had been virtually impossible to tolerize T cells *in vitro*, whereas B cells could be readily tolerized in similar situations. Successful systems have now been established with T cell clones using high doses of a peptide fragment of influenza A virus haemagglutinin or antigen on chemically fixed presenting cells. The unresponsive state induced shows the same specificity of MHC restriction as activation and does not require the continuing presence of antigen. Recognition *in vitro* by T cells of antigen + Ia molecules in the absence of other accessory molecules or signals leads to an unresponsive state resembling tolerance *in vivo*. A critical biochemical event seems to be intracellular accumulation of Ca^{++} leading to an impairment of interleukin-2 production. Since induction is prevented by cycloheximide the implication is that tolerance is an alternative activation pathway.

There are a number of instances where it has been shown that tolerance is maintained by Ts cells. Generally these are cases where suppression is generated in adult life and they contrast with the normal self-tolerance induced in neonatal life which is maintained by TH cell deletion. There is evidence that in different conditions Ts cells may act in different ways. In some cases they interfere with the process of T cell–B cell cooperation, in others they act directly on functioning TH, Tc and other Ts populations. Some antigens are so immunogenic that they can induce tolerance only if administered along with potent immunosuppressive measures such as X-irradiation or the drug cyclophosphamide. These forms of suppression are maintained by Ts cells (Fig. 12.17).

evidence for clonal deletion in antigen-induced T cell tolerance

- fully H-2 tolerant neonatal chimaeras lack anti-donor T cells and Ts cells
- radiation chimaeras possess reciprocally tolerant donor cells, no Ts cells
- loss of tolerance by terminating chimaerism is prevented by thymectomy – implying that recovery involves recruitment
- germ line encoded T cell receptors for self-antigens disappear during ontogeny

Fig. 12.16 Evidence for clonal deletion in antigen-induced T cell tolerance: evidence from transplantation models. The tolerance produced in these experimental models cannot be due to suppressor T cell activity. It is concluded that T cell clones have been deleted.

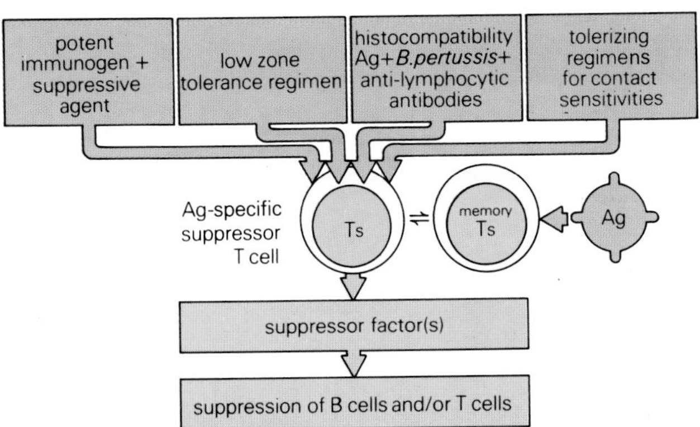

Fig. 12.17 Tolerance induced in adult life attributable to suppressor T cells. Antigen may be presented in a number of special ways to induce Ts cells specific to that antigen. Examples include the combination of a potent immunogen with a suppressive agent (e.g. the drug cyclophosphamide); sufficiently low levels of tolerogen to produce low zone tolerance; suppression of immunity to histocompatibility (MHC) antigens by administering the antigen together with a microorganism (e.g. *Bordetella pertussis*) and anti-lymphocytic serum. Certain tolerizing regimens for contact sensitivities selectively activate Ts cells when the antigen is introduced via a different route to that which induces skin sensitization. Ts cells may become memory cells in the same way as all other types of T cell. Memory Ts cells are reactivated following a subsequent contact with antigen. Suppressor cells release factors responsible for suppressing the activity of B cells or other T cells.

TOLERANCE ENHANCED BY IMMUNOSUPPRESSIVE DRUGS

Immunosuppressive drugs administered alone cannot produce antigen-specific tolerance since they act equally on all susceptible clones. Certain immunosuppressive drugs act preferentially against different lymphocyte subsets – for example, cyclosporin A acts preferentially on T cells. Immunosuppressive drugs can only be rendered antigen-specific by including an antigen-specific element in the tolerizing regimen, thus the drugs act as cofactors in tolerogenesis. An experiment which demonstrates the effect of cyclophosphamide in promoting antigen-induced tolerance is described in Fig. 12.18. There is evidence that immunosuppressive drugs may act in one of the following two ways:

1. by lowering the threshold for tolerance induction
2. by blocking differentiation sequences in cells triggered by antigen.

The commonly used immunosuppressive drug cyclophosphamide acts on both T and B cells. It increases B cell sensitivity to tolerogenesis by the normal mechanisms, and this action may be related to the inability of B cells treated with cyclophosphamide to regenerate their cell surface immunoglobulin receptors for antigen at the normal rate. It is noteworthy that neonatal B cells are also unable to regenerate their surface receptors after contact with antigen, and following capping. Capping is a procedure in which surface immunoglobulin aggregates, when coated with anti-immunoglobulin. The cap so formed is internalized by the cell, leaving the membrane free of immunoglobulin receptors (Fig. 12.19).

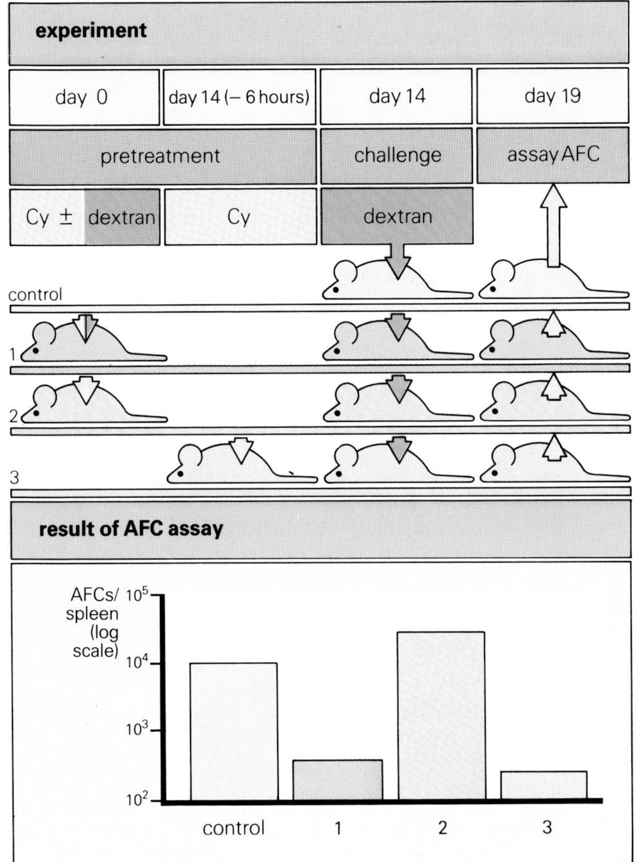

Fig. 12.18 Promotion of antigen-induced tolerance by cyclophosphamide (Cy). Four groups of mice are used. One group is a control and the three others receive different pretreatments as follows:
(1) Cy and a normally immunogenic dose of antigen (dextran) on day 0
(2) Cy only on day 0
(3) Cy only, 6 hours prior to antigen challenge on day 14.
The immune response is assessed on day 19 by AFC assay, and the results are shown in the bar diagram.
Cy administered together with antigen promotes long-lasting antigen-specific tolerance, but if administered immediately prior to antigen challenge it leads to a temporary generalized unresponsiveness.

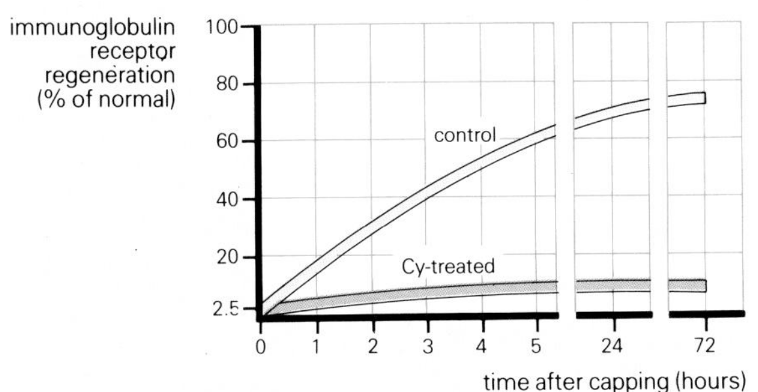

Fig. 12.19 Effect of cyclophosphamide on the ability of B cells to regenerate their immunoglobulin receptors. B cells are capped using anti-immunoglobulin, either in the presence (Cy-treated) or absence (control) of cyclophosphamide, and the time taken to regenerate the receptors is measured. Cy-treated cells regenerate their receptors very slowly.

ANTIBODY-INDUCED TOLERANCE

The antibody combining site may itself act as an antigen and induce the formation of specific antibody. Such antibodies, directed to the combining sites (idiotypes) of other antibodies, are termed anti-idiotypic antibodies (see Chapter 10). This type of antibody will bind specifically to the idiotypes which induced their formation, and if they bind to cell surface idiotypes, leading to cross-linking of the surface immunoglobulin receptors, they are effectively mimicking the action of antigen, and so may produce specific tolerance (or immunity in appropriate circumstances). These anti-idiotypic antibodies act only on cells bearing the idiotype.

In some animals the immune response to particular antigens produces antibodies of which the majority carry a particular idiotype. Suppression of this idiotype by blocking cell surface receptors with anti-idiotype can fundamentally alter the character of the immune response to that antigen. In this case tolerance to the antigen is partial, and other antibodies to this antigen carrying a different idiotype are still present. Furthermore, administration of an anti-idiotype in the neonate seriously impairs the response of that idiotype resulting in prolonged tolerance. The effect of anti-idiotype on adult and neonatal mice is illustrated in Fig. 12.20.

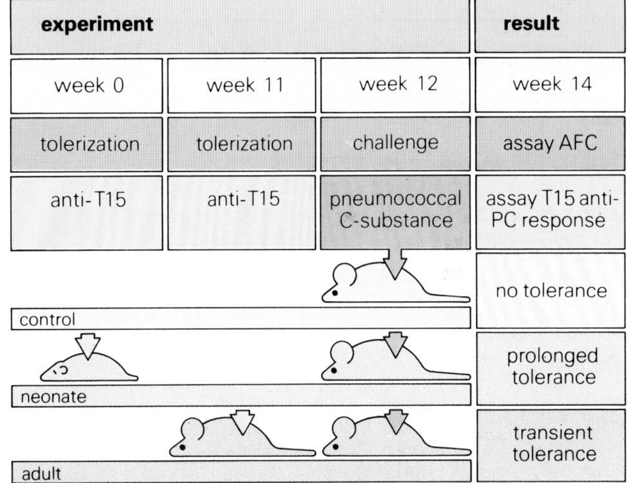

Fig. 12.20 The passive induction of tolerance by anti-idiotype. Three groups of BALB/c strain mice were used in this experiment: two adult and one neonate. BALB/c mice normally produce a particular antibody carrying the T15 idiotype to the phosphorylcholine (PC) determinant on the antigen, pneumococcal-C-substance (control). In the first week (week 0) the neonates were administered antibody to the T15 idiotype (anti-T15). A group of adults were similarly treated in week 11. In week 12 all mice were challenged with pneumococcal-C-substance and the production of anti-PC antibody of the T15 idiotype was assayed in week 14. It is found that exposure of the neonates to the anti-idiotype produces prolonged tolerance of the T15 anti-PC response, whereas exposure in the adults leads to transient tolerance. It is presumed that the prolonged tolerance is due to clonal abortion, and the transient adult tolerance to AFC blockade and B cell exhaustion. The tolerance is passively induced in this example since the tolerizing agent (anti-T15) is not actively generated by the individual but is received passively by injection.

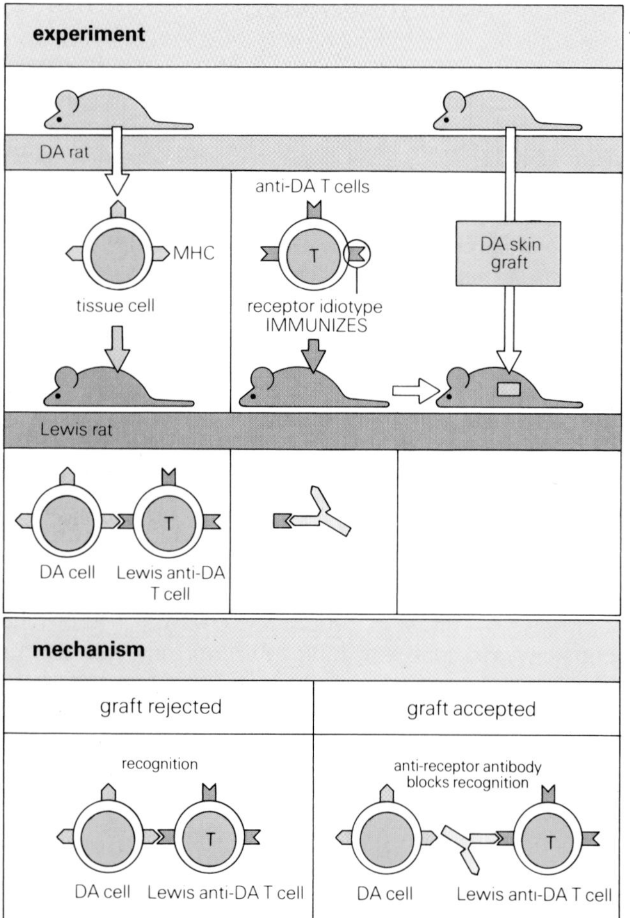

Fig. 12.21 Active induction of tolerance by anti-idiotype. In this experiment Lewis strain rats receive a tissue implant from rats of a different strain, DA. The Lewis rat's T cells (TH and Tc) recognize the MHC antigens carried on the DA rat cells, by anti-DA receptors (anti-DA idiotype). These receptors may be isolated and administered to the Lewis rat in an immunogenic form. Antibody is raised to the receptor idiotype and it is then found that Lewis rats will accept skin grafts from a DA rat. According to the normal mechanism of graft rejection, Lewis rats' T cells recognize DA tissue antigens (by their anti-DA receptor idiotype) to initiate an immune response. In the experimental situation however, antibody raised against the receptor idiotype blocks recognition of the DA cell by Lewis T cells, thereby preventing them from recognizing and rejecting DA tissue grafts.

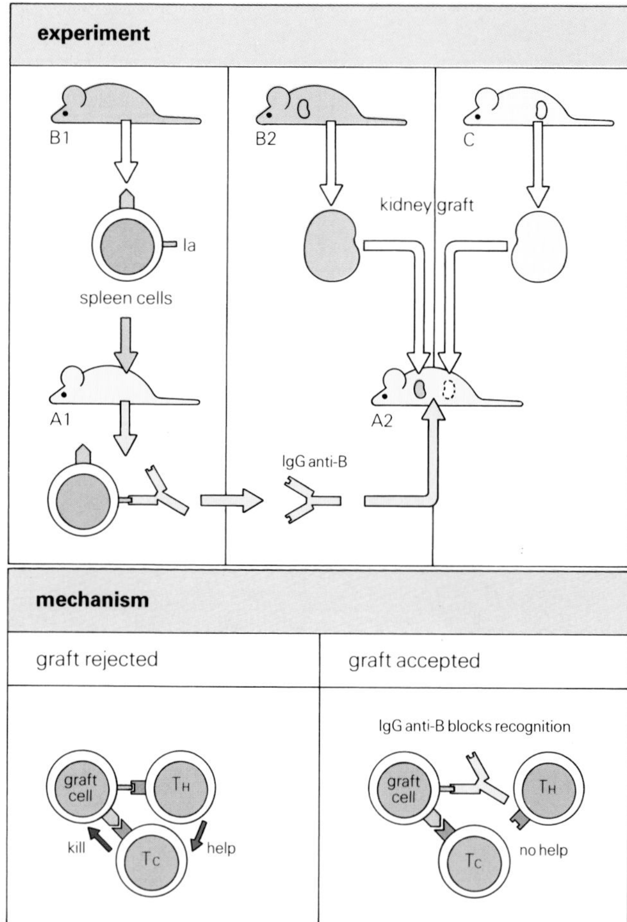

Fig. 12.22 Passive enhancement of graft survival by donor strain-specific alloantisera. Spleen cells are transferred from a B strain mouse (B1) to an A strain mouse (A1) where an antiserum is raised against these cells' Ia antigens. The antibody produced (IgG anti-B) is transferred to a second strain A mouse (A2). When kidneys from another individual of strain B (B2) and an individual of a third strain (C) are grafted into the A2 mouse, the C graft is rejected but the B graft survives. According to the normal mechanism of graft rejection the host TH cells recognize the graft cell antigens and help the host Tc cells kill the graft cell. In this experiment however, alloantisera blocks the normal TH recognition of the graft and consequently no help is given to the Tc cell.

In other conditions, animals can themselves be induced to generate anti-idiotypes; these are called auto-anti-idiotypes and lead to tolerance by blockading the animal's own idiotype. If the idiotype is on a receptor involved in the recognition of foreign tissue antigens, the blockade of this receptor idiotype will lead to the animal becoming tolerant of tissue grafts from animals of that tissue type, as illustrated in Fig. 12.21. A similar mechanism operates in the phenomenon termed passive enhancement. Alloantisera raised to H-2I region antigen determinants of a foreign tissue interfere with graft rejection in a recipient animal. The anti-I region antibodies bind to the graft I region determinants and block recognition of these determinants by the recipient's TH cells involved in graft rejection (Fig. 12.22) (see Chapter 24).

SELF-TOLERANCE

The fundamental basis of the immune system is tolerance to self tissues and lack of tolerance to foreign antigens, marked by an appropriate immune response. Failure of the appropriate response may be marked by a failure to respond against foreign antigens, or a hypersensitivity reaction. The original hypothesis of Burnet and Fenner, dealing with unresponsiveness to self-antigens, stated that all anti-self lymphocytes were eliminated before maturity. This view is untenable since anti-self B cells are found in normal adult animals. At present it is believed that anti-self B cells are normally present, but quiescent due to lack of associative recognition of the self-antigens by TH cells (functional deletion) (see Chapter 23). In this hypothesis the Ts cell system is seen as a back-up mechanism to the primary mechanism of deletion of anti-self TH cells in maintaining self-tolerance. Although tolerance due to the action of Ts cells is known to operate, whether it constitutes a major mechanism depends upon its importance with respect to the TH cell deletion mechanism – the two are not mutually exclusive.

An alternative fail-safe mechanism mediated by T cells has been termed the 'veto cell' effect, that is, potential self-reactive T cells are 'vetoed' by other T cells. This concept is based on the observation that MHC class I incompatible T cells induce reciprocal tolerance of each other persisting long after elimination of incompatible donor cells. Thus self MHC expression by haemopoietic cells is essential for maintenance of self-tolerance.

Depletion of Ts cells during ontogeny by exposure to anti-I–J[k] antibodies leads to an increase in self-reactive B cells, but not TH cells. It seems that the immune system relies primarily on TH cell deletion (effective from neonatal life onwards), and secondarily on Ts cell or veto cell generation, which is required particularly to deal with self-antigens encountered later in life, for example, antigens appearing at puberty. Ts cells are also probably involved in immunoregulation of normal immune responses. These three possible mechanisms of maintaining self-tolerance are summarized in Fig. 12.23.

	maintenance of self-tolerance	breakdown of self-tolerance
historical	self antigen; TH; B	self antigen; help; mutant TH; mutant B
TH deletion	self antigen; TH; B	foreign antigen; help; TH; B
suppression	self antigen; TH; B; suppression; Ts; suppression	self antigen; help; TH; B; Ts

Fig. 12.23 Self-tolerance: three alternative explanations. **Historical.** The original hypothesis of Burnet and Fenner, that all self-antigens induce the elimination of anti-self T and B lymphocyte clones in the neonate, is untenable. Loss of self-tolerance leading to autoimmunity would occur by mutation in adult life, producing new clones of anti-self lymphocytes. **TH deletion.** According to this hypothesis, B cell clones are unable to respond to antigens due to lack of T help resulting from clonal deletion of anti-self TH cells. This tolerance may be circumvented by foreign antigen cross-linking the B cells with TH cells of a different specificity, which are able to substitute for the deleted TH clone. Alternatively, adjuvants and B cell mitogens circumvent the need for T cell help. **Suppression.** This hypothesis proposes continual suppression of TH and B cell function by Ts cells. Loss of Ts cells means loss of tolerance. This possibility may be considered fail-safe suppressing any autoantibodies produced following failure of clonal deletion. A similar end result could be attained by 'veto' T cells which preclude potential autoreactive TH cells from responding to antigen.

TOLERANCE IN AREAS OF POTENTIAL THERAPEUTIC APPLICATION

A highly desirable objective would be the ability to promote a patient's tolerance to a foreign tissue graft, or to control an inappropriate hypersensitivity reaction. Suppression of transplant rejection can either be aimed at mimicking self-tolerance, for example by inducing tolerance in perinatal life, or at activating the Ts population. Unfortunately, perinatal tolerance induction, which offers the best hope of success, cannot by its nature be performed on adult graft recipients. Suppression of allergic responses is aimed primarily at causing a switch in the antibody isotype produced by the B cell's response, rather than in blocking recognition of the sensitizing agent (Fig. 12.24). A better understanding of the mechanism of isotype switching could lead to improved approaches to the therapy of these ailments.

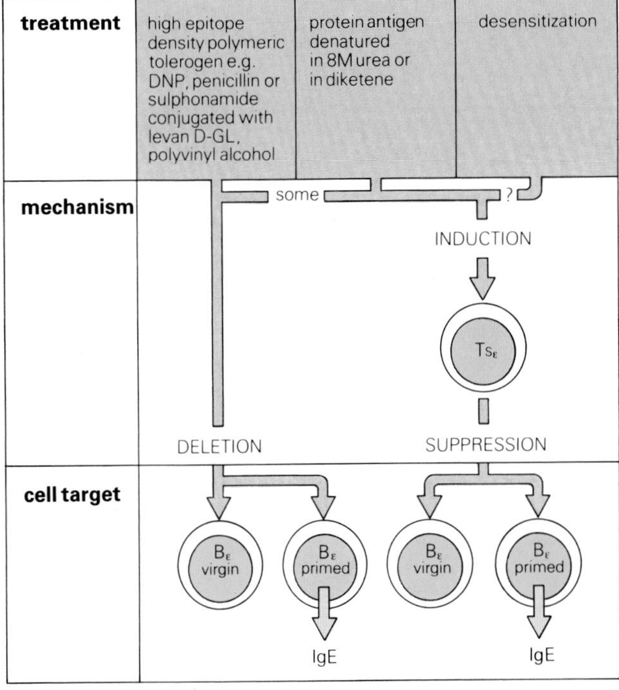

Fig. 12.24 Immunosuppression of the allergic response. An overvigorous IgE response to antigen (allergen) causes the allergic response. The aim of treatment is to delete the B cells producing IgE specific to the allergen, or to promote IgE class-specific Ts cells. The treatments in the box on the left delete both newly-formed virgin IgE-producing B cells (B_ε) and primed B cells. Some of these agents, as well as denatured protein antigen, can induce Ts cells which specifically suppress B_ε cells. An allergic individual can also be desensitized to specific allergens by administering the allergen under a carefully controlled regimen to limit the danger of anaphylactic reaction; this may operate by inducing Ts cells. The diagram is based on animal studies only.

FURTHER READING

Howard, J.G. (1979) Immunological Tolerance. In *Defence and Recognition*. Vol. 22 – *Cellular Aspects*. Edited by E.S. Lennox. Baltimore: University Park Press.

Howard, J.G. & Mitchison, N.A. (1975) Immunological Tolerance. In *Progress in Allergy*, **18**, 43. Edited by B.H. Waksman. Basel: Karger.

Humphrey, J.H. *et al* (1976) Immunological Tolerance. *British Medical Bulletin*, **32**, 99.

Nossal, G.J.V. (1983) Cellular mechanisms of immunological tolerance. *Annual Review of Immunology*, **1**, 33.

Nossal, G.J.V. & Pike, B.L. (1981) Functional clonal deletion in immunological tolerance to major histocompatibility complex antigens. *Proceedings of the National Academy of Science USA*, **78**, 3844.

13 Complement

INTRODUCTION

HISTORY

The term, complement, was originally applied by Ehrlich to describe the activity in serum which, combined with specific antibody, would cause lysis of bacteria. The discovery of this heat-labile activity in serum is usually attributed to Bordet (1895), although Nuttall, had described a similar activity some years earlier. In 1907, Ferrata demonstrated that complement could be fractionated into two components by dialysis of serum against acidified water to yield a euglobulin precipitate and a water-soluble fraction. Complement activity could only be demonstrated in the presence of both of these fractions C′1 and C′2. Subsequently Sachs and Omorokow showed that cobra venom inactivated another component (C′3) while Gordon found that a further component was destroyed by ammonia (C′4). The order of discovery of these components of complement does not correspond to their order of reaction; this explains some of the illogicality of the complement nomenclature system. Further analysis of the components of the haemolytic pathway of complement largely depended on the development of new techniques of protein purification. A major advance in this direction was the purification of the plasma protein, β1c, by Muller-Eberhard in 1960 and his demonstration that it corresponded to C′3. Subsequently Linscott and Nishioka, and Nelson and his collaborators were able to purify functionally the nine components now recognized to participate in the sequence of haemolysis by the complement classical pathway.

An antibody-independent pathway of complement activation was first suggested by Pillemer and his colleagues in the early 1950s who identified the properdin system of activation of the complement pathway by yeasts and certain bacteria. The existence of this independent activation pathway for complement was not readily accepted by other scientists and caused acrimonious debate.

Similarly the role of complement proteins in mediating the adherence reactions of certain bacteria and parasites to receptors on leucocytes and erythrocytes was neglected for many years. Thus, although it was known by 1930 that trypanosomes treated with antibody and complement would bind to erythrocytes from primates, it was not until the 1950s that this phenomenon was thoroughly investigated. This led to the discovery of specific receptors for complement proteins.

NOMENCLATURE

Study of the complement system is not assisted by the arcane nomenclature of its constituent proteins, an inevitable consequence of the manner of their discovery. The proteins of the classical pathway and membrane attack complex are each assigned a number and react in the following order: C1q, C1r, C1s, C4, C2, C3, C5, C6, C7, C8, C9. Many of the proteins are zymogens, that is, proenzymes requiring proteolytic cleavage in order to gain enzyme activity. The enzymatically-active form is distinguished from its precursor by a bar drawn above its symbol, for example, $C\overline{1r}$. The cleavage products of complement proteins are distinguished from the parent molecules by suffix letters, a, b, etc. Conventionally the small initial cleavage fragment is designated the 'a' fragment and the large, the 'b' fragment, for example, C3a and C3b. However, the small fragment of C2 was originally designated C2b and the large fragment, C2a. In this chapter, a uniform approach to fragment nomenclature is adopted; the small fragment of C2 is called C2a.

The proteins of the alternative pathway are assigned letters preceded by the letter F (factor). Regulatory proteins are symbolized by abbreviations, usually derived from a name related to the functional activity of the molecule. Complement receptors are named either according to their ligand, for example C5a receptor; or by using a numbering system for receptors for the major fragments of C3, that is complement receptor types 1 to 4 (CR1 to CR4); or using the Cluster of Differentiation (CD) system. The unfortunate consequence of this nomenclature is that some receptors have three names in current usage: for example, the receptor for C3b, iC3b and C4b is variously called 'the C3b receptor', 'CR1' and 'CD35'.

ACTIVITIES OF COMPLEMENT PROTEINS

The complement system is one of the major effector pathways of the process of inflammation. Its physiological activities *in vivo* are best illustrated by studying the deleterious effects of hereditary and acquired deficiencies of individual complement proteins. Individuals with such deficiencies have an increased susceptibility to recurrent infections by pyogenic bacteria, and illnesses characterized by the production of autoantibodies and immune complexes, suggesting a role for the complement system in defence against bacteria and in the handling of immune complexes, which has been confirmed by studies *in vitro*.

The physiological consequences of complement activation are:

1. opsonization
2. cellular activation
3. lysis (Fig. 13.1).

Opsonization is accomplished by the fixation of certain complement proteins to particles. Specific cellular receptors for these complement proteins then mediate the binding and uptake of the opsonized particles. Cellular activation also follows from the interaction of complement-derived ligands with specific cell surface receptors. The activation of the complement system results in the proteolytic cleavage of small fragments from complement proteins which are able to diffuse readily.

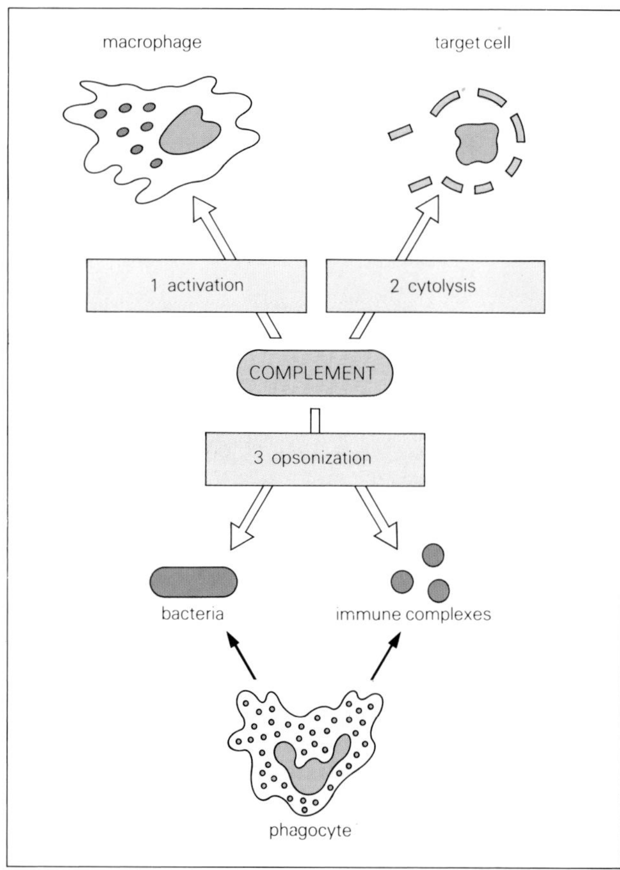

Fig. 13.1 The three major biological activities of the complement system. (1) Activation of phagocytes including macrophages and neutrophils, (2) cytolysis of target cells, and (3) opsonization of microorganisms and immune complexes for cells expressing complement receptors.

There are specific receptors on polymorphs and macrophages for some of these fragments; ligation of these causes directed cellular movement (chemotaxis) and activation. Similar receptors on lymphocytes and antigen-presenting cells bind complement-opsonized antigens (in the form of immune complexes) and enhance specific immune responses. The third physiological consequence of complement activation, lysis, is caused by the insertion of a hydrophobic 'plug' into lipid membrane bilayers, allowing osmotic disruption of the target.

PHYLOGENY OF COMPLEMENT

It is clear from biochemical and protein sequence data that many proteins may be assigned to 'superfamilies' whose members share close structural and functional homology, for example the immunoglobulin supergene family (see Chapter 4). Many of the proteins of the complement system may be assigned to such families (Fig.13.2). The molecular basis of relationships within families has become apparent with the cloning and sequencing of many genes. During evolution it seems probable that exons have been duplicated and 'shuffled' between different genes. These duplicated genes evolved in parallel and have often maintained closely related structures and functions, although in some cases the activities of particular exons have been lost or new activities have been acquired. Analysis of many proteins has shown that they consist of a 'mosaic' of exons derived from different families. C1s, an enzyme of complement which cleaves C4 and C2 is an example of such a mosaic, containing exons from the serine esterase, LDL receptor and C3b binding superfamilies.

Classification of complement proteins into superfamilies is still at a relatively early stage, but already provides a framework for understanding the structural

	families of complement molecules								
structural features	**FI**	**C1r C1s**	**FB C2**	**C4bp, FH CR1, CR2 DAF**	**C3 C4 C5***	**C6, C7 C8 C9**	**CR3 p150, 95**	**C1 inh**	**related molecules**
serine esterase domain	+	+	+						trypsin chymotrypsin
short consensus repeats		+	+	+					IL-2 receptor β_2 glycoprotein 1 F XIII
thioester group					+				α_2-macroglobulin
pore forming molecules						+			polyperforin eosinophil cationic protein
CD18$^+$ adherence molecules and receptors							+		LFA-1
serine protease inhibitor								+	anti-thrombin III α_1-anti-trypsin α_1-anti-chymotrypsin
LDL receptor domains	+	+				+			LDL-receptor

Fig. 13.2 Families of complement molecules. Structurally similar complement components are grouped together (green) and their major structural features indicated (left). Some non-complement molecules which also have these features are listed (right). *C5 has structural homologies to C3 and C4, but lacks the internal thioester group.

and functional relationships between certain complement proteins. This is illustrated by an apparently structurally disparate family of molecules which share a domain of approximately 60 amino acids. Factor H, C4-binding protein (C4-bp), decay accelerating factor (DAF) and complement receptor type 1 (CR1) are respectively an elongated globular plasma protein, an hexameric plasma protein with a 'spider-like' configuration visualized by electron microscopy, a membrane protein attached by an unusual glycolipid 'foot' and a cellular receptor with a transmembrane domain. However, despite these apparently dissimilar structures, these four proteins share similar functions and are encoded by closely linked genes on chromosome 1. The structural scaffold of each consists of tandem homologous repeats (short consensus repeats) of the 60 amino acid domain whose sequence is strongly conserved both within and between the proteins comprising the family.

Factor H, C4-bp, DAF and CR1 have in common the important function of inhibiting the stable formation of the C3 convertase enzymes, $\overline{C4b2b}$ and $\overline{C3bBb}$. They share overlapping, though not identical, functions which include:

1. inhibition of the association of C2 with C4b and B with C3b
2. acceleration of the decay of C2b from C4b and Bb from C3b
3. acting as cofactors to Factor I, the enzyme responsible for the catabolism of C3b and C4b.

The same 60 amino acid domain has also been identified in the C2a portion of C2 and in the Ba portion of Factor B (FB). (C2 and FB are themselves closely homologous in structure and function and are encoded by tandem genes located in the MHC.) It is the 'a' region of these molecules that allows their binding to C4b and C3b respectively. This allows the obvious speculation that the domain mediates the binding reaction to C4b and to C3b, but this awaits experimental verification.

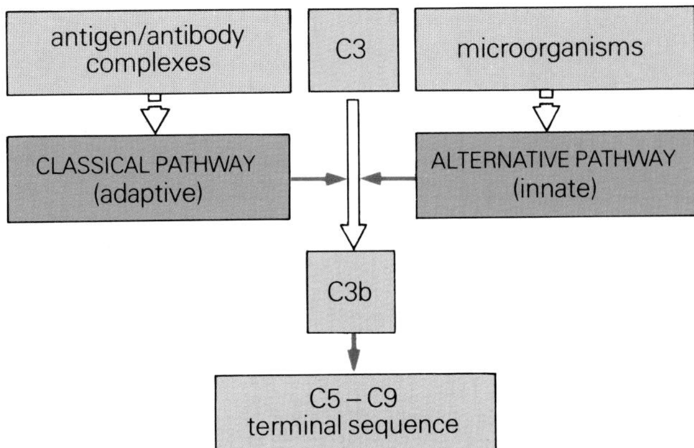

Fig. 13.3 Comparison of the classical and alternative complement pathways. Both generate a C3 convertase, which converts C3 to C3b, the central event of the complement pathway. C3b in turn activates the terminal lytic complement sequence, C5-C9. The first stage leading to C3 fixation by the classical sequence is the complexing of an antigen with its specific antibody. C3 fixation by the alternative pathway does not require complexed antibody since it can be promoted by the sugar component of the microorganism's cell membrane. The alternative pathway provides non-specific 'innate' immunity, whereas the classical pathway probably represents a more recently evolved adaptive mechanism.

ACTIVATION OF COMPLEMENT

The essence of immunity is the discrimination between 'self' and 'non-self'. It is widely recognized that antibodies represent the specific humoral system that recognizes non-self. In contrast, it is not well appreciated that the complement system subserves a similar discriminatory function.

The key step in distinction of self from non-self by complement is the covalent binding of C3 to particles. This bound C3 functions as an opsonin and as a nidus for deposition of the lytic membrane attack complex. Self surfaces contain molecules that effectively limit C3 deposition, whereas non-self surfaces act as sites that allow the rapid deposition of many molecules of C3. Activation of C3 generates a metastable binding site, transiently allowing the formation of a covalent bond between a glutamic acid residue within C3 and adjacent nucleophilic groups. As will be described below, there is a constant slow turnover of C3 in plasma which allows the non-specific binding of C3 and initiates the process of deposition of C3 on to surfaces.

Complement was discovered as an activity in serum which led to the lysis of bacteria coated with antibody. This illustrates the second mechanism whereby complement distinguishes between self and non-self. Interaction of certain classes and subclasses of antibodies with antigens activates the classical pathway of activation of complement. This is a potent mechanism for specifically directing C3 deposition on to foreign substances (Fig. 13.3).

C3 AND THIOESTER-CONTAINING PROTEINS

The major constituent of the complement system is C3, present in plasma at a concentration of approximately

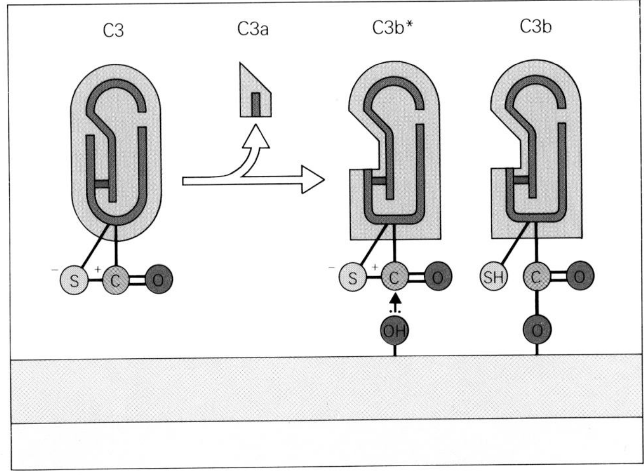

Fig. 13.4 Activation of the C3 thioester bond. The α chain of C3 contains a thioester bond formed between a cys and a gln residue. Following cleavage of C3 into C3a and C3b*, the bond becomes unstable and susceptible to nucleophilic attack by electrons on $-OH$ and $-NH_2$ groups, allowing the C3b to form covalent bonds with proteins and carbohydrates. In this diagram and subsequently, the polypeptide chains are shown in dark green and interchain disulphide bonds in red.

1 g/litre. The activation of the C3 by spontaneous hydrolysis or by proteolytic cleavage by a C3 convertase enzyme is the pivotal step in the process of complement activation.

C3 belongs to a family of proteins containing an unusual post-translational structural modification – an internal thioester bond consisting of a glutamine whose terminal $-CONH_2$ group is bound to the $-SH$ group of a nearby cysteine. This bond is metastable and the electrophilic (electron-acceptor) carbonyl group ($-C^+=O$) of the glutamine is susceptible to attack by adjacent nucleophilic groups (electron-donors) (Fig. 13.4). This reaction allows the glutamine residue to bind covalently to other molecules and is the mechanism for the covalent fixation of C3 to other molecules.

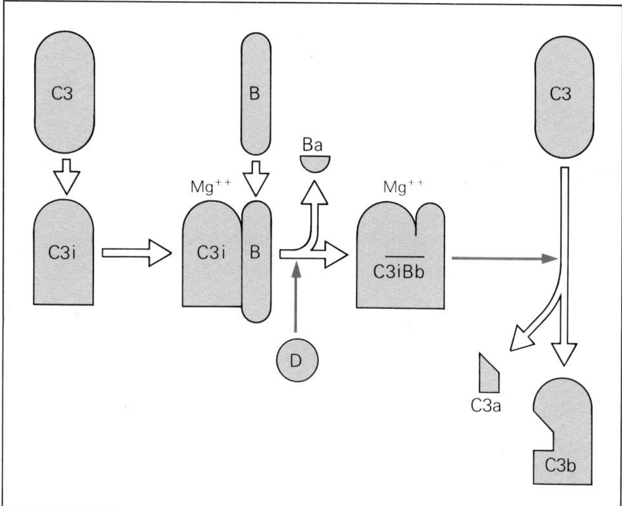

Fig. 13.5 C3 tickover. The thioester bond of native C3 becomes hydrolysed by water forming C3i (C3(H_2O)) which binds to Factor B in the presence of Mg^{++}, and following cleavage of B by Factor D forms a C3 convertase which can directly cleave C3 into C3a and C3b.

The thioester bond within native C3 in plasma is susceptible to very slow cleavage by water; this is the basis for the 'tick-over' mechanism of C3 activation (Fig.13.5) Cleavage of the C3a peptide from the *N*-terminus of the α-chain by C3-convertase enzymes results in a conformational change which greatly decreases the stability of the internal thioester bond. This becomes a nascent binding site within C3b* (*denotes the metastable state of the molecule in which the nascent binding site is activated) which is extremely susceptible to interaction with adjacent nucleophils. The majority of C3b* interacts with water, but a small percentage binds to hydroxyl and amine groups in adjacent proteins and carbohydrates.

The complement protein C4 also contains an internal thioester bond within a sequence closely homologous to that of C3. Two isotypes of C4 exist, C4A and C4B, encoded by tandem genes within the major histocompatibility complex (MHC). C4A preferentially binds to amine groups, forming an amine bond, whereas C4B binds mainly to hydroxyl groups producing an ester linkage. Thus C4A binds mainly to amino groups within proteins and C4B to hydroxyl groups within carbohydrates.

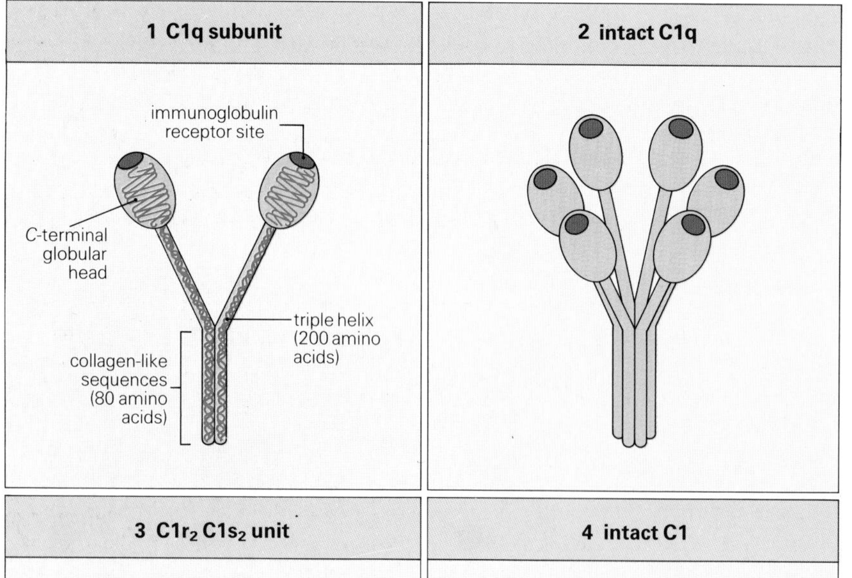

Fig. 13.6 Structure of C1. C1q is formed from 18 polypeptide chains formed into 3 subunits of 6 chains each (1). Each subunit consists of a Y-shaped pair of triple helices joined at the stem and ending in a globular head. The receptors for Ig Fc regions are in the globular heads, which appear in a ring in the entire C1q molecule (2). A $C1r_2C1s_2$ unit (3) lies across the C1q molecule, with the catalytic sites of C1r in apposition at the centre of the ring (4).

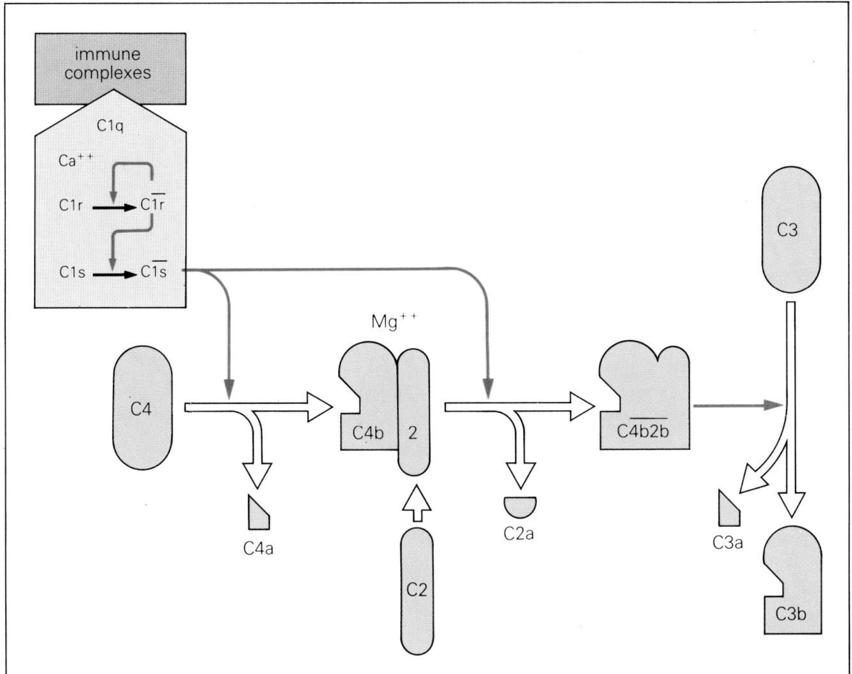

Fig. 13.7 Summary of the classical pathway. Following binding of C1q to immune complexes, C1r catalyses its own activation and that of C1s. C1s cleaves C4a from C4, which now binds C2 in the presence of Mg^{++}. C1s cleaves from C2a from this complex to leave a classical pathway C3 convertase C4b2b.

CLASSICAL PATHWAY

The classical pathway of complement is the main antibody-directed mechanism for the triggering of complement activation. It is initiated by the binding of two or more of the six globular domains of C1q, a subcomponent of C1, to its ligands. C1q binds with high avidity to the C$_{H}$2 domains of aggregated IgG molecules, as contained in an immune complex, or to the C$_{H}$3 domains of a single IgM molecule whose conformation has been modified from a 'planar' to a 'staple' configuration by binding to antigen. C1q is also capable of binding directly to certain microorganisms including some retroviruses (though not HIV) and to some mycoplasmas.

C1 is a pentamolecular Ca^{++}-dependent complex consisting of a single C1q molecule, two C1r and two C1s molecules (Fig. 13.6). The multivalent binding of the globular domains of C1q is believed to lead to a conformational change in the C1 complex. Consequently a single C1r molecule autocatalytically activates and cleaves the other C1r zymogen; the two C1s molecules are then cleaved by C1r into active serine esterases.

The next steps in classical pathway activation both amplify the response and concentrate the site of activation to the particle that initiated complement activation. C1s cleaves the thioester-containing protein, C4, into C4a and the unstable intermediate, C4b*, which undergoes nucleophilic attack within a few milliseconds by amine or hydroxyl groups in its immediate vicinity forming covalent amide (mainly C4A) or ester bonds (mainly C4B), as described above. Only about 1% of such cleaved C4 binds to proteins or to carbohydrates, the rest reacts with adjacent water molecules to form the intermediate iC4b which is rapidly catabolized. Surface-bound C4b now acts as a binding site for the zymogen C2, which, combined with C4b, becomes a substrate for C1s and is cleaved to C2a and C2b. $\overline{\text{C4b2b}}$ is the classical pathway C3 convertase enzyme and C2b in this form is the serine esterase that cleaves C3 into C3a and the unstable intermediate, C3b* in a manner closely analogous to the cleavage of C4 by C1s. C3b* too is susceptible to nucleophilic attack, mainly by hydroxyl groups, and a small percentage binds to the activating surface, acting as a focus for further complement activation (Fig. 13.7).

REGULATION OF CLASSICAL PATHWAY ACTIVATION

Classical pathway activation is regulated very efficiently in the fluid phase by two mechanisms: by the serine proteinase inhibitor (serpin), C1 inhibitor, which binds and inactivates C1r and C1s, and by inhibition of the formation of the classical pathway C3 convertase enzyme, $\overline{\text{C4b2b}}$. The formation of $\overline{\text{C4b2b}}$ is inefficient in the fluid phase due to the presence of plasma proteins which catabolize C4b (Factor I and C4 binding protein), and promote the dissociation of C2b from $\overline{\text{C4b2b}}$ (C4 binding protein).

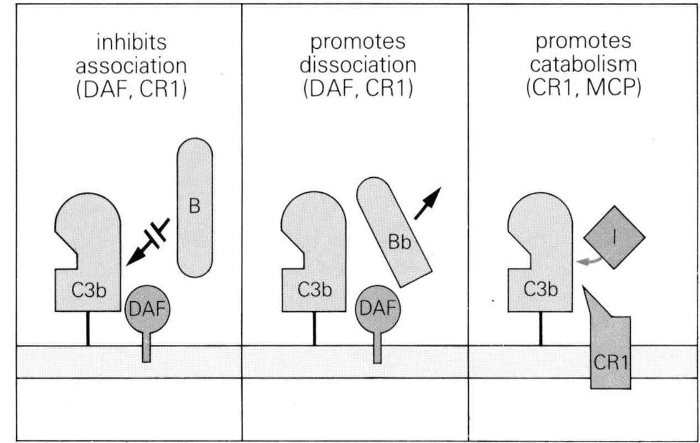

Fig. 13.8 Regulation of C3 convertases. Decay accelerating factor (DAF) and CR1 inhibit the association between C3b and B, and promote dissociation of the C3bBb complex. CR1 and membrane cofactor protein (MCP) promote Factor I (FI) mediated cleavage of C3b. These molecules control the interactions between C4b and C2 similarly. In the fluid phase Factor H promotes FI-mediated inactivation of C3b and C4bp promotes inactivation of C4b by FI.

There are also important molecules on autologous cell surfaces that regulate classical pathway activation: decay accelerating factor (DAF), CR1, and probably also a recently described protein, membrane cofactor protein (MCP). These molecules between them:

1. inhibit the binding of C2 to C4b and of Factor B to C3b
2. promote the catabolism of C4b and C3b by Factor I (Fig. 13.8).

The physiological activities of these regulatory proteins have been clearly illuminated by studies of patients suffering from isolated deficiencies of individual proteins, and are considered below.

ALTERNATIVE PATHWAY ACTIVATION

There are close structural and functional homologies between the proteins participating in the activation of the classical and alternative pathways of the complement system (Fig. 13.9). Native C3 in plasma undergoes continuous low grade hydrolysis of the internal thioester bond and the product, C3i, acts as a binding site for Factor B (FB), analogous to the binding of C2 to C4b (Fig. 13.5). FB, bound to C3i is cleaved by Factor D to Ba and Bb. Fluid phase C3iBb is a C3 convertase enzyme that cleaves further C3 to C3b*, some of which covalently binds to adjacent surfaces. This surface-bound C3b can then act as a binding site for more FB and initiates the amplification loop described below. It is clear that this system of activation results in the indiscriminate binding of C3 to any adjacent surfaces; however, there are molecules on autologous cell surfaces that prevent the formation of stable C3 convertase enzymes.

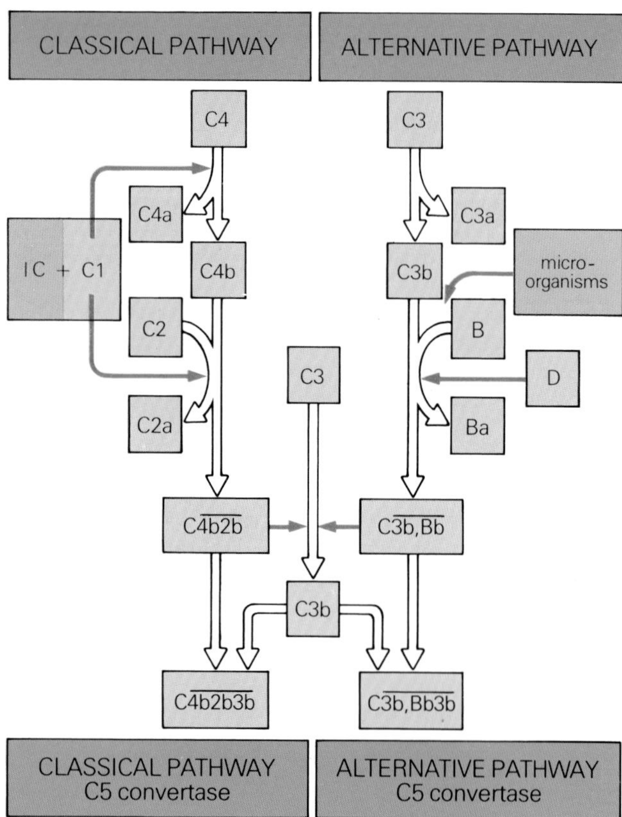

Fig. 13.9 Analogous action of the classical and alternative pathways. Both pathways generate a C3 convertase: C4b2b (classical pathway) and C3bBb (alternative pathway). In the classical sequence, C1 activated by complexed antibody splits C4 and C2 with the loss of the small fragments C4a and C2a: the major components form C4b2b. In the alternative route, pre-existing C3b binds Factor B, which is split releasing a small fragment, Ba. The major fragment, Bb, remains bound to form C3bBb. This converts more C3 so continuing the feedback cycle. Activator surfaces, on microorganisms for example, facilitate the combination of Factor B and C3b, and promote alternative pathway activation. The C3 convertases of both pathways may bind further C3b to yield the enzymes which activate the next component of the complement system, C5: classical pathway C5 convertase, C4b2b3b, and alternative pathway C5 convertase C3bBb3b. (IC = immune complexes)

AMPLIFICATION LOOP

On surfaces which are good activators of complement, initial binding of a few molecules of C3b by one of the two mechanisms outlined above is followed by an amplification step which results in the binding of many more molecules of C3b to the same surface. Factor B (FB), structurally and functionally homologous to C2, binds to C3b and in this form is a substrate for the serine esterase, Factor D, which is unusual amongst complement enzymes in that it circulates at very low concentration in an active form. The cleavage of FB results in the release of a small fragment Ba and the formation of the C3 convertase enzyme, C3bBb, which cleaves many more C3 molecules, some of which bind covalently to the activating surface (Fig. 13.10). The C3bBb enzyme dissociates fairly rapidly unless it is stabilized by the binding of properdin (P), forming the complex, C3bBbP. This amplification mechanism for the cleavage of C3 is a positive feedback system which will cycle until all the C3 is cleaved unless it is regulated adequately. Indeed, the nature of the amplification pathway was originally clarified by the analysis of serum from a patient with a hereditary deficiency of the regulatory enzyme, Factor I, in whom the amplification loop had cycled to exhaustion; that is, all the C3 in his serum was converted to C3b.

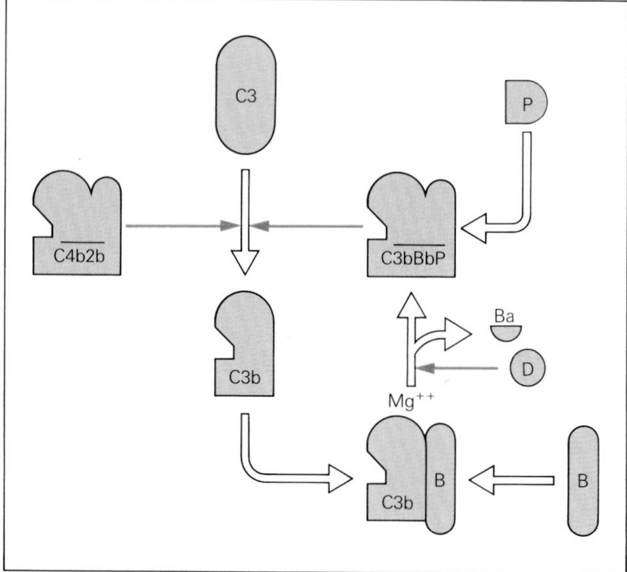

Fig. 13.10 The alternative pathway amplification loop. C3b binds to Factor B in a Mg^{++} – dependent complex and is acted on by Factor D releasing Ba and generating the alternative pathway C3 convertase C3bBb. This in turn can act on more C3 to generate further C3b, a positive feedback loop, which may amplify the initial complement activation.

REGULATION OF ALTERNATIVE PATHWAY AND AMPLIFICATION LOOP ACTIVATION

Fluid-phase activation of the alternative pathway is an inefficient process and is regulated by proteins similar or identical to those which inhibit classical pathway activation. Factor H (FH), homologous with, and closely linked to, C4 binding protein, promotes the dissociation of Bb from C3i and C3b, and also functions as a cofactor to Factor I (FI) for the catabolism of C3i and C3b (Fig. 13.11).

Regulation of the fate of C3b bound to surfaces is the critical step enabling the non-specific distinction of self from non-self by the complement system. The two possible outcomes for bound C3b are:

1. C3b acts as a binding site for Factor B (FB), forms a convertase enzyme, and focuses the deposition of more C3b to the same surface – amplification
2. C3b is catabolized by FI using one of three cofactors FH, CR1 or MCP – that is, inhibition.

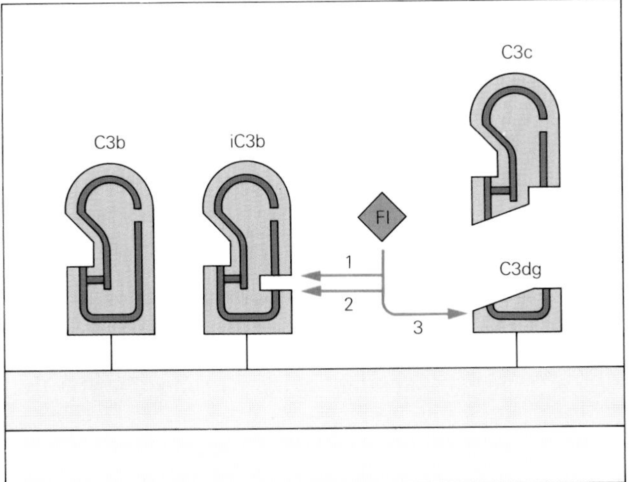

Fig. 13.11 Breakdown of C3b. Factor I cleaves C3b in three places to release C3c, leaving C3dg, a fragment of the α chain still bound to the substrate. The first two cleavages are promoted by Factor H and CR1 and the third cleavage is promoted by CR1.

The nature of the surface to which the C3b is bound regulates which of these two outcomes is most likely (Fig. 13.12).

Self surfaces, particularly the cell membranes, contain intrinsic molecules such as CR1 and/or MCP that bind to C3b, and also promote the binding of FH rather than FB to C3b. This effectively limits the formation of C3 convertase enzymes on autologous cell membranes. On the other hand non-self surfaces, for example bacterial cell membranes, act as a protected site for C3b since they do not contain intrinsic regulatory proteins and, more importantly, Factor B has a higher affinity for C3b than FH at these sites. Thus the deposition of a few molecules of C3b on to a non-self surface is followed by the formation of relatively stable $\overline{\text{C3bBbP}}$ C3 convertase enzymes which focus more C3 deposition in the near vicinity.

Aggregated immunoglobulins, for example in immune complexes, also function as the 'protected sites' for C3b. Although the precise structural requirements for a 'protected surface' are not understood, the carbohydrate composition seems to be important; membrane sialic acid seems to be one of the components protecting autologous cell membranes from amplified C3b deposition.

MEMBRANE ATTACK COMPLEX

The final phase in the activation of the complement cascade is the formation of the membrane attack complex (MAC).

The initial phase in the formation of the MAC is the enzymatic cleavage of C5, which is a protein homologous to C3 and C4 but lacking the internal thioester bond. C5 requires to be bound to C3b in order to be susceptible to cleavage by the C5 convertase enzymes.

Recent evidence suggests that the classical pathway C5 convertase enzyme is a trimolecular complex composed of $\overline{\text{C4b2b3b}}$ in which C3b is covalently bound to the C4b. The selective binding of C5 to this complex is explained by the high binding constant of C5 to C4b3b dimers relative to its binding constant to C3b bound to other cell surface molecules. Probably the alternative pathway C5 convertase enzyme will by analogy

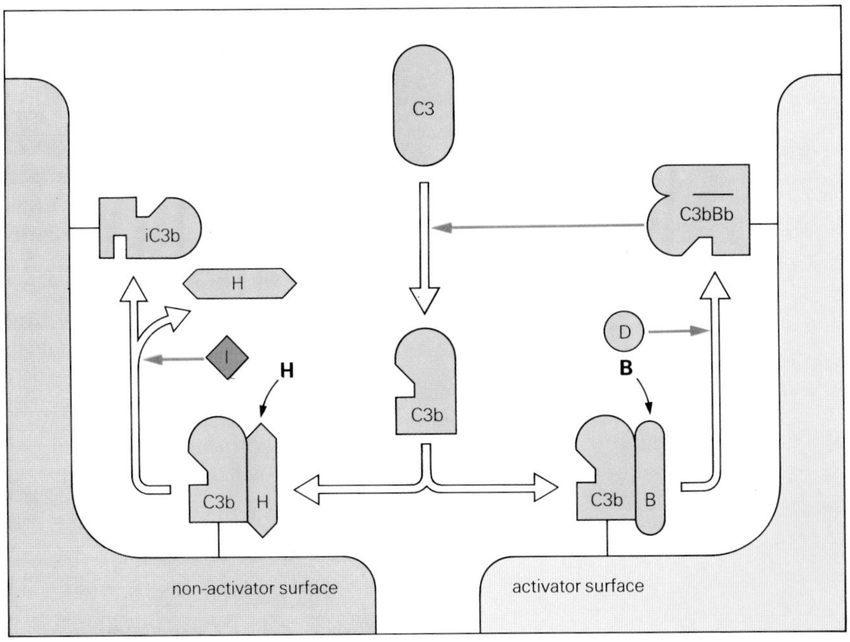

Fig. 13.12 Regulation of the amplification loop. Alternative pathway activation depends on the presence of activator surfaces. C3b which has bound to an activator surface binds Factor B and an alternative pathway C3 convertase, $\overline{\text{C3bBb}}$, is generated which drives the amplification loop. However on non-activator surfaces the binding of Factor H is favoured and C3b becomes inactivated by Factor I. Thus the binding of Factor B or Factor H controls the development of alternative pathway reactions.

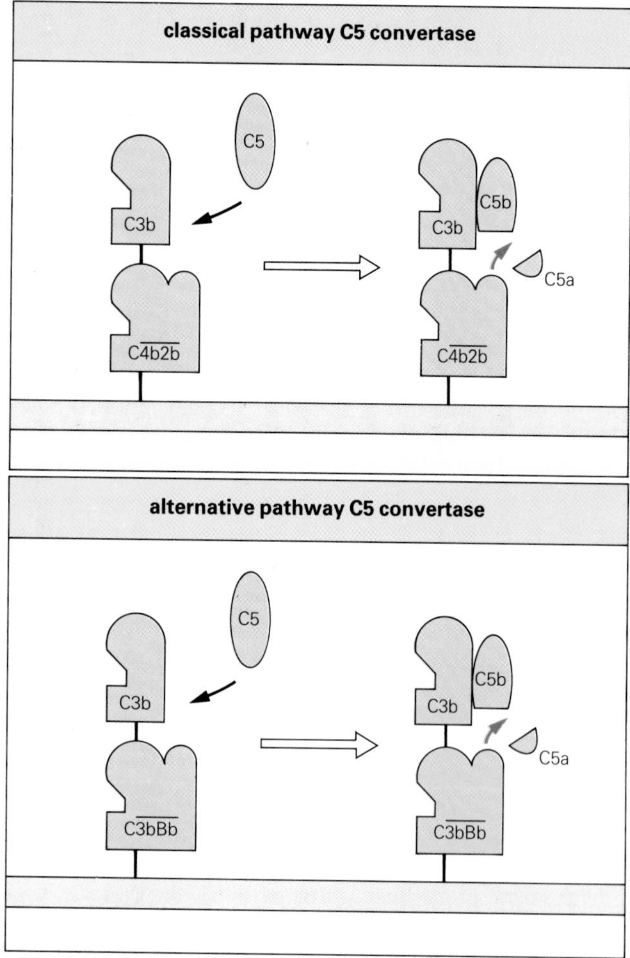

Fig. 13.13 Generation of C5 convertases. It is thought that C3b becomes covalently attached to either a classical pathway or alternative pathway C3 convertase, to form C5 convertases. This can then bind C5 which is acted on by either C2b or Bb to release C5a (anaphylatoxin) generating C5b, the first component of the lytic pathway.

turn out to be a trimolecular $\overline{C3bBb3b}$ trimer containing a covalent dimer of C3b (Fig. 13.13).

The subsequent formation of the MAC is non-enzymatic and follows the successive binding of C6 and C7 and C5b to form a C5b67 complex (Fig. 13.14). The binding of C7 is associated with a transition of the complex from a hydrophilic to a hydrophobic state that preferentially inserts into lipid bilayers. C8 and C9 then sequentially bind to this complex resulting in the formation of the lytic 'plug', first observed in electronmicrographs by Humphrey and Dourmashkin (Fig. 13.15). C9 forms a polymeric complex containing up to 14 C9 monomers. Although a small amount of lysis occurs when C8 binds to C5b67, it is polymerized C9 that causes most lysis.

Hydrophobic molecules that polymerize to form pores may be a common mechanism for cellular cytotoxicity. It has recently been shown that T lymphocytes may kill target cells by inserting into their membranes a pore forming molecule, perforin, which has structural homology to C9. Similar molecules are found in the granules of eosinophils.

REGULATION OF ACTIVATION

The release of C5b6 from C3b bound to cell membranes and subsequent binding of C7 to form the hydrophobic C5b67 complex allows the insertion of membrane attack complex (MAC) into other cell membranes in the vicinity of the primary surface on which complement activation is focused. This is the process of 'reactive lysis' and could have potentially damaging consequences to autologous tissues. There are a number of proteins that inhibit this process by binding to fluid phase C5b67. The most abundant is S protein, also known as vitronectin, and the SC5b67 complex is unable to insert into lipid bilayers. There are specific receptors for S protein, but is it not known whether these have a physiological role in the clearance of SC5b67 from plasma. The binding of C8 β chain to C5b67 in the fluid phase also forms a complex incapable of membrane insertion as does binding of LDL.

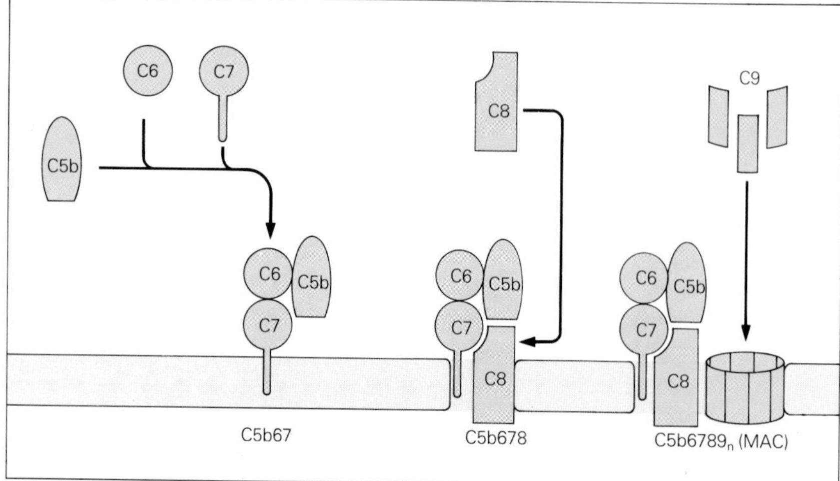

Fig. 13.14 The lytic pathway. C5b binds C6 and C7, which has a membrane binding site allowing the complex to attach to plasma membranes in the immediate vicinity of the reaction site. C8 binds to a site on C5b and inserts into the membrane, where it can subsequently polymerize the assembly of a number of molecules of C9 to generate the characteristic membrane attack complex (MAC).

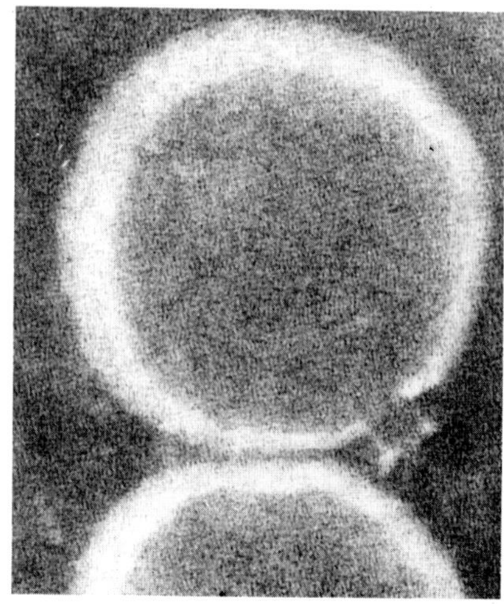

Fig. 13.15 Electronmicrograph of the membrane attack complex. The funnel-shaped lesion is due to a human C(5b-9) complex reincorporated into lecithin liposomal membranes. x234,000. (Courtesy of Professor J. Tranum-Jensen and Dr S Bhakdi).

Autologous cells also have a protein that protects them against lysis by the MAC. This explains the old observations that erythrocytes are poorly lysed by homologous complement, but readily lysed by complement derived from other species. The protein mediating this species restriction has recently been partially characterized and named homologous restriction factor (HRF) or C8-binding protein. It inhibits the insertion of C8 and C9 into cell membranes bearing C5b67.

Nucleated cells are much more resistant than erythrocytes to lysis by complement. They are able to remove actively MAC from their cell membranes by a process of exocytosis of fragments of membrane containing MAC.

COMPLEMENT RECEPTORS

The interaction of activation fragments of complement proteins with specific cell surface receptors is an important mechanism for the mediation of the physiological effects of complement. The two main consequences of ligation of these receptors are the uptake of particles opsonized by complement, and activation of the cell bearing the occupied receptors.

C3 RECEPTORS

Four receptors for the major split products of C3 (C3b, iC3b and C3dg, shown in Fig. 13.11) have been characterized and named complement receptor types 1 to 4 (CR1, CR2, CR3 and CR4); their ligand binding properties and cellular distribution are shown in Fig. 13.16.

CR1 The first recognition of a complement-dependent binding reaction to cells was the description of the phenomenon later named 'immune adherence'. Trypanosomes opsonized with antibody and complement were shown to adhere to the platelets of rodents and to the erythrocytes of primates.

The receptor mediating these binding reactions has been characterized and named complement receptor type 1 (CR1, the immune adherence receptor, the C3b/C4b receptor, CD35). CR1 is thought to have four physiological activities:

receptor	ligands	cellular distribution
CR1	C3b > iC3b C4b	B cells, neutrophils, monocytes, macrophages, erythrocytes, follicular dendritic cells, glomerular epithelial cells
CR2	iC3b, C3dg Epstein-Barr virus	B cells, follicular dendritic cells, epithelial cells of cervix and nasopharynx
CR3	iC3b zymosan certain bacteria	monocytes, macrophages, neutrophils, NK cells, follicular dendritic cells
p150, 95 (CR4)	iC3b	neutrophils, monocytes, tissue macrophages

Fig. 13.16 Complement receptors for opsonic fragments of C3.

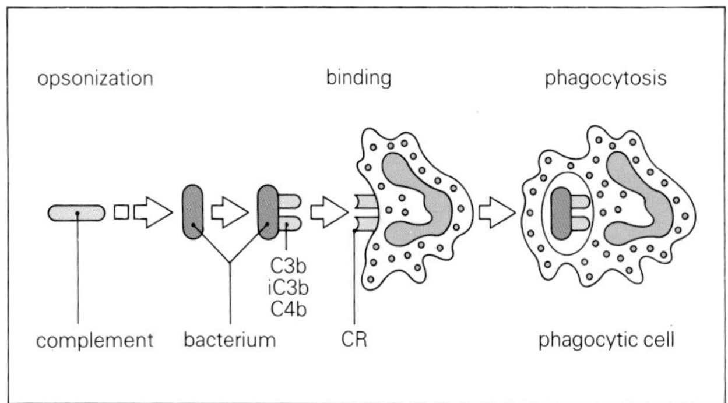

Fig. 13.17 Opsonization and phagocytosis. The diagram illustrates the steps in the uptake of a particle such as a bacterium opsonized by either C3b or C4b.

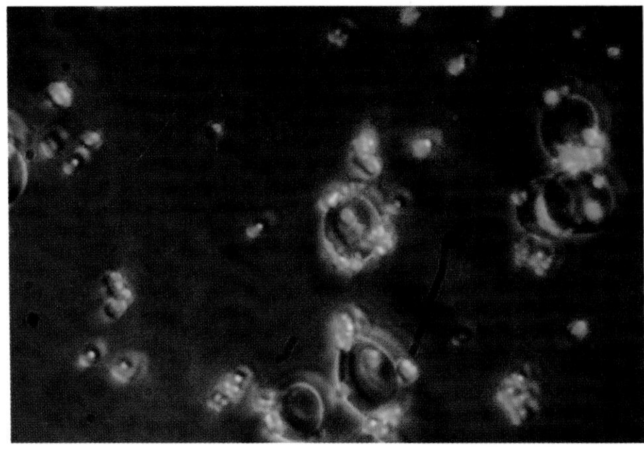

Fig. 13.18 Immune adherence. Fluoresceinated bacteria opsonized with antibody and complement are seen adhering to human erythrocytes. This reaction is mediated by C3b and iC3b and C4b on the bacteria binding to CR1. (Courtesy of Professor G. D. Ross.)

1. it is an opsonic receptor on neutrophils, monocytes and macrophages mediating endocytosis and phagocytosis by appropriately primed cells (Fig. 13.17)
2. it is a cofactor to the serine esterase Factor I for the cleavage of C3b to iC3b plus C3f and for the subsequent cleavage of iC3b to C3c plus C3dg (Factor H is physiologically probably more important than CR1 as a cofactor for the C3b to iC3b cleavage but CR1 is probably the sole cofactor for the cleavage of iC3b to C3dg)
3. CR1 on erythrocytes or platelets may serve as a receptor mediating the attachment and transport of opsonized immune complexes or bacteria to the cells of the fixed mononuclear phagocytic system (Fig. 13.18)
4. on B lymphocytes, CR1 may serve with CR2 as a receptor mediating lymphocyte activation.

CR2 CR2 is located on B lymphocytes, follicular dendritic cells and certain epithelial cells;its ligands are iC3b, C3dg and the Epstein-Barr virus (EBV). The physiological activity of CR2 on B cells is not established with certainty, though ligation of CR2 *in vitro* results in B cell activation in some experimental protocols. In view of observations that show a role for C3 in the efficient induction of secondary antibody responses and in the localization of immune complexes to antigen presenting cells, it seems likely that the main physiological activity of CR2 is as an accessory receptor for the stimulation of antibody responses. The main pathophysiological activity of CR2 follows from its role as the receptor for EBV. The *in vivo* tissue distribution of this virus parallels the locations of this receptor and it seems very likely that EBV gains intracellular access by binding directly to this receptor in a complement-independent manner.

CR3 CR3 is distributed on cells of myeloid lineage and is an important receptor mediating phagocytosis of particles opsonized with iC3b. CR3 is also a lectin and binds certain carbohydrates. Some yeasts, including *Saccharomyces cerevisiae,* bind directly to CR3 without the mediation of complement as do other microorganisms, such as *S.epidermidis* and *Histoplasma capsulatum.*

CR3 belongs to a family of three cell surface molecules which are heterodimers containing a common β chain and three different α chains. The other members of this family are lymphocyte function-associated antigen type 1 (LFA-1) and p150-95 (CR4).

These three molecules belong to a superfamily of structurally-related cell surface receptors and adhesion molecules which includes the fibronectin and vitronectin (S protein) receptors, and the fibrinogen receptor on platelets. These receptors bind their ligands in a calcium-dependent fashion and seem to have a common binding specificity for the tripeptides arg-gly-asp (RGD), although additional sequence or conformational determinants influence their individual ligand-binding specificities.

CR4 CR4 (p150-95) is the least well characterized of this group of receptors but has been shown to bind to iC3b in a calcium-dependent manner. CR4 is distributed on cells of the myeloid and lymphoid lineages and is strongly expressed on tissue macrophages, where it may be an important receptor for particles opsonized with iC3b.

ANAPHYLATOXIN RECEPTORS

The effect of the anaphylatoxins (C3a, C5a) are mediated by binding to specific receptors. These have been partially characterized for C5a only; there are 50,000–113,000 receptors on neutrophils and their estimated molecular size is 40–60 kD. Following receptor-binding, C5a is internalized and degraded to inactive peptide fragments; this appears to be an important mechanism for regulating and limiting C5a activity.

OTHER RECEPTORS

A 70 kD molecule has been identified which binds to the collagenous tail of C1q. This receptor is located on polymorphonuclear leucocytes, monocytes, macrophages, B lymphocytes, platelets and endothelial cells. Its physiological function is uncertain, but it may augment the uptake of immune complexes opsonized with C1q. A receptor for Factor H has also been partially characterized, and is found on B cells, monocytes and neutrophils; it may similarly enhance immune complex uptake.

ACTIVATION OF COMPLEMENT RECEPTORS

Little is understood at present about the mechanisms of the cellular events occurring after the ligation of complement receptors. There is evidence that CR1, CR2 and CR3 undergo a reversible activation step of phosphorylation in order to prime them to mediate activities, such as phagocytosis or the generation of a respiratory burst. The cooperative ligation of other cell surface receptors, such as those for laminin or fibronectin, may stimulate this activation step.

BIOLOGICAL EFFECTS OF COMPLEMENT

COMPLEMENT, INFLAMMATION AND ANAPHYLATOXINS

Activation of the complement system is a potent mechanism for initiating and amplifying inflammation. Activation products of complement proteins stimulate chemotaxis and activation of leucocytes. The anaphylatoxins, C3a and C5a (Fig. 13.19), stimulate chemotaxis of neutrophils, and degranulation of basophils and mast cells. The net effects of these activities are histamine- and leukotriene-mediated contraction of vascular smooth muscle, increased vascular permeability, and emigration of neutrophils and monocytes from blood vessels (Fig. 13.20). Bound C3 and C4 fragments act as opsonins, enhancing phagocytosis. In addition to inducing phagocytosis, ligation of complement receptors on neutrophils, monocytes and macrophages may also stimulate exocytosis of granules containing powerful proteolytic enzymes and free radical production mediated via the respiratory burst (Fig. 13.21). The complement cascade interacts with each of the other major triggered enzyme cascades that is, coagulation, kinin generation and fibrinolysis (see Fig. 13.21), and similarly the regulatory protein, C1 inhibitor, inhibits not only C1r and C1s, but also Factor XIIa of coagulation, kallikrein of the kinin system and plasmin of the fibrinolytic cascade.

The production of anaphylatoxins follows from complement activation and from activation of enzyme systems which may directly cleave C3, C4 and C5 at similar sites to the reactive complement convertase enzymes. Such enzymes include plasmin, kallikrein, tissue and leucocyte lyosomal enzymes, and bacterial proteases.

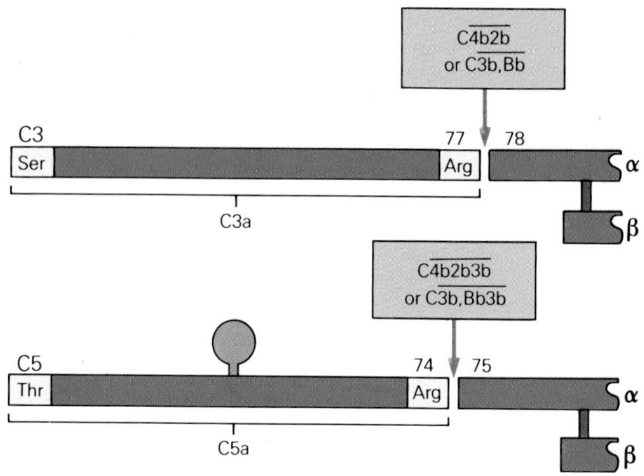

Fig. 13.19 Anaphylatoxin formation. The *N*-terminal ends of C3 and C5 α chains are shown. A 77 amino acid peptide, C3a, is split from the C3 molecule, revealing a carboxy-terminal arginine, by the C3 convertase $\overline{C4b2b}$ (classical pathway) or $\overline{C3bBb}$ (alternative pathway). In the case of C5, a 74 amino acid peptide, C5a, is split from C5 also revealing a carboxy-terminal arginine, by the C5 convertase, $\overline{C4b2b3b}$ (classical pathway) or $\overline{C3bBb3b}$ (alternative pathway). C5a contains a carbohydrate moiety indicated by a blue circle.

The anaphylatoxins have powerful effects on blood vessel walls, causing contraction of smooth muscle and an increase in vascular permeability. These effects show specific tachyphylaxis and can be blocked by antihistamines; they are probably mediated indirectly via release of histamine from mast cells. C5a is the most powerful agonist and is approximately 100-fold more effective than C3a and 1000-fold more effective than C4a and C5a-des-Arg. C5a is extremely potent at stimulating neutrophil chemotaxis, adherence, respiratory burst generation and degranulation. Ligation of the neutrophil C5a receptor is followed by mobilization of membrane arachidonic acid which is metabolised to prostaglandins and leukotrienes including LTB4, a further potent chemotactic agent for neutrophils and monocytes. Another powerful mediator released following ligation of monocyte C5a receptors is IL-1. Thus the local synthesis of C5a at sites of inflammation has powerful pro-inflammatory properties. The role of complement in the development of inflammatory reactions and immune reactions is summarized in Fig. 13.22.

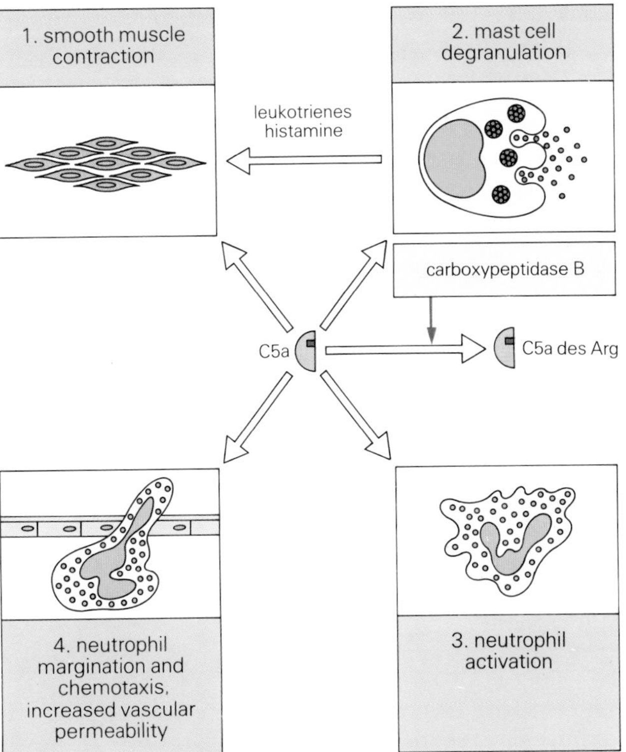

Fig. 13.20 Biological effects of C5a and C5a des Arg. C5a causes (1) smooth muscle contraction, (2) mast cell degranulation, (3) neutrophil activation and (4) margination and chemotaxis of neutrophils. Smooth muscle is further affected by histamine and leukotrienes released following mast cell degranulation or activation. Loss of the *C*-terminal arginine residue, following cleavage by carboxypeptidase B, produces C5a des Arg, which possesses weak cell-activating properties.

effects of C3b and C4b
facilitate binding of bacteria, viruses and immune complexes to neutrophils, monocytes and macrophages
mediate endocytosis, phagocytosis and generation of respiratory burst by CR receptor-mediated activation
augment IgG-induced phagocytosis, IgG-mediated cytotoxicity (ADCC) and NK-mediated cytotoxicity
binding to erythrocyte CR1 facilitates clearance of immune complexes from the circulation
focus immune complexes on antigen-presenting cells
disrupt lattices of immune complexes to increase their solubility

Fig. 13.21 Effects of C3b and C4b.

COMPLEMENT AND INDUCTION OF IMMUNE RESPONSES

Complement plays an important accessory role in the induction of antibody responses. It enhances the localization of antigen to both antigen-presenting cells and to B lymphocytes, and the localization of antigen–antibody complexes which efficiently elicit immune responses to the germinal centres of lymph nodes has been shown to be a complement-dependent process (Fig. 13.23). B lymphocytes carry two receptors for C3: CR1 which binds C3b and iC3b, and CR2 which binds iC3b and C3dg. Similarly antigen-presenting cells bear complement receptors; follicular dendritic cells are the only cells which have been shown to bear all three receptors, CR1, CR2 and CR3. Humans with hereditary deficiency of C3 do not show overt evidence of impaired antibody production. However primary and secondary

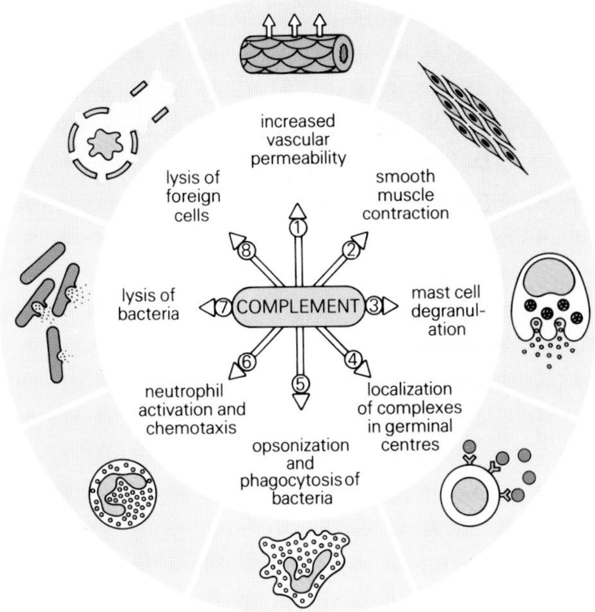

Fig. 13.22 Summary of the actions of complement and its role in the acute inflammatory reaction. Note how the elements of the reactions are induced: increased vascular permeability (1) due to the action of C3a and C5a on smooth muscle (2) and mast cells (3) allows exudation of plasma protein. C3 facilitates both the localization of complexes in germinal centres (4) and the opsonization and phagocytosis of bacteria (5). Neutrophils, which are attracted to the area of inflammation by chemotaxis (6) phagocytose the opsonized microorganisms. The membrane attack complex, C5-9, is responsible for the lysis of bacteria (7) and other cells recognized as foreign (8).

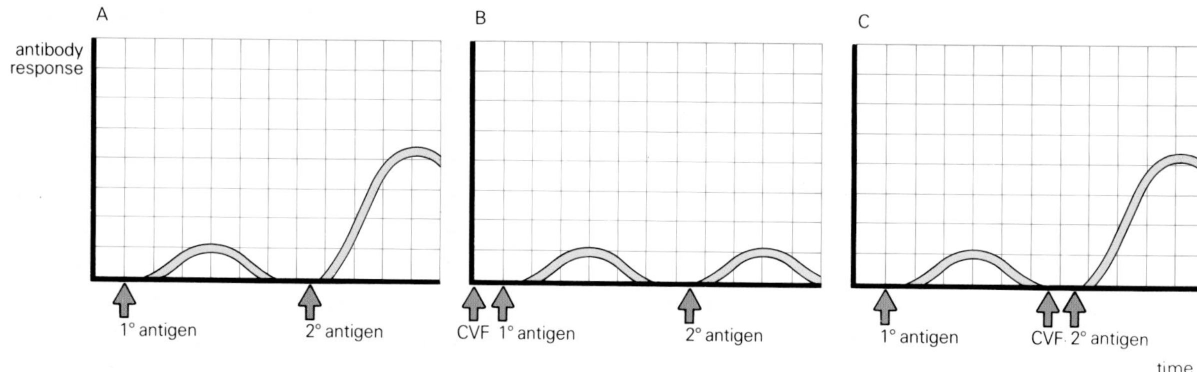

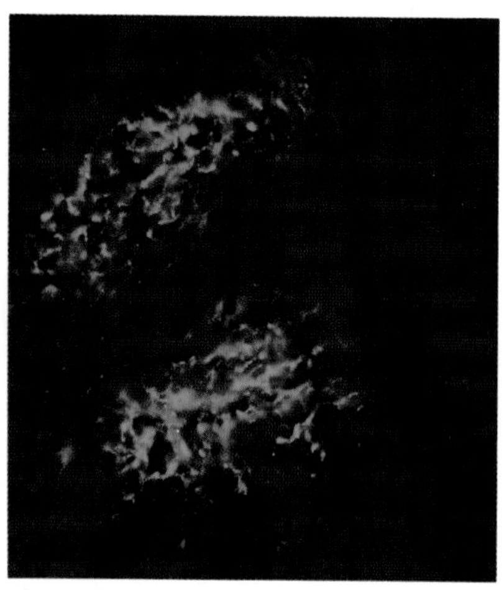

Fig. 13.23 Effect of complement depletion on the IgG response. Injection of priming (1°) and boosting (2°) doses of antigen produces a classical primary and secondary immune response (A). If the animal is complement-depleted by the addition of cobra venom factor (CVF) prior to the primary response, immunological memory fails to develop, and on subsequent antigen challenge the animal produces another primary response (B). The effect of CVF is only produced if complement is depleted prior to the primary response – depletion subsequent to the primary response does not hinder a normal secondary response (C). The effect of depletion is thought to be related to poor localization of antigen–antibody complexes in the germinal centres of complement-depleted animals. The immunofluorescence picture shows antigen localized in the germinal centres of mouse spleen (24 hours after injection of 1 mg of aggregated human IgG, here acting as antigen) and bound predominantly to the dendritic cells. This localization does not occur in complement-depleted mice. (Courtesy of Professor John Holborow.)

antibody responses of the C2-, C4- or C3-deficient guinea-pigs to low immunizing doses of Tcell-dependent antigens is markedly impaired. Present evidence therefore suggests that complement plays an accessory, but not necessary, role in the efficient induction of antibody responses.

COMPLEMENT AND IMMUNE COMPLEXES

Complement was first observed to inhibit the formation of precipitating antigen–antibody lattices by Heidelberger in the early 1940s. Immune complex lattice size is influenced by many factors which include:

1. concentration of reactants, antibody and antigen
2. the affinity of antibody for antigen
3. the valency of both antibody and antigen, high valency favouring large lattice formation.

The classical pathway of complement inhibits the formation of precipitating immune complexes in plasma, and alternative pathway activation solubilizes preformed precipitates of immune complexes, including complexes located in tissues. The mechanism of these effects involves the covalent incorporation of C3 into immune complex lattices. C3-binding may disrupt immune complex lattices by reducing the valency of both the antigen and antibodies, thus reducing the possibilities for forming large lattices (see Chapter 21).

The consequences of complement activation by immune complexes are normally beneficial. Immune complexes bearing C3 are efficiently removed from the tissues and circulation by cells of the mononuclear phagocytic system, enabling degradation of the complexed antigens. Similarly antigen in the form of complexes is extremely efficient in the induction of antibody responses by the mechanisms reviewed above. However, there are circumstances in which continuing immune complex production occurs *in vivo* when complement activation by immune complexes may prove deleterious. For example, the inflammatory effects of immune complexes in diseases such as subacute bacterial endocarditis and SLE may be mediated largely by the complement system.

COMPLEMENT AND DEFENCE AGAINST INFECTION

Microorganisms can activate complement via the classical or alternative pathways (Fig. 13.24). Nevertheless an important determinant of the pathogenicity of many bacterial strains is the ability to resist complement-mediated destruction. Many mechanisms mediating such resistance have been described and these include:

1. the direction of C3b and membrane attack complex (MAC) deposition to sites on the bacterial surface where they are unable to mediate opsonization and lysis
2. the possession of surface molecules which resist alternative pathway activation and amplification of C3 deposition.

Conversely bactericidal antibody may function by directing complement activation to sites on the bacteria which result in effective opsonization or lysis. The complex structure of bacterial cell walls, coupled with efficient facilities for membrane repair and rapid division, confers considerable resistance to complement-mediated damage.

The possession of a capsule rich in sialic acid

	immuno-globulins	microorganisms			other
		viruses	bacteria	other	
classical pathway	complexes containing IgM, IgG1, IgG2, IgG3	murine retroviruses, vesicular stomatitis virus		*Mycoplasma*	polyanions, esp. when bound to polycations, PO_4^{---} (DNA, lipid A, cardiolipin), SO_4^{--} (dextran sulphate, heparin, chondroitin sulphate)
alternative pathway	complexes containing IgG, IgA, IgE (less efficiently)	some virus - infected cells (e.g. EBV)	many strains of Gram-positive and Gram-negative organisms	trypanosomes, *Leishmania*, many fungi	dextran sulphate, heterologous erythrocytes, carbohydrates (e.g. agarose)

Fig. 13.24 Activators of complement. The diagram summarizes the activators of the classical and alternative pathways. Note that a number of microorganisms can activate complement independently of antibody.

distinguishes some pathogenic Gram-positive bacterial strains from their non-pathogenic counterparts. On such a capsule, the binding of Factor H rather than Factor B to C3b is favoured, leading to catabolism of C3b.

The physiological role of complement as opsonin and bacteriolysin is elegantly illustrated by two different hereditary deficiency states in humans. A similar spectrum of pyogenic bacterial infections follows either a deficiency of classical pathway components and C3, or a deficiency in the family of cell surface receptors comprising CR3, p150-95 (CR4) and LFA-1. This demonstrates convincingly that complement plays an important role in the destruction of pyogenic bacteria by allowing their phagocytosis and intracellular destruction. In contrast, deficiencies of components of the MAC are associated almost exclusively with recurrent infections with *Neisseria meningitidis* or *N. gonorrhoeae*. Thus host defence against these bacteria, which are characterized by their ability to survive in the intracellular milieu, depends on their lysis in plasma by complement.

Complement seems to be less important in host defence against viral infections; T-lymphocytes play a more important role. Complement deficiency is not associated with undue susceptibility to viral infections. However there are a number of links between viruses and the complement system of which the most striking is the use of the CR2 by the Epstein-Barr virus as the receptor for gaining intracellular access. Some viruses may gain access to cells indirectly via immunoglobulin and C3 fixed to the virus. Examples of this include antibody-enhanced uptake of flaviviruses (including Dengue virus) via macrophage Fc receptors, and CR3-mediated uptake of West Nile virus (a flavivirus) by C3 fixed to virus particles (shown in mice).

Molecules with Fc receptor activities on microorganisms have been known for some time, for example staphylococcal protein A, and the Fc receptor present on many *Herpes* viruses. A recent finding is that *Herpes simplex* expresses a molecule with complement receptor activity. Such molecules may protect bacteria and viruses from the normal consequences of the binding of antibody and complement proteins to their surfaces; for example, such bound IgG or C3 may be blocked from recognition by opsonic receptors on host phagocytes.

COMPLEMENT AND PATHOGENESIS OF DISEASE

Under some circumstances the consequences of complement activation *in vivo* may be deleterious rather than beneficial. The state of shock that may follow bacteraemia with Gram-negative organisms may, in part, be mediated by the extensive intravascular activation of complement by endotoxin. The resulting activation and cleavage of C3 and C5 leads to the production of large quantities of C3a and C5a which cause activation and degranulation of neutrophils, basophils and mast cells. These anaphylatoxins may also stimulate intravascular neutrophil aggregation and embolization to the pulmonary micro-vasculature, where neutrophil products including elastase and free radicals may cause the condition of shock lung; in this condition there is interstitial pulmonary oedema due to damage to small blood vessels, exudation of neutrophils into alveoli, and arterial hypoxaemia. Extracorporeal blood circulation, for example through the bulb oxyenators of heart-lung bypass machines, or over cuprophane dialysis membranes, may similarly cause activation of complement, and transient leucopenia thought to be caused by aggregation of neutrophils in the lungs has commonly been observed.

Complement activation is also an important cause of tissue injury in diseases mediated by antigen–antibody complexes. Such complexes may form *in situ* in tissues, for example in glomeruli of patients with autoantibodies to glomerular basement membrane (Goodpasture's syndrome) or at motor end-plates in patients with autoantibodies to acetylcholine receptors (myasthenia gravis) (see Chapter 20). Alternatively, immune complexes may become trapped in blood vessel walls having travelled through the circulation as occurs, for example, in bacterial endocarditis in which an infected heart valve provides the source of immune complexes which travel to the renal and other microvascular beds, and in systemic lupus erythematosus, a disease mediated by immune complexes composed of intracellular antigens complexed with autoantibodies. Complement mediates inflammation in these diseases by two major pathways:

1. by activated leucocytes attracted to sites of immune complex deposition by locally-produced anaphylatoxins, which bind via their cell surface complement receptors to C3 and C4 fixed to the complexes

2. by the membrane attack complex (MAC), which causes cell lysis and stimulates prostaglandin synthesis from arachidonic acid mobilized from perturbed cell membranes.

These two mechanisms of damage are well exemplified by considering two types of glomerular disease. Autoantibodies to glomerular basement membrane cause inflammation which can be inhibited by either complement depletion or neutrophil depletion. In contrast, membranous nephritis, which may be induced experimentally by antibodies to subepithelial antigens, is unaffected by neutrophil depletion, but almost totally abrogated in animals deficient in C5. In this disease the basement membrane is presumed to act as a physical barrier to cellular exudation and the heavy proteinura that accompanies membranous nephritis seems to be caused by deposition of MAC.

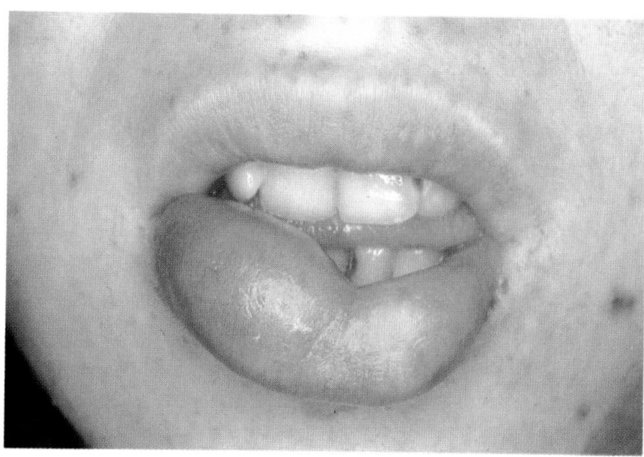

Fig. 13.25 C1 inhibitor deficiency and angioedema. The picture illustrates the appearance of angioedema in a patient suffering from acquired C1 inhibitor deficiency.

DEFICIENCIES OF COMPLEMENT PROTEINS AND THEIR RELATIONSHIP TO DISEASE

Much has been learnt about the physiological activities of the complement systems *in vivo* by studying patients with hereditary or acquired deficiencies of complement proteins. Although patients with these deficiencies are very uncommon, their identification and detailed study has proved enormously worthwhile. Deficiencies of complement proteins are frequently associated with an immunodeficiency state similar to that associated with immunoglobulin deficiency. These patients suffer from recurrent bacterial infections with organisms that are normally susceptible to opsonization or lysis by complement. The second major disease association of complement deficiency is with syndromes closely resembling SLE and other vasculitides. Although the mechanism for this association has not been established, it is likely that failure of normal mechanisms of complement-mediated enhancement of the uptake of the immune complexes by cells of the mononuclear phagocytic system may play a role, causing disease susceptibility.

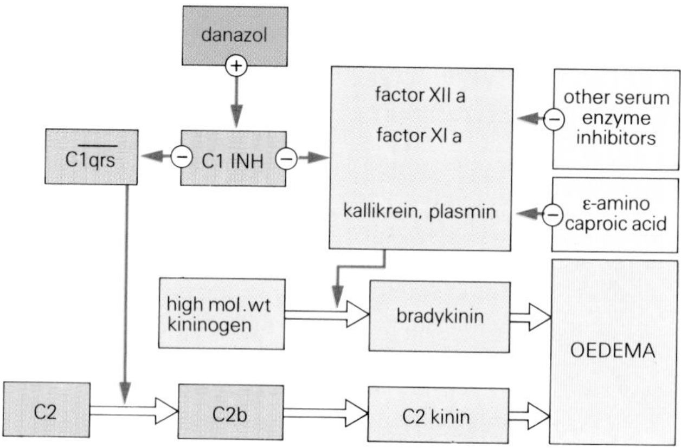

Fig. 13.26 Molecular pathways in angioedema. In patients with hereditary angioedema the levels of C1 inhibitor (C1 INH) are low, and may become locally exhausted by consumption via different plasma enzymes such as Hageman factor XIIa. In this case kallikrein may become activated with the generation of bradykinin. There is no serpin available to control C1r and C1s. In this case a pathological factor C2 kinin may be generated by the action of plasmin on C2b. This, in association with bradykinin produces oedema. Therapy is aimed at increasing C1 INH (e.g. with danazol) or reducing activity of enzymes including plasmin (ε-aminocaproic acid).

DEFICIENCIES OF COMPLEMENT REGULATORY PROTEINS

C1 Inhibitor Deficiency Reduced levels of C1 inhibitor are characterized clinically by recurrent attacks of angioedema affecting the skin and mucosae (Fig. 13.25). Angioedema of the oropharynx may cause life-threatening upper airway obstruction, and of the gastrointestinal tract may lead to abdominal pain which may easily be misinterpreted resulting in inappropriate and potentially dangerous surgery. Two types of C1 inihibitor deficiency occur: hereditary and acquired. The hereditary form is unusual in that it is inherited in an autosomal dominant fashion. The physiological rate of C1 inhibitor turnover appears to frequently exceed the capacity for synthesis by a single functional gene. Therefore, under conditions of increased protease activation, when a single C1 inhibitor gene is dysfunctional, the C1 inhibitor produced by the remaining gene may be exhausted. Subsequently, unregulated activity of protease enzymes leads to the production of mediators which cause increased local vascular permeability and exudation of oedema fluid. The protease responsible for producing the vasoactive mediator has not been identified; the two main candidates are kallikrein (cleaving high molecular weight kininogen to produce bradykinin) and C1s (cleaving C2 to produce a kinin-like peptide) (Fig. 13.26). Androgens have a therapeutic effect by increasing the rate of C1 inhibitor synthesis by the single functional gene in the liver; the impeded androgens, danazol and stanozolol, are of most clinical value in hereditary angioedema as they have relatively minor virilizing side-effects. A small proportion of patients with hereditary angioedema have normal levels of C1 inhibitor when detected antigenically due to inheritance of a gene encoding a dysfunctional product.

The complement profile of patients with hereditary C1 inhibitor deficiency shows normal levels of C1q, reduced levels of C1r, C1s, C4 and C2, and relatively normal levels of C3 (illustrating the inefficiency of fluid phase conversion of C3 by the classical pathway). In contrast to this profile of complement component levels, patients who have acquired C1 inhibitor deficiency have reduced levels of C1q; this is an important clue to the diagnosis and aetiology of this condition, which is due to the consumption of C1 inhibitor by interaction with activated C1r and C1s consequent on C1q binding. Acquired C1 inhibitor deficiency usually occurs as an accompaniment to B cell lymphoproliferative disease; the precise mechanism of C1 activation in this disease has not been established although anti-idiotypic antibodies to the surface immunoglobin on the lymphoma have been implicated.

Abnormalities of Regulation of the Amplification Loop Deficiencies of Factor I or Factor H, or the presence of molecules increasing the stability of the $\overline{C3bBb}$ C3 convertase enzyme, result in a similar pattern of complement activation in which C3 is turned over at an extremely high rate, and no measurable native C3 may be detected in plasma. The few patients described with hereditary deficiencies of Factor H or I provided the initial clue to the identification of the 'tickover' mechanism of complement activation. In normal plasma, only very slow activation of C3 occurs, as the fluid phase C3 convertase enzyme is efficiently regulated by Factor H and Factor I. Deficiency of either of these proteins allows the amplification loop to cycle to complete exhaustion of C3. The pathological effects of Factor H and I deficiency are similar to those of primary C3 deficiency and are considered together.

The autoantibody, C3 nephritic factor, is similarly associated with unregulated activation of the amplification loop. This antibody binds to $\overline{C3bBb}$ and stabilizes the enzyme by inhibiting the dissociation of Bb from C3b by Factor H. It is associated with the disfiguring condition of partial lipodystrophy, in which subcutaneous fat is lost from parts of the body, and also mesangiocapillary glomerulonephritis.

Abnormalities of Cell-surface Complement Regulatory Proteins Paroxysmal nocturnal haemoglobinuria (PNH) is an acquired clonal disorder of haematopoietic cells in which there is monoclonal proliferation of a haematopoietic stem cell deficient in the expression of several molecules which share an unusual type of anchor to cell membranes. These molecules are attached via a glycolipid tail to a membrane phospholipid, phosphatidyl inositol. Such membrane proteins lack a transmembrane domain and are believed to be able to move laterally within the cell membrane with great ease. The variant surface glycoproteins (VSG) of trypanosomes were the first proteins characterized with this type of membrane anchor. Human membrane proteins with this type of anchor include decay accelerating factor (DAF), homologous restriction factor (HRF), LFA-3, 5′-nucleotidase and erythrocyte acetylcholinesterase; each of these proteins has been shown to be deficient from the clones of haematopoietic cells in PNH. Erythrocytes from patients with PNH show two major abnormalities of defence against homologous complement. They are abnormally susceptible to the deposition of C3b following either classical pathway or alternative pathway activation. This sensitivity illustrates the normal role of DAF in inhibiting formation and increasing dissociation of $\overline{C4b2b}$ and $\overline{C3bBb}$ on autologous cell membranes. Some PNH erythrocytes also show markedly increased susceptibility to reactive lysis, with increased C8 and C9 deposition; preliminary evidence suggests that this abnormality may be due to deficiency of homologous restriction factor. Patients with PNH suffer from recurrent attacks of complement-mediated intra- and extravascular haemolysis.

COMPLEMENT DEFICIENCY AND IMMUNODEFICIENCY

The disease associations of complement deficiencies are shown in Fig. 13.27. Deficiencies of proteins of the classical and alternative pathways including C3 deficiency are commonly associated with recurrent infections with pyogenic organisms. Such infections are not associated with deficiencies of proteins of the membrane attack complex (MAC). This emphasizes that the role of the complement system in host defence against the majority of pyogenic organisms depends on opsonization for phagocytosis, rather than lysis by the MAC. In contrast, deficiencies of proteins of the MAC, with the exception of C9 deficiency, are associated with increased susceptibility to infection with *Neisseria meningitidis* (often recurrent), and with *N. gonorrhoeae*. This illustrates that an important component of host defence against these organisms, capable of intracellular survival, is lysis by complement. Subtotal C9 deficiency is common amongst Japanese and has no disease associations; lysis mediated by C8 or by the low concentrations of C9 present in these individuals may be sufficient to protect them against *Neisseria* infections.

component	disease associations
classical pathway C1–C4	SLE pyogenic infections
C3, FH, FI	disseminated infections particularly with pyogenic bacteria, vasculitis, nephritis
lytic pathway C5–C8	disseminated neisserial infections, occasionally SLE
C9	none
CR3, p150, 95 LFA-1	gingivitis, delayed umbilical cord separation, recurrent pyogenic infections

Fig. 13.27 Diseases associated with complement deficiencies.

DEFICIENCIES OF COMPLEMENT RECEPTORS

Hereditary deficiency of the family of cell surface molecules comprising CR3, CR4 (p150,95) and LFA-1 causes an immunodeficiency syndrome with distinctive clinical features. Affected infants have delayed separation of the umbilical cord, followed by recurrent ulcerating cutaneous infections, gingivitis, and abnormal 'paper-thin' scar formation. The severity of the disease is variable and related to the degree of deficiency of the surface expression of these molecules. Infants with less than 1% expression of the normal levels of these molecules usually die of sepsis in infancy; whereas 5% expression is associated with a milder syndrome compatible with survival into adulthood. The sites of infection are marked by an absence of neutrophil infiltration and most of the pathological features of the disease may be explained by severe neutrophil dysfunction. Neutrophils show severely impaired adhesion, chemotaxis and phagocytosis of particles opsonized with iC3b. These patients are susceptible to infection by the same species of bacteria that cause disease in patients with C3 deficiency. This observation again emphasises the importance of opsonization and phagocytosis in host defence against pyogenic bacteria.

COMPLEMENT DEFICIENCY AND IMMUNE COMPLEX DISEASE

Immune complex diseases closely resembling systemic lupus erythematosus are predominantly associated with deficiencies of classical pathway components. The mechanism of this association is not established with certainty. One hypothesis follows from the activities of the classical pathway in:

1. the modification of the lattice of immune complexes to prevent the formation of large immune complexes and
2. the opsonization of immune complexes for phagocytosis.

Failure of these activities may lead to failure of the fixed mononuclear phagocytic system to remove immune complexes from the circulation efficiently. Such complexes could deposit in tissues causing inflammation with the release of autoantigens which may stimulate autoantibody production. A second hypothesis is that complement deficiency allows the establishment of chronic viral infections, which may stimulate the development of autoimmunity.

FURTHER READING

Anderson, D.C. & Springer, T.A. (1987) Leukocyte adhesion deficiency: an inherited defect in the Mac-1, LFA-1, and p150,95 glycoproteins. *Annual Review of Medicine*, **38**, 175–194.

Arlaud, G.I., Colomb, M.G. & Gagnon, J. (1987) A functional model of the human C1 complex. *Immunology Today*, **8**, 106–111.

Atkinson, J.P. & Ferries, T. (1987) Separation of self from non-self in the complement system. *Immunology Today*, **8**, 212–215.

Bhakdi, S. & Tranum-Jensen, J. (1984) Mechanism of complement cytolysis and the concept of channel-forming proteins. *Philosophical Transactions of the Royal Society of London (Biology)*, **36**, 311–324.

Campbell, R.D., Caroll, M.C. & Porter, R.R. (1986) The molecular genetics of components of complement. *Advances in Immunology*, **38**, 203–244.

Carrell, R.W. & Boswell, D.R. (1986) Serpins: the superfamily of plasma serine proteinase inhibitors. In *Proteinase Inhibitors*. Edited by A. Barrett & G. Salveson, pp 403–420. Amsterdam: Elsevier.

Colten, H.R. (1987) Hereditary angioneurotic edema, 1887 to 1987. *New England Journal of Medicine*, **317**, 43–45.

Colten, H.R., Strunk, R.C., Perlmutter, D.H. & Cole, F.S. (1986) Regulation of complement protein biosynthesis in mononuclear phagocytes. In *Ciba Symposium 118: Biochemistry of Macrophages*. Edited by D. Evered, J. Nugent & M. O'Connor, pp 141–151. London: Pitman Ltd.

Cooper, N.R. (1985) The classical complement pathway: activation and regulation of the first complement component. *Advances in Immunology*, **37**, 151–216.

Couser, W.G., Baker, P.J. & Adler, S. (1985) Complement and the direct mediation of immune glomerular injury: a new perspective. *Kidney International*, **28**, 879–890.

Fearon, D.T. (1984) Cellular receptors for fragments of the third component of complement. *Immunology Today*, **5**, 105–110.

Frank, M.M., Gelfand, J.A. & Atkinson, J.P. (1976) Hereditary angioedema: the clinical syndrome and its management. *Annals of Internal Medicine*, **84**, 580.

Holers, V.M., Cole, J.L., Lublin, D.M., Seya, T. & Atkinson, J.P. (1985) Human C3b and C4b regulatory proteins: a new multi-gene family. *Immunology Today*, **6**, 188–192.

Klaus, G.G.B. & Humphrey, J.J. (1986) A re-evaluation of the role of C3 in B-cell activation. *Immunology Today*, **7**, 163–165.

Lachmann, P.J. (1986) A common form of killing. *Nature*, **321**, 560.

Lachmann, P.J. & Walport, M.J. (1987) Deficiency of the effector mechanisms of the immune response and autoimmunity. In *Ciba Foundation Symposium 129: Autoimmunity and Autoimmune Diseases*. Edited by J. Whelan, pp 149–171. Chichester: Wiley.

Law, S.K.A. & Reid, K.B.M. (1988) *Complement in Focus*. Edited by D. Male. Oxford: IRL Press.

Muller-Eberhard, H.J. (1986) The membrane attack complex of complement. *Annual Review of Immunology*, **4**, 503–528.

Muller-Eberhard, H.J. & Schreiber, R.D. (1980) Molecular biology and chemistry of the alternative pathway of complement. *Advances in Immunology*, **29**, 1–53.

Porter, R.R. & Reid, K.B.M. (1978) The biochemistry of complement. *Nature*, **275**, 699–704.

Reid, K.B.M. & Porter, R.R. (1981) The proteolytic activation system of complement. *Annual Review of Biochemistry*, **50**, 433–464.

Ross, S.C. & Densen, P. (1984) Complement deficiency states and infection. *Medicine (Baltimore)*, **62**, 243–273.

Ross, G.D. (ed.) (1986) *Immunobiology of the Complement System*. New York: Academic Press.

Ross, G.D. & Medof, M.E. (1985) Membrane complement receptors specific for bound fragments of C3. *Advances in Immunology*, **37**, 217–267.

Rother, K. & Rother, U. (eds) (1986) Hereditary and acquired complement deficiencies in animals and man. *Progress in Allergy*, **39**.

Schifferli, J.A., Ng, Y.C. & Peters, D.K. (1986) The role of complement and its receptor in the elimination of immune complexes. *New England Journal of Medicine*, **315**, 488–495.

Whaley, K. (ed.) (1987) *Complement in Health and Disease*. Lancaster: MTP Press.

14 Development of the Immune System

An efficient immune system depends upon the interaction of many cellular and humoral components which develop at different rates during fetal and early postnatal life. Many of the cells involved in the immune response are derived from undifferentiated haemopoietic stem cells (HSCs) and are thought to differentiate into the various cell lineages under the influence of different microenvironmental factors (Fig. 14.1).

In the chicken, HSCs originate from blood islands in the yolk sac and later in the bone marrow. In mammals, the HSCs are found in the fetal liver, spleen and bone marrow, but after birth and throughout adult life they are normally found only in the bone marrow. These 'self-renewing' HSCs, through the action of various growth and differentiation factors within the sites of haemopoiesis, give rise to most or all cells involved in the immune response. The HSCs give rise to four major cell lineages: erythroid (erythrocytes); megakaryocytoid (platelets); myeloid (granulocytes and monocytes); lymphoid (lymphocytes). The latter two lineages are critical to the functioning of the immune system. We will first deal with development of granulocytes and monocytes.

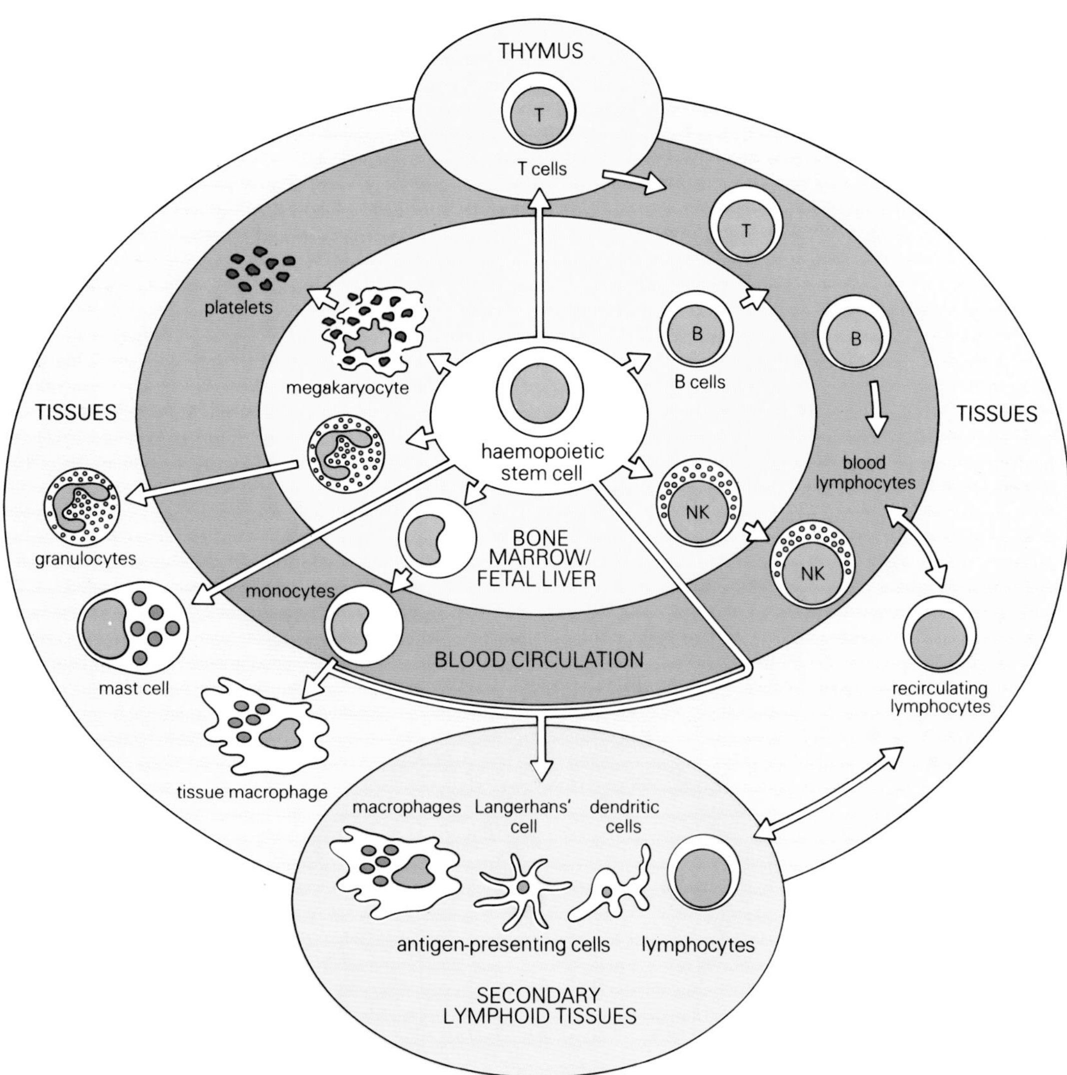

Fig. 14.1 Origin of the cells of the immune system. All of these cells arise from the haemopoietic stem cell. Platelets produced by megakaryocytes are released into the circulation, granulocytes pass from the circulation into the tissues. Mast cells are identifiable in all tissues. B cells mature in the fetal liver and bone marrow in mammals while T cells mature in the thymus. The origin of the large granular lymphocytes with NK activity is uncertain. Both lymphocytes and monocytes (which develop into macrophages) can recirculate through secondary lymphoid tissue. Langerhans' cells and dendritic cells act as antigen-presenting cells in secondary lymphoid tissues.

MYELOID CELLS

Myelopoiesis commences in the fetal liver at about 6 weeks of gestation in man. From experiments *in vitro*, where it is possible to grow 'colonies' from individual stem cells, it has been shown that the first progenitor cell derived from the HSC is the 'colony forming unit' which can give rise to granulocytes (G), erythrocytes (E), monocytes (M) and megakaryocytes (M) (CFU-GEMM). Further development of these into mature cells occurs under the influence of 'colony stimulating factors' (CSFs) and several interleukins including IL-1, IL-2, IL-3 and IL-5 (Fig. 14.2). These factors which are important in the regulation of haemopoiesis are derived mainly from stromal cells, but they are also produced by mature forms of the differentiated myeloid cells and lymphoid cells.

GRANULOCYTE DEVELOPMENT

Induction of CFU-GM along the granulocyte pathway gives rise to distinct morphological stages of development. Promyelocytes develop into myelocytes and are released into the circulation as mature neutrophils, basophils or eosinophils. The 'one-way' differentiation of cells from the CFU-GM into mature granulocytes is probably the result of the acquisition of specific growth/differentiation factor receptors at different stages of the developmental process.

Surface differentiation markers disappear or appear on the cells as they develop into granulocytes (Fig. 14.3). For example the CFU-GM carries MHC class II molecules and CD34 on its surface. These molecules are absent on mature neutrophils. A number of surface molecules are acquired during the differentiation process. These include CD13, CD14 (low density; activated?), the leucocyte function antigens CD11a, b and c, complement receptors and Fc receptors for IgG (see Fig. 2.11).

Although it is difficult to assess the functional activity of different developmental stages of granulocytes it is likely that the full functional potential is only achieved after mature forms are produced. There is some evidence that neutrophil function, as measured by phagocytosis or chemotaxis is lower in fetal than in adult life. This may be due to the lower opsonization ability of the fetal serum rather than endogenous functional activity. Since functioning of neutrophils is dependent on direct interaction of the mature effector cells with microorganisms and/or with the cytokines generated as a consequence of exposure of the animal to an antigenic insult, this could be a limiting factor in early life.

MONOCYTE DEVELOPMENT

CFU-GM give rise to proliferating monoblasts which then differentiate, into promonocytes and finally into mature circulating monocytes which are thought to represent a replacement pool for tissue-fixed macrophages. Several different forms of these macrophages comprise the 'reticuloendothelial' system (see Chapter 2).

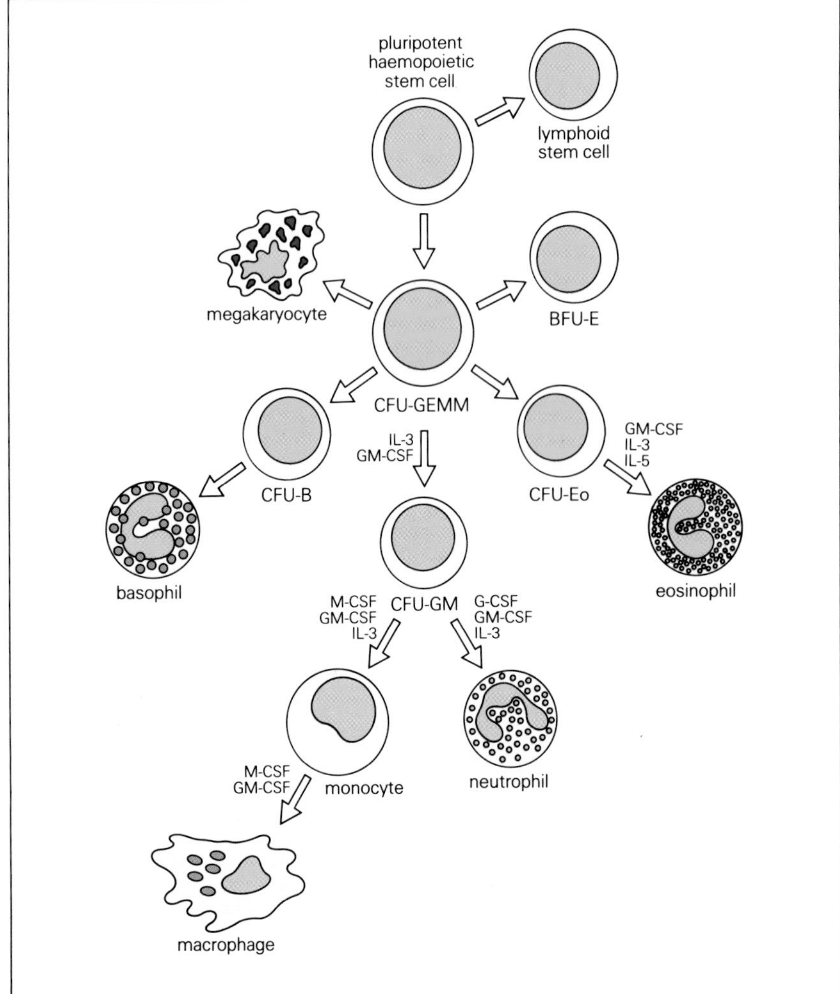

Fig. 14.2 Development of granulocytes and monocytes. Pluripotent haemopoietic stem cells generate CFU-GEMMs which have the potential to give rise to all blood cells except lymphocytes. IL-3 and GM-CSF are required to induce this stem cell into one of five pathways (i.e. to give rise to megakaryocytes, erythrocytes via 'burst-forming units' (BFU-E), basophils neutrophils or eosinophils) and are also required during further differentiation of the granulocytes and monocytes. Eosinophil differentiation from CFU-Eo is promoted by IL-5. Neutrophils and monocytes are derived from the CFU-GM through the effects of G-CSF and M-CSF respectively. Both GM-CSF and M-CSF, and other cytokines, promote the differentiation of monocytes into macrophages.

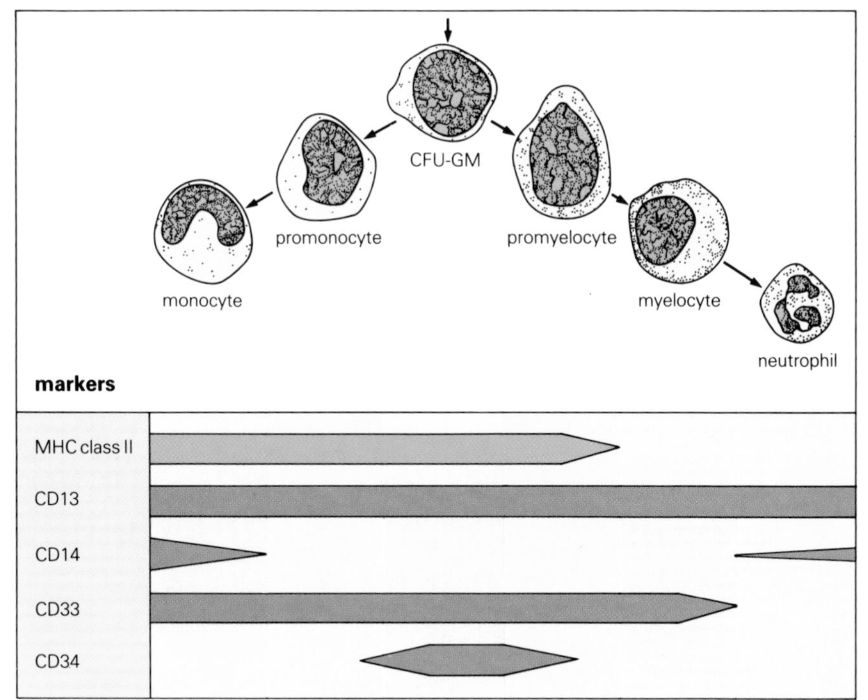

Fig. 14.3 Morphology and markers on developing granulocytes and monocytes. Cells of the monocyte and granulocyte lineages develop from a common CFU-GM. Differentiation along either pathway results in loss of CD34. CD33 is maintained on monocytes but is lost from mature neutrophils, as are MHC class II molecules. CD14 is expressed on monocytes but only weakly on some granulocytes (possibly activated).

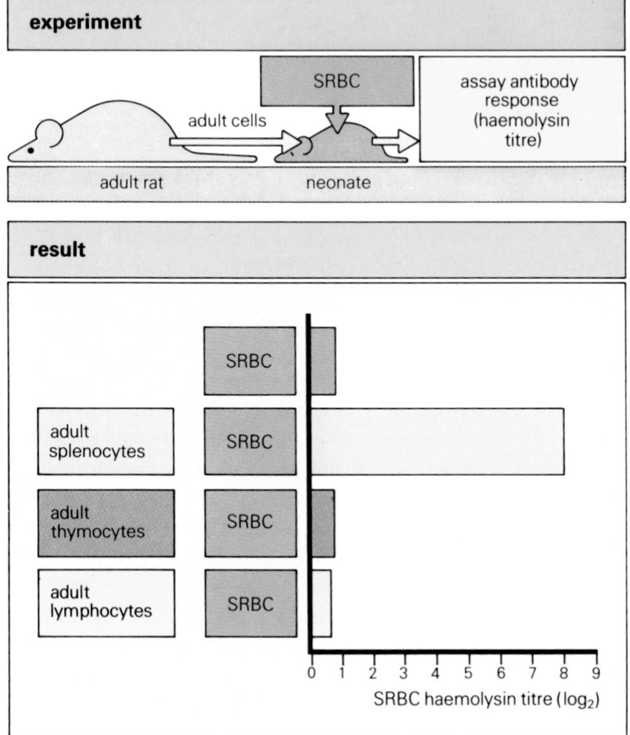

Fig. 14.4 Development of macrophage function: antigen processing and presentation. In this experiment neonatal rats are injected with sheep red blood cells (SRBCs) and cells (splenocytes including antigen-presenting cells (APCs), thymocytes or lymphocytes) from an adult of the same strain. The antibody response following each injection schedule is assayed and the results are shown in the bar diagram. Neonatal rats injected with SRBCs do not make an antibody response to this antigen but if the animals are given adult APCs with the antigen, they can make a response. Neither adult thymocytes nor adult lymphocytes can perform this function. Thus neonatal APCs are unable to present this antigen effectively.

Like the mature neutrophils, mature monocytes and macrophages lose CD34. However, unlike neutrophils they maintain MHC class II molecules in their membrane (see Fig. 14.3). The latter are clearly important for their role in the presentation of antigen to T cells. They also acquire many of the same surface molecules as mature neutrophils.

Like granulocytes, it is difficult to assess the functional potential of different stages of monocyte development. However, studies on myeloid tumour cell lines *in vitro*, believed to represent distinct stages of monocyte differentiation, indicate that both phagocytic efficiency and Fc receptor-mediated cytotoxicity of nucleated cells is optimal in mature macrophages. Generation of the cytokine IL-1 by monocytes is equally good at birth as in adults. Like that of granulocytes, the function of these cells is enhanced by interaction with cytokines.

DEVELOPMENT OF ANTIGEN-PRESENTING CELLS

In addition to macrophages, most of the 'classical' antigen-presenting cells (APCs) which include the follicular dendritic cells, Langerhans' cells and interdigitating follicular cells are present at birth. Their origin is at present unclear but it is likely that they are all derived from bone marrow stem cells. One school of thought is that they are derived from the same stem cell. Morphological, cytochemical and functional differences would then be due to local microenvironmental influences. The other school believes that they are derived from different stem cells and represent separate lineages of differentiation. APCs are present in the thymus very early in development and their function in MHC restriction and selection indicates that at least some APCs must be fully mature at this time.

However, the functional activity of cells involved in processing and presenting exogenous antigens is clearly suboptimal early in life. For example, neonatal rats fail to make a normal antibody response to sheep red blood cells unless they are also injected with adult APCs (Fig. 14.4).

THE COMPLEMENT SYSTEM

The complement system is another important component of the innate immune system, and plays a major role in protection against microorganisms. At least 20 distinct plasma proteins have been identified as belonging to the system (see Chapter 13). These proteins appear during fetal development and are detectable before circulating IgM (Fig. 14.5). They are present in the neonate at 50–60% of the adult serum levels. The appearance of complement components before IgM synthesis reflects the fact that complement, together with phagocytic cells, provided the main protection of animals before the evolutionary development of antibodies. Thus ontogeny recapitulates phylogeny.

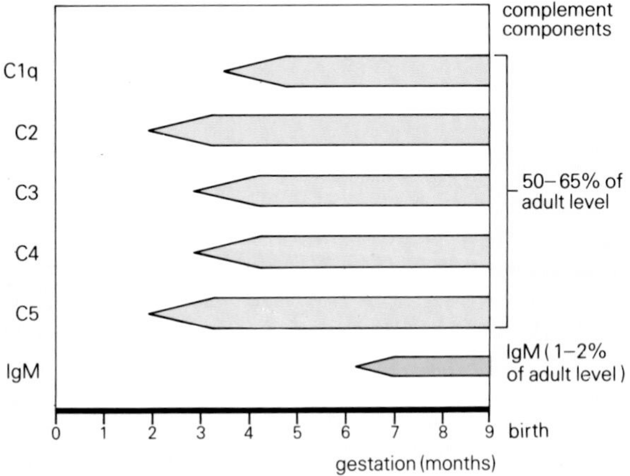

Fig. 14.5 Development of the complement system. The bar diagram shows the earliest times at which the components of the complement system can be detected in human fetal tissue. The levels of most complement components reach more than 50% of their adult value by birth. By comparison endogenously produced immunoglobulin develops later.

LYMPHOID CELLS

Lymphocytes develop in the primary lymphoid organs – T cells in the thymus and B cells in the avian bursa of Fabricius or, for mammals, in the fetal liver and bone marrow. These cells then migrate to the secondary lymphoid tissues where they can respond to antigen.

T CELLS

The thymic rudiment develops from the third (and in some species the fourth) pharyngeal pouch as an outpushing of the gut entoderm which then becomes seeded with blood-borne lymphoid stem cells. Few stem cells appear to be needed to give rise to the repertoire of mature T cells with diverse antigen binding specificities.

Migration of stem cells into the thymus is not a random process. In birds, at least, it has been shown that they enter in two or possibly three waves. This has been demonstrated using chicken and quail chimaeras (Fig. 14.6). Attraction factors released by the thymus have

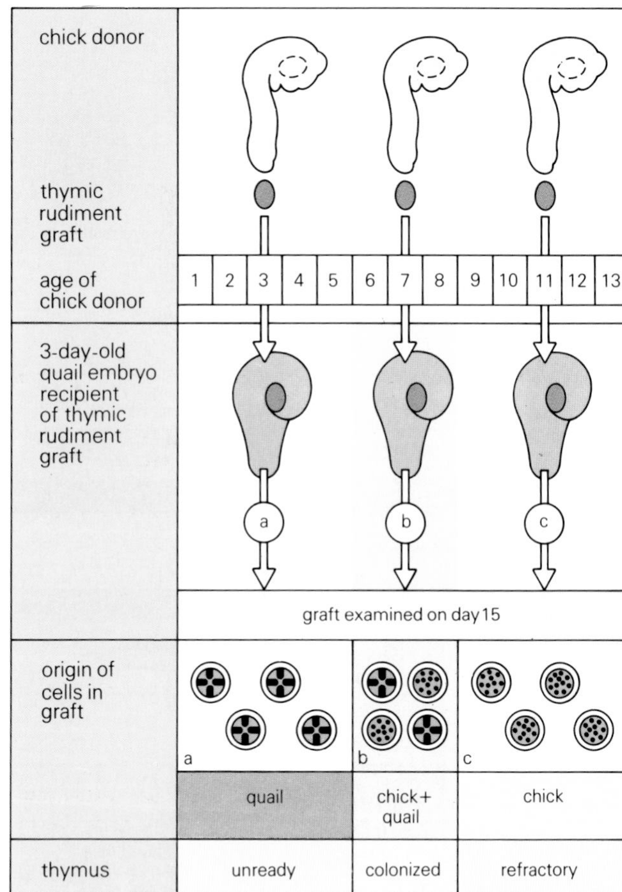

Fig. 14.6 Stem cell colonization of the chick thymus. The thymic rudiment from a chick embryo of different ages was grafted onto a 3-day old quail embryo and examined later to determine the origin of cells in the thymus. Quail cells can be distinguished from chicken cells by the appearance of condensed chromatin in the resting cell. If the graft was less than 6 days old it had not yet become colonized with chick stem cells and on subsequent examination was found to contain quail cells only (a). If the graft was older than 8 days it was found to be colonized with chick lymphocytes (c). Grafts transferred between day 6 and day 8 contained both chick and quail cells (b). The interpretation is that before 6 days the chick thymus is not ready to receive stem cells. There follows a window of colonization after which (from day 8) the thymus becomes refractory to further colonization. Further studies indicate that there may be additional windows open later in embryogenesis.

been proposed to explain the immigration of thymic stem cells. Once there the stem cells begin to differentiate into thymic lymphocytes under the influence of the thymic epithelial microenvironment. Whether or not the stem cells are pre-committed to becoming T cells, that is, pre-T cells, before they arrive in the thymus is controversial. Specialized epithelial cells in the peripheral areas of the cortex (thymic 'nurse' cells) contain intracytoplasmic thymocytes in vesicles and may be involved in the process of thymic education.

The thymocytes become organized into well-defined lobules forming a cortex and a medulla (see Chapter 3) where epithelial cells and bone marrow-derived dendritic cells rich in MHC class II antigens are important in the differentiation of the T lymphocytes (Fig. 14.7). It has

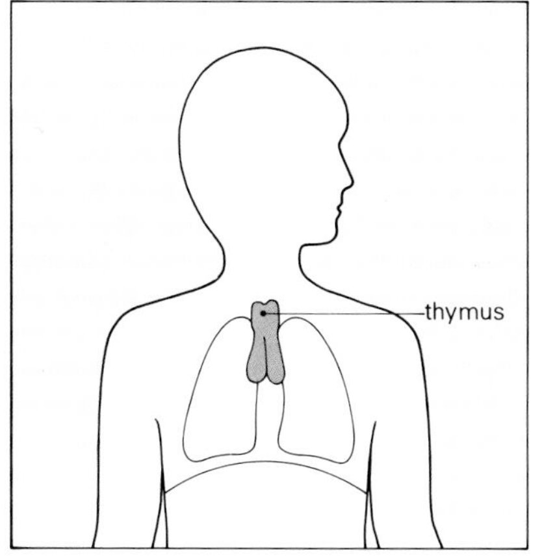

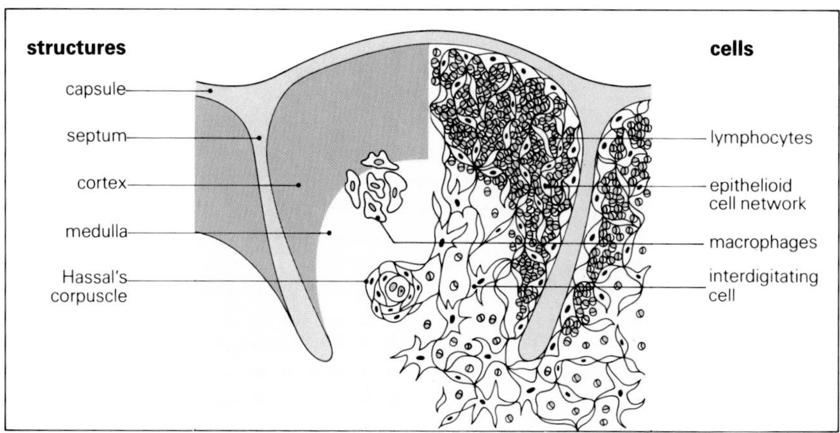

Fig. 14.7 Structure of the thymus. The bilobed thymus is an encapsulated organ divided into lobules by septa. The cortex contains densely packed dividing lymphocytes in a network of epithelial cells which extends into the medulla. The medulla contains fewer lymphocytes, but there are more bone marrow-derived interdigitating cells. Note the close association of the developing lymphocytes with epithelial and interdigitating cells. The function, if any, of the whorled epithelial structures termed Hassal's corpuscles is unknown.

been shown that stem cells surrounding the human thymic rudiment already express the pan-T marker, CD7.

Cortical cells represent 85–90% of the thymocytes whilst the remainder are medullary cells. Studies of their function and cell surface markers have indicated that cortical thymocytes are less mature than medullary thymocytes. It has been found that cortical cells are more sensitive to high levels of corticosteroids *in vivo* and this may be reflected by the decrease in this cell population which occurs during pregnancy in mice. Some cortical cells migrate to, and mature in, the medulla.

Mature medullary T cells leave the thymus via post-capillary venules located at the cortico-medullary junction. However, other routes of exit may exist including lymphatic vessels. These cells possess 'homing' receptors which allow their migration into specific areas (T-dependent) of the peripheral or secondary lymphoid tissues where they carry out their function.

As in the development of granulocytes and monocytes, a number of 'differentiation' antigens of functional significance appear and are lost during the change from the T stem cell into mature T cells. Analyses of the rearrangement of genes encoding for the two presently known T cell receptors (TCR), the γ/δ (TCR-1) and the α/β (TCR-2), and phenotypic studies of surface membrane antigens, suggest that at least two pathways of T cell differentiation occur in the thymus. Whether these pathways are distinct, or whether they diverge from an early common pathway is not known. Most thymocytes differentiate into TCR-2^+ cells, which account for the majority of T lymphocytes found in the secondary lymphoid tissues and in the circulation. In these cells the rearrangement of genes encoding the TCR-2 β chain precedes that of genes encoding the α chain (see Chapter 6). Phenotypic analyses of surface membrane antigens have delineated a continuum of changes in surface membrane antigens during T cell maturation. A summary of these changes is shown in Fig. 14.8. The phenotypic variations can be simplified in a three-stage model.

Stage I or Early Thymocytes express CD7 (see above) together with CD2 (the sheep erythrocyte receptor) and

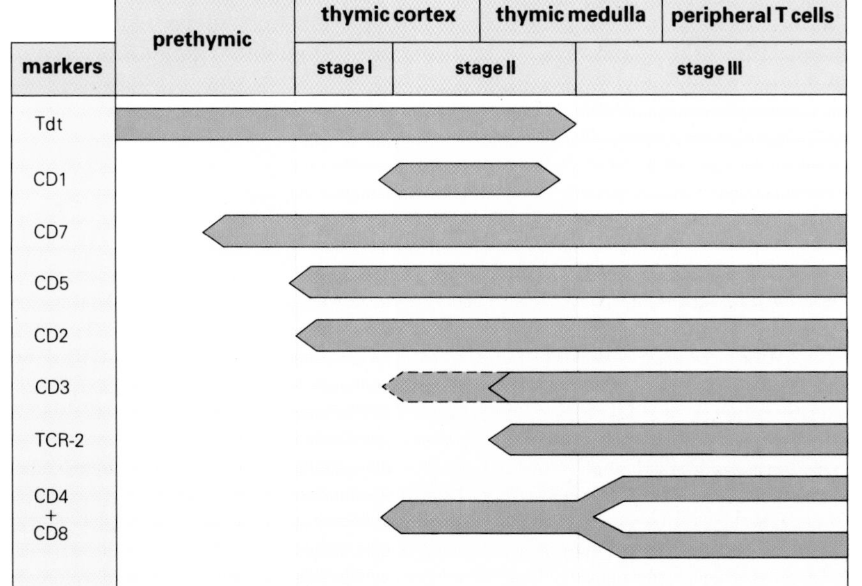

Fig. 14.8 Human T cell differentiation. The development of markers on human T cells is shown. Tdt (terminal deoxynucleotidyl transferase) is an enzyme present in thymic stem cells through to stage III and is lost in the medulla. Several surface glycoproteins appear during differentiation. CD1 is found in cortical stage II thymocytes, but is lost in the medulla. CD2 and CD7 appear very early in differentiation and are present on mature T cells. CD5 appears at an early stage and is also present on mature cells. CD3 appears in the cytoplasm in early stage II cells (dotted line) and is expressed on the cell surface simultaneously with TCR-2. CD4 and CD8 are found together on stage II cells, and one is lost during differentiation into stage III cells.

CD5. Proliferation markers such as the transferrin receptor and CD38 (a marker common to all early haemopoietic precursors) are also expressed at this stage. It is of note that none of these molecules are T lineage-specific. However, the T commitment of early thymocytes is shown by the TCRβ chain gene rearrangements and by expression of the TCR-associated complex, CD3, in the cytoplasm but not on the membrane.

Stage II, Intermediate or Common Thymocytes are characterized by the appearance of additional surface markers such as CD1, and by the co-expression of CD4 and CD8 on the same cell. Genes encoding the α chain of TCR-2 are rearranged in intermediate thymocytes.

Stage III or Mature Thymocytes show major phenotypic changes – namely loss of CD1, presence on the cell membrane of CD3 associated with the α/β TCR-2, and the distinction of two subsets of cells expressing CD4 (T-helpers), or CD8 (T-cytotoxic cells). The majority of thymocytes at this stage lack CD38 and the transferrin receptor, and are virtually indistinguishable from mature, circulating T cells.

The intrathymic pathway of TCR-1$^+$ (γ/δ) cell differentiation has not been fully defined thus far. These cells represent a minority of both the thymic and the circulating T cells (<5%). The following maturational events are of note:

1. during ontogeny the genetic changes leading to γ chain gene rearrangements precede those of ß and α chain genes
2. the differentiation pathway of TCR-1$^+$ cells is probably distinct from that of TCR-2$^+$ cells and does not usually involve the expression of CD1, CD4 and CD8
3. the mature product of this differentiation pathway is a TCR-1$^+$/CD3$^+$ cell which expresses neither CD4 nor CD8.

Additional features of TCR-1$^+$ cells are represented by their exquisite characteristics of homing into peripheral tissues, particularly into the epidermis and mucosal epithelium where, upon activation, they may acquire the CD8 marker. A major role of these intraepithelial lymphocytes may be that of mediating cytotoxic functions, thus contributing to the surface defence barriers.

Thymic hormones or factors may play a role in development of T cells in the thymus and their maintenance within the secondary lymphoid tissues. Fig. 14.9 lists some of the better studied preparations and their properties. It seems likely that different hormones or factors act on T cells at different stages of their development. Whereas some may act within the thymus and induce thymic cell maturation, others could act at peripheral sites. They have, in fact, been found in thymic epithelial cells and in the circulation where they decrease with age concomitantly with thymic atrophy. Many of the thymic factors or hormones have now been sequenced and synthesized. Since a number of endogenous pharmacologically active agents have been shown to have similar effects to thymic factors/hormones, for example cyclic AMP and epinephrine, their exact physiological relevance needs to be established.

B CELLS

In the chicken, primary B cell lymphopoiesis occurs in a discrete lympho-epithelial organ, the bursa of Fabricius. The bursal rudiment develops as an outpushing of the hindgut entoderm and becomes infiltrated with blood-borne stem cells. Studies on chicken/quail chimaeras have indicated that there is a window for the immigration of stem cells into the bursa between days 10 and 14 (see Chapter 15). Pyroninophylic cells, the putative stem cells, are seen in contact with epithelial cells. Bursal cell proliferation gives rise to the cortex and the medulla in each bursal follicle, which, like the thymus lobules, may be seeded by one or a few stem cells (Fig. 14.10).

Mammals do not have a specific discrete organ for B cell lymphopoiesis; instead these cells develop directly from lymphoid stem cells in the haemopoietic tissue of the fetal liver (Fig. 14.11) from 8–9 weeks of gestation in man and by about 14 days in mice. The function of the fetal liver as a site of B cell production wanes and the site of production transfers into the bone marrow where it is continued into adult life. This is also true of the other haemopoietic lineages giving rise to erythrocytes, granulocytes, monocytes and platelets. The microenvironment of the fetal liver is important in the differentiation of B cells.

The characteristic marker of the B lymphocyte lineage is the expression of immunoglobulins which act as the cell surface antigen receptor. Lymphoid stem cells (probably expressing Tdt) proliferate and differentiate and following immunoglobulin gene rearrangements (see Chapter 6), pre-B cells emerge which express μ heavy chains in the cytoplasm. Allelic exclusion of maternal or paternal immunoglobulin genes has already

Fig. 14.9 Thymic hormones and factors. All preparations, except FTS, were originally extracted from bovine thymus. FTS was derived from pig serum but has now been shown to be present in the thymus. (Ubiquitin, a 74 amino acid protein with a molecular weight of 8457, has similar properties to the other factors and at one time was thought to be a thymic hormone; however it is present not only in thymus but also in many other animal and plant tissues, bacteria and yeasts.) * Preparations which have been synthesized artificially.

name	chemistry	comment
thymosin (fraction 5)*	α, β and γ polypeptides α-1-sequenced: 28 amino acids mol. wt 3108	some produced in thymic epithelial cells
thymopoietin 1, 2 and 3	sequenced: 49 amino acids mol. wt 5562	produced only in thymus, activity in pentapeptide (TP-5) *
thymic humoral factor (THF)	31 amino acids mol. wt 3220	partially sequenced
thymostimulin (TP-1)	group of peptides	least well characterized
facteur thymique serique (FTS)*	9 amino acids	present in serum, disappears after thymectomy

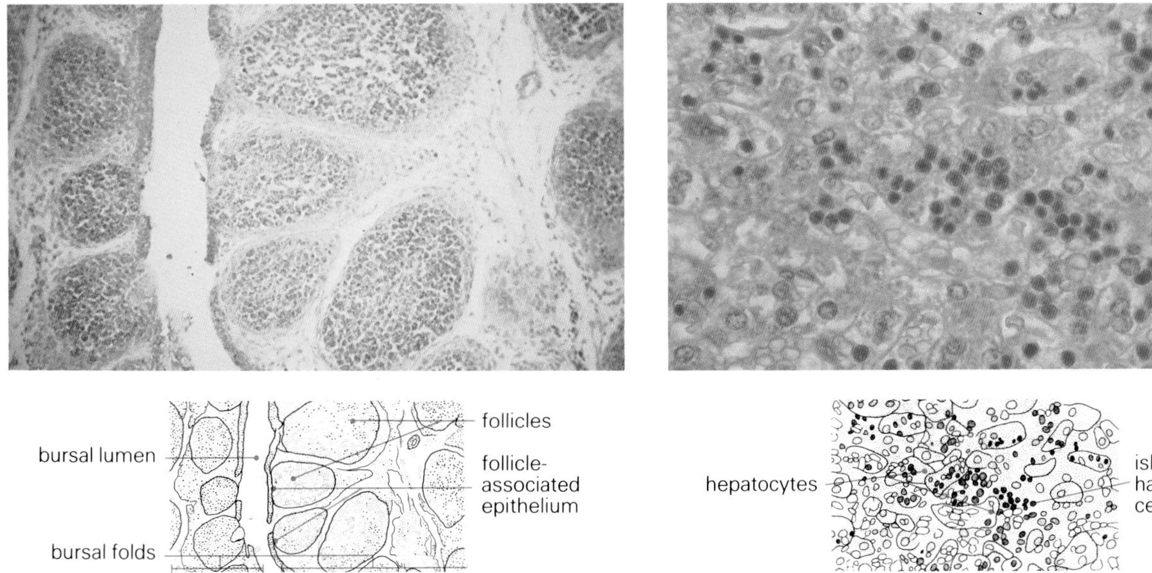

Fig. 14.10 Section of a bursa showing B lymphocytes developing in follicles. Like the fetal liver, the bursa is a site of haemopoiesis as well as myelopoiesis. H&E stain, ×50.

Fig. 14.11 Section of human fetal liver showing islands of haemopoiesis. HSCs give rise to islands of differentiating lineage-specific cells, including B lymphocytes.

occurred by this time. The proliferating pre-B cells are thought to give rise to smaller pre-B cells. On synthesis of light chains, which may be either of κ or λ type but not both, the B cell assembles surface immunoglobulins (sIg) and each B cell is then committed to the antigen binding specificity of the sIg for the rest of its life. Thus one B cell can only make one specific antibody and this forms the basis of the clonal selection theory for antibody production. A summary of B cell differentiation with expression of immunoglobulins and other relevant molecules is shown in Fig. 14.12.

Similar to that described for T cells (see above and Chapter 6), a sequential hierarchy of immunoglobulin gene rearrangements and of phenotypic changes takes place during B cell ontogeny. Heavy chain gene rearrangements occur in B cell progenitors and represent the earliest indication of B lineage commitment. This is followed by light chain gene rearrangements which occur at later pre-B cell stages. Certain B cell surface markers are expressed prior to immunoglobulin detection, namely class II MHC molecules, CD19, CD20 and the CD10 (CALLA) antigen. The latter marker is transiently expressed on early B progenitors that precede the pre-B cell (cytoplasmic μ-positive) stage. A number of

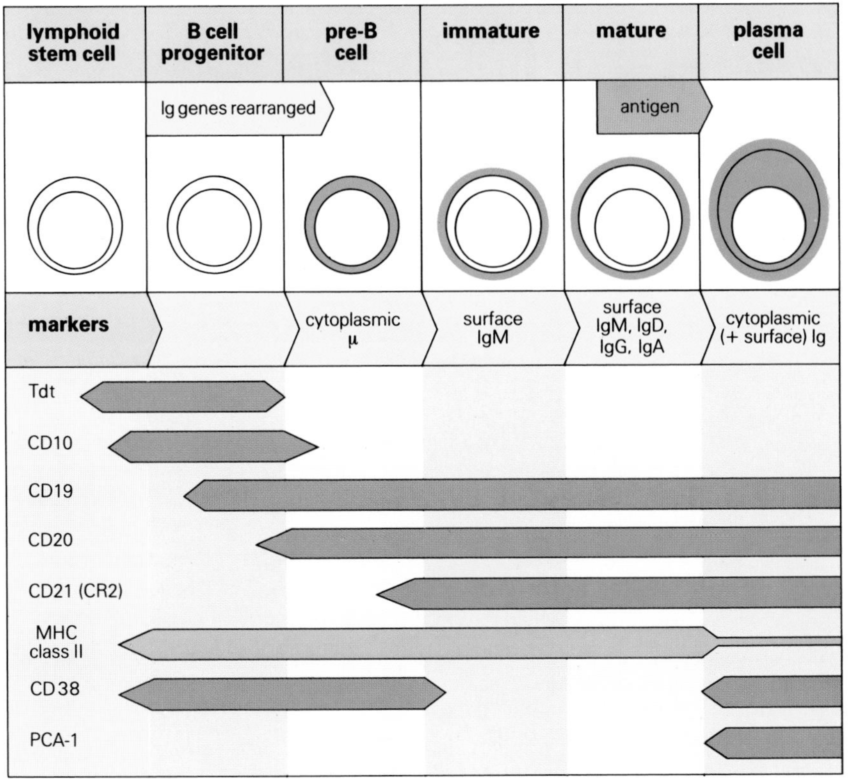

Fig. 14.12 B cell differentiation. B cells differentiate into plasma cells from lymphoid stem cells. Only the final stage is antigen driven. The cellular location of immunoglobulin is shown in yellow. The genes coding for antibody are rearranged in the course of progenitor cell development. Pre-B cells express cytoplasmic μ chains only. The immature B cell has surface IgM and the mature B cell other immunoglobulin isotypes. On antigen stimulation the B cell proliferates and develops into a plasma cell. Tdt is expressed very early in ontogeny. The diagram also shows the sequence of appearance of other B cell surface markers. PCA-1 is found only on plasma cells. Note that CD38 is an example of a molecule found on early progenitors that is lost and reappears on the fully differentiated plasma cells.

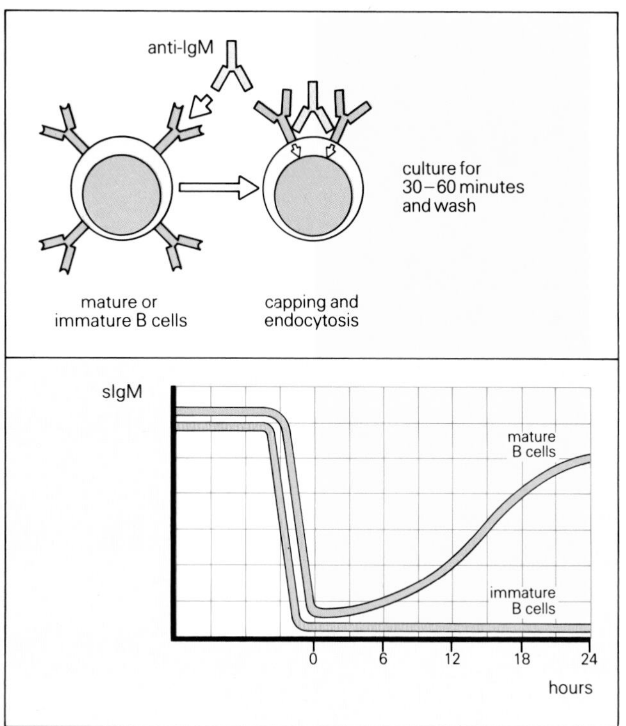

Fig. 14.13 Differentiation of B cells: differential modulation of surface immunoglobulin (sIg) on mature and immature B cells. Mature (adult) and immature (neonatal) B cells are incubated at 37°C together with antibody to their sIgM (anti-Ig) for 30–60 minutes; this causes capping of the sIgM and its internalization by endocytosis. The cells are then washed free of anti-Ig. As shown in the graph, mature B cells resynthesize their sIgM over the following 24 hours, but immature B cells do not.

growth and differentiation factors are required to drive the B cells through early stages of development. These include IL-3 and the newly described IL-7.

Following their production in the fetal liver, B cells migrate and function in the secondary lymphoid tissues. Early immigrants into fetal lymph nodes (17 weeks in man) are sIgM$^+$ and also carry a T cell marker (CD5) (Ly1$^+$ and sIgM$^+$ in mice). These B cells are present in small numbers in secondary follicles of adult lymph nodes and are involved in autoantibody formation.

Following maturation, the B cells, on antigen stimulation, can develop into antibody-forming plasma cells. sIg is usually lost by this stage since its function as a receptor is finished. Immature B cells respond differently to antigens than mature B cells. Treatment of both mature and immature B cells with anti-IgM antibodies or antigen results in loss of sIgM by capping and endocytosis. Mature, but not immature, cells resynthesize sIgM in culture (Fig. 14.13). This property of sIgM modulation explains why immature B cells can be more easily switched off resulting in central tolerance.

DIVERSITY OF ANTIBODY CLASS

It is presumed that class diversity in the antibody response evolved to cope in different ways and at different anatomical sites with the multitude of non-self antigens. Mature plasma cells produce only one class of antibody, thus immature B cells making only IgM are switched to other classes before reaching terminal differentiation as a plasma cell. A model for class switching within one clone is shown in Fig. 14.14. Some of the progeny of the immature B cells synthesize antibodies of other immunoglobulin classes, including IgG and IgA. Further differentiation results in synthesis of surface IgD – an antibody class that is almost exclusively found on B cell membranes. All three classes of sIg on the same cell will have the same antigen specificity, that is to say that they express the same V region genes, although additional diversity within a single clone may be generated by somatic mutation following class switching.

From this point on in clonal differentiation, antigen drives the cell into a fully mature plasma cell and/or a memory cell. Since there is a similar sequence of sIg expression on B cells of vertebrates raised in gnotobiotic environments it seems likely that class diversity develops independently of extrinsic antigen. Furthermore, it is probable that class switching can occur independently of T cells, although these play a significant role in switching to IgG, IgA and IgE. Indeed it has recently been shown that IL-4 and IL-6, which are involved in B cell maturation, are required for class switching. It is probable that all class switching events have taken place before the B cell matures into a plasma cell. Occurrence of different classes of immunoglobulin on the surface of a single cell is probably related to the persistence

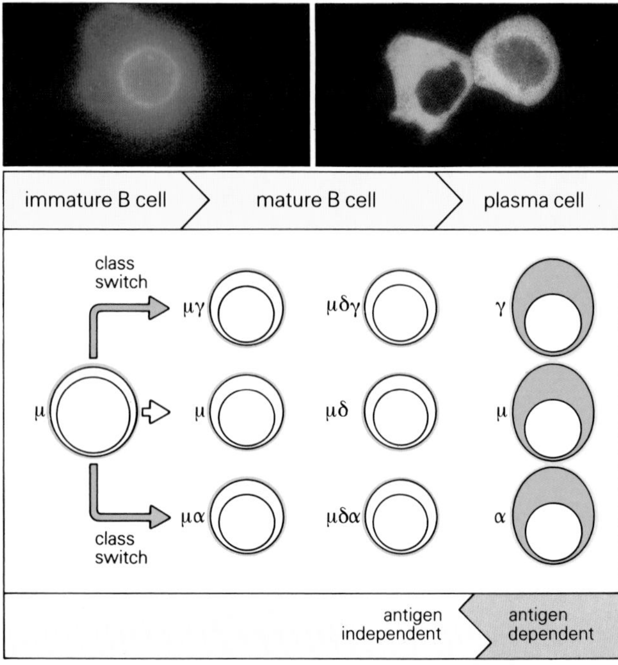

Fig. 14.14 B cell differentiation: class diversity. Immature B cells produce IgM only, but mature B cells can express more than one cell surface antibody, since mRNA and cell surface immunoglobulin remain after a class switch. IgD is also expressed during clonal maturation. Maturation can occur in the absence of antigen, but the development into plasma cells, which have little cell surface, but much cytoplasmic immunoglobulin requires antigen and (usually) T cell help. The photographs show B cells stained for surface IgM (green, left) and plasma cells stained for cytoplasmic IgM and IgG (green and red, right). IgM is stained with fluorescent anti-μ chain, and IgG with rhodaminated anti-γ chain.

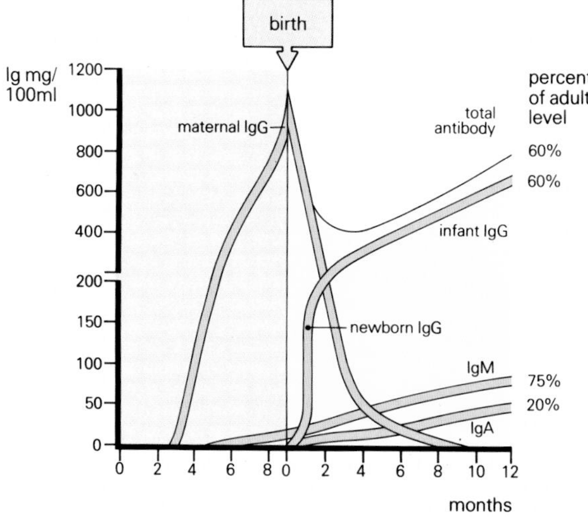

Fig. 14.15 Immunoglobulins in the serum of the fetus and newborn child. IgG in the fetus and newborn infant is derived solely from the mother. This maternal IgG has disappeared by the age of 9 months when the infant is synthesizing its own IgG. The neonate produces its own IgM and IgA: these classes cannot cross the placenta. By the age of 12 months, the infant produces 60% of its adult level of IgG, 75% of its adult IgM level and 20% of its adult IgA level.

of different antibodies on their surface and the generation of mRNA for different antibody isotypes by differential splicing of long nuclear RNA transcripts.

The sequence of appearance of immunoglobulin classes on the cell surface is reflected in detection of serum immunoglobulin in the human fetus and neonate. Fig. 14.15 shows that IgM is synthesized before birth whilst IgG and IgA begin to appear around birth. Serum IgG does not reach adult levels until 1–2 years after birth, whilst IgA takes even longer.

DIVERSITY OF ANTIBODY SPECIFICITY

There are tens of thousands of natural antigenic shapes and since one B cell can make only one antigen-specific antibody many B cells with specific antibody receptors have to be generated from B lymphocyte stem cells. Thus multiple V_H and V_L genes have to be expressed on different cells. It is thought that the earliest antigen-specific IgM^+ B cells appear in a programmed sequence through selected expression of germ line genes, and that later specificities are due to combination of different sets of V, D and J segments. Fig. 14.16 shows the sequential appearance of antigen binding cells with specificity for keyhole limpet haemocyanin, (T,G)-A--L and sheep erythrocytes in the chicken bursa of Fabricius. The same temporal sequence is found in chickens of different strains and occurs after the $sIgM^+$ B cells appear, when they are proliferating within the bursa. A similar sequence of antigen-binding cells is seen in mice and rats, and is reflected in the serum antibodies of neonatal rats (Fig. 14.17). Antibody production, as distinct from antigen recognition by B cells, is dependent on both T cells and APCs.

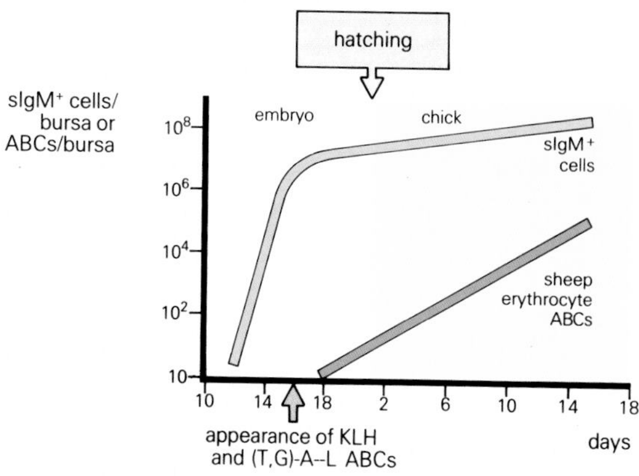

Fig. 14.16 Sequence of appearance of B cells and antigen-binding cells (ABCs) in the avian bursa of Fabricius. Cells which carry surface IgM ($sIgM^+$) are detectable by day 12 of incubation and increase at an exponential rate consonant with a generation time of about 10 hours. An abrupt change in growth rate occurs near the time of hatching corresponding to the onset of substantial seeding to the periphery. Cells binding keyhole limpet haemocyanin (KLH) and (T,G)-A--L appear by day 16. Cells binding sheep erythrocytes are not detectable in significant numbers before the 18th day of incubation, after which they increase at a rate that is significantly different from the total $sIgM^+$ population. This chronological appearance of $sIgM^+$ and ABCs is consistent with a programmed sequence of appearance of the earliest B cells with different antibody specificities during embryogenesis.

age (days)	*Brucella*	SRBC	DRBC	KLH	SSS_{III}
0	4.7	0	0	0	0
1	5.3	0	0	0	0
2		0	0		
3	7.3	2.9	0	0	0
4		5.4	0		
7			0.6	0	0
10–11			3.0	7.7	0
14–15			4.3	10.4	16%
20–22					70%
28					88%

Fig. 14.17 Development of immune responsiveness. The antibody responses to five different antigens – *Brucella abortis*, sheep red blood cells (SRBC), donkey red blood cells (DRBC), keyhole limpet haemocyanin (KLH) and type III pneumococcal polysaccharide (SSS_{III}) – were measured after injection into neonatal rats of different ages. The responses to the first four antigens are expressed as $\log_2$ antibody titres. The response to SSS_{III} is expressed as a percentage of animals responding. Blank boxes indicate not tested.

FURTHER READING

Adkins, B., Mueller, C., Okada, C.Y., Reichert, R.A., Weissman, I.L. & Spangnide, G.J. (1987) Early events in T cell maturation. *Annual Review of Immunology*, **5**, 325.

Dorshkind, K. (1987) Bone marrow stromal cells and their factors regulate B cell differentiation. *Immunology Today*, **8**, 191.

Hood, L.E., Weissman, I.L., Wood, W.B. & Wilson, J.H. (1984) *Immunology*. 2nd edition, p.243. The Benjamin/Cummings Publishing Co. Inc.

Kyewski, B.A. (1986) Nurse Cells: possible sites of T cell selection. *Immunology Today*, **7**, 374.

LeDouarin, N.M., Dieterlen-Lievre, F. & Oliver, P.D. (1984) Ontogeny of primary lymphoid organs and lymphoid stem cells. *American Journal of Anatomy*, **170**, 261.

Owen, J.J.T. & Jenkinson, E.J. (1984) Early events in T lymphocyte genesis in the fetal thymus. *American Journal of Anatomy*, **170**, 301.

Welte, K., Bonilla, M.A., Gabrilove, J.L., Gillio., A.P., Potter, G.K., Moore, M.A., O'Reilley, R.J., Boon., T.C. & Sauza, L.M. (1987) Recombinant human granulocyte-colony stimulating factor: *in vitro* and *in vivo* effects on myelopoiesis. *Blood Cells*, **13(1–2)**, 17–30.

15 Evolution of Immunity

An evolutionary progression towards the sophisticated mammalian immune system is apparent from detailed studies on a range of vertebrate organisms. In contrast, the phylogenetic origins of the vertebrate adaptive immune system, particularly at the molecular level, remain uncertain, despite extensive research into invertebrate immunity.

There is certainly much to be learned about the origins of vertebrate 'non-specific' immunity, for example phagocytosis, from examination of invertebrates. Since invertebrates comprise single or colonial animals, and those that are solid-bodied (acoelomate) or have body cavities (coelomate), with or without blood systems, there is no shortage of choice of suitable experimental animals.

INVERTEBRATE IMMUNITY

Fig. 15.1 presents a simplified evolutionary tree of the animal kingdom; the coelomate invertebrates are divided into two main evolutionary lines based principally upon embryological differences. One line, comprising molluscs, annelids and arthropods (the Protostomes) diverged early in evolution from the pathway that led to the echinoderms, tunicates and vertebrates (Deuterostomes). Since most research into invertebrate immune systems has concentrated on the Protostomes because the arthropods and molluscs are of major economic importance, work directed towards understanding the evolution of the vertebrate immune response has been rather limited.

The extent to which certain immunopotentialities found in vertebrates are also in existence in diverse invertebrate phyla is shown in Fig. 15.1. This approach simply serves to focus attention on possible evolutionary origins of certain cellular and humoral immune phenomena found in vertebrates.

THE MOST PRIMITIVE 'DEFENCE': WOUND HEALING

The highly specific immune response of vertebrates is superimposed upon a more basic protective response. The defence cells of all living multicellular organisms are capable of recognizing and responding to wounded 'self'. Since, in all vertebrates and nearly all invertebrates that have been studied, the response results in aggregation of defence cells at the wound site, a fundamental aspect of cell behaviour must be involved – the locomotory and adhesive behaviour of the cells must be modulated, and cells must adhere only at the wound site.

In mammals, components of the plasma-clotting and complement systems become activated on contact with damaged tissue and play an intermediary role in cell wound interactions; it is very likely that soluble molecules have a similar mediating role in invertebrates with fluid-filled compartments. However, in solid-bodied animals (sponges to Platyhelminthes),

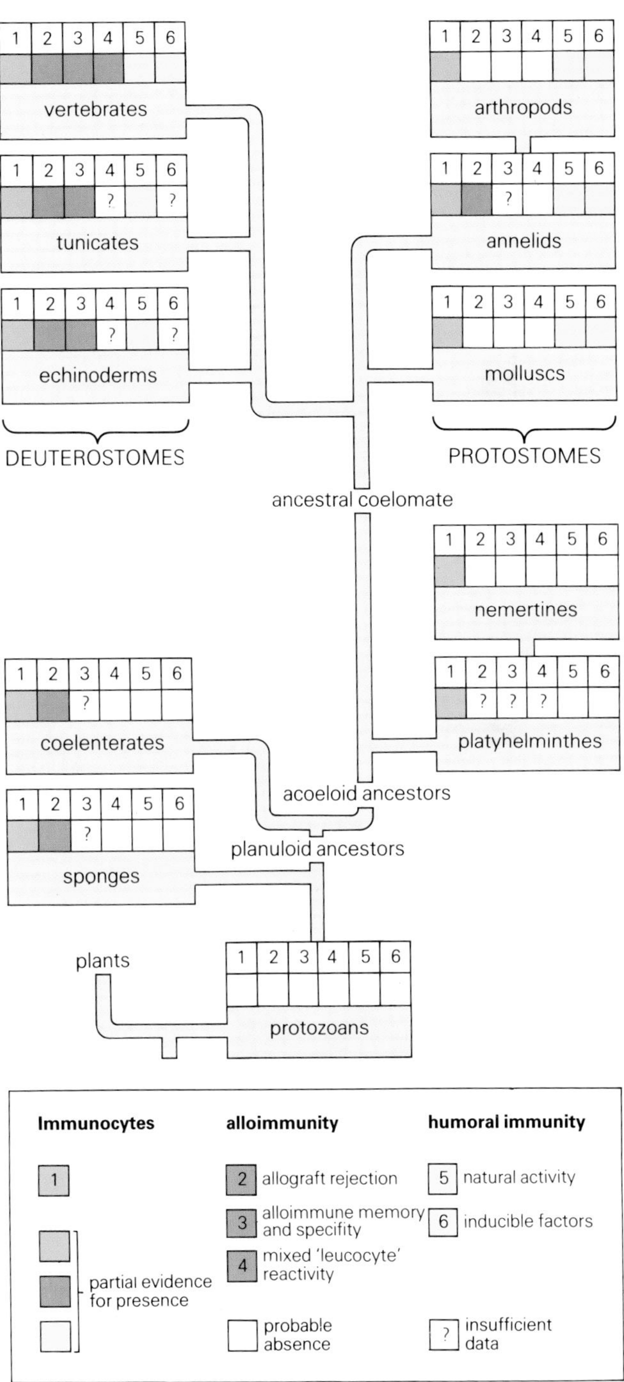

Fig. 15.1 Immunopotentialities of vertebrate and invertebrate phyla. The numbered boxes represent immunocyte activity (1), aspects of alloimmunity (2–4) and humoral immunity (5,6).

aggregation may be based on direct recognition of damage by migrating defence cells. Recognition of 'modified-self' in the form of wounds is but a short step towards recognition of more subtle differences.

IMMUNOCYTE DIVERSITY

The invertebrate response to non-self is primarily cellular and a variety of immunocyte types are found, from the primitive phagocytic amoebocytes of the acoelomate phyla to the haemocytes of molluscs and arthropods, the coelomocytes of annelids and echinoderms, and the blood leucocytes of tunicates.

In the coelomates, immunocytes are subdivided into morphologically distinct classes. Density gradient centrifugation has permitted separation of immunocyte classes within arthropods, echinoderms and tunicates. Subpopulations have been identified within these classes by several criteria, which include the cells' ability to bind various lectins and monoclonal antibodies, the enzymic content of intracellular granules, and behavioural characteristics such as adhesion, locomotion and phagocytosis. Wounding, and to a greater extent, immunological challenge, stimulate behavioural changes in particular subpopulations.

The persistence of immune reactivity must be influenced by the longevity of the reactive cell subpopulations, but information on this topic is surprisingly scant. Mechanisms for the production of immunocytes are, not unexpectedly, diverse; leucopoietic tissue, which undergoes proliferation upon immunological challenge, has been found in the nemertines, insects, molluscs, annelids, echinoderms and tunicates. Mitogens for mammalian T cells stimulate mitosis of annelid and echinoderm cells, but the immunocytes of other phyla tested cannot be stimulated to proliferate *in vitro*; maintenance of short-term enhanced immunocompetence may depend on enhanced reactivity of a particular subpopulation.

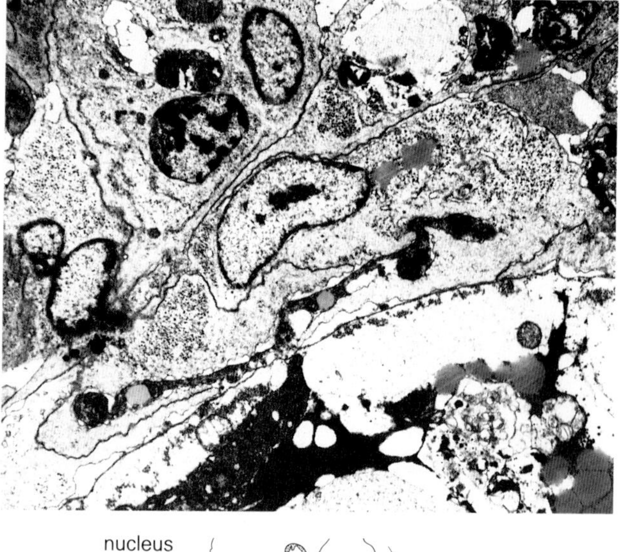

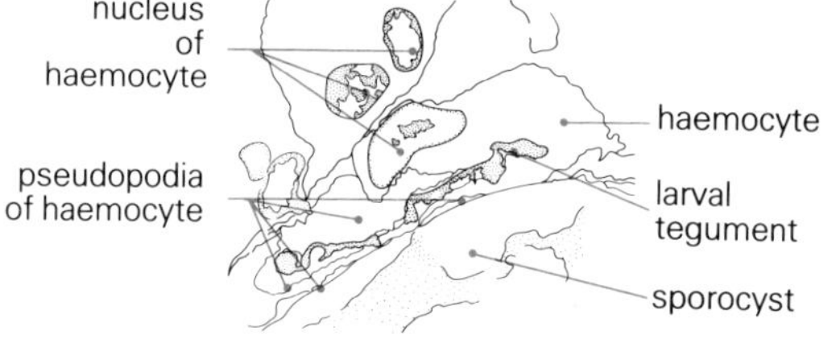

Fig. 15.2 Killing of schistosome larvae (intramolluscan stage) by snail haemocytes. Haemocytes from resistant snails adhere to sporocysts *in vitro*; haemocyte peroxidase is released onto the surface of the larva (not shown here) and the larval tegument is destroyed and engulfed by the adherent cells. ×5000. (Courtesy of Dr C.J. Bayne.)

PHAGOCYTOSIS AND AGGREGATION

Phagocytic cells are found throughout the animal kingdom, serving a nutritive function in lower invertebrates and becoming progressively more specialized towards internal defence in the higher phyla.

Objects too large to be phagocytosed are sequestered within multicellular aggregates that show some similarities to mammalian granulomata, particularly when different classes of immunocyte are involved. In arthropods, the core of the aggregates becomes melanized and, in nearly all phyla examined, such aggregates, whether around foreign objects or at the site of wounds or rejected transplants, become fibrous and/or coated with glycosaminoglycan-like (GAG) material.

Killing mechanisms, either within individual phagocytic cells or within aggregates, are not well understood. A system based on peroxidase and the production of reactive oxygen species has been found in snail haemocytes, and may also kill encapsulated parasites (Fig. 15.2). However, a peroxidase-type system is apparently absent from arthropods and the evidence for other phyla is inconclusive.

HUMORAL IMMUNITY AND COMPLEMENT

Although lacking immunoglobulins, invertebrates have a variety of agglutinins (lectins), and lytic and antimicrobial factors, of various degrees of specificity. Some of these are produced by cells other than immunocytes, and many, for example lysozyme, are continuously present in low concentrations. In general, however, any stimulus — which often includes wounding — tends to increase the concentration of antimicrobial molecules. There is no clear evolutionary trend in the types of molecules produced, other than the ubiquitous lysozyme. The only well-characterized and sequenced inducible antimicrobial factors are the cecropins and attacins and their family of related molecules found in insects.

In vertebrates, the main humoral lytic system is due to complement. Complement-like factors or C3b receptors have been demonstrated in a variety of protostome and deuterostome invertebrates, but evidence for the phylogenetic precursor of the vertebrate complement system is indirect and largely circumstantial. However, phagocytes bearing C3b-like receptors, and a humoral lytic system with many characteristics similar to complement, have been demonstrated in an echinoderm. Interestingly, cell-free insect haemolymph reacts with bound cobra venom factor (cobra C3b) to produce C3-convertase activity that cleaves bovine C3 to give a molecule similar to C3b. It is tempting to speculate that forerunners of the alternative complement pathway arose within the higher invertebrates. The enzymic sequence that activates haemolymph prophenoloxidase in arthropods, resulting in the phenoloxidase-catalyzed production of melanin at the core of haemocytic aggregates, possibly shares some analogous function with the complement system; so far, however, there is no evidence of molecular homologies.

CYTOKINE-LIKE FACTORS

There are a variety of immunocyte-derived 'cytokine-like' factors found in invertebrates that affect mammalian leucocytes *in vitro*. Sea-star factor, produced by the axial organ of echinoderms (a haemopoietic centre in which cells with reputedly T and B lymphocyte-like properties regarding their stimulation by lymphocyte mitogens are found), is mitogenic for mammalian lymphocytes, and an inducible lectin from flies stimulates mouse macrophages to produce tumour necrosis factor. The significance of these findings with regard to the phylogeny of immune systems is not clear; cross-linking of certain surface ligands is likely to have this effect. More important, however, these cytokine-like factors do not seem to be able to stimulate immunocytes from their own species.

TRANSPLANTATION IMMUNOLOGY

Tissue transplantation has been extensively and successfully used as an experimental indicator of the recognition capabilities of invertebrate immune systems. It should be noted that naturally occurring 'grafts' are found in both colonial and sessile invertebrates. Testing for allogeneic or xenogeneic recognition by grafting presents some formidable technical problems, particularly because of the hard skeletons at or near the surface of the animal, and the extreme flexibility of muscular body walls. Most deuterostomes are aquatic and, in all invertebrates, the rate of graft rejection depends on the ambient temperature.

Despite these difficulties, it appears that all invertebrates tested recognize and destroy xenografts, though to varying degrees. However, xenorecognition is often lacking between closely related species of insects (Fig. 15.3). Allogeneic recognition has been demonstrated in all multicellular invertebrates tested, except the nemertines, arthropods and molluscs (Figs 15.1, 15.4, 15.5 and 15.6). Interestingly, a high incidence of tumours has been reported in arthropods and molluscs; this could support the concept that efficient allorecognition is related to competent immune surveillance, but might also merely reflect the large number of investigators working in the medical and agricultural areas, on all aspects of mollusc and arthropod biology. It may be relevant,

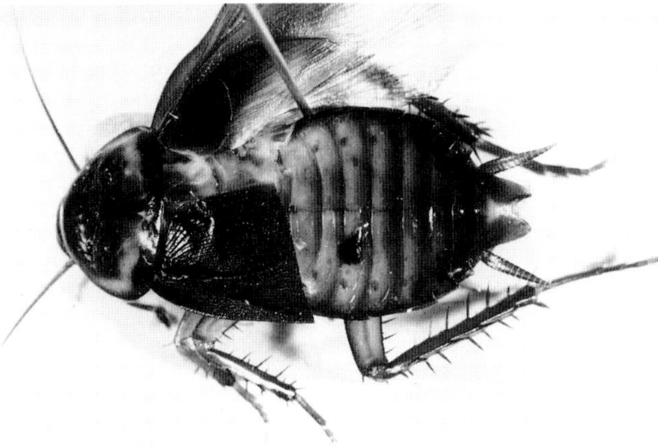

Fig. 15.3 Non-rejection of xenogeneic grafts between related insect species. Recipient *Periplaneta* were grafted pre-moult with donor *Blatta* cuticle. The donor epidermis, which healed in and moulted in synchrony with the recipient, is visible as a dark patch on the dorsal surface.

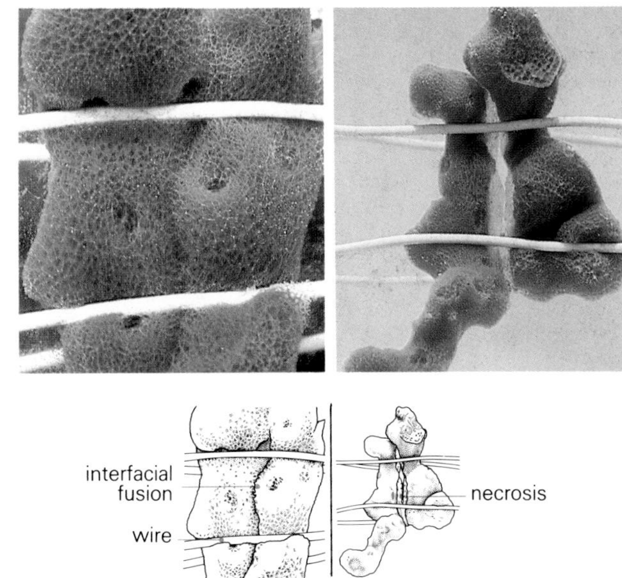

Fig. 15.4 Demonstration of cell-mediated immunity in sponges: allogeneic incompatibility and isogeneic compatibility. Two intact fingers of sponge *(Callyspongia)* from different colonies and two from the same colony are parabiosed (fused circulation) by being held together with vinyl-covered wire. The interfacial fusion between isogeneic parabionts (intracolony) persists indefinitely (left, ×0.5). Incompatibility between allogeneic parabionts (intercolony) results in a cytotoxic interaction; soft tissue necrosis is clearly seen after 7–9 days at 24–27°C (right, ×0.25). (Courtesy of Dr W.H. Hildemann.)

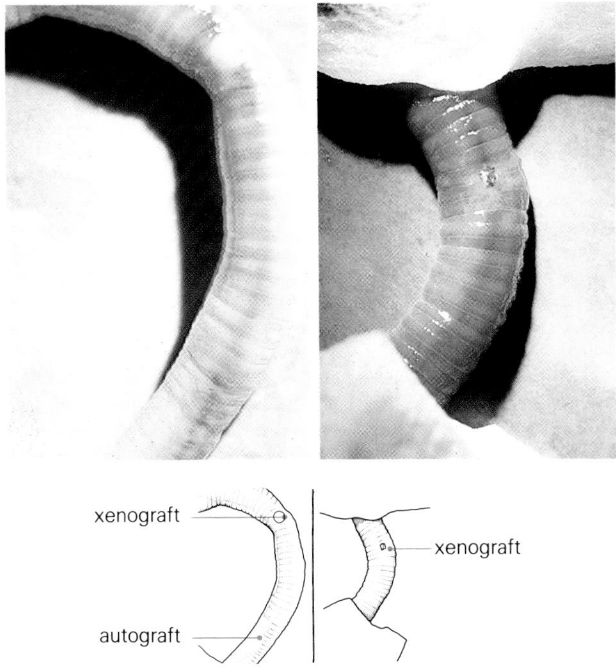

Fig. 15.5 Demonstration of transplantation immunity in annelids: graft rejection in the earthworm *Lumbricus*. Body wall tissue from the earthworm *Eisenia* is grafted onto the body wall of *Lumbricus*. This xenograft shows complete blanching, swelling and oedema 20 days later (15°C) (left); an autograft in the same worm persists indefinitely. At 50 days the xenograft has been destroyed, leaving a collagen pad overlain by necrotic pigment (right). Coelomocytes effect graft rejection in earthworms. (Courtesy of Dr E.L. Cooper.)

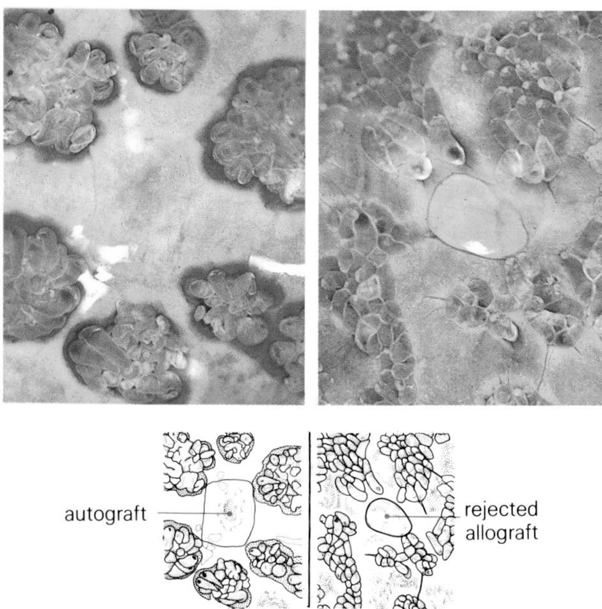

Fig. 15.6 Demonstration of transplantation immunity in echinoderms: allograft rejection in starfish *(Dermasterias).* An autograft remains in perfect condition 300 days after transplantation (left). An allograft rejected at 287 days (14–16°C) is blanched and contracted (right). Rejection involves lymphocyte-like cells and larger phagocytic cells. ×4. (Courtesy of Dr W.H. Hildemann.)

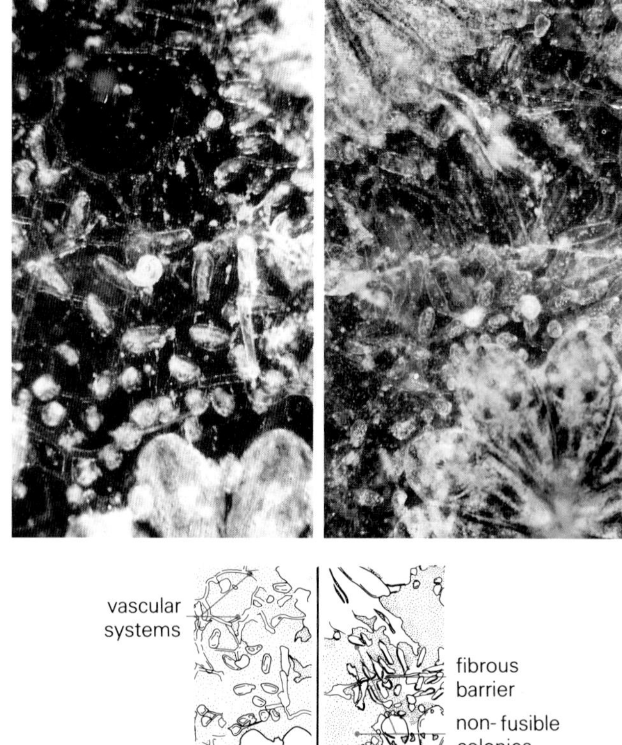

Fig. 15.7 Fusion or rejection between colonies of the colonial tunicate *Botryllus.* In the picture on the left, the ampullae of two colonies have fused and their vascular systems have re-modelled to form a contiguous blood system. In the picture on the right, a fibrous barrier has been deposited in the rejection zone between two non-fusible colonies. Allorecognition in this tunicate is controlled by a single gene locus. ×1500. (Courtesy of Dr V.J. Scofield.)

however, that these phyla contain the majority of the intermediate hosts and vectors of parasitic protozoans and helminths.

Failure to demonstrate allograft rejection may be related to the fact that the animals tested express similar 'self' determinants. Analysis of the frequency of allorecognition within a species has often been hampered by the need to use wild-caught, and thus genetically undefined, individuals. However, experiments using pairs of newly-metamorphosed oozoids of a colonial tunicate, produced by *in vivo* or *in vitro* crosses, have shown that both allorecognition and the control of fertilization are linked characters, controlled by a single gene locus with multiple alleles (Fig. 15.7).

It has been suggested that allograft destruction in many invertebrate phyla, for example sponges, coelenterates, annelids and echinoderms, leads to a 'short-term' anamnestic (memory) response. This interpretation is contentious however, since in all cases second-set grafts were applied while the response to first-set grafts was continuing. Longer-term, specific, memory has been convincingly demonstrated for allografts on tunicates and for xenografts on echinoderms. In contrast, insects display short-term, non-specific enhancement of xenograft rejection.

It is an interesting reflection that the chronic or absent allorecognition and xenorecognition observed in some invertebrates is not necessarily a good indicator of the overall efficacy of their immune system. For example, many arthropods and molluscs are long-lived and can respond quickly and efficiently to most natural immunological insults.

MHC, IMMUNORECOGNITION AND THE 'IG-SUPERFAMILY'

Although transplantation immunology reveals that many invertebrate phyla are capable of allogeneic recognition, there is no evidence to date that invertebrate cells express molecules that are structurally and functionally homologous to either major histocompatibility complex (MHC) glycoproteins or dimeric cell receptors for alloantigen. One possibility is that the MHC evolved within the vertebrates themselves (see below); absence of mixed 'leucocyte' reactivity (one functional marker of MHC in vertebrates) in invertebrates is consistent with this suggestion. On the other hand, the existence of cellular cytotoxicity that can be specifically induced in protochordates suggests that these animals possess a functional equivalent of the vertebrate MHC.

Although not encoded by the MHC genes, β_2-microglobulin in mammals is associated with MHC class I antigens at the cell surface, and shares a degree of structural homology with class I heavy chains, class II β chains and immunoglobulin C region domains. It may thus provide an ancestral link between the MHC and the immunoglobulin system. β_2-microglobulin has been identified in a variety of invertebrates using immunofluorescent techniques but sequence homology has not been investigated. These β_2-microglobulin-like molecules do not appear to be concerned with graft recognition, since they are also found in the arthropods, where allorecognition is lacking.

β_2-microglobulin also shares homology with the glycoprotein Thy-1, a molecule found in the brain of a protostome, the squid. Thy-1 is a member of the 'Ig-superfamily', an ever-enlarging group of molecules that share some structural and genetic homology, but not immunological function, with the immunoglobulins. It has recently been suggested that the Ig-superfamily originated from molecules which evolved to mediate interactions between cells, and that the vertebrate immune system developed from these molecules. How these recognition-mediating interactions became 'turned outwards' to produce an immune system recognizing 'non-self' remains unanswered.

Intuitively, it is plausible that the fine-tuning of invertebrate immunorecognition systems should be based on carbohydrate specificities, via cell-surface glycoproteins or, as suggested for sponges, glycosaminoglycans. Such a system would require the involvement of lectins of different specificities and avidities. So far, evidence for this role for invertebrate lectins is controversial and largely circumstantial; only for molluscs and tunicates are there convincing demonstrations that lectins mediate phagocyte-particle recognition. Ongoing studies on tunicate lectins reveal that their carbohydrate-binding molecules share some common determinants with intact immunoglobulins (or their isolated polypeptide chains) from elasmobranchs, whereas molluscan lectins do not show any serological relationships. This suggests that invertebrate and protochordate lectins contain phylogenetically different proteins.

VERTEBRATE IMMUNITY

Compared with the immense variety of forms seen within the panorama of invertebrate phyla, all vertebrates possess a fairly uniform basic plan of organization, being members of just one phylum – the Chordata. It is therefore to be expected that the basic cellular and molecular components of immunity will be common throughout vertebrate evolution, though increasing specialization of lymphoid tissues, T and B cell functions, histocompatibility antigens, immunoglobulins and other molecules of the immune system, for example complement proteins, appear to be associated with more complex grades of organization. Thus the more sophisticated immune systems of anuran amphibians compared to those of fishes and urodeles (Figs 15.8–15.10) may well relate to physiological and morphological changes, for example improved circulation of body fluids, which are necessary for the emergence of frogs and toads onto land. Immunoglobulin isotype diversity, MHC class I and II glycoproteins, and a full complement of lymphomyeloid tissues are found for the first time in the tetrapods. The most complex structural and functional immune systems are undoubtedly seen in mammals.

T CELL FUNCTIONS AND EVOLUTION OF THE MHC

The evolutionary relationships amongst vertebrates are illustrated in Fig. 15.8, which also summarizes experimental findings, *in vivo* and *in vitro*, of responses to allogeneic cells ('T cell functions'). Acute graft rejection and strong mixed lymphocyte reactions (MLR) are two of the functional markers of disparity between individuals and are associated with the major histocompatibility complex (MHC). These markers are present in 'advanced' amphibians (anurans), 'advanced' fishes (teleosts), birds ('advanced' reptiles?) and mammals, but absent in 'primitive' amphibians (urodeles and apodans), 'primitive' fishes, for example chondrichthyans and chrondrosteans, and reptiles; this suggests that the MHC may have evolved independently on four separate occasions during vertebrate phylogeny, reflecting convergent gene evolution. However, perhaps the MHC, or at least components of the MHC, have been lost from 'primitive' phyla which have evolved from the common ancestor of vertebrates.

Mammals, birds and anuran amphibians have all been shown to possess an MHC by both functional criteria and biochemical and genetic characterization.

In the clawed frog, *Xenopus,* helper and cytotoxic T cell subsets are MHC-restricted. The class I molecules of this anuran are polymorphic, map to the MHC, are noncovalently bound to non-MHC-coded β_2-microglobulin, and are expressed on all tissues. *Xenopus* class II molecules are composed of α and β chains, both of which are 30–35 kD transmembrane glycoproteins, encoded by the MHC; class II molecules are expressed on a limited range of adult cells, including thymic and peripheral leucocytes, antigen-presenting cells and thymic epithelial cells.

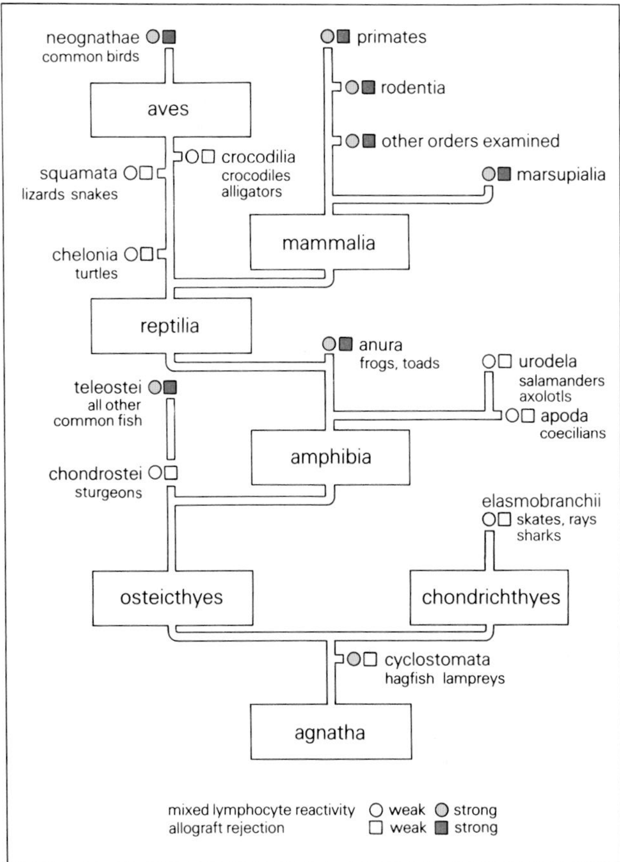

Fig. 15.8 Evolutionary tree illustrating aspects of alloimmunity amongst vertebrates. This tree shows the development of acute allograft rejection and mixed lymphocyte reactivity (MLR) in the vertebrates. These two aspects of MHC function are present in anurans, teleostei, birds and mammals, but absent in the phyla from which they evolved, suggesting either that the MHC evolved independently on four separate occasions, or that the system has been lost from the 'primitive' phyla which have evolved from the common ancestor of vertebrates.

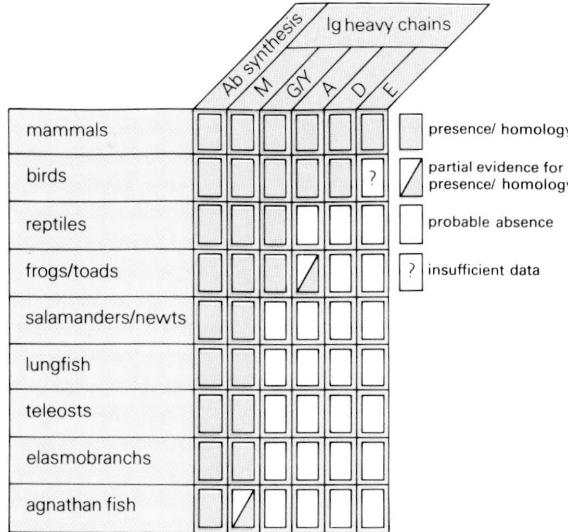

Fig. 15.9 Evolution of immunoglobulin isotypes (Ig heavy chains) in vertebrates.

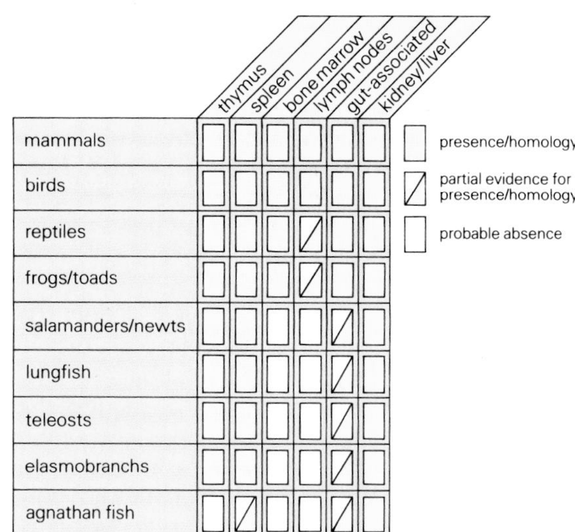

Fig. 15.10 Evolution of lymphomyeloid tissues in vertebrates.

Recent studies on the axolotl, which displays a poor alloimmune response, reveal that components of the MHC (class II molecules which are not very polymorphic), have in fact evolved in this urodele, but there are no class I glycoproteins. Furthermore, the axolotl displays MHC-encoded erythrocyte antigens similar to the polymorphic class IV molecules found on the nucleated erythrocytes of chickens and *Xenopus*; these are not found in mammals.

To date, experiments on both jawed and agnathan fish have failed to provide biochemical evidence for even MHC class II molecules, which may be the first MHC markers to appear in phylogeny. Lack of class II molecules in agnathans is particularly interesting in view of the recent findings of a distinct MLR afforded by hagfish leucocytes.

B CELLS AND IMMUNOGLOBULIN EVOLUTION

Immunoglobulins exist in all vertebrates (see Fig. 15.9). In fishes, the only immunoglobulin isotype is IgM, or at least 'IgM-like'; the immunoglobulins of agnathan fishes, however, lack the stabilized disulphide bonding patterns of higher vertebrate immunoglobulins. Anuran amphibians are the first group to possess a diversity of immunoglobulin isotypes; *Xenopus* possesses three heavy chain isotypes, namely IgM, IgY, and IgX; IgX is possibly the equivalent of mammalian IgA since this isotype is found exclusively in the gut. It is interesting that fish (and amphibians) lack IgE, since teleosts display anaphylactic type I hypersensitivity reactions, which in mammals are particularly associated with this immunoglobulin isotype.

Anuran B cells, and also the B cells of certain urodele amphibians and teleost fish, can readily be distinguished from T cells by the use of anti-immunoglobulin and anti-T cell monoclonal antibodies, respectively. The possibility that immunoglobulin might be the only type of antigen receptor used by 'primitive' fishes was suggested by studies showing that all leucocytes stained with polyclonal anti-immunoglobulin reagents; however, subsequent analysis with monoclonal anti-immunoglobulins has revealed both immunoglobulin-positive and immunoglobulin-negative leucocytes in hagfish.

In contrast to other vertebrates, birds possess a unique site for the differentiation of B cells – the cloacal bursa of Fabricius (Fig. 15.11). Transplantation experiments between quail and chicken embryos have shown that the bursa is colonized by a small number of stem cells over a few days during early embryonic

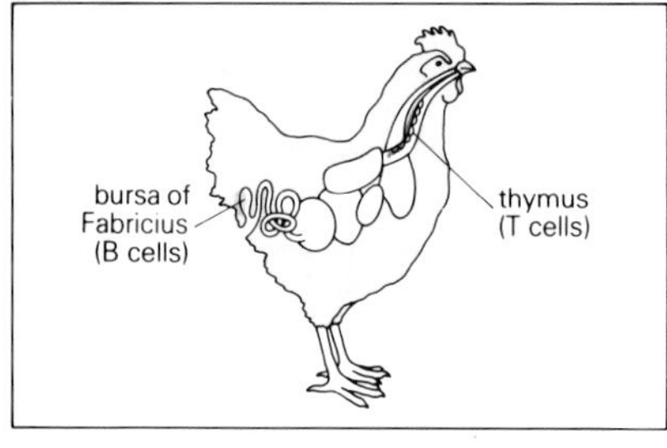

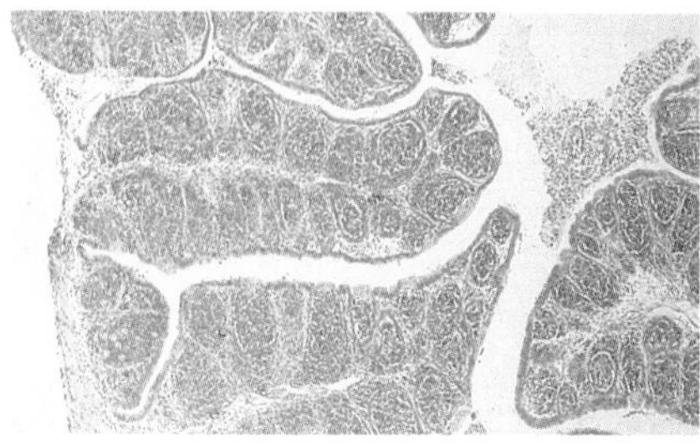

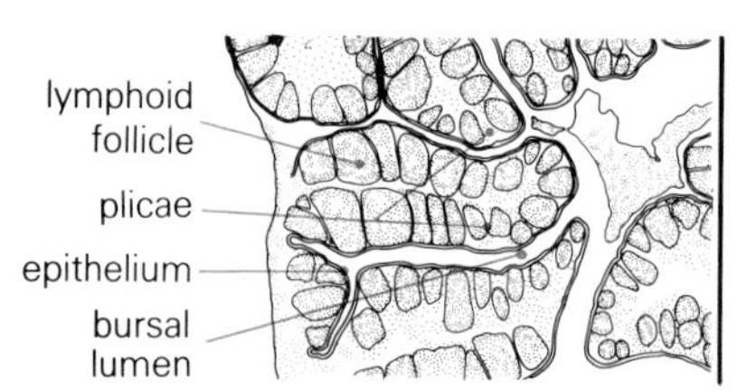

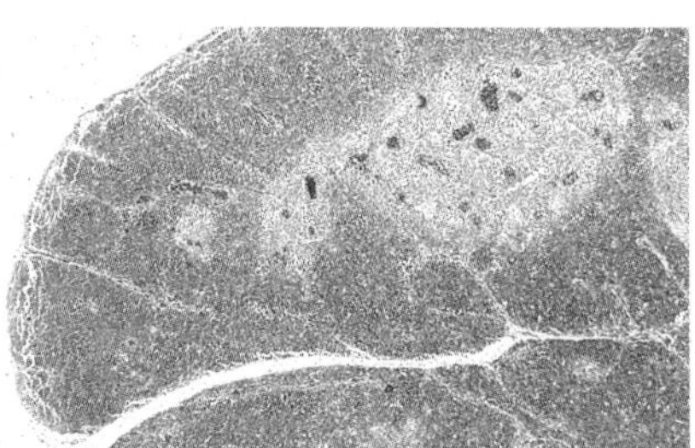

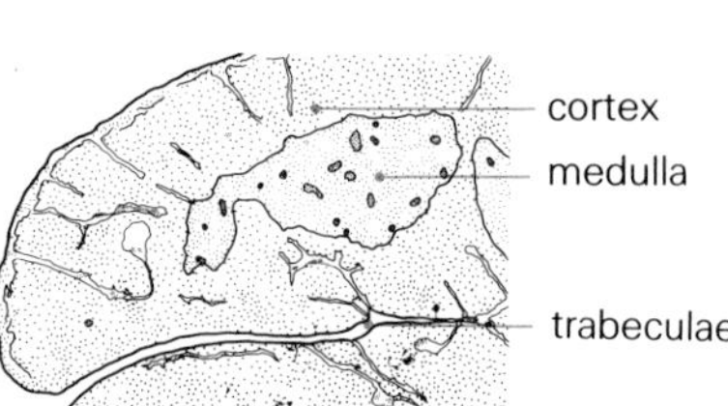

Fig. 15.11 The bursa of Fabricius. The two central organs in the avian immune system are the thymus (right) and the bursa of Fabricius (left). Lymphocytes developing in the thymus are termed T cells and those in the bursa, B cells. H&E stain, ×20.

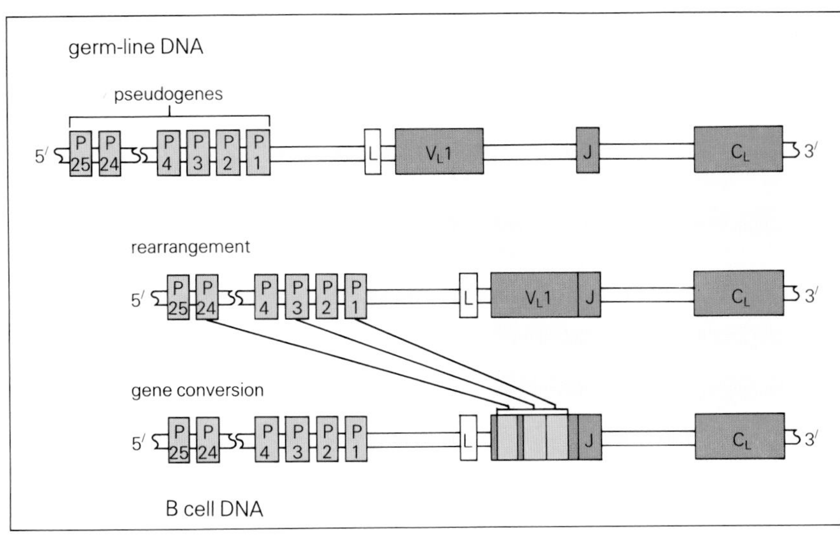

Fig. 15.12 Genetic basis of antibody diversity in chickens. The gene organization of the chicken germ-line immunoglobulin light chain locus (top) comprises less than 30 kbP of DNA. A single functional V gene (V_L) lies 2 kbP upstream from a single JC unit, with an adjacent cluster of 25 pseudogenes (P) in a 19 kbP region. Rearrangement of the V_L gene takes place briefly during early B cell development. Antibody diversity is achieved by subsequent gene conversion between the pseudogenes and the rearranged sequence. The rearrangement shown (P_1, P_3 and P_{24}) is illustrative; the converted segments do not necessarily lie in order in the V gene segment.

development. The stem cells then proliferate and differentiate to form the B lymphocytes of the bursal follicles. It has recently been revealed that the generation of antibody diversity in birds is approached differently to that occurring in mammals. Thus, in chickens the single functional V_L gene is initially rearranged and joined to a single JC unit (Fig. 15.12). This takes place for only a limited period at the beginning of colonization of the bursa; in mammalian B cell precursors, immunoglobulin gene rearrangements occur throughout life. Subsequently, in the chicken, stretches of nucleotide sequences from 'pseudogenes' lying adjacent to the single V gene, replace 10–120 base pair (bP) segments within the rearranged immunoglobulin gene sequences; such a high frequency gene conversion mechanism operates throughout the time B cells proliferate in the bursa.

Immunoglobulin gene structure in *Xenopus* resembles the situation in mammals, although the expressed diversity is much lower. It appears that the overall organization of the immunoglobulin heavy chain gene cluster was similar in a common ancestor of amphibians and

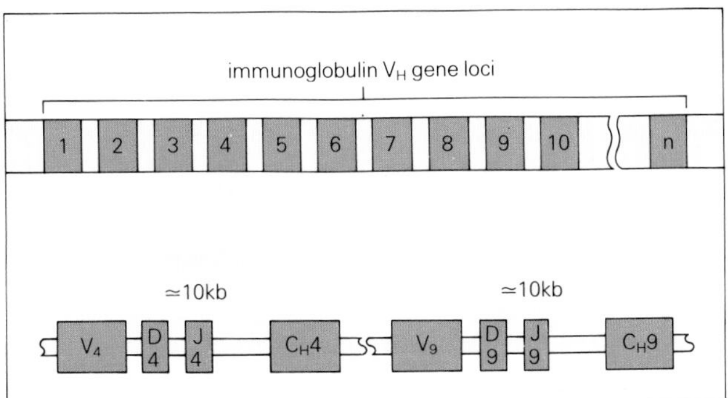

Fig. 15.13 Elasmobranch immunoglobulin V_H loci. In the shark there are a series of heavy chain gene loci, each with a single V, D, J and C gene segment. The fourth and ninth loci are shown expanded. V_H, D_H and J_H segments are closely linked and occur within approximately 1.3 kilobases (kb), and with the C_H segment, occupy only approximately 10–15 kb. Recombination appears to occur selectively only within each group of genes, which may account for the lack of inter-individual variation associated with the immune response of this species. (Based on data of Dr G.W. Litman.)

mammals some 300 million years ago. The situation with respect to shark immunoglobulin is somewhat different. Here multiple, closely-linked V-D-J-C subunits have been described, and limited combinatorial diversity may explain the restricted nature of the shark antibody response (Fig. 15.13). The elasmobranch immunoglobulin gene arrangement may be representative of a common ancestral gene family. Alternatively this arrangement may be a unique adaptation of this lower vertebrate.

NON-SPECIFIC MEDIATORS OF IMMUNITY

With the exception of the agnathan fishes, which may possess only the terminal complement components, both classical (antibody-mediated) and alternative pathways of complement activities have been demonstrated in all vertebrate classes. Genes coding for the full complement system and the 2H–2L chain immunoglobulin molecule therefore appear to have arisen at about the same time in evolution. Considerable homology appears to exist between the gene for C3 in *Xenopus* and the gene for mammalian C3. Basic properties of mammalian complement (thermolability, requirements for Ca^{2+}, and Mg^{2+}) are shared by fish and amphibian complement, although the temperature range over which poikilotherm complement remains active is greater (activity remains at 4°C) and heat-inactivation can be achieved at a lower temperature, for example *Xenopus* serum is completely decomplemented by treatment at 45°C for 40 minutes. Guinea-pig complement may be used successfully in haemolytic antibody assays *in vitro* in adult amphibians, whereas in most fish species and in larval *Xenopus*, isologous complement, or complement from a closely-related species, must be used.

Leukotrienes and other lipid mediators (collectively known as eicosanoids) are known to be involved in a variety of inflammatory processes in mammals. There is now evidence that leukotrienes are produced in fishes (and amphibians) and play an important role in inflammatory (non-specific) responses in fish; for example leukotriene B_4 enhances the migration of fish leucocytes.

There is currently considerable interest in the evolution of cytokines within the vertebrates. For example, T cell growth factors functionally like IL-2 and able to promote the proliferation of T cell lymphoblasts *in vitro*

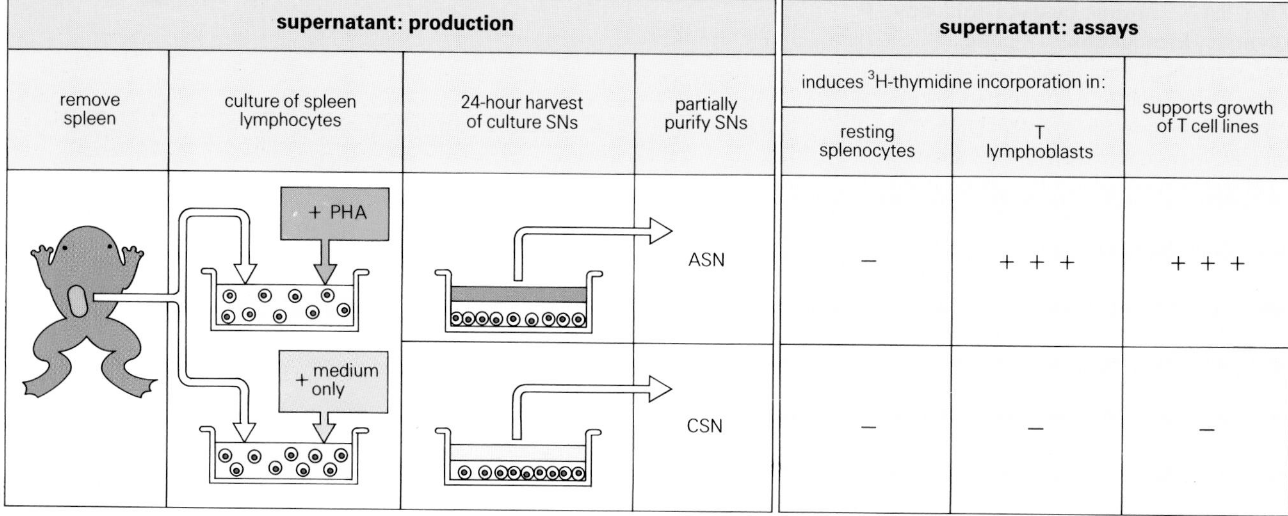

Fig. 15.14 T cell growth factors in *Xenopus*. Active culture supernatants (ASNs) are harvested from PHA-stimulated *Xenopus* splenocytes and compared with supernatants from control cultures (CSNs). The supernatants are partially purified by ammonium sulphate precipitation, dialysis and 'removal' of any PHA by incubation with chicken erythrocytes. The ASNs induce proliferation of T lymphoblasts (but not resting splenocytes) and support the growth of alloreactive T cell lines; CSNs have no comparable effects. A similar but reduced level of activity can be generated in MLC supernatants and may be attributable to molecules functionally homologous to mammalian T cell growth factor (i.e. IL-2).

have now been identified and partially characterized from supernatants of stimulated lymphocytes taken from teleost fish and anuran amphibians (Fig. 15.14). The extent to which IL-2 and its lymphocyte surface receptor molecules are evolutionarily conserved requires molecular and genetic analysis. IL-1-like activity has recently been detected in teleost and anuran macrophages. Furthermore, migration inhibition factors and leucocyte chemotactic factors also appear to play a role in the amphibian's immune system.

STRUCTURE AND FUNCTION OF LYMPHOID TISSUES IN LOWER VERTEBRATES

The lymphomyeloid system produces and stores lymphocytes, granulocytes and other blood cells. In mammals, lymphoid tissues, for example thymus, lymph nodes, spleen and mucosal-associated lymphoid tissue (MALT), containing predominantly lymphocytes, are anatomically separate from myeloid tissues, for example bone marrow, where granulocytes and a variety of other blood cell types predominate. However, in lower vertebrates, for example fishes and amphibians, lymphoid and myeloid compartments are more intermingled.

An incomplete complement of lymphomyeloid tissue is seen in fishes (see Fig. 15.10), in the sense that they lack bone marrow, lymph nodes and nodular MALT. However, a well-developed thymus, spleen and lymphomyeloid tissue associated with the kidney and liver is found at this level of evolution (Fig. 15.15), though it should be noted that hagfish do not possess a true thymus and have only a rudimentary spleen.

One particularly noticeable feature concerning piscine lymphomyeloid tissue is the abundance of melano-macrophage centres within the liver of 'primitive' forms and also within the spleen and kidney of teleosts (Fig. 15.16). These centres are heavily laden with

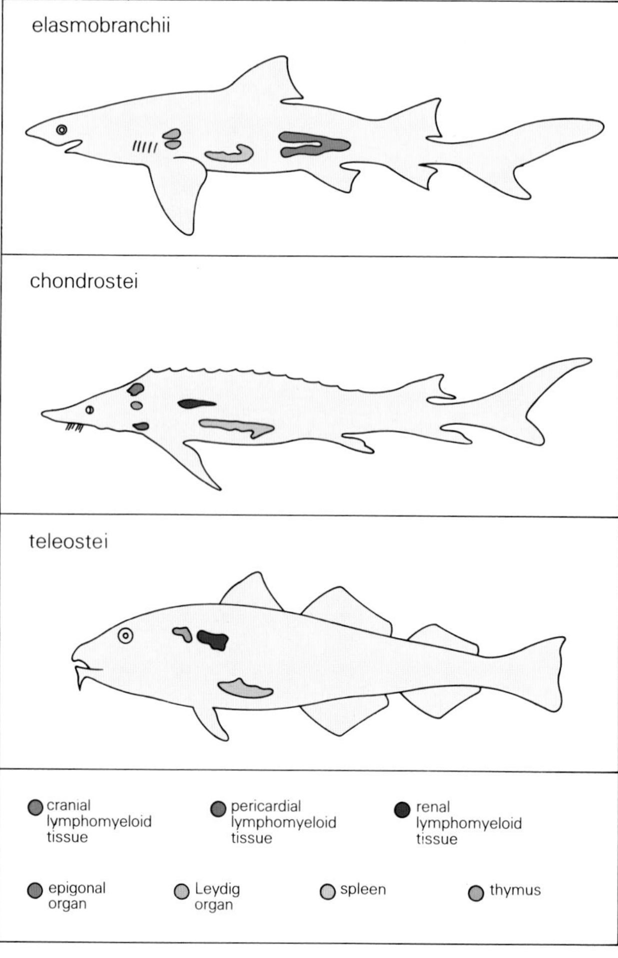

Fig. 15.15 Lymphomyeloid tissues in different types of fishes. Note that the intestine of elasmobranchs and chondrosteans is rich in lymphomyeloid tissue (in the spiral valve); neither this tissue nor the thymus are shown here. (Courtesy of Dr R. Fänge.)

pigments, for example haemosiderin, ceroid, melanin and, in particular, lipofuscin. It has been suggested that these melano-macrophage centres represent a primitive analogue of the germinal centres first found in avian lymphoid tissues. Pigment accumulation in the fish 'macrophage aggregates' may, in part, relate to the high levels of unsaturated fats present in fish for membrane fluidity purposes at low temperatures; these fats are particularly prone to peroxidation and formation of lipofuscin.

Two anuran amphibian species – the leopard frog, *Rana pipiens* and the clawed frog, *Xenopus laevis* – are used to illustrate the general histological features of lymphoid tissues found in poikilothermic vertebrates.

THYMUS

The adult frog thymus lies just under the skin, posterior to the middle ear. Detachment of the thymus from the pharyngeal epithelium occurs early in development as in most other vertebrates except teleost fish. The thymus is differentiated into an outer cortex and a central (paler-staining) medulla. The rapidly-proliferating cortical lymphocytes are particularly sensitive to irradiation (Fig. 15.17).

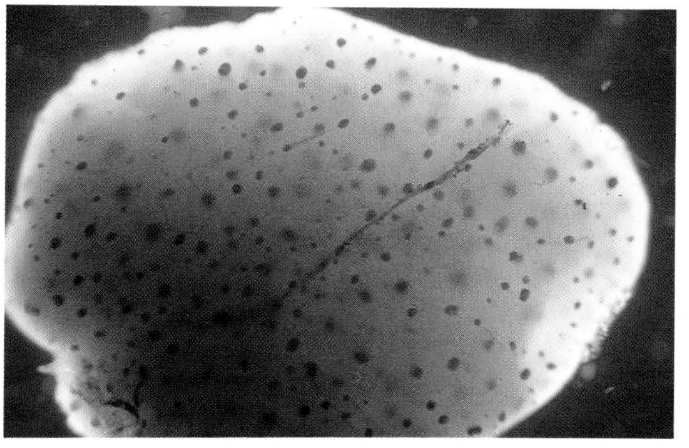

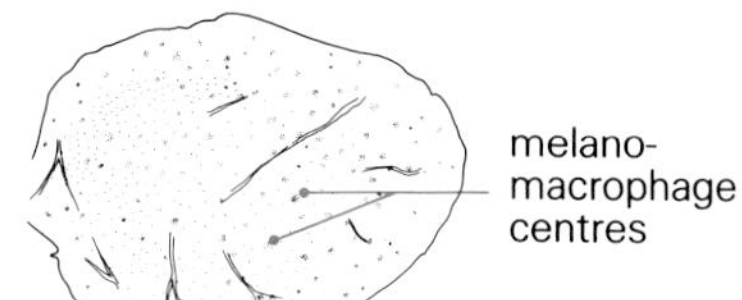

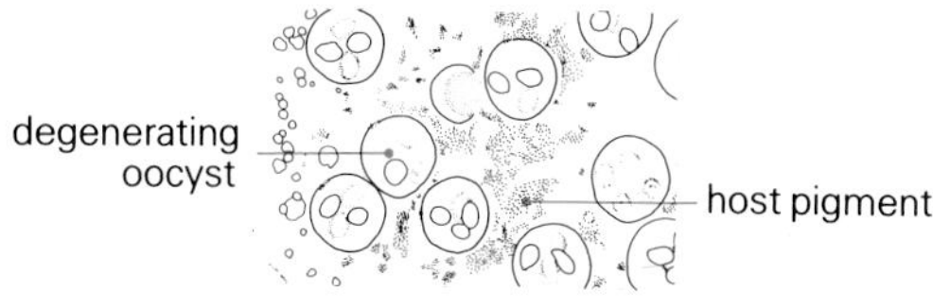

Fig. 15.16 Melano-macrophage centres in fish liver. Gross and microscopic views of liver of a cyptinodontid fish *(Rivulus marmoratus)* experimentally infected with the coccidian parasite *Calyptospora funduli*, to show formation of melano-macrophage centres (MMCs). At 60 days post-infection, distinct MMCs (arrowed) have appeared (left; ×60). The squash preparation (right, ×600) shows that these MMCs are comprised of degenerating oocysts of the parasite and associated host pigment. Histological studies have revealed that mononuclear phagocytes play a dominant role in MMC formation. (Courtesy of Dr W. K. Vogelbein.)

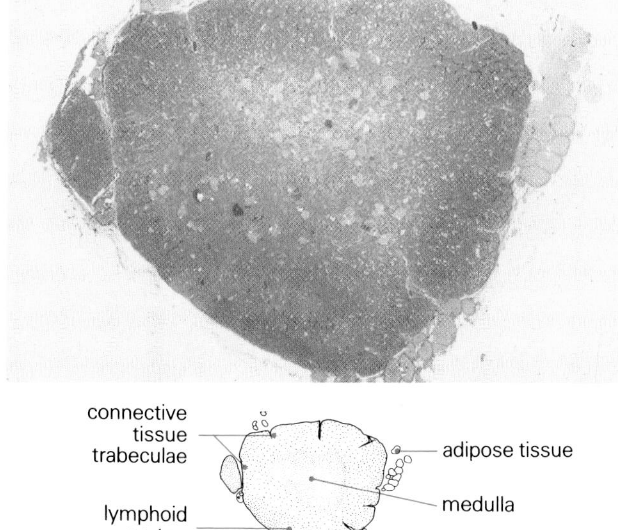

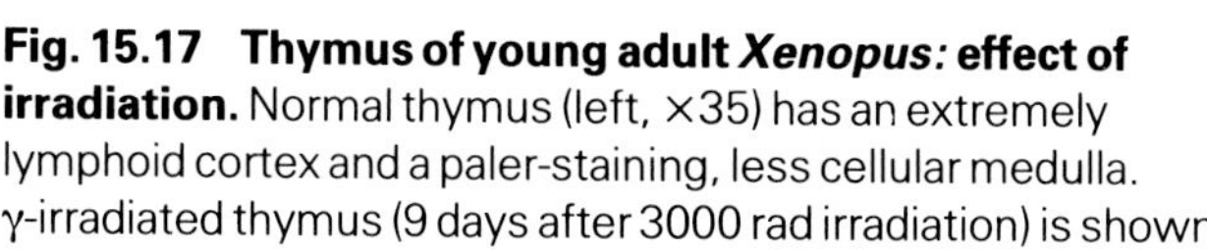

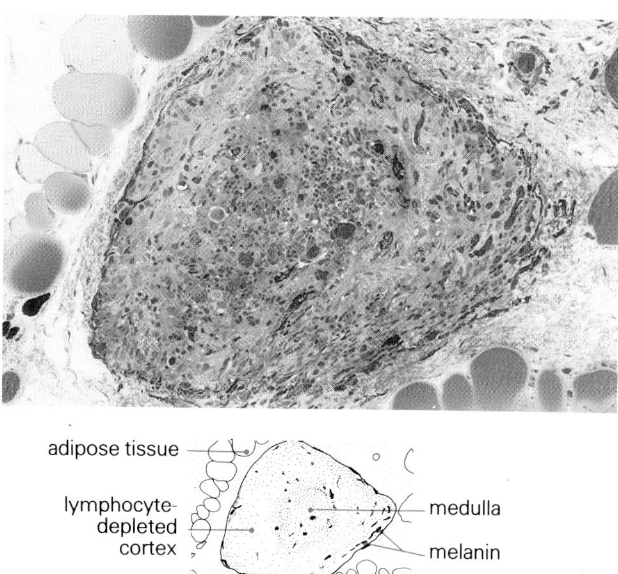

Fig. 15.17 Thymus of young adult *Xenopus:* effect of irradiation. Normal thymus (left, ×35) has an extremely lymphoid cortex and a paler-staining, less cellular medulla. γ-irradiated thymus (9 days after 3000 rad irradiation) is shown on the right (×90). Note the dramatic loss of lymphocytes from the cortex following irradiation, but retention of some lymphocytes in the medulla. The irradiated thymus is reduced in size. Toluidine-blue stain.

There is considerable evidence that the poikilotherm thymus, like its counterpart in endotherms, produces lymphocytes with T cell functions. The ultrastructure of thymic lymphocytes and neighbouring epithelial cells is shown in Fig. 15.18. Several other stromal cell types are found within the thymic medulla, though some, for example the granular cells, appear only after metamorphosis. Myoid cells have been found in the thymus of mammals, reptiles and several amphibian species (see Fig. 15.18); it has been suggested that they are involved in promoting the circulation of tissue fluids within the thymus, or that they may provide a source of self-antigen. These cells, along with thymic epithelial cells and interdigitating cells must be included as candidates for educating T-lineage cells to become tolerant of self-antigens and to be preferentially restricted to interacting with cells expressing self-MHC.

B cells have also been found in the thymus of diverse vertebrate species and can be readily demonstrated in the amphibian thymus (Fig. 15.19), though this organ does not seem to be involved in the production of these lymphocytes.

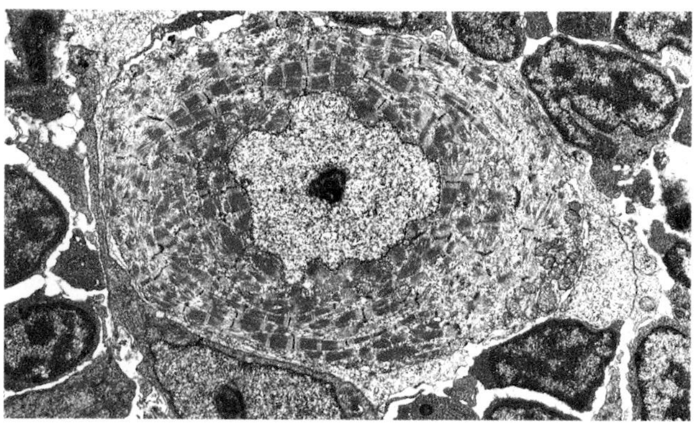

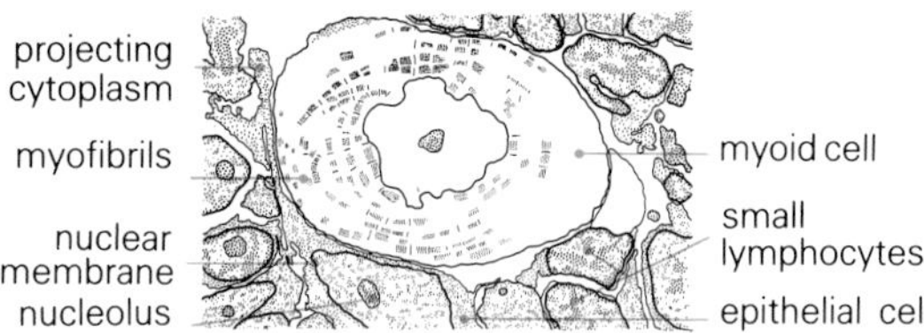

Fig. 15.18 Electronmicrograph of thymus medulla of larval *Xenopus laevis.* The ultrastructure of a myoid cell, small lymphocytes and an epithelial cell is shown.
Myoid cell – the nucleus is surrounded by concentric rings of striated myofibrils resembling those of skeletal muscle.
Small lymphocytes – the nuclear chromatin is organized into a series of electron-dense zones with a thin margin of dense chromatin adjacent to the nuclear membrane; the cytoplasm is scant with few organelles.
Epithelial cells – the nuclei possess evenly-dispersed chromatin and prominent nucleoli; the cytoplasm is extensive and projections extend in an interdigitating fashion between lymphocytes and other cell types to form a supportive network. ×700. (Courtesy of Dr J.J. Rimmer.)

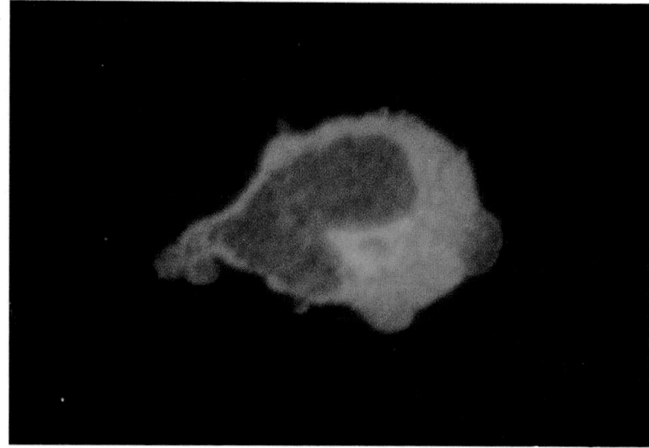

Fig. 15.19 B-lineage cells in the *Xenopus* thymus. Cytocentrifuge preparation of a 7-day thymocyte culture treated with the B cell mitogen, LPS. Stained using rabbit IgG anti-*Xenopus* μ chain antiserum, followed by goat IgG anti-rabbit IgG, conjugated with FITC. One B-lineage lymphoid cell with cytoplasmic IgM is seen in this field. Most thymic lymphocytes are immunoglobulin-negative, but express a T cell differentiation antigen, XT-1. ×1600.

SPLEEN

The spleen is a major peripheral lymphoid organ in all jawed vertebrates. Together with 'lymph nodes' and kidney it traps antigen, houses proliferating lymphocytes after their stimulation by antigen and provides for the appropriate release of these cells and their products. Thymus-dependent and thymus-independent lymphoid zones within the spleen have been demonstrated in *Xenopus* (Fig. 15.20). The white pulp follicles are rich in B cells, as shown by selective staining of this region with anti-immunoglobulin monoclonal antibodies. Splenic T cells found in the perifollicular regions are surface immunoglobulin-negative, but a population will bind with a monoclonal

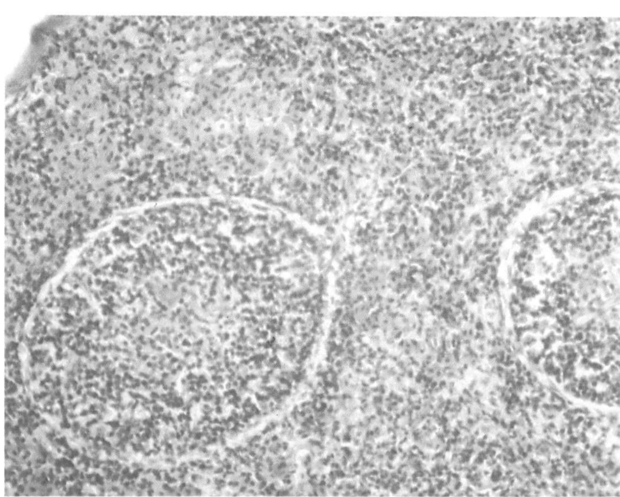

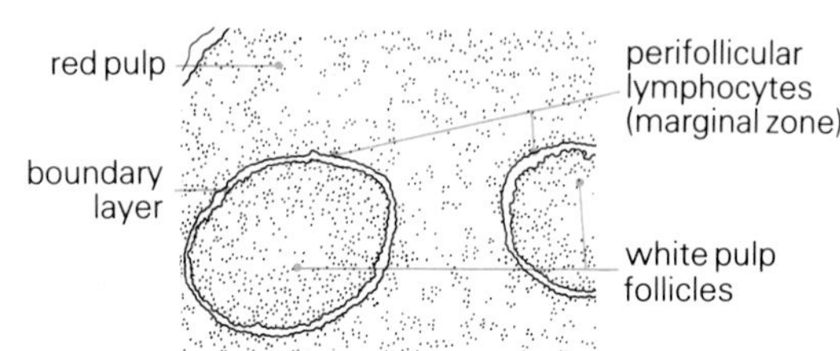

Fig. 15.20 Spleen section of adult *Xenopus.* Thymus-dependent (perifollicular red-pulp) and thymus-independent (white-pulp) areas are shown. In *Xenopus* (unlike many other poikilotherms) the white pulp is clearly separated from the surrounding red pulp by lightly-staining boundary layer cells. Concentrations of lymphocytes are also seen in the red pulp. H & E stain, ×80.

antibody (XT-1) raised against thymocytes. Blood vessels enter the spleen through the white pulp from where capillaries leave and empty into the surrounding red pulp. Experimental studies with India ink and fluoresceinated antigens reveal that it is the red pulp that initially receives material circulating in the blood. Circulating antigens are later trapped within the white pulp follicles, that is, they are closely associated with potential antibody-producing cells, as illustrated in Fig. 15.21. Antigen is held on the surfaces of large dendritic cells whose cytoplasmic processes extend pseudopods through the boundary layer and into the T-lymphocyte rich marginal zone. The overall arrangement of the white pulp is not very dissimilar from that of the mammalian spleen.

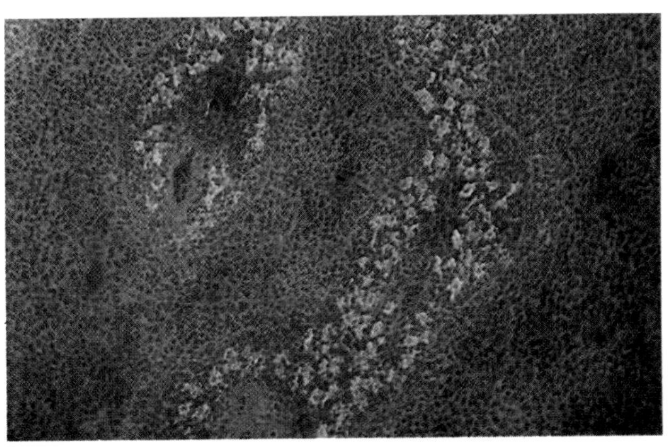

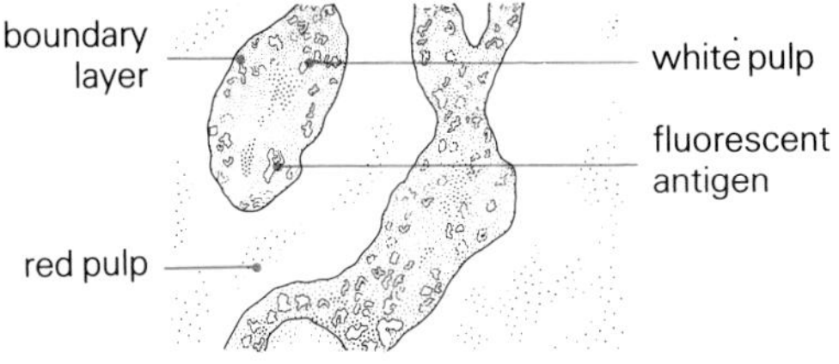

Fig. 15.21 Immunofluorescence of adult *Xenopus* spleen showing antigen trapping. The toad has been injected with a soluble protein antigen (human IgG) 3 weeks before the preparation of frozen sections and their incubation with fluorescein-labelled antiserum (anti-human IgG). The bright apple green fluorescence indicates the presence of antigen within white pulp follicles. The antigen is trapped in a dendritic pattern which is similar to that seen in mammals and birds where it appears to be held on reticular cell surfaces. ×35.

LYMPHOMYELOID NODES

Lymphomyeloid nodes bearing superficial functional resemblance to the lymph nodes of endothermic vertebrates are seen for the first time in vertebrate evolution in certain anuran amphibians. Histologically, these anuran nodes are very different from their mammalian counterparts (Fig. 15.22). The lymphomyeloid nodes are mainly blood-filtering organs (contrast with mammalian lymph nodes) although trapping of material from surrounding lymph is also believed to occur. These lymph glands do not have the clearly defined architecture of mammalian lymph nodes but appear as aggregations of lymphoid and myeloid cells lying within lymph channels. In the adult frog, 'lymph nodes' of similar structure to the larval lymph gland shown in Fig. 15.22 are found in the neck and axillary regions.

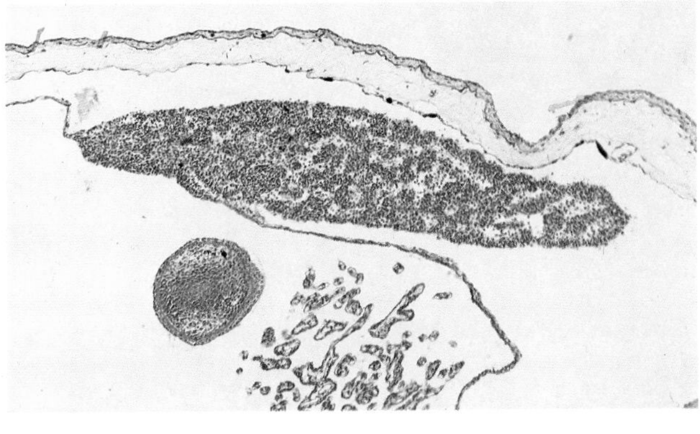

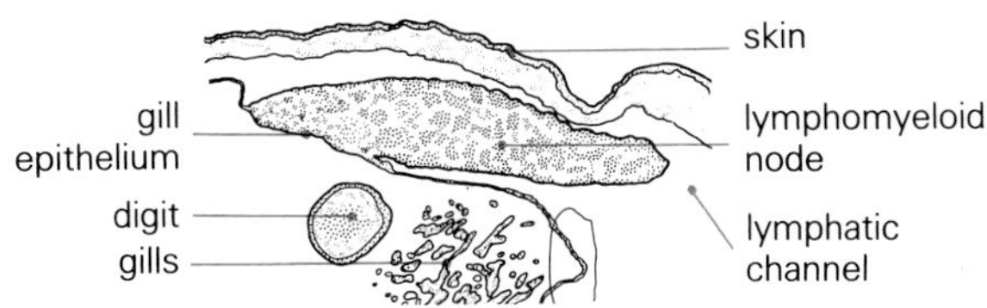

Fig. 15.22 Lymph gland section of larval *Rana*. The elongated (paired) lymphomyeloid node is seen attached ventrally to the epithelium of the gill chamber and projects into a large lymphatic channel. Gills, and a digit of the anterior limb lying in the gill chamber are seen medially, the larval skin lies laterally. The lymph gland consists of an extensive lymphoid parenchyma with phagocytes and intervening sinusoids (pale staining). H&E stain, ×25.

GUT-ASSOCIATED LYMPHOID TISSUE

Nodular gut-associated lymphoid tissue (GALT), analogous to the mammalian MALT system, occurs throughout the small intestine in frogs (Fig. 15.23). Smaller accumulations of lymphocytes loosely associated with the gut are found throughout vertebrate evolution. GALT is conveniently situated to form a first-line of defence against antigens in the gut. In *Xenopus*, IgX is exclusively associated with GALT, and may represent the equivalent of mammalian IgA.

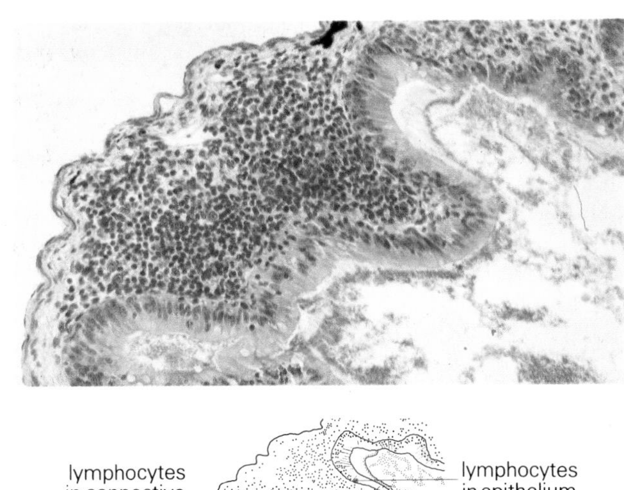

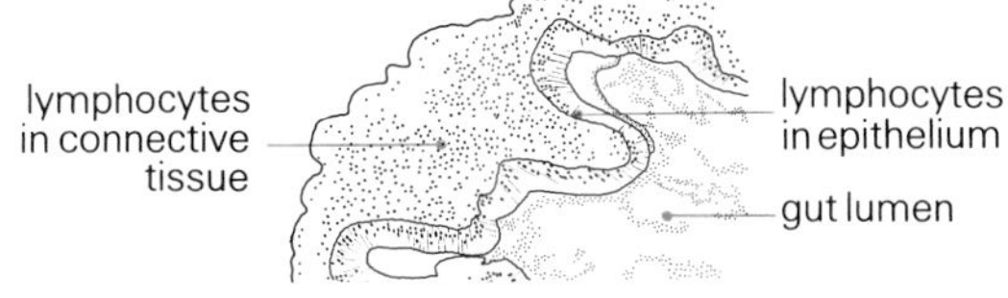

Fig. 15.23 Section of nodular gut-associated lymphoid tissue in adult *Rana*. Lymphocytes are seen in the subepithelial connective tissue and in the overlying gut epithelium. H&E stain, ×50.

KIDNEY AND LIVER

The kidney is a major lymphomyeloid organ in fishes and amphibians, but this function wanes in the kidneys of amniotes. In anurans, the kidney, and liver appear as the initial site of B lymphocyte development in ontogeny. The kidney is, in fact, intimately involved with the early differentiation of erythroid, lymphoid and myeloid cells in diverse vertebrates. A section of *Rana* kidney (Fig. 15.24) shows the haemopoietic tissue.

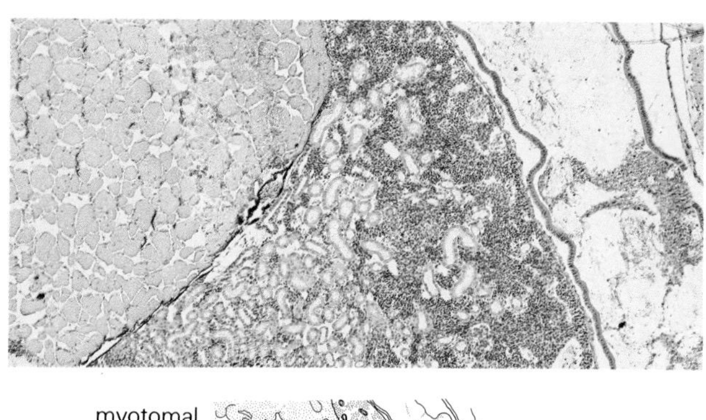

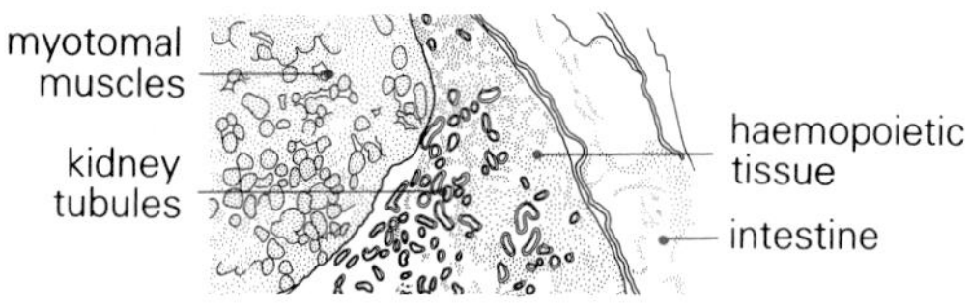

Fig. 15.24 Kidney section in larval *Rana* showing haemopoietic tissue. Haemopoietic tissue is extensive in the intertubular regions where lymphocytes, granulocytes and other developing blood cell types are found. Myotomal muscles and a loop of the intestine lie adjacent to the mesonephros. H&E stain, ×25.

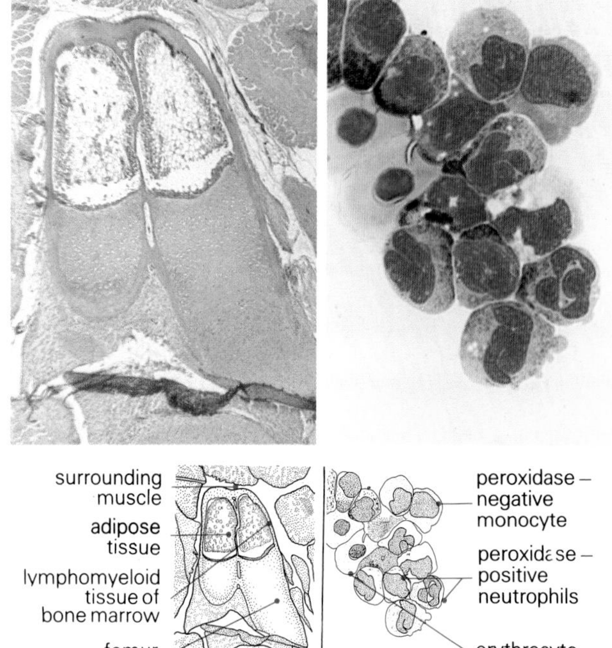

Fig. 15.25 Bone marrow. Lymphomyeloid tissue in bone marrow from *Rana* is shown on the left. H&E stain, ×20. On the right, a bone marrow cytocentrifuge preparation from *Xenopus*, shows several peroxidase-positive neutrophilic granulocytes. ×700. (Cytocentrifuge preparation, courtesy of Dr I. Hadji-Azimi.)

BONE MARROW

Although bone marrow makes its first appearance in amphibians, its immunological role at this level of evolution still awaits clarification. In adult *Rana pipiens* bone marrow lymphomyeloid tissue is readily evident (Fig. 15.25). In *Xenopus*, on the other hand, bone marrow appears more rudimentary; the femoral marrow is mainly a site for the differentiation of neutrophilic granulocytes (see Fig. 15.25).

ASPECTS OF AMPHIBIAN IMMUNOLOGY

Anuran amphibians, particularly *Xenopus*, are proving to be excellent models for studying ontogenetic aspects of immunity, some of which are reviewed below. Histocompatible strains of several amphibian species have been developed and, in recent years, several isogeneic and inbred families of *Xenopus* have become available for immunological research.

The technique for producing isogeneic *Xenopus* involves the use of hybrid *Xenopus*. For example, *X. laevis/X. gilli* hybrids lay some diploid eggs (due to endoreduplication of chromosomes during oöcyte development), and gynogenetic development of these eggs results in a clone; members of the clone are identical when tested by a variety of criteria, including mixed leucocyte reactivity and allograft responsiveness (Fig. 15.26). Different *Xenopus* clones, that are either MHC compatible (but express minor histocompatibility differences) or possess one or two MHC haplotype differences, are proving invaluable for a whole range of immunological investigations.

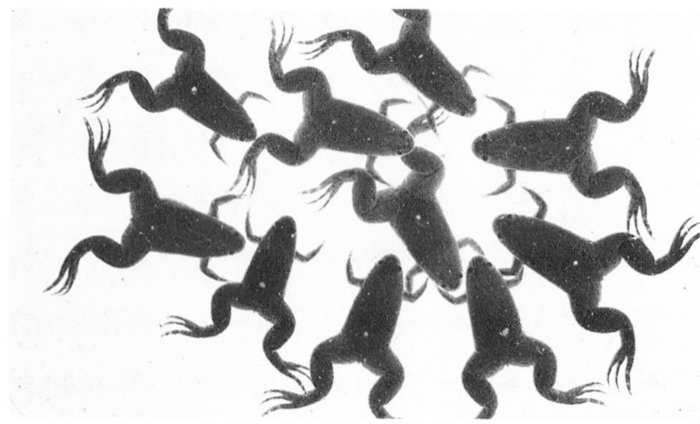

Fig. 15.26 A 'family' of genetically identical *Xenopus*. The white spot on the back of each animal is a piece of belly skin grafted from another animal of the same family or clone. (Courtesy of Dr L. Du Pasquier.)

THYMUS DEVELOPMENT AND THYMECTOMY EXPERIMENTS

Xenopus is ideally suited for investigating the role of the thymus in the development of the immune system since the free-living larva can be thymectomized very early in life (when the thymus is still at a rudimentary stage of its histogenesis) without the animal runting (Figs 15.27 and 15.28). Different pairs of gill pouches yield the thymic buds in different vertebrates. In anurans the paired thymus develops from the dorsal epithelium of the second pharyngeal pouches. Experimental studies

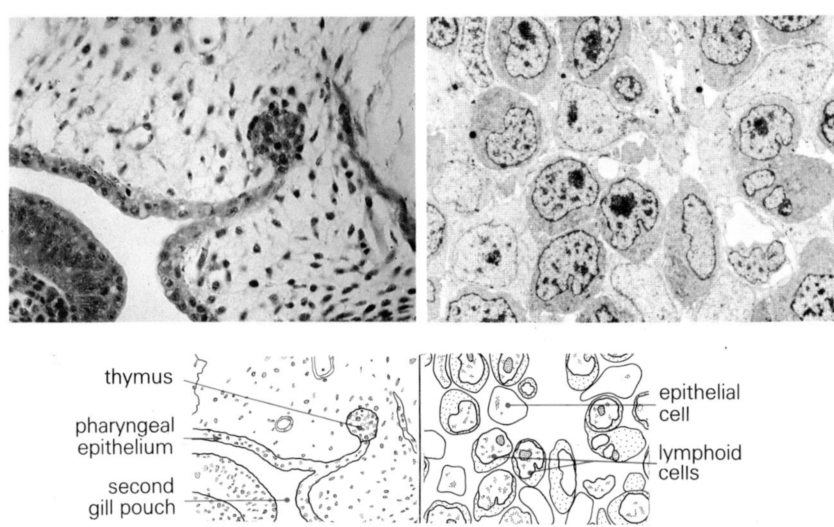

Fig. 15.27 *Xenopus* thymus at 3 days and 7 days. At 3 days (left, H&E stain, ×100), the developing thymus is still attached to the pharyngeal epithelium and comprised mostly of epithelial cells. At 7 days (right, electronmicrograph, ×500), the thymus consists of less than 1000 cells of two major types. The epithelial cells have a prominent nucleolus, dispersed chromatin and pale-staining cytoplasm. Lymphoid cells possess large amounts of densely-staining cytoplasm with an abundance of free ribosomes and mitochondria. At 7 days, the XT-1 marker begins to appear on the thymic lymphoid cell population.

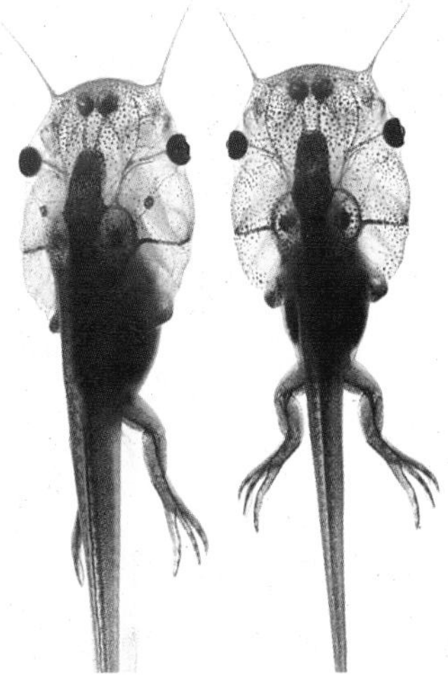

Fig. 15.28 *Xenopus* thymus at 38 days. The pigmented paired thymus lies posterior to the eyes (left); its absence is readily apparent in the sibling thymectomized at 7 days (right).

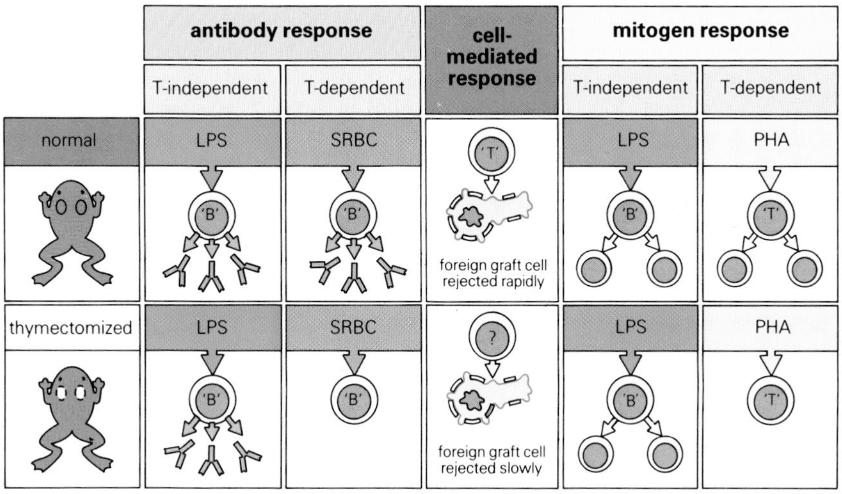

	antibody response: T-independent	antibody response: T-dependent	cell-mediated response	mitogen response: T-independent	mitogen response: T-dependent
normal	LPS → 'B'	SRBC → 'B'	'T' — foreign graft cell rejected rapidly	LPS → 'B'	PHA → 'T'
thymectomized	LPS → 'B'	SRBC → 'B'	? — foreign graft cell rejected slowly	LPS → 'B'	PHA → 'T'

Fig. 15.29 Effect of thymectomy in *Xenopus*. *Xenopus*, thymectomized at 4–8 days of age are assessed for antibody response, cell-mediated response and mitogen response *in vitro*. The treatments may be classified as T-dependent or T-independent according to whether or not thymectomy impairs the response to the treatment. Antibody response – *Escherichia coli* lipopolysaccharide (LPS, a T-independent antigen and B cell mitogen) induces antibody production in a T-independent manner, whereas the normal antibody response to sheep red blood cells (SRBC) is impaired in the absence of T (T-helper?) cells. Cell-mediated response – the normal cell-mediated response is T-dependent, but chronic allograft rejection can sometimes still occur in thymectomized *Xenopus*. Mitogen response – lymphocytes may be stimulated by mitogens in two ways. LPS stimulates B cells polyclonally. A second group of mitogens, including phytohaemagglutinin (PHA), stimulates T lymphocytes polyclonally.

reveal that lymphoid precursor cells enter the thymic epithelial rudiments at 3–4 days of age. A T cell differentiation antigen (the XT-1 marker recognized by an anti-thymocyte mouse monoclonal antibody) begins to appear on the thymic lymphoid cell population at 7 days, before the emergence of XT-1^+ T cells in the periphery.

Thymectomy of *Xenopus* from 4–8 days of age has clearly demonstrated the existence of T-dependent and T-independent components of immunity (Fig. 15.29). Following 5-day thymectomy, XT-1^+ T cells are no longer found in larval and adult lymphoid organs, whereas surface immunoglobulin-positive B lymphocytes are plentiful. The possibility of an extrathymic maturation pathway for alloreactive cells in *Xenopus* is suggested, however, since frogs thymectomized when only 4–7 days old can sometimes be shown to chronically reject MHC-disparate skin grafts and, following rejection, their splenocytes become positive when tested in mixed lymphocyte culture (MLC), but not when stimulated with the T cell mitogen, PHA.

Thymectomy of anuran larvae at sequential times during development suggests that different T cell functions require the presence of the thymus for varying periods in

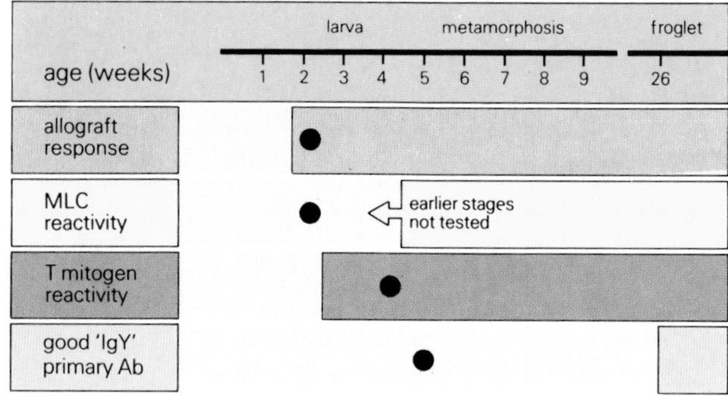

Fig. 15.30 Ontogeny of immune reactivity and the effect of sequential thymectomy in *Xenopus*. The allograft response, mixed lymphocyte reactivity and T-mitogen reactivity appear early and are followed by T-helper cells, particularly helper cells involved in the 'IgY' primary antibody response. ● Indicates the age until which thymectomy still impairs function.

order to become established in the periphery (Fig. 15.30). Studies on the ontogeny of T cell-dependent immunity in intact animals reveal that alloimmune reactivity *in vivo* and *in vitro*, together with the ability of splenocytes to respond to T cell mitogens, develops early in larval life, whereas good IgY primary antibody responses are only seen in the froglet.

THYMIC EDUCATION

Implantation of thymus, which may be either lymphoid or lymphocyte-depleted following γ-irradiation, to early-thymectomized *Xenopus* reveals that foreign thymus grafts can promote the differentiation of host precursor cells along a T cell pathway (Fig. 15.31). The *in vivo* construction of thymuses with MHC-disparate epithelial and lymphoid compartments can readily be achieved by a different surgical approach which is feasible with the amphibian embryo. This approach involves joining the anterior part of one 24-hour embryo (containing the thymic epithelial buds) to the posterior portion of an MHC-incompatible embryo (from which the haemopoietic stem cells, including lymphocytes, arise) (Fig. 15.32).

These two experimental systems are currently being used to explore the rôle which is played by thymic stromal cells in establishing tolerance of T-lineage lymphocytes to self- and alloantigens, and in restricting the MHC antigen specificities with which helper and effector T cell populations preferentially interact, during recognition and/or destruction of non-MHC antigens. Overall, the experiments have indicated involvement of the foreign thymus epithelium in inducing tolerance (? by clonal deletion) towards skin grafts of thymus MHC type, although interestingly this tolerance does not appear to prevent a mixed lymphocyte reaction towards donor cells.

In mammals, it is currently thought that thymic interdigitating (dendritic) cells, which are a stromal population of extrinsic origin, rather than intrinsically-derived epithelial cells, play a critical role in inducing thymocyte tolerance to MHC antigens. A role of the amphibian thymus in establishing the MHC type with which T cells preferentially interact has been suggested from *in vivo* experiments with chimeric *Xenopus*.

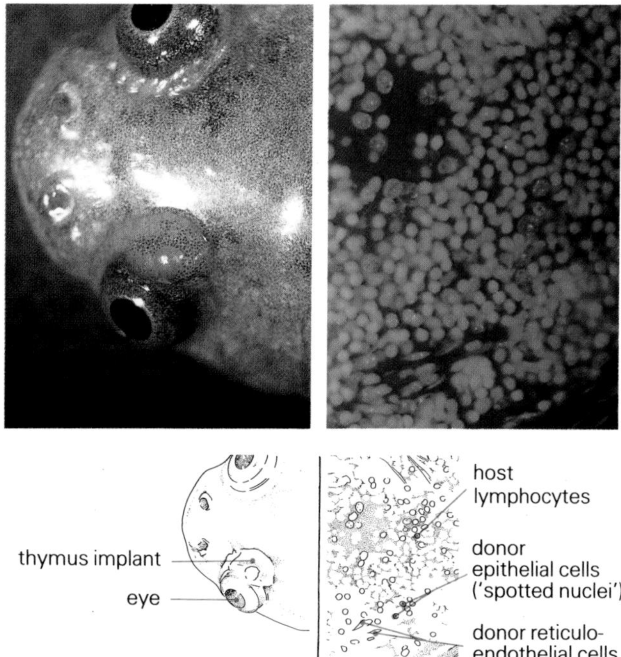

Fig. 15.31 Thymus implantation to thymectomized *Xenopus*. The frog *(X. laevis)* shown on the left was thymectomized at 7 days of age and a thymus from a larval *X. borealis* donor was then implanted subcutaneously in late larval life. This thymus implant grows well and lies adjacent to the left eye following metamorphosis. A section of this thymus, stained with quinacrine and examined by fluorescence microscopy, is shown on the right. ×300. Donor-derived cells can be distinguished from host cells, because *X. borealis* nuclei display brightly fluorescent spots, whereas *X. laevis* cells stain homogeneously dull green. The thymus is now repopulated with host lymphocytes, whereas many stromal cell types remain 'spotted' (i.e. they are of donor origin). The role played by these stromal cells in T cell education is being explored.

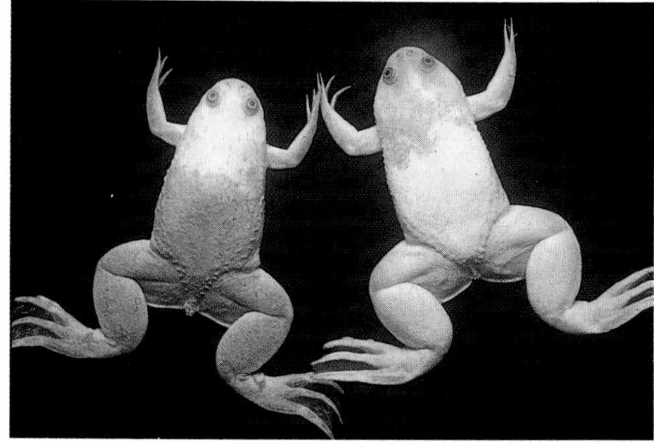

Fig. 15.32 Chimeric frogs *(Xenopus)*. Chimeric *Xenopus* were made by exchanging the anterior and posterior regions of two embryos at 24 hours after fertilization. At this stage, the thymic anlage (e.g. thymic epithelium) is in the anterior region, whereas all the lymphocyte precursors are in the posterior region. One embryo was from an albino variant with white skin and red eyes, the other embryo was from a normal *Xenopus*. These chimeras are proving useful for studying thymic education. (Courtesy of Dr Martin Flajnik and Dr Louis DuPasquier.)

ONTOGENY OF ALLOIMMUNITY, ALLOTOLERANCE AND ANTIBODY DIVERSITY

Onset of alloimmunity (to MHC antigens) in the anuran larva correlates with the lymphoid maturation of the thymus and, presumably, the appearance of the necessary T cell populations in the periphery (Fig. 15.33). Later in development a more vigorous alloimmune response is seen, concomitant with a rapid phase of lymphoid organ differentiation. Immunocompetent larvae (but not adults) can, nevertheless, be rendered tolerant of allogeneic skin; allotolerance induction is particularly easy at metamorphosis (Fig. 15.34). The size of grafts applied and the degree of histoincompatibility appear to be critical in this respect – for example, minor histoincompatibility-disparate skin grafts are always tolerated by larval and peri-metamorphic *Xenopus*. These alloimmune 'deficiencies' of anuran larvae may well relate to the recent finding that MHC class I molecules (against which mammalian cytotoxic T cells are particularly effective) are not expressed prior to metamorphosis.

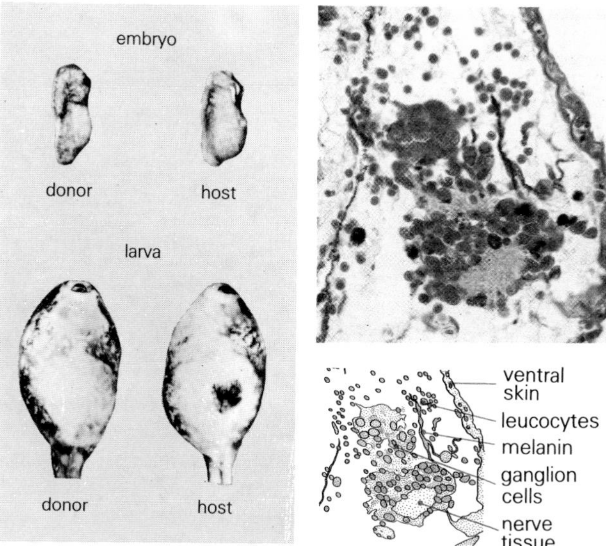

Fig. 15.33 Transplantation of embryonic tissue in *Rana* – ontogeny of alloimmunity. A piece of neural fold removed from one embryo (tail-bud stage, top left) is transplanted to the mid-ventral surface of another embryo (host). Intimately associated with the neural folds are the neural crest elements which are precursors of diverse cell types, including pigment cells. The pigment cells that differentiate provide an externally visible means of following the progress of the embryonic transplant. The host larva has developed a distinctive mass of graft-derived pigment cells. The section on the right shows differentiated graft elements (large ganglion cells with prominent nucleoli, other nervous tissue and melanin), 15 days after transplantation. Despite the earliness of the transplantation, lymphocytes and granulocytes are invading the graft. H&E stain, ×100. (Courtesy of Dr E.P. Volpe.)

Larval and adult *Xenopus* also possess distinct differences in their expression of antibody repertoires. It is postulated that two waves of rearrangements of the genes for variable immunoglobulin heavy chains (V_H) occur, one early and one only after metamorphosis. A few cells generate only the larval repertoire and do not express the total repertoire of possible V_H rearrangements. More cells contribute to the repertoire after metamorphosis and offer a wider spectrum of antibody specificities.

IMMUNOLOGY OF METAMORPHOSIS

Immunologists are intrigued to know how amphibians escape the risk of dying from an autoimmune disease at metamorphosis since there is a need for the immunocompetent animal to become tolerant of adult-specific determinants that are first expressed at this time. The involvement of suppressor cell populations in allotolerance generated at metamorphosis seems likely. On the other hand, high plasma corticosteroid levels are found during the metamorphic climax, and such hormonal alterations may directly impair cell-mediated immunity, possibly by inhibiting interleukin-2 production.

Amphibian metamorphosis is a fascinating period for probing the interplay between endocrine and immune systems in the regulation of cellular and humoral immunity; such investigations will undoubtedly have significance outside purely phylogenetic considerations.

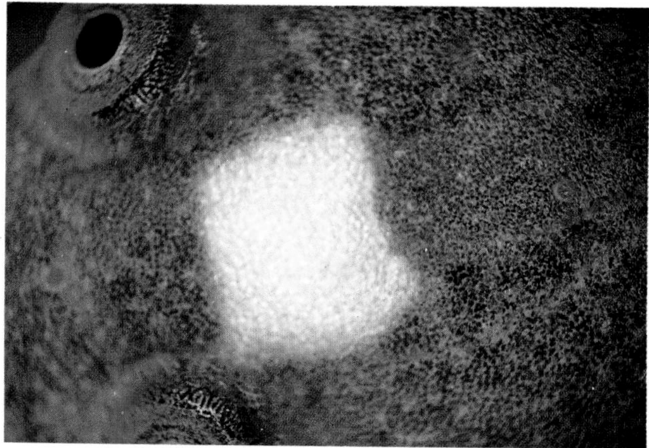

Fig. 15.34 Skin graft tolerance in *Xenopus*. Allogeneic skin, even from an MHC-disparate donor, may be tolerated by a larval or metamorphosing recipient. Subsequent skin grafts (here a piece of white belly skin) from the same donor are similarly retained by the adult frog whereas third-party skin is rejected within 3 weeks at 25°C.

MODELS FOR THE STUDY OF LYMPHOID CELL ORIGINS

Embryonic transplantation of ploidy-marked gill buds in *Rana pipiens* and *Xenopus laevis* some years ago revealed that thymic lymphocytes develop from precursor cells which colonize the thymus (Fig. 15.35). In *Xenopus*, lymphoid precursor cells destined for the thymus have now been shown to arise from both ventro-lateral plate mesoderm (ventral blood islands) and dorso-lateral plate mesoderm of the embryo. Transplantation experiments using varying numbers of cytogenetically distinct (triploid/diploid) ventral mesoderm cells have recently revealed that thymocyte and B lymphocyte lineage specific precursors differentiate in this embryonic layer by 20 hours of development. These experiments illustrate the usefulness of amphibian embryos for exploring the embryonic origins of T and B lymphocytes.

SUMMARY OF IMMUNOEVOLUTION

Salient features of immunological phylogeny in vertebrates and invertebrates are summarized in Fig. 15.36.

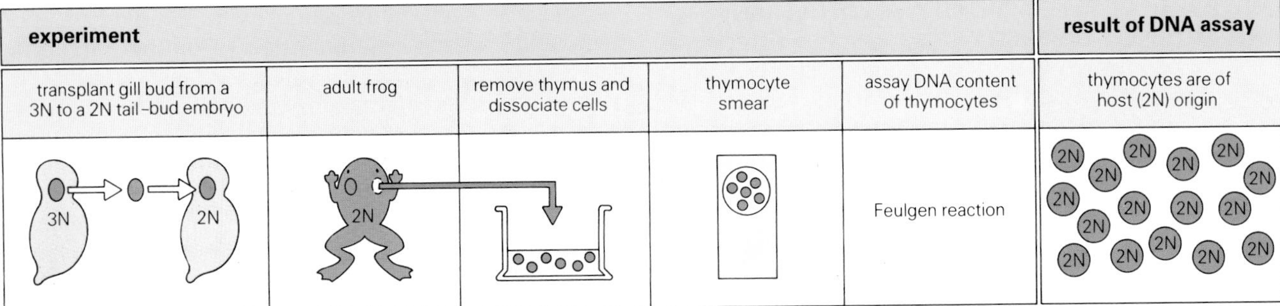

Fig. 15.35 Experimental demonstration of the extrinsic (stem cell) origin of thymic lymphocytes in amphibians. A gill bud (containing the thymus precursor tissue) of an artificially induced triploid (3N) tail-bud stage embryo was transplanted into a normal, diploid (2N) tail-bud stage embryo. When the embryo developed into a normal adult frog the transplanted thymus was removed, and the thymus cells were dissociated. A cell smear was prepared and the cell's DNA content was determined by the Feulgen reaction. The thymus cells were found to be diploid and lead to the conclusion that amphibian thymocytes are derived from cells external to the thymus, as occurs in birds and mammals.

invertebrates	vertebrates
phagocytosis/encapsulation important in eliminating non-self material	all display cell-mediated and humoral immunity
cell-mediated immunity evident early in evolution	all have IgM with 'higher' forms possessing different heavy chains
different classes and subclasses of immunocyte in coelomates	all possess T and B lymphocytes and lymphoid tissues; these tissues become more complex in 'higher' forms
inducible humoral immunity in some coelomates, but immunoglobulins absent from all phyla	functional lymphocyte heterogeneity demonstrated in fish/amphibians and birds/mammals
lectins involved in recognition of self/non-self in at least some phyla	molecular and genetic characterization of immunoglobulins, MHC glycoproteins, complement and cytokines of lower vertebrates is in progress

Fig. 15.36 Summary of the immune responses found in invertebrate and vertebrate phyla.

FURTHER READING

Brehélin, M. (ed.) (1986) *Immunity in Invertebrates*. Heidelberg: Springer-Verlag.

Cohen, N. (ed.) (1987) First international symposium on the immunology of ectothermic vertebrates. *Developmental and Comparative Immunology*, **11**, 435.

Cohen, N. & Sigel, M. M. (eds) (1982) *The Reticuloendothelial System. Ontogeny and Phylogeny*. New York: Plenum.

Cooper, E. L., Langlet, C. & Bierne, J. (eds) (1987) *Developmental and Comparative Immunology*. New York: A. R. Liss.

Cooper, E. L. & Wright, R. K. (eds) (1984) Aspects of developmental and comparative immunology. II. *Developmental and Comparative Immunology*, Suppl. 3.

Flajnik, M., Hsu, E., Kaufman, J. F. & DuPasquier, L. (1987) Changes in the immune system during metamorphosis of *Xenopus*. *Immunology Today*, **8**, 58–63.

Horton, j. D. (ed.) (1980) *Development and Differentiation of Vertebrate Lymphocytes*. Amsterdam: Elsevier.

Horton, J. D. (1988) *Xenopus* and developmental immunobiology: a review. *Developmental and Comparative Immunology*, **12**, 219.

Lackie, A. M. (ed.) (1986) Immune mechanisms in invertebrate vectors. *Zoological Society of London Symposia*, **56**. Oxford: Oxford University Press.

Langlet, C., Bierne, J. & Cooper, E. L. (eds) (1986) Third international congress of developmental and comparative immunology. *Developmental and Comparative Immunology*, **10**, 93.

Litman, G. W., Hinds, K & Kokubu, F. (1988) The structure and organisation of immunoglobulin genes in lower vertebrates. In *Immunoglobulin Genes*. London: Academic Press.

Manning, M. J. & Tatner, M. F. (eds) (1985) *Fish Immunology*, London: Academic Press.

Manning, M. J., Tatner, M. F. & Secombes, C. J. (eds) (1987) Immunology and disease control mechanisms of fish. *Journal of Fish Biology*, **31**, Suppl. A.

Manning M. J. & Turner, R. J. (1976) *Comparative Immunobiology*. Glasgow: Blackie.

Ratcliffe, N. A. & Rowley, A. F. (eds) (1981) *Invertebrate Blood Cells. Vols. 1 & 2. London: Academic Press.*

Rowley, A. F. & Ratcliffe, N. A. (eds) (1988) Vertebrate Blood Cells. Cambridge: Cambridge University Press.

Solomon, J. B. (ed.) (1981) *Aspects of Developmental and Comparative Immunology*. I. Oxford: Pergamon Press.

Solomon, J. B. (1986) Invertebrate receptors and recognition molecules involved in immunity and determination of self and non-self. In *Receptors in Cellular Recognition and Developmental Processes*. London: Academic Press.

CYTOTOXIC T CELLS AND MHC RESTRICTION

There is evidence for Tc cells in some virus infections. Vaccination of man with killed whole influenza A results in an increased ability to mount an *in vitro* HLA-restricted Tc cell response against cells infected with the same or different strains (a virus subunit vaccine had little effect). The lack of strain specificity agrees with several reports that, in mice, Tc cells generated by one variant can protect against serologically distinct variants (Fig. 16.10). This may prove important; influenza A virus avoids the antibody response by changing its surface haemagglutinin and neuraminidase glycoproteins every few years. Antibodies to these glycoproteins are type-specific and so do not block infection with antigenic variants. Note that HLA restriction implies that Tc cells are involved unlike the K cell activity described above.

Immunity in man appears to be virus strain-specific but this does not rule out a role for cross-reactive Tc cells in the recovery phase of influenza infection. Although rapid boosting of Tc cell memory during an established infection may be essential for rapid recovery, this boosted response is short-lived and may not be able to block reinfection with another strain.

Other evidence for T cell activity is provided by studies involving human volunteers, in which it is found that high Tc cell activity before challenge with live influenza correlates with low or absent subsequent shedding of virus.

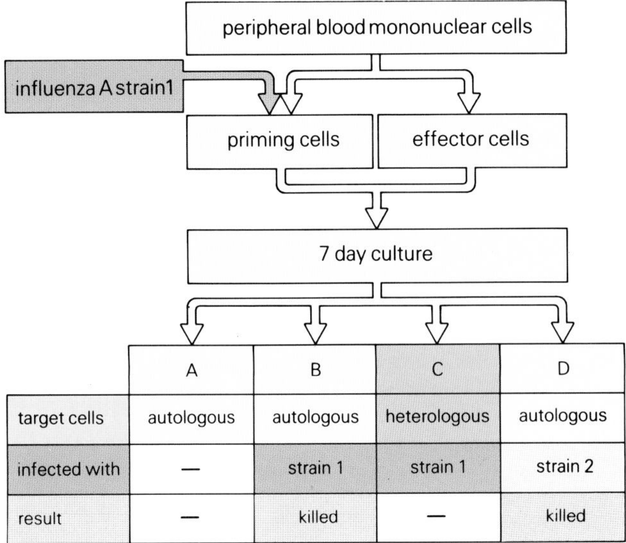

Fig. 16.10 Experiments to show cytotoxic T cell activity to influenza A in man. Peripheral blood lymphocytes from a person vaccinated 28 days previously with killed influenza A virus (strain 1) were harvested and divided into two aliquots. One aliquot (10% of the total) was incubated with influenza A strain 1 for 90 minutes ('priming cells'). These were then mixed with uninfected (effector) cells and cultured for 7 days. The aim is to keep the effector cell population free from infection. Cytotoxic T cells generated in the culture were tested on either autologous HLA identical cells (yellow) or heterologous HLA mismatched cells (red) infected with strain 1 or strain 2 virus. The effector cells kill HLA matched infected targets (B) but not uninfected (A) or mismatched infected targets (C). The cytotoxic T cells are not virus-strain specific (D). Tc cells are implicated in these experiments since the cytotoxicity is restricted to infected autologous cells only.

DELAYED HYPERSENSITIVITY TO VIRAL ANTIGENS

In the murine influenza model, delayed type hypersensitivity (DTH) responsiveness – a measure of T cell sensitization – can be transferred to syngeneic recipients by either $CD4^+$ I-region restricted T cells, or by $CD8^+$ K- or D-region restricted T cells. However only the $CD8^+$ cells are protective in transfer experiments. Indeed the $CD4^+$ cell type results in accelerated death following challenge with live virus (Fig. 16.11). This result illustrates the heterogeneity of the phenomena included under the 'umbrella' term 'delayed hypersensitivity'. Thus the presence of a positive delayed skin test response to viral antigen is unlikely to prove a reliable correlate of any one mechanism. Since T cells can have several actions, DTH responsiveness is not necessarily a corollary of protective immunity.

INTERFERON

The term interferon (IFN) is used for several unrelated classes of proteins, which have antiviral effects. Some of them are glycosylated. The classification of these molecules is constantly changing as new classes and subtypes are described.

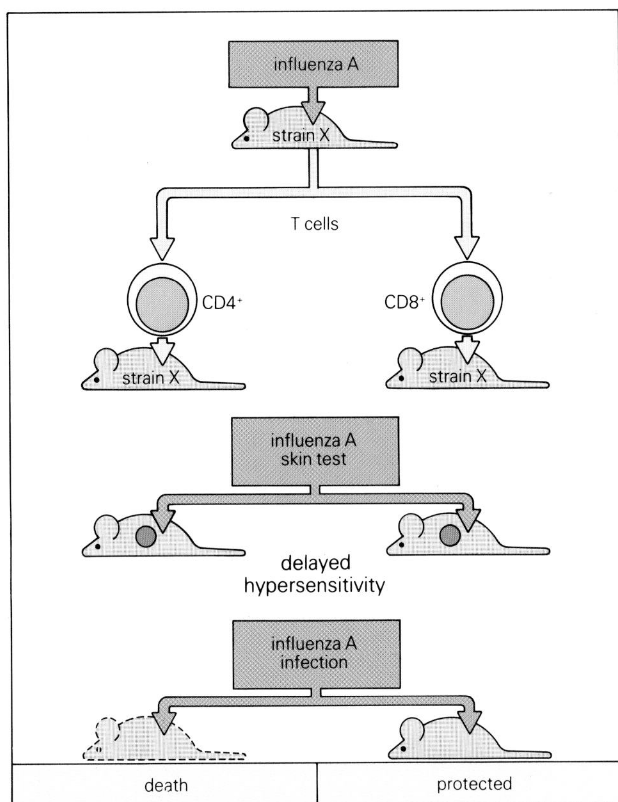

Fig. 16.11 Lack of correlation between delayed hypersensitivity and protection in murine influenza. A strain X mouse is infected with influenza A virus. T cells are later removed and divided into those carrying the CD4 surface phenotype and those carrying CD8. These are injected into other strain X mice. A delayed hypersensitivity response is then induced in both mice by skin testing with influenza A. Subsequent infection of the mice with virus results in the accelerated death of the mouse which received $CD4^+$ T cells. The mouse which received $CD8^+$ T cells is protected from the virus. Thus the capability to produce a delayed hypersensitivity response to a virus does not necessarily imply protective immunity.

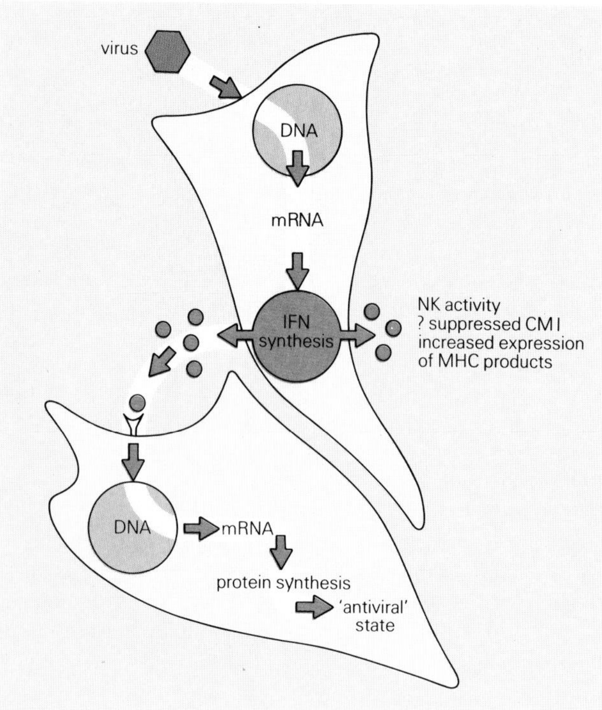

Fig. 16.12 The action of interferon. Virus infecting a cell induces the production of interferon. This is released and binds to interferon receptors on other cells. Interferons are species specific and this is probably determined by the receptor specificity. The interferon induces production of antiviral proteins which are activated if virus enters the second cell. Interferon also has other actions, which may be effected by common molecular pathways.

IFNα exists as at least 15 subtypes, the genes for which show 85% homology. IFNβ, which together with IFNα formed the original Type 1 IFN, is now known to represent two quite unrelated molecules. IFNβ1 shows 30% homology with the IFNα family, while IFNβ2 shows no homology with either IFNβ1 or IFNα, and has been found to be identical to the B cell differentiation factor BSF-2. It is now also known as interleukin-6 (IL-6). IFNϒ is the original Type II or 'immune' IFN, and shows no homology with any of the other types. Like IFNβ2, IFNϒ is a lymphokine as well as an IFN. There are two main types of IFN receptors – one for IFNϒ; the other for IFNα and IFNβ1.

IFNs are released from many cell types in response to virus infection, double-stranded RNA, endotoxin, and mitogenic and antigenic stimuli. In general IFNϒ differs from the others as it is released as a lymphokine from activated T cells, though under some circumstances macrophages also appear to secrete it.

The antiviral effects of IFNs are exerted via several pathways (Fig. 16.12) which include the following.

1. Increased expression of Class I and Class II MHC glycoproteins facilitating recognition of viral antigens by the immune system.
2. Activation of cells with the ability to destroy virus-infected targets; these include NK cells and macrophages. IFNβ also stimulates B cells.
3. Direct inhibition of viral replication.

Several mechanisms contribute to the third pathway. Released IFN binds to receptors on neighbouring cells and induces synthesis of antiviral proteins. These include a protein kinase and a 2′,5′-adenyl synthetase, both of which are activated by double-stranded RNA which is produced during metabolism. The kinase inactivates an enzyme needed for ribosome assembly, and the synthetase catalyzes a cascade of enzymes resulting in cleavage of RNA. These and other mechanisms result in inhibition of protein synthesis, with some selectivity for the viral proteins. However this selectivity is not absolute, which may account for the ability of IFN to inhibit cell growth (including some anti-tumour activity), and for the decrease in cell-mediated responses seen early in virus infections.

There are also reports that IFNs can inhibit other viral processes such as penetration of cells, uncoating of the viral nucleic acid, and budding from infected cells.

The clearest evidence for the antiviral efficacy of IFNs *in vivo* comes from experiments which show that mice treated with antibody to murine IFNs can be killed by several hundred times less virus than that needed to kill control animals.

ANTIVIRAL EFFECTS OF TUMOUR NECROSIS FACTOR

Tumour necrosis factor (TNF) exerts several antiviral activities which are similar to those of IFNϒ, but apparently work through a separate pathway. Thus pretreatment of cultured cells with TNF for 24 hours before addition of vesicular stomatitis virus (VSV) profoundly inhibits virus yield, whereas IFNϒ has no effect. In contrast IFNϒ is more effective than TNF when encephalomyocarditis virus (EMCV) is used. However when added together TNF and IFNϒ show synergistic inhibition of both these RNA viruses and also of DNA viruses such as herpes simplex (HSV). It is possible that in some cases this antiviral effect of TNF is a secondary result of its ability to induce IFNβ2 (IL-6) production. However, it is active on cells which do not make this mediator, the antiviral activity of which is also controversial. If TNF is added to cells after virus infection, it can selectively kill them, even when the cell line is normally TNF-resistant. This effect is also synergistic with that of IFNϒ. The likely relevance of these pathways *in vivo* is highlighted by the fact that HSV will trigger TNF release from human peripheral blood mononuclear cells, and from the promonocytic line HL60.

IMMUNOPATHOLOGY

The immune response to viruses can cause damage to the host via the formation of immune complexes, or by direct damage to infected cells. Complexes can form in the fluid phase, or following capping and stripping of virus expressed on cell surfaces. Chronic immune complex glomerulonephritis can occur in mice infected neonatally with lymphocytic choriomeningitis virus (LCM) as shown by the experiment described in Fig. 16.13. Direct damage to infected cells by a T cell-dependent mechanism is responsible for most of the tissue damage in LCM infection of adult mice. A similar mechanism has been postulated for chronic active hepatitis in man. Thus the *in vitro* 'correlate' of cell-mediated immunity, leucocyte migration inhibition, is positive in a proportion of patients with chronic active hepatitis, but negative in asymptomatic carriers.

Viruses may also evoke autoimmunity, possibly by release of sequestered antigens, derepression of developmental antigens, inhibition of suppressors, or proliferative stimulation of autoreactive cells.

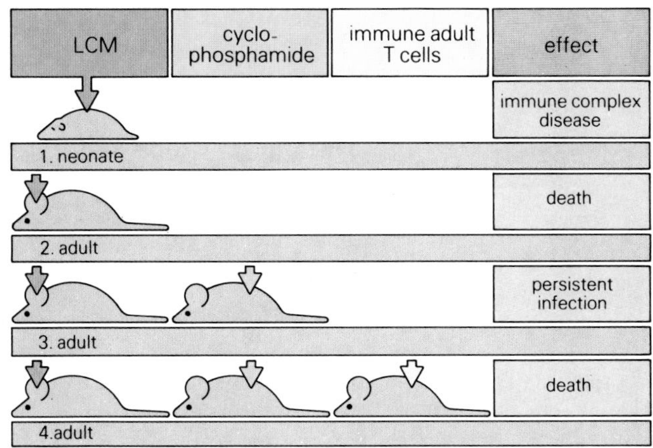

Fig. 16.13 Effects of lymphocytic choriomeningitis virus (LCM) in mice. The different effects of LCM are related to differences in immune status. Infection of neonatal mice (1) produces chronic virus shedding and immune complex disease, manifesting itself as glomerulonephritis and vasculitis. Intracerebral infection of adult mice (2) results in death. This is due to a T cell reaction, since suppression of immunity with cyclophosphamide (3) leads to persistent infection, but prevents death. The effect produced by cyclophosphamide can be reversed by T cells from an immune animal (4).

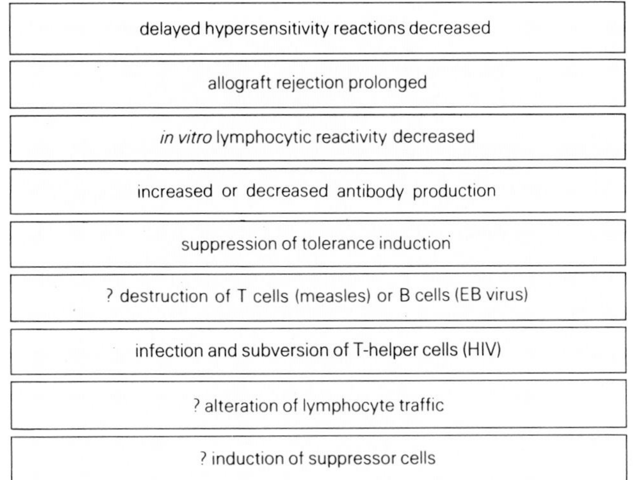

Fig. 16.14 Effects of virus on the host's immune response.

Virus infection may have profound effects on the immune system (Fig. 16.14). The classical observation is the loss of tuberculin test positivity during measles infections. The tuberculin test is a DTH reaction and in this instance is used as a marker of T cell reactivity. Some of these effects may be due to infection of the lymphoid and phagocytic cells; others may be secondary to release of mediators with powerful non-specific activities.

IMMUNITY TO BACTERIA

The body's defence against pathogenic bacteria consists of a variety of specific and non-specific mechanisms. Thus the skin and exposed epithelial surfaces have protective systems which limit the entry of potentially invasive organisms (Fig. 16.15). Very few organisms can breach intact skin, and the effectiveness of this barrier is made evident when considering the infections which frequently occur following skin loss, for example, following burns. Therefore, only a minute proportion of the huge numbers of potentially pathogenic organisms ever gain access to the body.

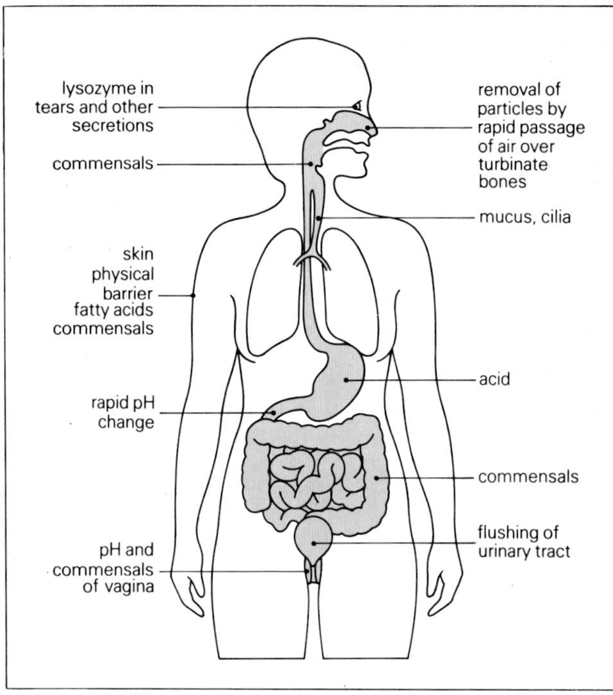

Fig. 16.15 Non-specific barriers to infection, before entry into the tissues. Invasion by potentially pathogenic organisms is limited by a variety of non-specific mechanisms.
1. The intact skin is impenetrable to most bacteria. Additionally fatty acids produced by the skin are toxic to many organisms. The pathogenicity of some strains correlates with their ability to survive on the skin.
2. Epithelial surfaces are cleansed, for example, by ciliary action in the trachea or by flushing of the urinary tract.
3. pH changes in the stomach and vagina lead to destruction of many bacteria – both are acidic. In the case of the vagina, the epithelium secretes glycogen which is metabolized by particular species of commensal bacteria producing lactic acid. This also limits pathogen invasion.
4. Commensals occupy particular ecological niches and so stop pathogens gaining access to it. Thus *Candida* or *Clostridium difficile* can occur when the normal flora is disturbed by antibiotics.

BACTERIAL CELL WALLS

When bacteria do gain access to the tissues the mechanisms involved in immunity to them depend on the particular species involved; the effectiveness of an immune response depends to a large degree on the host's ability to damage the components of the bacterial cell wall. From the pathological point of view there are four main types of bacterial cell wall (Fig. 16.16), namely:
1. Gram-positive
2. Gram-negative
3. mycobacterial
4. spirochaetal.
The outer surface of the bacterium may also contain fimbriae or flagellae, or be covered by a protective

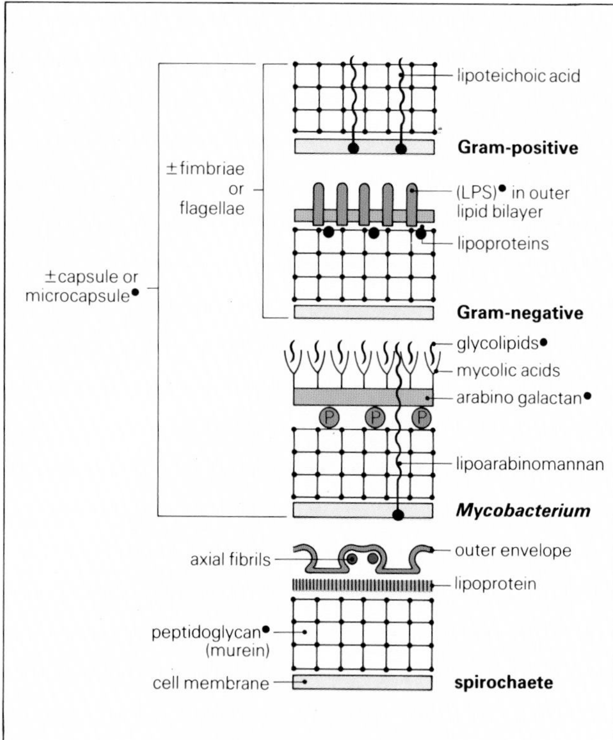

Fig. 16.16 Bacterial cell walls. The cell wall structure of the different groups of bacteria predetermines the type of mechanism which is able to destroy them. All types have an inner cell membrane and a peptidoglycan wall. Gram-negative bacteria also have an outer lipid bilayer in which lipopolysaccharide (LPS) is sometimes found. Lysosomal enzymes and lysozyme are active against the peptidoglycan layer, while cationic proteins and complement are effective against the outer lipid bilayer of the Gram-negative bacteria. The compound cell wall of the *Mycobacterium* is extremely resistant to breakdown, and it is likely that this can only be achieved with the assistance of the bacterial enzymes working from within. The different types may also have fimbriae or flagellae, which can provide targets for the antibody response. Some bacteria have an outer capsule which renders the organisms more resistant to phagocytosis. The components indicated with a black spot (•) all have adjuvant properties.

triggering of inflammatory mechanisms
activation of complement (alternative pathway)
activation of macrophages
T cell-dependent or T cell-independent polyclonal B cell activation
polyclonal T cell activation via interleukin-1 release from macrophages
disturbance of lymphocyte traffic
modification of antigen processing possibly by macrophages and dendritic cells

Fig. 16.17 Some known effects of the adjuvant-active components of the mycobacterial cell wall.

capsule. Proteins and polysaccharides in these structures can act as targets for the antibody response. However, although antibodies may interfere with bacterial functions and interact with other systems in the development of the immune response, ultimately destruction of the bacteria requires synergistic action with phagocytic cells.

ADJUVANTICITY AND OTHER NON-SPECIFIC MECHANISMS

The cell walls of most bacteria and the capsular substances of some of them have adjuvant properties. These probably represent phylogenetically ancient 'broad spectrum' recognition mechanisms for common microbial components, which evolved before antigen-specific T cells and immunoglobulins. The response to a pure bacterial antigen, without adjuvant is, for some bacteria, an artefact created in the laboratory. Although adjuvanticity is therefore an adaption of the host, some organisms may 'exploit' it to disturb immunoregulation. The non-specific effects of the mycobacterial cell wall are given as an example in Fig. 16.17. Many organisms, such as non-pathogenic cocci, are probably removed from the tissues without the need for a specific immune component (Fig. 16.18).

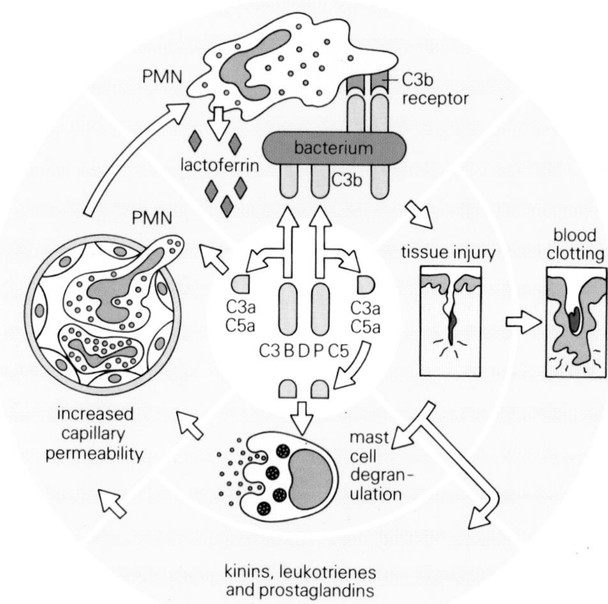

Fig. 16.18 Some non-specific mechanisms involved in immunity. Activation of the alternative complement pathway (Factors C3, B, D, P, C5) by components of the bacterial cell surface produce complement deposition (C3b) on the bacterial surface, which promotes opsonization by polymorphonuclear neutrophils (PMNs) via C3b receptors. PMNs are also stimulated to release free lactoferrin which takes up available iron and thus inhibits bacterial growth: it is noted that the ability of many bacteria to grow depends on the availability of free iron. C5a acts as a chemotactic agent for PMNs and macrophages as well as triggering mast cell degranulation. Tissue injury caused by the bacteria activates the clotting system and fibrin formation, which limits bacterial spread. Kinins, leukotrienes, prostaglandins and products of mast cell degranulation produce increased blood flow in the local capillary beds and increased capillary permeability.

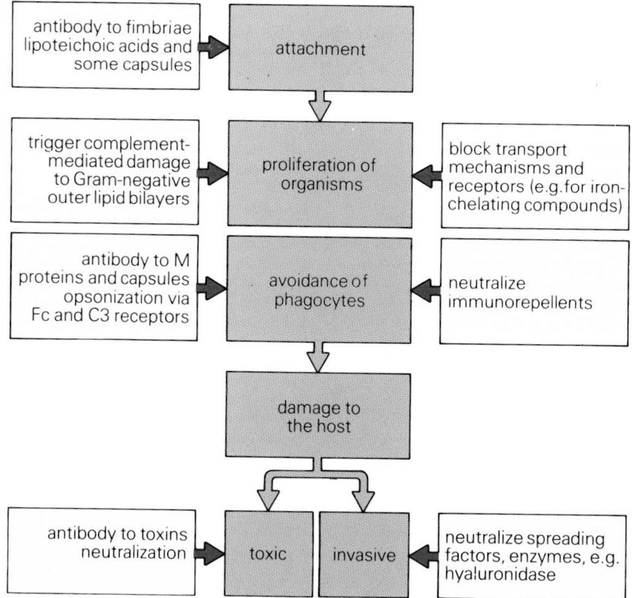

Fig. 16.19 The antibacterial roles of antibody. This diagram lists the stages of bacterial invasion (blue) and indicates the antibacterial effects of antibody that operate at different points (yellow). Antibody to fimbriae, lipoteichoic acid and some capsules block attachment of the bacterium to the host cell membrane. Proliferating bacteria trigger complement-mediated damage to Gram-negative outer lipid bilayers. Antibody directly blocks bacterial surface proteins which pick up useful molecules from the environment and transport them across the membrane. Antibody to M proteins and capsules opsonizes the bacteria via Fc and C3 receptors for phagocytosis. Immunorepellents – factors which interfere with normal phagocytosis and may be toxic for leucocytes – are neutralized. Following host cell damage the bacterial toxins may be neutralized by antibody, as may be bacterial spreading factors, which facilitate invasion, for example, by the destruction of connective tissue or fibrin.

THE ROLE OF ANTIBODY AND COMPLEMENT

Antibody, if present, may enhance opsonization. However, the triggering by 'procidins' of intracellular killing by phagocytes appears to be a separate event from opsonization. C3 at the concentrations likely to be achieved in inflammatory exudates is an effective procidin *in vitro*, as well as producing opsonization by alternative pathway activation.

Some organisms, such as Group A streptococci, and some gut pathogens have receptors for epithelial surfaces which can be blocked by antibody. The effects of streptococcal M-proteins, which inhibit phagocytosis, can be neutralized by antibody, giving type-specific immunity. The same is true for many capsules for example that of the meningococcus.

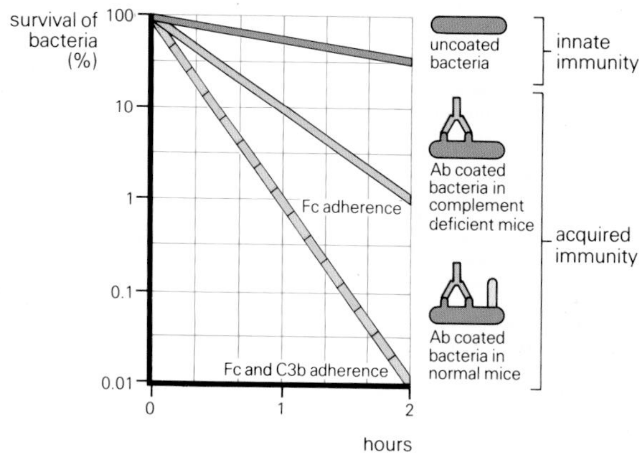

Fig. 16.20 Effect of opsonizing antibody and complement on rate of clearance of virulent bacteria from the blood. The uncoated bacteria are phagocytosed rather slowly but on coating with antibody, adherence to phagocytes is increased many-fold. The adherence is somewhat less effective in animals temporarily depleted of complement.

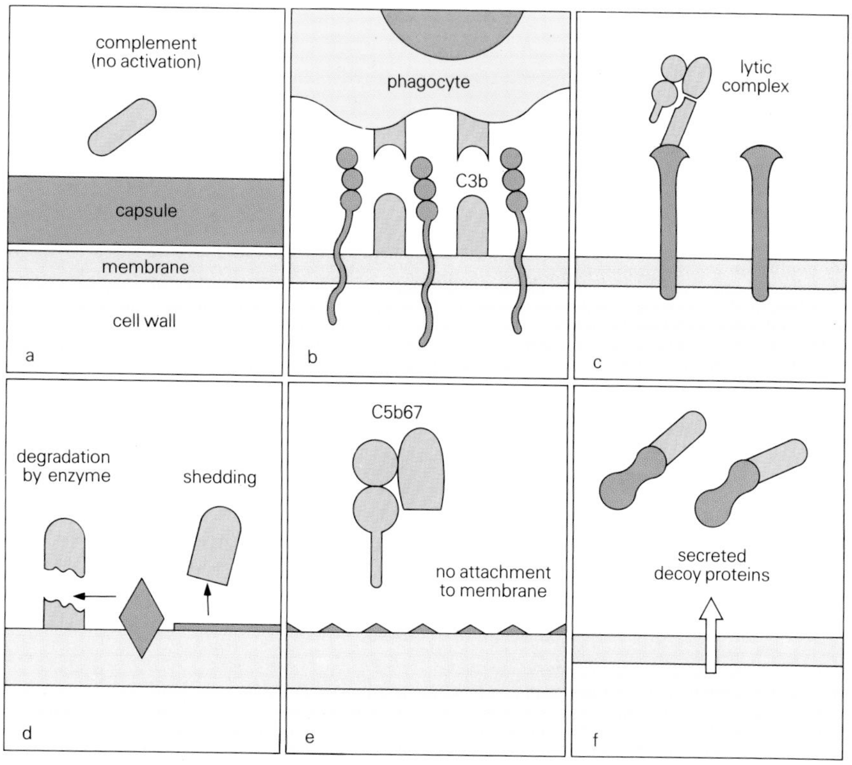

Fig. 16.21 Avoidance of complement-mediated damage. Bacteria avoid complement-mediated damage by a variety of strategies which include: a) having outer capsules or coats which prevent complement activation; b) having an outer surface configured so that complement receptors on phagocytes cannot obtain access to the fixed C3b; c) expressing structures which divert attachment of the lytic complex (MAC) from the cell membrane; d) enzymatically degrading fixed complement or causing its shedding; e) having an outer membrane which resists the insertion of the lytic complex; f) secreting decoy proteins which cause complement to be deposited on them and not on the bacterium itself.

Antitoxin antibodies can neutralize toxins such as those of tetanus and diphtheria, thus preventing the major damaging effect of these bacteria. The effects of antibody are summarized in Fig. 16.19.

Opsonization can be more rapid in the presence of antibody, even when the organism activates the alternative pathway, since phagocytes have Fc as well as C3b receptors (Fig. 16.20). In general Gram-negative organisms activate the alternative complement pathway and are killed, perhaps by lytic components acting on the outer lipid bilayer. Gram-positive organisms, while not being killed by complement, are opsonized by it. However both groups of organisms have developed mechanisms to avoid these effects (Fig. 16.21).

INTERACTION WITH PHAGOCYTES

Ultimately almost all bacteria are killed by phagocytes. This process involves several steps, summarized in Fig. 16.22.

1. Chemotaxis, in which bacterial components, such as f-Met.Leu.Phe and complement components such as C5a attract the phagocytes.
2. Attachment of the organism to the phagocyte surface, which is the first stage in the intracellular killing of an organism. This is an important interaction which may determine whether subsequent uptake occurs, and whether killing mechanisms are triggered during uptake. The binding can be mediated by:

a) lectins on the organism, such as the mannose-binding lectin on the fimbriae of *Escherichia coli*.

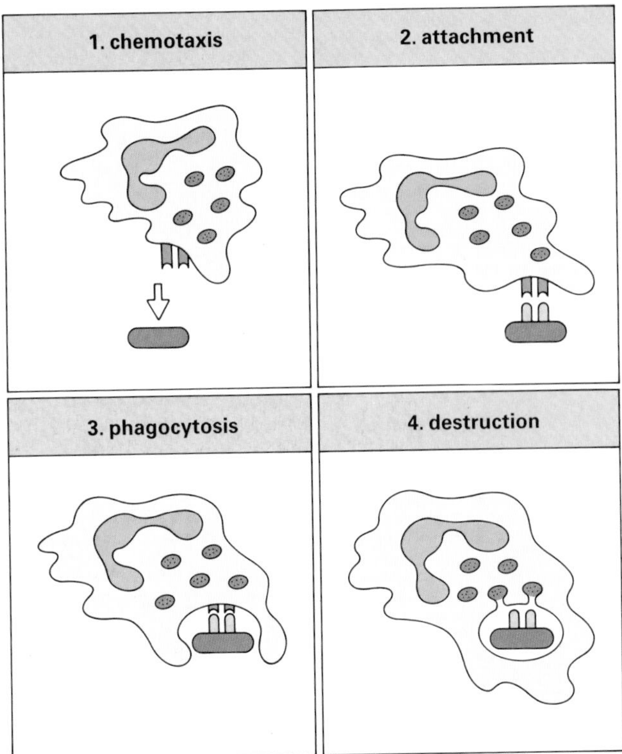

Fig. 16.22 The main stages of bacterial killing by phagocytes (polymorphs and macrophages). Phagocytes are attracted chemotactically to a bacterial infection. The phagocytes attach to the bacteria via C3b receptors, Fc receptors and lectins on the organism or the phagocyte. The organism is phagocytosed. Finally lysosomes fuse with the phagosome to release microbicidal chemicals and proteins into the phagolysosome.

b) lectins on the phagocyte. (Of particular interest in this respect are the complement receptors CR3 and p150,95 and the related molecule LFA-1, which have multiple binding sites with different specificities and can bind to β-glucans and to the endotoxin (LPS) of Gram-negative bacteria.)

c) complement deposited via the alternative or classical pathways, or following binding to the organism of a recently recognized complement-fixing mannose-binding lectin present in serum.

d) antibody Fc receptors, which link to antibody bound to the bacteria.

3. Triggering of uptake. The binding of an organism to a receptor on the macrophage membrane does not always lead to its uptake. For example zymosan particles bind via the glucan-recognizing lectin-like site on CR3 and are taken up, whereas erythrocytes coated with C3bi are not.
4. Triggering of microbicidal activity. Just as binding of an organism to membrane receptors does not guarantee uptake, so uptake does not guarantee the triggering of killing mechanisms. It seems that interaction with CR3 is particularly likely to trigger killing.

KILLING MECHANISMS

Once the organism has been internalized lysosomes fuse with the phagosome to form a phagolysosome and various killing mechanisms are activated. Monocytes possess a number of oxygen-dependent and independent anti-microbial mechanisms. The oxygen-independent mechanisms may be more important than previously thought. Many organisms can be killed by cells from patients with chronic granulomatous disease which cannot produce reactive oxygen intermediates, or from patients with myeloperoxidase deficiency, which cannot produce hypohalous acids. Similarly many organisms can be killed under anaerobic conditions.

Non-Oxygen-Dependent Killing Mechanisms Following lysosome fusion there is a transient rise in pH, before acidification of the phagolysosome takes place. Some organisms may be killed by the acidification itself which occurs within 10–15 minutes, although this is more likely to be related to the pH optima of lysosomal enzymes, which themselves kill some species. Certain Gram-positive organisms with readily exposed peptidoglycan may be killed by lysozyme. Also important are the defensins and cationic proteins. These are cysteine- and arginine-rich cationic peptides of 32–34 amino acids, found in the macrophages of rabbits and human neutrophils. They can kill organisms as diverse as *Staphylococcus aureus*, *Pseudomonas aeruginosa*, *Escherichia coli*, *Cryptococcus neoformans* and even the enveloped virus herpes simplex. They may act by damaging membranes and are most active during the transient rise in pH which occurs before acidification.

A variety of other substances, such as lactoferrin (neutrophils) have also been implicated in killing. Lactoferrin can bind iron and render it unavailable to bacteria even at an acid pH; thus the ability of polymorphs to kill some bacteria is lost if they are loaded with iron. These mechanisms may all require phagolysosome fusion (Figs 16.23 and 16.24).

Oxygen-Dependent Killing Mechanisms There may have been too much emphasis in the past on the oxygen-dependent pathways, since release of oxygen reduction products may be partly a by-product of the rapid activation of an electron transport chain, to provide energy for cell movement, phagocytosis and digestion (Fig. 16.25). However, cells from patients with chronic granulomatous disease lack this pathway, and are unable to kill some microorganisms; the disease is characterized by chronic inflammatory lesions involving pyogenic organisms, for example staphylococci.

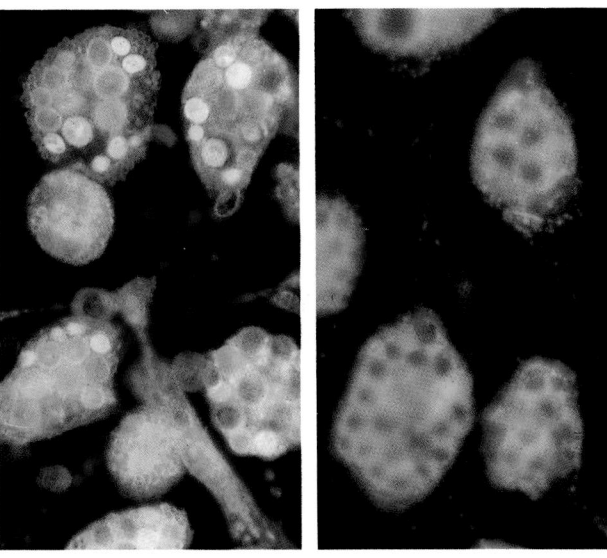

Fig. 16.23 Inhibition of fusion of secondary lysosomes with yeast-containing phagosomes by the addition of ammonium chloride. Mouse peritoneal macrophages were incubated in acridine orange which concentrates in secondary lysosomes. Live baker's yeast was then added – this assumes the appearance of 'holes' in the cell. In the absence of ammonium chloride the secondary lysosome fuses normally with the phagosome, into which the acridine orange enters and fluoresces green, yellow or orange depending on the concentration (left). However, in the presence of ammonium chloride fusion does not occur and the 'holes' remain dark (right). Such blocking of lysosomal fusion may be employed by *Mycobacterium tuberculosis* and some *Leishmania* which secrete ammonia. Some polyanions such as polyglutamic acid or suramin can also do this. (Courtesy of Mr R. Young and Dr P.D. Hart.)

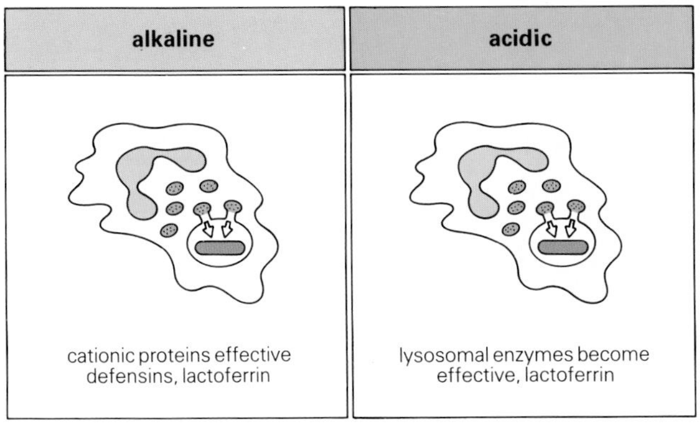

alkaline	acidic
cationic proteins effective defensins, lactoferrin	lysosomal enzymes become effective, lactoferrin

Fig. 16.24 Mechanisms involved in bacterial killing. After phagocytosis there is a transient increase in pH when cationic proteins may be effective. Subsequently the pH falls and lysosomal enzymes become effective. Lactoferrin acts by chelating free iron. Lysozyme digests the peptidoglycan of bacterial cell walls.

The ability to produce reactive oxygen intermediates and the content of myeloperoxidase decline rapidly in culture. The same may be true of some oxygen-independent mechanisms. Consequently many cells which are killed by monocytes are not killed by cultured macrophages (Fig. 16.26).

ACTIVATION OF MACROPHAGES

Killing mechanisms can be enhanced, and the decline which normally occurs as the cells mature can be abrogated by culture with suitable activating stimuli (Fig. 16.26). It is also likely that new mechanisms not present in monocytes can be activated.

Activation by Microbial Products A number of microbial products cause activation or triggering of monocytes and macrophages. These effects are partly responsible for the 'adjuvant' effects of bacteria, and probably represent phylogenetically ancient broad-spectrum recognition mechanisms for common microbial components. The best characterized are listed below but it is likely that there are many others.

1. Formyl-methionyl-leucyl-phenylalanine and related peptides.
2. Muramyl dipeptide (MDP), a derivative of bacterial peptidoglycan.
3. Trehalose dimycolate (TDM), which is derived from mycobacteria.
4. Endotoxin (LPS), which is derived from Gram-negative bacteria.
5. Various carbohydrate polymers, such as β-glucans.

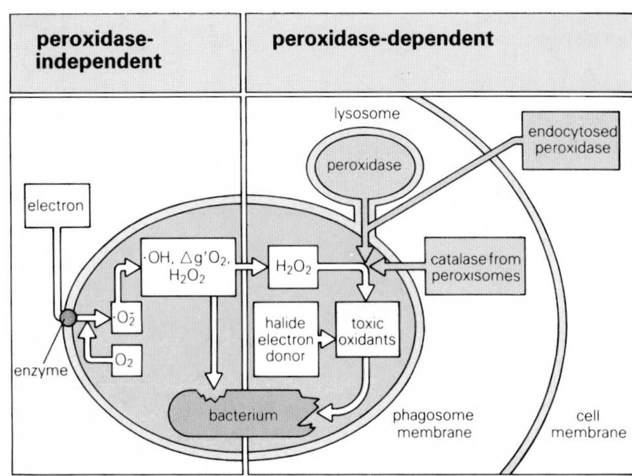

Fig. 16.25 Oxygen-dependent microbicidal activity. An enzyme in the phagosome membrane (possibly an oxidase, or a cytochrome b), reduces oxygen to the superoxide anion $\cdot O_2^-$. This can give rise to hydroxyl radicals (·OH), singlet oxygen, (Δg^1O_2) and hydrogen peroxide (H_2O_2), all of which are potentially toxic. Lysosome fusion is not required for these parts of the pathway, and the reaction takes place spontaneously following internalization of the phagosome. If lysosome fusion occurs, myeloperoxidase may enter the phagosome. In the presence of peroxidase (or under some circumstances, catalase from peroxisomes) plus halides, additional toxic oxidants such as hypohalite are generated. The monocytes of individuals with congenital myeloperoxidase deficiency may show defective microbicidal activity. However, it remains unclear whether sufficient halide (preferably iodide) is available in phagosomes *in vivo*. Tissue macrophages do not contain peroxidase.

	source and preparation of monocytes or macrophages			
	day 0	cultured > 7 days		
bacteria	**no stim**	**no stim**	**IFNϒ**	
Escherichia coli	yes	yes		
Salmonella typhimurium	yes	no	yes	
Listeria monocytogenes	yes	no	yes	this effect of IFNϒ is not blocked by glucocorticoids
Legionella pneumophila	no	no	yes	
Nocardia asteroides	yes	-	yes	this effect of IFNϒ is blocked by glucocorticoids
Mycobacterium tuberculosis	no	no	variable	some stasis, but no killing with cells from some donors; enhanced growth with others. 1,25(OH)$_2$ cholecalciferol is more active than IFNϒ in this system
Chlamydia	**no stim**	**no stim**	**IFNϒ**	
Chlamydia psittaci	yes	no	yes	
Chlamydia trachomatis	yes	yes		
Biovar lymphogranuloma venereum	yes	no	yes	

Fig. 16.26 Antibacterial function of human monocytes and macrophages. Many monocytes have an intrinsic ability to kill bacteria of different strains, indicated above. This may be partly lost after 7 days in culture, but can often be restored by treatment with IFNϒ.

Lymphokine-Mediated Activation *In vivo* the T cell response is frequently required for the full expression of phagocyte-mediated immunity. This response acts both by attracting phagocytes to the site of infection, and by activating them. The relative importance of these two components differs for different organisms. Thus for immunity to *Listeria monocytogenes,* which is readily killed by the baseline levels of oxygen-dependent mechanisms in both monocytes and neutrophils, it is the attraction of the cells to the lesion which is most important. In contrast, for *Mycobacterium tuberculosis,* which thrives inside neutrophils and monocytes, it is the activation of unidentified oxygen-independent mechanisms in the cells which is critical.

The lymphokine most often implicated is interferon-gamma (IFNϒ) which enhances both oxygen-dependent and-independent mechanisms, though there are sporadic reports implicating GM-CSF, TNF, and other often undefined lymphokines. As discussed in Chapter 9, activation of some functions requires combinations of lymphokines.

Mycobacteria illustrate the complexity of this topic. IFNϒ can induce total stasis of *M. tuberculosis* in murine macrophages, but it causes anything from feeble inhibition to significantly increased growth of it in human monocytes. On the other hand it causes human (but not murine) macrophages to express a 1-hydroxylase enzyme which converts the circulating inactive form of vitamin D3 (25(OH) vitamin D3) into the active 1,25-dihydroxy metabolite. This metabolite activates antimycobacterial mechanisms in the macrophages rather more efficiently than IFNϒ itself.

THE SHWARTZMAN REACTION

Shwartzman observed that if Gram-negative organisms were injected intracutaneously into rabbits, and then a second dose was given intravenously 24 hours later, haemorrhagic necrosis occurred at the prepared skin site. This is known as the Shwartzman phenomenon. He also noted that two *intravenous* injections 24 hours apart caused a systemic reaction commonly involving circulatory collapse and bilateral renal cortical necrosis. Sanarelli had made similar observations and this is now known as the 'Systemic Shwartzman or 'Sanarelli-Shwartzman' reaction. These reactions can also be accompanied by necrosis in the pancreas, pituitary, adrenals and gut. There is marked diffuse intravascular coagulation and thrombosis. Subsequently numerous other organisms have been shown to be able to 'prepare' the skin, including streptococci, mycobacteria, *Haemophilus*, corynebacteria and even vaccinia virus. Endotoxin (LPS) has been shown to be the relevant active component of the intravenous 'triggering' injection.

Early work implicated endothelial changes and neutrophil accumulation and degranulation. It now seems probable that TNF and IL-1 are major mediators of these reactions (see Chapter 9), and direct injection of TNF into 'prepared' sites causes a similar type of necrosis, substituting perhaps for arrival of TNF via the circulation following the intravenous dose of endotoxin (LPS).

THE RELATIVE IMPORTANCE OF THE VARIOUS DEFENCE MECHANISMS IN DIFFERENT BACTERIAL INFECTIONS

The major defence mechanisms in a bacterial infection can be related to the nature of the organism, and the disease caused (Fig. 16.27). The pathogenicity of some

infection	pathogenesis	major defence mechanisms
Corynebacterium diphtheriae	non-invasive pharyngitis–toxin	neutralizing antibody
Vibrio cholerae	non-invasive enteritis–toxin	neutralizing and adhesion-blocking antibodies
Neisseria meningitidis	nasopharynx → bacteraemia → meningitis	opsonized and killed by antibody and lytic complement
Staphylococcus aureus	locally invasive and toxic in skin etc.	opsonized by antibody and complement, killed by phagocytes
Mycobacterium tuberculosis	invasive, locally toxic, hypersensitivity	macrophage activation by T cells
Mycobacterium leprae	invasive, space-occupying and/or hypersensitivity	

Fig. 16.27 The major mechanisms of immunity in some important bacterial infections.

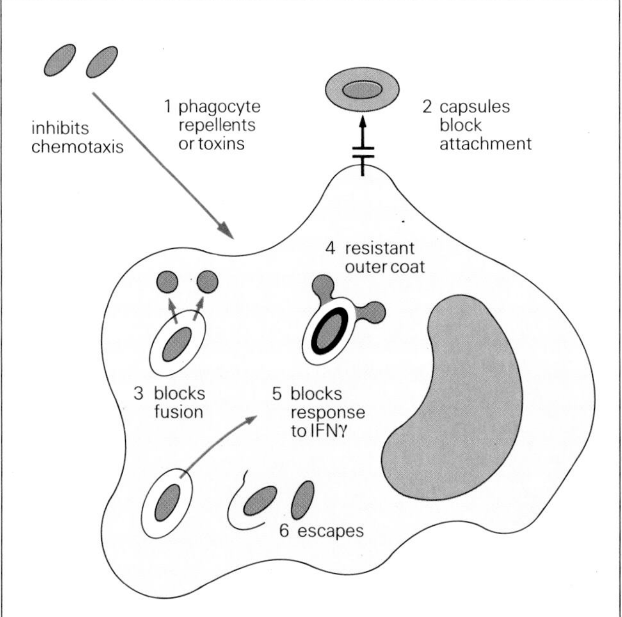

Fig. 16.28 Evasion of phagocytes. Bacteria have evolved to evade different aspects of phagocyte-mediated killing. Some can secrete repellents or toxins which inhibit chemotaxis (1). Others have capsules or outer coats which inhibit attachment to the phagocyte (2). Once ingested, some such as *Mycobacterium tuberculosis* secrete molecules which inhibit lysosome fusion (3). Organisms such as *M. leprae* have highly resistant outer coats. *M. leprae* surrounds itself with a phenolic glycolipid which scavenges free radicals (4). Mycobacteria also release a lipoarabinomannan which blocks the ability of macrophages to respond to the activating effects of IFNγ (5). Several organisms (e.g. *M. leprae*), can escape from the phagosome to multiply in the cytoplasm (6).

non-invasive infections of epithelial surfaces, for example *Corynebacterium diphtheriae* and *Vibrio cholerae* infection, depends on toxin production, and neutralizing antibody is probably sufficient for immunity, though antibody blocking adhesion to the epithelium may also be important.

The pathogenicity of most invasive organisms does not rely so heavily on a single toxin, so immunity requires killing of the organism itself. Organisms with an outer lipid membrane (Gram-negative) may be killed by antibody and the lytic pathway of complement, for example *Neisseria meningitidis*. Gram-positive organisms, for example *Staphylococcus aureus* are killed by phagocytic cells, and the role of the specific immune response is opsonization by antibody and complement. The lytic pathway is probably irrelevant. Organisms which are resistant to the killing mechanisms of polymorphs and monocytes, for example *Mycobacterium tuberculosis*, or obligate intracellular parasites, for example *M. leprae*, are killed by additional poorly understood mechanisms which are induced in macrophages by T cell products.

The importance of phagocytes in protection against bacterial infection is reflected in the numerous ways in which different organisms attempt to evade the actions of these cells. Pathogens have developed ways of blocking every point in the pathway from the initial attraction of the phagocyte to the final intracellular killing (Fig. 16.28).

IMMUNITY TO FUNGI

Little is known about the precise mechanisms involved in immunity to fungal infections, but it is thought that they are essentially similar to those involved in resistance to bacterial infections. The fungal infections of man fall into four major categories.

1. Superficial mycoses – dermatophytes usually restricted to the non-living keratinized components of skin, hair and nails.
2. Subcutaneous mycoses – saprophytic fungi which can cause chronic nodules or ulcers in subcutaneous tissues following trauma, for example chromomycosis, sporotrichosis, mycetoma.
3. Respiratory mycoses – soil saprophytes which produce subclinical or acute lung infections (rarely disseminated) or producing granulomatous lesions, for example histoplasmosis, coccidioidomycosis.
4. *Candida albicans* – ubiquitous commensal causing superficial infections of skin and mucous membranes, rarely systemic.

The cutaneous fungal infections are usually self-limiting and recovery is associated with a certain limited resistance to reinfection. Resistance is apparently based on cell-mediated immunity since patients develop DTH reactions to fungal antigens, and the occurrence of chronic infections is associated with a lack of these reactions. T cell immunity is also implicated in resistance to other fungal infections, since resistance can sometimes be transfered with immune T cells. It is presumed that T cells release lymphokines which activate macrophages to produce destruction of the fungi (Fig. 16.29). In respiratory mycoses, spectra of disease activity somewhat similar to the spectrum of activity in leprosy can be seen

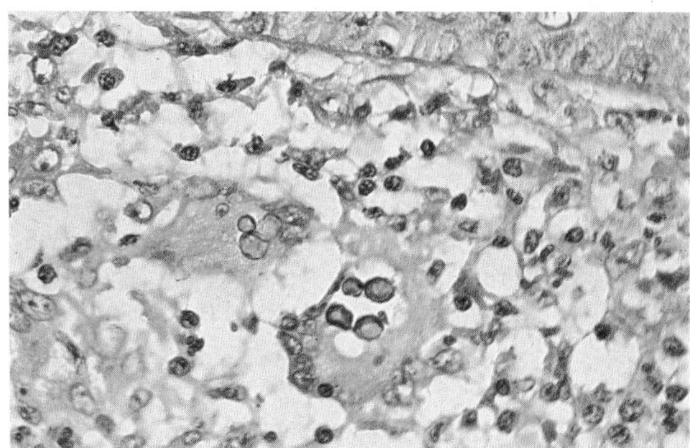

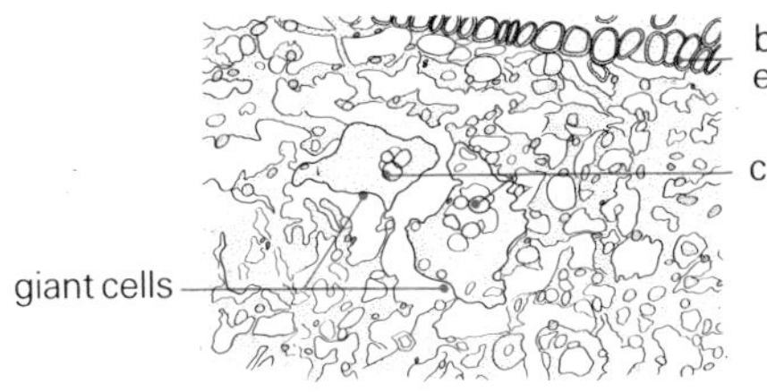

Fig. 16.29 Evidence for T cell immunity in chromomycosis. Pigmented cells of chromomycosis (a subcutaneous mycosis) are visible in giant cells in the dermis of a patient. The area is surrounded by a predominantly mononuclear cell infiltrate. H&E stain, × 400. (Courtesy of Dr R.J. Hay.)

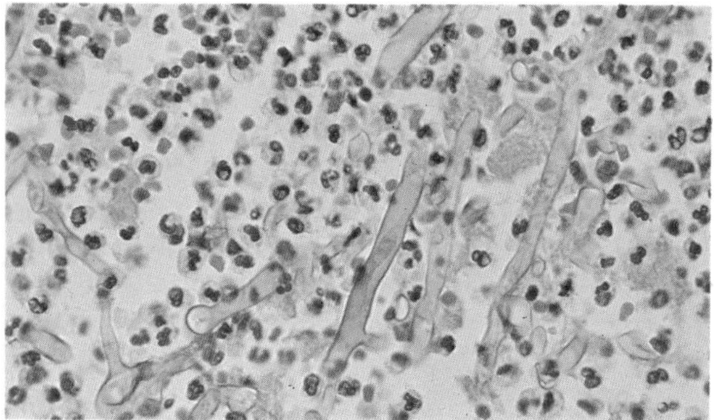

Fig. 16.30 Evidence for neutrophil-mediated immunity to mucormycosis. Section through a lung of a patient suffering from mucormycosis – an opportunistic infection in an immunosuppressed subject. The inflammatory reaction consists almost entirely of neutrophil polymorphs around the fungal hyphae. The disease is particularly associated with neutropenia. Silver stain, × 400. (Courtesy of Dr R.J. Hay.)

organism	source of monocytes/macrophages: normal	chronic granulomatous disease	myelo-peroxidase deficiency
Candida albicans	+	(+)	(+)
Candida parapsilosis	+	–	+
Cryptococcus neoformans	+		+
Aspergillus fumigatus conidia	+	+	
Aspergillus fumigatus hyphae	+	+	

Fig. 16.31 Monocyte/macrophage killing of fungi. Many fungi are killed by monocytes or macrophages. Since cells from patients with chronic granulomatous disease and individuals with myeloperoxidase deficiency can also effect killing, this shows the importance of non-oxygen dependent mechanisms.

(see Chapter 22). Disturbance of normal physiology by immunosuppressive drugs or of normal flora by antibiotics can predispose to invasion by *Candida*. *Candida* infections are also common in immunodeficiency diseases (severe combined immunodeficiency, thymic aplasia, etc.) implying that the immune system is involved in confining the fungus to its normal commensal sites.

There is also evidence for neutrophil involvement in immunity to some respiratory mycoses such as mucormycosis (Fig. 16.30). It is likely that the cationic proteins discussed earlier in relation to bacteria are important for protection from fungi, since cells from patients with defective oxygen reduction pathways usually kill yeast and hyphae with near normal efficiency (Fig. 16.31). As with bacterial infections different mechanisms are active against different organisms.

VACCINE DESIGN

In order to design a vaccine, the following knowledge is required.
1. The relevant protective antigen(s).
2. The anatomical site where the mechanism needs to be expressed.
3. The immunological mechanism required.
4. An adjuvant and immunization schedule which is safe to use and will evoke the relevant response in that site.

All four criteria are fulfilled by those organisms which owe their pathogenicity to a single identified immunogenic protein. Toxins such as those of *Corynebacterium diphtheriae* and *Clostridium tetani* lose their toxicity when heated, but retain their immunogenicity. Such a toxoid will evoke a systemic antibody response when injected with a simple adjuvant such as $Al(OH)_3$ or killed *Bordetella pertussis*. Thus adjuvants for systemic antibody responses are not a problem.

Relevant Antigens Organisms such as *Streptococcus pyogenes* and *Str. pneumoniae* have large numbers of serotypes, so that an effective vaccine becomes a complex mixture which is expensive to make and incomplete in its coverage. Problems are still greater when there are numerous toxic products, but there is little definitive information as to which ones are protective antigens, or even the mechanism of protection. *B. pertussis* is an example, where the efficacy of a crude killed vaccine is due to luck rather than science. Neither its action, nor its occasional association with brain damage are understood, so a truly rational and safe vaccine cannot yet be designed.

Localization of Effect The next type of problem is the need to achieve expression of immunity in certain sites such as the genito-urinary tract or gut. Experimentally direct intravaginal immunization with antigens of *Neisseria gonorrhoeae* is much more effective than systemic immunization at evoking a response in this site. Similarly the conventional *Vibrio cholerae* vaccine injected intramuscularly has a very limited protective effect, while experimental oral vaccines can be more effective. The answer probably lies in the development of stable mutants of pathogenic organisms which after ingestion initiate an infection, and invade the local epithelium or lymphoid tissue, but die after a limited number of replication cycles. Thus derivatives of *Salmonella typhimurium* have been constructed which carry stable mutations determining the period of survival in the gut-associated lymphoid tissue and spleen. Such mutations can be transferred to other species, or the genes for relevant antigenic determinants from other pathogens can be inserted into the mutant, in the hope that they will be expressed in a way which will evoke appropriate responses.

Immunological Mechanisms When the required mechanism of response is cell-mediated, there are two problems for the designer of vaccines. First, for bacteria such as *Mycobacterium leprae* or *M. tuberculosis* protective antigens have not been identified. Secondly, when an adjuvant is required which is acceptable for use in man and will evoke a cell-mediated response rather

organism	antigen	mechanism	adjuvant	site
Corynebacterium diphtheriae / *Clostridium tetani*	toxin	neutralizing antibody	Al $(OH)_3$ or pertussis	systemic
Streptococcus pneumoniae	capsular polysaccharide but many serotypes	antibody		systemic
Bordetella pertussis	not certain various toxins	? antibody		systemic + secretory
Neisseria gonorrhoeae	pili, LPS	antibody	? recombinant commensal	GU tract
Vibrio cholerae	toxin, LPS	antibody	? recombinant organism	gut
Mycobacterium tuberculosis	not known	? T cell-dependent macrophage activation	BCG – but often fails, and is a live vaccine	systemic

Fig. 16.32 Requirements for vaccine design. Different organisms require different strategies for vaccine design. In general those further down this list present increasing problems.

than only antibody, there are a few alternatives to live BCG (Bacille Calmette Guérin) – an attenuated strain of *M. bovis* – though the orally ingested *Salmonella* mutants discussed above may have some ability to evoke cell-mediated immunity (CMI) and vaccinia virus has also been considered. Therefore even if we could identify and clone the genes for a manageable number of protective antigens, they would probably need to be expressed in BCG before they could be used to evoke CMI. The technology for doing this has now been developed and BCG derivatives expressing protective epitopes from, for instance, *Leishmania* species are an exciting prospect.

Adjuvants Attempts are being made to develop safe adjuvants derived from the concept of Complete Freund's Adjuvant. This is a water - in - oil emulsion containing killed mycobacteria, which has severe side effects in humans. It is possible that isolated or synthetic adjuvant-active components of bacteria, such as derivatives of muramyl dipeptide, in a metabolizable oil, such as squalene, will prove acceptable in man.

Ultimately we will need adjuvants for CMI which can direct the response preferentially towards particular subsets of cell-mediated mechanisms, for example cytotoxic T cells versus T cells mediating delayed hypersensitivity. At present we have no idea how to do this, though in some virus models activation of the wrong T cell subset can increase rather than decrease susceptibility to the infection. The problems associated with vaccine design are illustrated in Fig. 16.32.

FURTHER READING

VIRUSES

Borden, E.G., Rosenzweig, I.B. & Byrne, G.I. (1987) Interferons: from virus inhibitor to modulator of amino acid and lipid metabolism. *Journal of Interferon Research*, **7**, 591.

Denman, A.M. (1983) Viruses and immunopathology. In *Immunology in Medicine*. Edited by E.J. Holborrow & W.G. Reeves. Grune and Stratton.

Eckels, D.D., Lamb, J.R., Lake, P., Woody, J.N., Johnson A.H. & Hartzman, R.J. (1982) Antigen-specific human T lymphocyte clones. Genetic restriction of influenza virus-specific responses to HLA–D region genes. *Human Immunology*, **4**, 313.

Mandel, B. (1979) Interaction of viruses with neutralising antibodies. In *Comprehensive Virology*. Vol.15. Edited by H. Fraenkel-Contrat & R.R. Wagner. New York: Plenum Press.

McMichael, A.J., Gotch, F. & Noble, G.R. (1983) Cytotoxic T cell immunity to influenza. *New England Journal of Medicine*, **309**, 13.

Mims, C.A. & White, D.W. (1984) *Viral Pathogenesis and Immunology*. Oxford: Blackwell Scientific Publications.

Murray, K. (1988) Application of recombinant DNA techniques in the development of viral vaccines. *Vaccine*, **6**, 164.

Nash, A.A., Jayasuriya, A., Phelan, J., Cobbold, S.P., Waldman, H. & Prospero, T. (1987) Different roles for L3T4$^+$ and Lyt2$^+$ T cell subsets in the control of an acute herpes simplex virus infection of the skin and nervous system. *Journal of General Virology*, **68**, 825.

Sehgal, P.B., Pfeffer, L.M. & Tamm, I. (1982) Interferon and its inducers. In *Chemotherapy of Viral Infections*. Edited by P.E. Carne & L.A. Caliguiri. Berlin: Springer-Verlag.

Sissons, J.G. & Oldstone, M.B.A. (1980) Antibody-mediated destruction of virus-infected cells. *Advances in Immunology*, **31**, 1.

Stroop, W.G. & Baringer, J.R. (1982) Persistent, slow and latent viral infections. *Progress in Medical Virology*, **28**, 1.

Smith, G.L. & Moss, B. (1984) Uses of vaccinia virus as a vector for the production of live recombinant vaccines. *BioEssays*, **1**, 120.

Wiley, D.C., Wilson, I.A. & Skehel, J.J. (1981) Structural identification of the antibody binding sites of Hong Kong influenza haemagglutinin and their involvement in antigenic variation. *Nature*, **289**, 373.

Wraith, D.C. (1987) The recognition of influenza A virus-infected cells by cytotoxic T lymphocytes. *Immunology Today*, **8**, 239.

Zinkernagel, R.M. & Doherty, P.C. (1979) MHC-restricted cytotoxic T cells. Studies on the biological role of polymorphic major transplantation antigens determining T cell restriction, specificity, function and responsiveness. *Advances in Immunology*, **27**, 51.

BACTERIA

Catterall, J.R., Black, C.M., Leventhal, J.P., Rizk, N.W., Wachtel, J.S. & Remington, J.S. (1987) Nonoxidative microbicidal activity in normal human alveolar and peritoneal macrophages. *Infection and Immunity*, **55**, 1635.

De Libero, G. & Kaufmann, S.H.E. (1986) Antigen-specific Lyt2$^+$ cytolytic T lymphocytes from mice infected with the intracellular bacterium *Listeria monocytogenes*. *Journal of Immunology*, **137**, 2688.

Ganz, T., Selsted, M.E., Szklarek, D., Harwig, S.S., Daher, K., Bainton, D.F. & Lehrer, R.I. (1985) Defensins. Natural peptide antibiotics of human neutrophils. *Journal of Clinical Investigation*, **76**, 1427.

Hahn, H. & Kaufmann, S.H.E. (1981) The role of cell-mediated immunity in bacterial infections. *Review of Infectious Disease*, **3**, 1221.

Horwitz, M.A. & Silverstein, S.C. (1981) Activated human monocytes inhibit the intracellular multiplication of Legionnaires disease bacilli. *Journal of Experimental Medicine*, **154**, 1618.

Joiner, K.A., Brown, E.J. & Frank, M.M. (1984) Complement and bacteria: chemistry and biology in host defence. *Annual Review of Immunology*, **2**, 461.

Mims, C.A. (1977) *The Pathogenesis of Infectious Disease*. London: Academic Press.

Mitchell, G.F. (1988) The way ahead for vaccines and vaccination: symposium summary. *Vaccine*, **6**, 200.

Nahmias, A.J. & O'Reilly, J. (eds) (1981) *Comprehensive Immunology. Vol. 8. Immunology of Human Infection. Part 1: Bacteria, Mycoplasmae, Chlamydiae and Fungi*. New York: Plenum Medical Book Company.

Nathan, C.F., Murray, H.W., Wiebe, M.E. & Rubin, B.Y. (1983) Identification of interferon-γ as the lymphokine that activates human macrophage oxidative metabolism and antimicrobial activity. *Journal of Experimental Medicine*, **158**, 670.

Ofek, I. & Sharon, N. (1988) Lectinophagocytosis: a molecular mechanism of recognition between cell surface sugars and lectins in the phagocytosis of bacteria. *Infection and Immunity*, **56**, 539.

Rook, G.A.W. (1987) Progress in the immunology of the mycobacterioses. *Clinical and Experimental Immunology*, **69**, 1.

Rothstein, J.L. & Schreiber, H. (1988) Synergy between tumour necrosis factor and bacterial products causes haemorrhagic necrosis and lethal shock in normal mice. *Proceedings of the National Academy of Science of the USA*, **85**, 607.

Sibley, L.D. & Krahenbuhl, J.L. (1987) *Mycobacterium leprae*-burdened macrophages are refractory to activation by gamma interferon. *Infection and Immunity*, **55**, 446.

FUNGI

Bullock, W.E. & Wright, S.D. (1987) Role of the adherence-promoting receptors CR3, LFA-1, and p150, 95 in binding of *Histoplasma capsulatum* by human macrophages. *Journal of Experimental Medicine*, **165**, 195.

Calderon, R.A. & Hay, R.J. (1984) Cell-mediated immunity in experimental murine dermatophytosis. Adoptive transfer of immunity to dermatophyte infection by lymphoid cells from donors with acute or chronic infections. *Immunology*, **53**, 465.

Cox, R.A. (1979) Immunologic studies of patients with histoplasmosis. *American Review of Respiratory Disease*, **120**, 143.

Grayhill, J.R. & Drutz, D.J. (1979) Host defence in cryptococcosis in the nude mouse. *Cellular Immunology*, **40**, 263.

Nahmias, A.J. & O'Reilly, J. (eds) (1981) *Comprehensive Immunology. Vol.8. Immunology of Human Infection, Part 1: Bacteria, Mycoplasmae, Chlamydiae and Fungi*. New York: Plenum Medical Book Company.

Rogers, T.J. & Balish, E. (1980) Immunity to *Candida albicans*. *Microbiological Reviews*, **44**, 660.

17 Immunity to Protozoa and Worms

Parasite infections typically stimulate more than one immunological defence mechanism, and the response that predominates depends upon the identity of the parasite. In order to illustrate the general principles of immunity to the diseases caused by parasites some of the more important infections of man are considered here, together with the main defence mechanisms that control the multiplication and spread of the parasites within the host. This discussion will therefore be centred on the events that occur in nature, where a number of immunological effector mechanisms act simultaneously.

Parasitic protozoa which infect man include amoebae which live in the gut, those protozoa which live in the blood, either free, for example African trypanosomes, or in erythrocytes (*Plasmodium* spp.), and those which live in macrophages, either in the skin or lymphatics (*Leishmania*), or in the mononuclear phagocyte system of the liver, spleen and bone marrow, (for example, *Trypanosoma cruzi* and *Leishmania* spp.). *T. cruzi* also lives in both smooth and striated muscle.

Parasitic worms that infect man include trematodes, for example schistosomes, some cestodes (tapeworms) some nematodes such as *Trichinella spiralis*, hookworms, *Ascaris* and the filarial worms. Tapeworms and hookworms inhabit the gut while adult schistosomes live in the blood vessels. Other worms, for example *Filaria* live in lymphatics. Many parasitic worms pass through complicated life cycles involving migration through various parts of the host's body and development of different stages in different organs before they reach the site where they finally mature and spend the rest of their lives. Examples of these different parasites, their life cycles, vectors, geographical distribution and diseases they cause are described in Figs 17.30–17.35.

Parasites infect very large numbers of people and present a major medical problem, especially in tropical countries (Fig. 17.1). The diseases caused are diverse and the immune responses which are effective against the different parasites vary considerably. Parasitic infections do, however, share a number of common features.

parasites responsible	disease
protozoa	
Plasmodium vivax *Plasmodium falciparum* *Plasmodium ovale* *Plasmodium malariae*	malaria
Leishmania tropica *Leishmania donovani* *Leishmania braziliensis*	leishmaniasis (tropical sore, kala-azar, espundia)
Trypanosoma rhodesiense *Trypanosoma gambiense*	sleeping sickness
Trypanosoma cruzi	Chagas' disease
helminths	
trematodes (flukes) *Schistosoma mansoni* *Schistosoma haematobium* *Schistosoma japonicum*	schistosomiasis
nematodes (roundworms) *Trichinella spiralis*	trichinosis
Ancylostoma duodenale *Necator americanus*	hookworm
Wuchereria bancrofti *Brugia malayi* *Loa loa* *Dipetalonema perstaris* *Onchocerca volvulus*	filariasis

0 1 10 100 1000
millions of people infected (log scale)

Fig 17.1 Some important parasitic infections of man. Figures for leishmaniasis and sleeping sickness are unavailable.

GENERAL FEATURES OF PARASITIC INFECTIONS

Protozoan parasites and worms are larger than other infectious agents such as bacteria and viruses (Fig. 17.2).

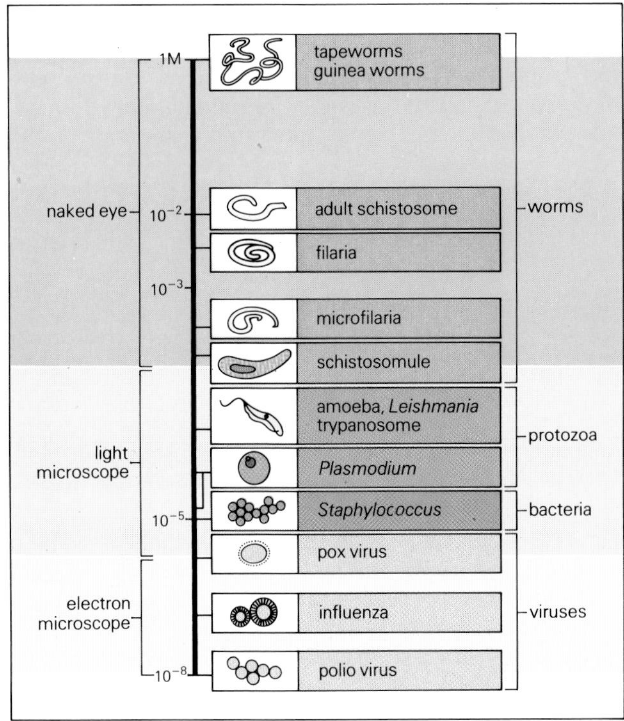

Fig. 17.2 Comparative size of various infective agents.

These parasites often have complicated life cycles and additionally some depend upon a vector to transmit them from one host to another. Larger size entails the existence of more antigens, both in number and kind. In the case of parasites which display more complicated life histories, some of these antigens may be specific to a particular stage of development. For example, the protein coat of the mosquito-borne stage of malaria is confined to that stage and antibodies against it do not react with parasites present in hepatocytes or erythrocytes. On the other hand, in some infections a state of 'concomitant immunity' may exist, whereby the presence of a pre-existing infection by an adult worm protects the host against invasion by fresh larvae of the same species; the mechanism is not known.

Parasitic infections are generally chronic. It is to the disadvantage of the parasite to kill its host and over millions of years of evolution the parasites that have survived are well adapted to their host and show marked host specificity. For example, the malarial parasite of birds, rodents or man can each multiply only in its own particular kind of host. There are some exceptions to this general rule, for example, the worm *Trichinella spiralis* that infects pigs is also able to infect man but cannot complete its life cycle in the incorrect host. Within a species, strains may vary in their resistance depending on a variety of immune response genes. Non-MHC genes are particularly important in this respect. For example, the innate resistance of mice to infection by *Leishmania donovani* and several other parasites is determined by the Lsh gene (see Chapter 11).

Among the consequences of chronic infection are the presence of circulating antigens, persistent antigenic stimulation and the formation of immune complexes (Fig. 17.3). Characteristically, levels of immunoglobulins are raised in some infections: IgM in trypanosomiasis and malaria; IgG in malaria and visceral leishmaniasis; IgE in worm infections. Splenomegaly is pronounced in most parasitic infections, and there is evidence that parasite antigens can act directly as polyclonal mitogens for lymphocytes. In addition to the immune responses directed against the parasite, immunosuppression and immunopathological effects are often observed.

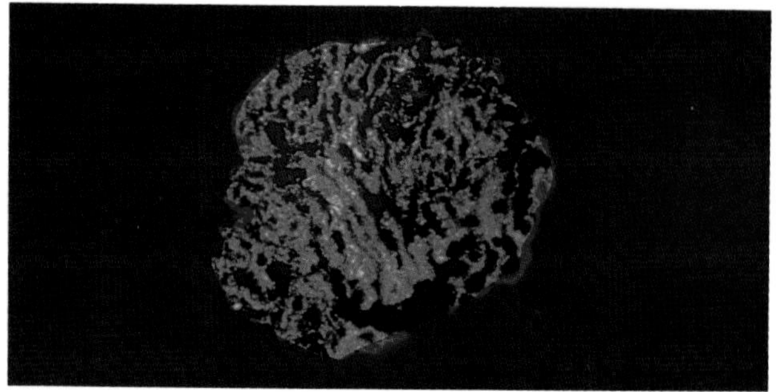

Fig. 17.3 Immune complex deposition in quartan malaria nephrotic syndrome. Low power fluorescence micrograph of a renal glomerulus in a biopsy specimen from a Nigerian child with the syndrome. People infected with *Plasmodium malariae,* as in this case, may develop glomerulonephritis as a result of the deposition of immune complexes in the renal glomerulus. The section was stained with FITC conjugated anti-human IgG and shows granular deposition of immunoglobulin throughout the capillary loops of the glomerulus. (Courtesy of Dr V. Houba.)

As a result of the close adaptation of the parasite to its host, a balanced relationship is set up. In the natural host no single immunological effector mechanism acts in isolation, there are always several, and in return parasites have evolved many different ways of evading the host's defences. In general terms, however, cell-mediated responses are more effective against intracellular protozoa while antibody is more effective against extracellular parasites, especially when acting in conjunction with certain effector cells. Thus even within a single infection, different immune responses may act against different developmental stages of the parasite. For example, in malaria cell-mediated immunity appears to prevent development within hepatocytes, while antibody against extracellular forms blocks their capacity to invade new cells. This has been shown in mice immunized with *Salmonella typhimurium* carrying the sporozoite surface antigen gene. The mice developed cell-mediated immunity to the sporozoite, but no antibody, and multiplication of the liver stage was inhibited.

EFFECTOR MECHANISMS

Various kinds of effector cells such as macrophages, neutrophils, eosinophils – and even platelets – help defend the host against invasion by parasites and act to control the multiplication and spread of parasites already in residence. The anatomical location of these effector cells is obviously important. For example, experimental depletion of the three types of nucleated cell from the cutaneous tissue of immune mice increased their susceptibility to infection by cercariae of *Schistosoma mansoni,* showing that in this case a cellular effector mechanism in the skin contributes to immunity.

Many of the anti-parasitic activities of effector cells are enhanced by interaction with cytokines released by other types of cell in response to infection; cytokines may also affect cell migration. Principally, cytokines are secreted by T lymphocytes and by macrophages, but some may be derived from such cells as B lymphocytes, fibroblasts and the endothelial cells of blood vessels. Some cytokines may themselves induce endothelial cells to release others, and many act synergistically with each other causing further amplification of inflammatory responses. Some cytokines can also induce endothelial cells to secrete reactive O_2 metabolites which are toxic to parasites but which may also damage the host's own tissues. Cytokines can also cause endothelial cells to secrete immunosuppressive molecules, for example prostaglandins.

T CELLS

T cells are fundamental to the control of parasite multiplication. In most parasite infections protection can be conferred on normal animals by the transfer of spleen cells, especially T cells, from immune animals. However, transfer of T cells from acutely infected animals can in some cases (for example infection caused by *Leishmania tropica*) suppress the protective response and cause death of the recipients.

The T cell requirement is demonstrable by the way in which nude (athymic) or T-deprived mice fail to clear otherwise non-lethal infections, for example rodent malaria or infections caused by *T. cruzi* (Fig. 17.4).

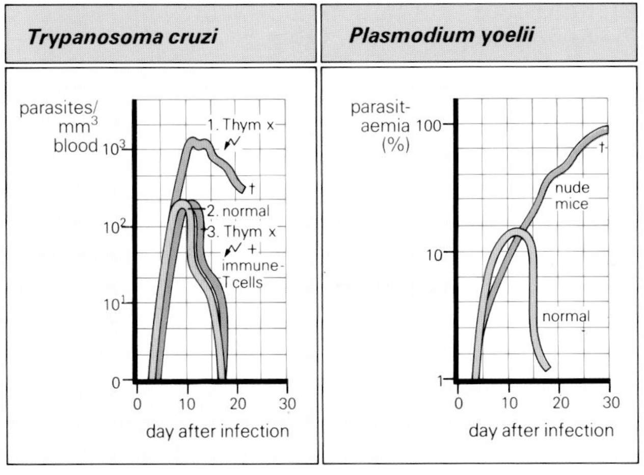

Fig. 17.4 Parasite infections in T-deprived mice. These graphs plot the increase in number of blood-borne parasites (parasitaemia) following infection of mice. *T. cruzi* multiplies faster (and gives fatal parasitaemia) in mice that have been thymectomized (Thym x) and irradiated (↯) to destroy T cells (1) than in normal mice, in which parasites are cleared from the blood by 16 days (2). Reconstitution of T-deprived mice with T cells from immune mice (immune-T) restores their ability to control the parasitaemia (3). In these experiments both experimental groups (1 and 3) were given fetal liver cells to restore vital haematopoietic function. *P. yoelii* causes a self-limiting infection in normal mice and the parasites are cleared from the blood by day 20. In nude mice (which lack T cells congenitally) the parasites continue to multiply, killing the mice after about 30 days.

The type of T cell involved in protection and how it acts depends upon the nature of the infection. T cells of the $CD4^+$ (helper) phenotype, for example, transfer protective immunity against *L. major* and *L. tropica*, the parasites that cause cutaneous leishmaniasis; monoclonal antibodies against the $CD4^+$ antigen enhance the size of skin lesions in resistant mouse strains and cause an increase in the number of parasites present. T cells of the same phenotype are necessary for the mouse to effect cure of the parasite *Giardia muris* which inhabits the gut lumen.

Cytotoxic T cells have a destructive effect against some intracellular parasites, such as *Theileria parvum*, which lives in the lymphocytes of cattle, and they may also play a role in *T. cruzi* infections, in which autoimmune destruction of parasitized heart cells and fibroblasts has been demonstrated.

Different T cell phenotypes may be required for protection at different stages of infections. Thus whereas $CD8^+$ T cells protect mice against the liver stage of infection by the rodent malarial parasite *Plasmodium berghei* (since immune mice depleted of such cells become susceptible to infection by sporozoites), it is the $CD4^+$ T cells which mediate immunity against the blood stage of *P. yoelii*. The mode of action of the different types of T cell is not clear. Although $CD4^+$ T cells may act partly as helper cells for antibody production, they also secrete various cytokines that interact with other effector cell types, and although $CD8^+$ cells may act as cytotoxic T cells, as they do against other intracellular pathogens such as viruses, they too can secrete cytokines.

Cytokine Secretion by T Cells Specific T cells respond to antigens by secreting several soluble factors which are required for the development of an effective immune response. Proliferating T cells secrete interleukin-2 (IL-2), and in some infections, for example malaria, African trypanosomiasis and Chagas' disease, IL-2 production is deficient. Both IL-2 production and expression of the IL-2 receptor have been found to be diminished when T cells from mice infected with *T. brucei* are stimulated with a mitogen. In mice infected with *T. cruzi*, injection of IL-2 restored helper cell activity, leading to an increase in the amount of parasite-specific IgM and IgG, reduced parasitaemia and increased host longevity.

Other T cell factors enhance the ability of effector cells to control parasite multiplication by increasing their number, as well as their activity. The monocytosis of malaria and the characteristic enlargement of the spleen, caused by an enormous increase in cell number, are T cell-dependent, as are the accumulation of macrophages in the granulomata that develop in the livers of individuals with schistosomiasis and the eosinophilia characteristic of worm infections. Activated T cells secrete cytokines of the family of molecules known as colony-stimulating factors, for example interleukin-3 (IL-3) and GM-CSF, which act on cells of the myeloid lineage (bone marrow precursors of neutrophils, eosinophils and macrophages) inducing an increase in their number, and then their differentiation and activation. Thus eosinophils activated by colony-stimulating factors, including IL-3 and GM-CSF, have an enhanced ability to kill schistosome larvae.

In some circumstances, however, secretion of a cytokine may harm the host. Administration of IL-3 to mice infected with *L. major*, for instance, leads to an exacerbation of the local infection and increases dissemination of the parasites, probably by enhancing proliferation of bone marrow precursors of the cells the parasites inhabit.

Interferon-γ Interferon-γ (IFNγ) is secreted by activated T cells (see Chapter 9). Although it inhibits the proliferation of many types of mammalian cell, it does not appear to have a directly inhibitory or cytotoxic effect on any parasites themselves. However, it does appear to be involved in some immune mechanisms that control parasite multiplication. Thus, in malaria, administration of IFNγ to chimpanzees infected with sporozoites of *P. vivax* diminished parasitaemia, and the ability of immune mice to withstand challenge by sporozoites of *P. berghei* can be overcome by treatment with a monoclonal antibody against recombinant IFNγ.

One effect of IFNγ is to inhibit the multiplication of the liver stages of the malarial parasite: hepatocytes express surface receptors for IFNγ and treatment of the cells *in vitro* prevents the development of *P. falciparum*, although the mechanism is not known. Similarly, treatment of macrophages with IFNγ renders them resistant to invasion by some intracellular parasites which multiply within them, for example *Toxoplasma gondii* and *Leishmania* spp., and may lead to the elimination of parasites already resident (Fig. 17.5). Conversely, the ability of crude lymphokine preparations to stimulate macrophages to kill these parasites is abolished by antibodies against IFNγ. Although the enhanced capacity of the cells to kill *T. gondii* is correlated with enhanced

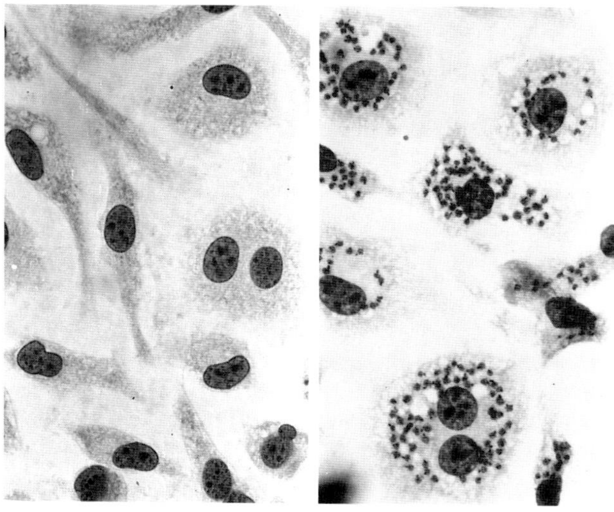

Fig. 17.5 Inhibition of parasite multiplication in macrophages treated with cytokines. Peritoneal macrophages from Balb/c mice infected 72 hours previously with 10^7 amastigotes of *Leishmania donovani* were treated with either a supernatant from activated T cells (containing lymphokines) or a control supernatant. Cells treated with cytokines do not contain any parasites following culture (left) whereas untreated macrophages contain many parasites (right). (Courtesy of Dr H. Murray, with permission from *Journal of Immunology*, **129**, 344–357, © by American Association of Immunologists, 1982.)

production of H_2O_2, an O_2-independent mechanism is also active. That these findings *in vitro* reflect events that occur *in vivo* has been confirmed by experiments which show that mice treated with a monoclonal antibody that blocks the binding of IFNY to its receptor succumbed to infection by an avirulent strain of *T. gondii*. Peritoneal macrophages taken from the treated mice were not activated and supported multiplication of the parasite, whereas those from control mice were activated and resistant.

MACROPHAGES

Apart from acting as antigen-presenting cells in the initiation of an immune response, macrophages affect the course of parasitic infections in two ways.

1. They secrete molecules which act to regulate the inflammatory response. Some, like the cytokines interleukin-1 (IL-1), tumour necrosis factor (TNF) and the colony-stimulating factors, may enhance immunity by activating other cells or stimulating their proliferation; others like prostaglandins may be immunosuppressive.
2. They act as effector cells which inhibit the multiplication of parasites or destroy them.

Activation of macrophages is a general feature of the early stages of infection. Both immunoregulatory and effector functions are enhanced when macrophages are activated, for instance, by cytokines. Factors secreted by T cells (for example IFNY, GM-CSF, IL-3 and IL-4) may be mainly responsible, but not all activation is mediated by T cells. Some products of parasites, such as of *T. brucei* and of malarial parasites, can cause activation independently of T cells, perhaps directly or by inducing macrophages to secrete TNF, for example, which then activates other macrophages in an autocrine fashion.

Granulomata Formation in Liver and Fibrous Encapsulation In some parasitic infections in which the immune system cannot completely eliminate the parasite, the body reduces damage by walling off the parasite behind a capsule of inflammatory cells. This reaction, which is T-dependent, is a chronic cell-mediated response to locally released antigen. Macrophages accumulate, release fibrogenic factors and stimulate the formation of granulomatous tissue and ultimately fibrosis. Granuloma formation around worm eggs which have become trapped in the liver is particularly marked in schistosome infections. This reaction may benefit the host, in that it insulates the liver cells from toxic products secreted by the worm eggs, but it is also responsible for pathology, including the development of irreversible changes in the liver and the loss of liver function. In the absence of T cells, there is no granulomata formation and no subsequent fibrous encapsulation (Fig. 17.6).

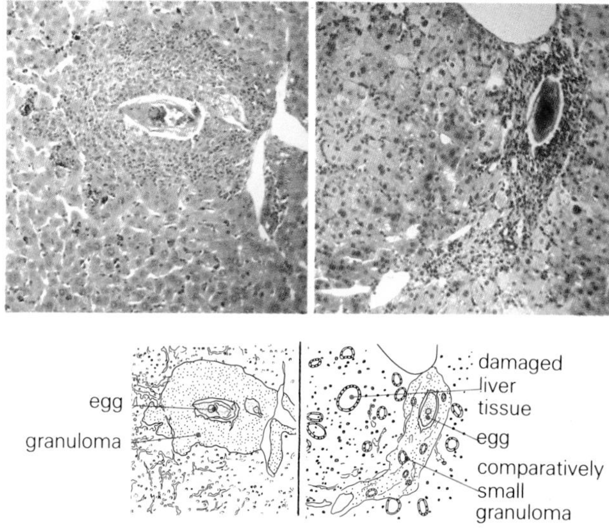

Fig. 17.6 T cell-dependence of granuloma formation around schistosome eggs in the liver. Many of the eggs of schistosome worms are carried to the liver where they become insulated behind a capsule of inflammatory cells. In normal mice, the granulomata consist predominantly of eosinophils and are the result of a T cell-dependent reaction (left). In T cell-deficient hosts, eggs of *Schistosoma mansoni* do not induce much granuloma formation and as a consequence of the lack of immune protection, toxic products of the eggs can diffuse out and cause damage to the surrounding liver tissue (right). (Courtesy Dr M. Doenhoff.)

Phagocytosis Phagocytosis is one of the primary functions of the macrophage important in host defence against the smaller parasite invaders and its effectiveness is markedly enhanced by opsonization of the organism to be ingested.

In addition, activated macrophages may express more Fc and C3 receptors, which also tend to enhance their phagocytic function. The rate of clearance of protozoan parasites from the blood is therefore greatly enhanced by the presence of specific antibody. Thus, African trypanosomes such as *T. brucei*, are quickly taken up by macrophages in the liver particularly when opsonized with antibody and C3b. Comparison of the resistance of strains of mice with various immunological defects to

T. rhodesiense infection shows that phagocytosis and destruction of parasites by macrophages is a major effector mechanism in trypanosomiasis.

Phagocytosis also provides a means of entry into macrophages for parasites that multiply inside those cells. Thus, promastigotes of *L. donovani,* the causative agent of visceral leishmaniasis, and of *L. major,* which causes cutaneous leishmaniasis, fix complement by the alternative pathway and then bind to CR3 receptors on the macrophage cell surface, which trigger their uptake by phagocytosis. Binding is blocked by monoclonal antibodies against the receptor. The parasites also bind to the mannose-fucose receptor on the macrophage surface, which acts similarly to facilitate their entry.

Parasite Killing Properties Macrophages secrete scores of soluble factors, many of which can be cytotoxic, and consequently they can also kill parasites by processes that do not depend upon ingestion; again, they have a greater capacity to do so when activated.

Activated macrophages are important in the control of infections, caused by, for example, *T. cruzi,* and *Leishmania* and *Plasmodium* spp. Macrophages are capable of killing not only relatively small extracellular parasites, such as the erythrocytic stages of the malarial parasite, but also, when activated, larger parasites such as the larval stages of schistosomes. They can also act as killer cells by antibody-mediated cytotoxicity; specific IgG and IgE, for instance, can enhance their ability to kill schistosomules.

When activated, macrophages are better able to resist infection by intracellular parasites which normally multiply within them, for example *Leishmania* and *T. cruzi,* and acquire the ability to eliminate already established parasites.

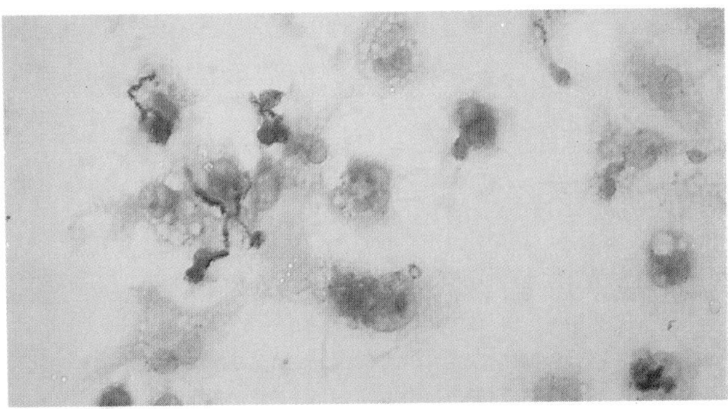

Fig. 17.7 The triggering of the respiratory burst of macrophages by *Leishmania donovani.* This picture shows a culture of resident peritoneal macrophages that have ingested promastigotes of *L. donovani* in the presence of nitroblue tetrazolium (NBT). The development of a black precipitate shows that the NBT has been reduced by products of the respiratory burst that was triggered by contact with the parasites, presumably by interaction with a specific receptor. More than 80% of promastigotes (the stages injected by the insect vector) are destroyed by normal macrophages but some escape from the phagolysosomes to become amastigotes. Amastigotes do not trigger the respiratory burst as effectively as promastigotes and survive well in normal macrophages. They can, however, be eradicated *in vitro* by incubation of the cells with lymphokines. Both stages are killed by H_2O_2 but not by the other O_2 metabolites. The promastigote is more sensitive to H_2O_2 than the amastigote. (Courtesy of Dr J. Blackwell.)

Perturbation of the membrane of macrophages, for instance during phagocytosis, can induce a respiratory burst, demonstrable by increased uptake of oxygen, activation of the hexose monophosphate shunt pathway and the production of oxygen metabolites (O_2^-, H_2O_2, OH·) that are cytotoxic and which kill bacteria and many parasites, including *T. cruzi, T. gondii, Leishmania* spp., malarial parasites, filarial worms and schistosomes (Fig. 17.7). Macrophages activated by cytokines release more superoxide and hydrogen peroxide than normal resident macrophages and their O_2-independent killing mechanisms are more potent; they also secrete various cytokines that interact with other types of cell to control parasite infections. For example, IL-1 and TNF (like IFNY) render hepatocytes resistant to the liver stage of infection of malarial parasites, and TNF can also decrease parasitaemia. Macrophages secrete other cytokines too which, like TNF and GM-CSF, increase the cytotoxicity of eosinophils for schistosomules.

GRANULOCYTES

Neutrophils Like macrophages, neutrophils are phagocytic cells that can kill a variety of parasites, large and small, and many of their effector properties are similar. They can kill by both O_2-dependent and independent mechanisms; they produce a more intense oxidative burst than macrophages and their secretory granules contain highly cytotoxic proteins. They too can be activated by cytokines, for example, producing more superoxide anion when pretreated with IFNY or TNF, and even more when pretreated with both factors together. Similarly, neutrophils when pretreated with GM-CSF kill the parasite *T. cruzi* more rapidly. Extracellular destruction in this case is mediated by an O_2-dependent mechanism that depends upon H_2O_2, since it is inhibited by catalase, whereas granule components are involved in intracellular destruction. Neutrophils are present in parasite-infected inflammatory lesions and probably act to clear parasites from bursting cells. Their membranes bear Fc receptors and receptors for complement that render them effective participants in antibody-dependent cytotoxic reactions. Thus they can kill the larvae of *S. mansoni* by mechanisms that are enhanced in the presence of antibody or complement and they may be more destructive than eosinophils against several species of nematode, including *T. spiralis,* although the relative effectiveness of the two types of cell may vary with the source of antibody.

Eosinophils Eosinophilia, and the production of high levels of IgE, are the common consequences of infection by parasitic worms and the eosinophil appears to be a major effector cell against helminths. It has been argued that the eosinophil has evolved especially as a defence against the tissue stages of parasites that are too large to be phagocytosed (for example, helminths) and that the IgE-dependent mast cell reaction has evolved primarily to localize eosinophils near the parasite and then enhance their anti-parasitic functions. The increase in the number of eosinophils in worm infections like schistosomiasis and ascariasis is T-dependent, and the cells show an enhancement in their state of activity; T cells also recruit eosinophils into the gut mucosa in worm infections of the gastrointestinal tract. The recruitment is mediated by a specific factor, eosinophil stimulation promoter (ESP) (Fig. 17.8). The importance of these effector cells *in vivo* has been shown by experiments using antiserum against eosinophils, in which, for example, mice infected with *T. spiralis* and treated with the antiserum developed more cysts in their muscles than controls; without protection by eosinophils the mice cannot eliminate the worms but encyst the parasites to minimize damage. Similarly, treatment of immune mice

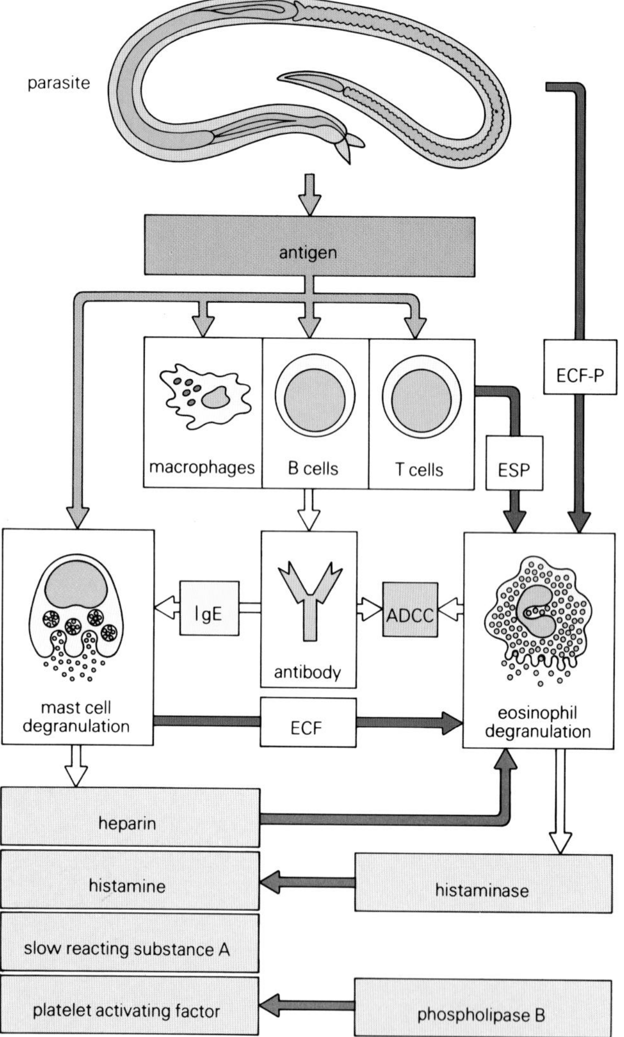

Fig. 17.8 The interaction of cells in response to a worm infection. Antigens released by the parasite stimulate T cells and macrophages to interact with B cells to produce specific antibody. IgE-specific antibody sensitizes local mast cells so that they degranulate when they come into contact with antigen, releasing a variety of effector molecules. The mast cells also release eosinophil chemotactic factors (ECF). Eosinophils are attracted towards the worm by parasite-derived chemotactic factors (ECF-P) and are stimulated to proliferate by eosinophil stimulation promotor (ESP) derived from antigen-stimulated T cells. The eosinophils act in two main ways:

1. in association with specific antibody they kill the worm by antibody-dependent cytotoxicity (ADCC)
2. enzymes released from the eosinophil granules exert a controlling effect on the substances released from the mast cells.

The mast cell-derived factors are important in controlling the permeability of local blood vessels and inflammation at the site of infection. Heparin inhibits eosinophil degranulation. (Green arrows indicate stimulation, and red arrows inhibition.)

with antiserum to eosinophils abrogated their ability to resist infection by *S. mansoni.*

Eosinophils are less phagocytic than neutrophils, but like neutrophils they can kill parasites by both O_2-dependent and independent mechanisms. They degranulate in response to perturbation of their surface membrane, so that their binding to the surface of the larvae of worms (for example *S. mansoni, T. spiralis*), especially when the larvae are coated with IgE or IgG, causes deposition of granule contents onto the surface of the worms and consequent destruction of the parasites. The antigens released cause local IgE-dependent degranulation of mast cells and the release of mediators which selectively attract eosinophils to the site and further enhance their activity. Other products of eosinophils later block the mast cell reactions.

MAST CELLS

Mast cell mediators appear to enhance the activity of other effector processes in worm infections. They interact with eosinophils as described above, and also play an important (though not essential) role in accelerating the expulsion of nematodes from the gut (Fig. 17.9). In response to local release of antigens, T cells induce a vast increase in the number of inflammatory

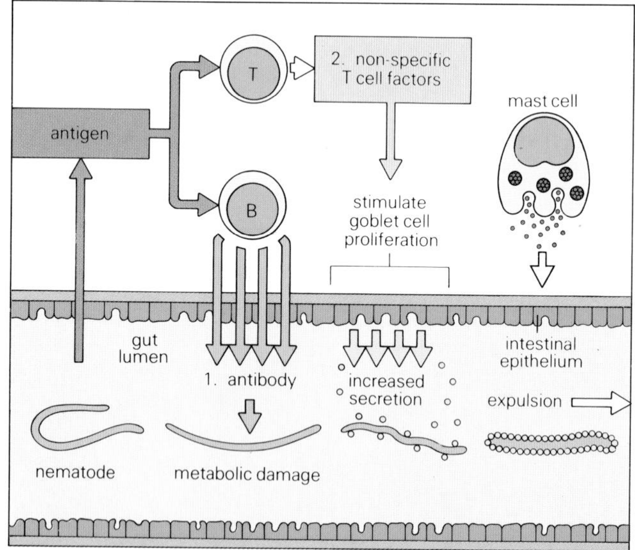

Fig. 17.9 Two-stage expulsion of nematodes from the gut. The expulsion of some intestinal nematodes occurs spontaneously a few weeks after a primary infection. It depends upon two sequential steps, following antigen sensitization of specific T cells and B cells.

1. The production of antibody which damages the worms but is not itself sufficient to cause their elimination,
2. A T cell-dependent secretory response. The T cells do not adhere directly to the worms but cause their expulsion through the release of non-specific factors acting on mucus-secreting goblet cells in the intestinal epithelium. The antigen-specific effector T cells are generated early in infection and the rate-limiting step is the onset of antibody damage. The numbers of goblet cells in the jejunal epithelium and the secretion of mucus increase in proportion to the worm burden.

Mast cells also accumulate in the jejunal mucosa during infection and secrete factors that accelerate expulsion but worms can be eliminated by mice deficient in mast cells.

cells, including monocytes, and of mucosal mast cells and goblet cells. They also promote enhanced secretion of mediators and of mucus, and provide help for the local accumulation of IgG, IgA and IgE. Mast cell products, including a proteinase, cause changes in the permeability of the gut and shedding of the epithelium which may help eject some protozoan parasites, for instance. In intestinal infections caused by nematodes, worms become embedded in mucus just before expulsion (Fig. 17.10). In a new host, the worms may bind to the gut wall, but in an immune animal they are trapped in mucus and fail to do so. Antibody and complement appear to promote mucus trapping and the effect of mast cell mediators in altering mucosal permeability allows leakage of serum antibodies and complement into the gut lumen. The mediators can also act on intestinal smooth muscle.

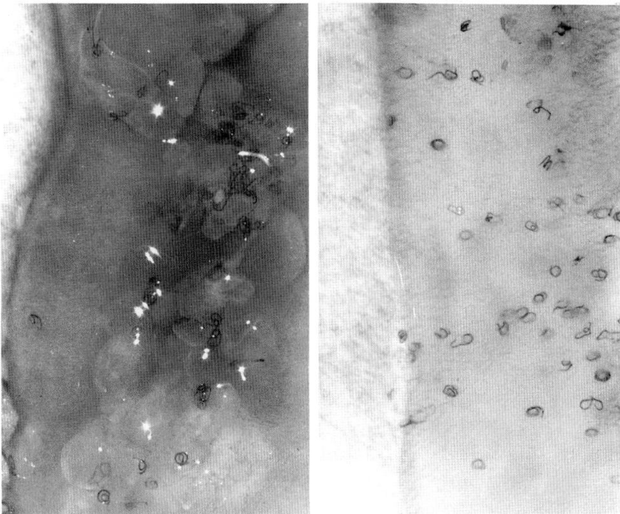

Fig. 17.10 Effect of mucus secretion on worm expulsion. Stereomicrographs of the intestine of rats challenged with 1000 intestinal worms (*Nippostrongylus brasiliensis*), 2 hours previously. Animals on the left were primed 18 days previously with a subcutaneous injection of the parasite; in these animals the worms become enveloped in globules of mucus. In unimmunized rats (right) the worms become attached to the wall of the intestine and there is no mucus production. (Courtesy of Dr H.R.P. Miller; with permission from *Immunology* 1981, **44**, 419–429.)

PLATELETS

Platelets are capable of killing various types of parasite, including schistosomules, *T. gondii* and *T. cruzi,* and like other effector cells their cytotoxic activity is enhanced by treatment with cytokines (for example, IFNγ, TNF). Platelets become activated to be larvacidal during infection of rats with *S. mansoni,* before antibody can be detected but when acute phase reactants appear in the serum, and incubation of normal platelets in such serum can cause their activation. Furthermore, they also bear Fc receptors for IgE on their surface membrane, by which they mediate antibody-dependent cytotoxicity.

ANTIBODIES

In addition to the rise in specific antibodies, many parasite infections provoke a non-specific hypergammaglobulinaemia. While specific responses are mostly T cell-dependent, much of the non-specific antibody production is probably due to antigens released from the parasites acting as B cell mitogens. Specific antibody is particularly important in the control of extracellular parasites. Thus, antibody is effective in preventing the reinvasion of cells by blood-borne parasites but is ineffective once the parasite has entered its host cell. The importance of antibody-dependent relative to antibody-independent varies with the infection (Fig. 17.11). The mechanism by which specific antibody controls parasite

parasite and habitat		antibody-dependent			antibody-independent	
		importance	mechanism	means of evasion	importance	mechanism
T. brucei free in blood		++++	lysis with complement which opsonizes for phagocytosis	antigenic variation	–	
Plasmodium inside red cell		+++	blocks invasion, opsonizes for phagocytosis	intracellular antigenic variation	liver stage +++ blood stage +++	cytokines macrophage activation
T. cruzi inside macrophage		++	limits spread in acute infection, sensitizes for ADCC	intracellular habitat	+++ (chronic phase)	macrophage activation by cytokines and killing by metabolites of O_2
Leishmania inside macrophage		+	limits spread	intracellular habitat	++++	

Fig. 17.11 Relative importance of antibody-dependent and -independent responses in protozoal infections. This table summarizes the relative importance of the two immune responses, the mechanisms involved and, for antibody, the means by which the protozoan can evade damage by antibody. Antibody is the most important part of the immune response against those parasites that live in the bloodstream, such as African trypanosomes and malarial parasites, whereas cell-mediated immunity is active against those like *Leishmania* that live in the tissues. Antibody can damage parasites directly, enhance their clearance by phagocytosis, activate complement or block their entry into their host cell and so limit the spread of infection. Once inside, the parasite is safe from its effects. *Trypanosoma cruzi* and *Leishmania* are both susceptible to the action of oxygen metabolites released by the respiratory burst of macrophages. Treating macrophages with cytokines enhances release of these products and diminishes entry and survival of the parasites. Malarial parasites within the red cell may be destroyed by some products of activated macrophages, including hydrogen peroxide and other cytotoxic factors; their importance in immunity to the disease is still under investigation.

infections and its effects are summarized in Fig. 17.12 and are as follows.

1. Antibody can act directly on protozoa to damage them, either by itself or by interacting with the complement system (Fig. 17.13).

2. Antibody can neutralize a parasite directly by blocking its attachment to a new host cell. This effect can be observed in the case of *Plasmodium* spp.; the merozoites enter red blood cells through a special receptor and their entry is inhibited by specific antibody (Fig. 17.14). Antibody may also act to prevent spread, for example in the acute phase of infection with *T. cruzi*.

3. Antibody can enhance phagocytosis mediated by Fc receptors on macrophages. Phagocytosis (mediated by C3 receptors) of the parasites is increased even more by addition of complement. Both Fc and C3 receptors may themselves be increased in number as a result of macrophage activation. Phagocytosis plays an important role in the control of infections with *Plasmodium* and *T. brucei*.

4. Antibody is also involved in antibody-dependent cytotoxicity, for example, in infections caused by *T. cruzi, T. spiralis, S. mansoni* and filarial worms. Cytotoxic cells such as macrophages, neutrophils and eosinophils adhere to worms coated with antibody by means of Fc and C3 receptors (Fig. 17.15). Damage to schistosomes is caused by the major basic protein (MBP) of the eosinophil crystalloid core (Fig. 17.16). Destructive effects are non-specific but the release of the MBP into a small space between the eosinophil and the schistosome surface localizes its action and minimizes damage to bystanding host cells (Fig. 17.17). The cells damage the tegument of the worms and kill them. Different kinds of cell and of antibody may act at different stages in the life cycle. For example, eosinophils are more effective at killing the newborn larvae of *T. spiralis* than other cells, macrophages are more effective against the microfilariae, and in each case antibody mediating the reaction is stage-specific. IgG can mediate killing by eosinophils, and IgE, killing by macrophages. Killing of *S. mansoni* by eosinophils is enhanced by mast cell products and eosinophils from patients with schistosomiasis are more effective than those from normal subjects. The importance of these effector mechanisms *in vivo* has been shown in monkeys, in which schistosome killing is associated with eosinophil accumulation (Fig. 17.18).

parasite	*Plasmodium* sporozoite, intestinal worms, trypanosome	*Plasmodium* sporozoite, merozoite, *T. cruzi* *T. gondii*	*Plasmodium*, trypanosome	schistosomes, *T. spiralis*, filarial worms
mechanism	1	2 *Plasmodium* schizonts in red cells merozoites released invasion of new red cell	3	4 larval worm
effect	direct damage or complement-mediated lysis	prevents spread by neutralizing attachment site, prevents escape from lysosomal vacuole, prevents inhibition of lysosomal fusion	enhancement of phagocytosis	antibody-dependent cytotoxicity (ADCC)

Fig. 17.12 Control of parasite infections by specific antibody. 1. Direct damage caused by antibody activating the classical pathway of complement causes damage to the parasite membrane and increased susceptibility to other mediators. 2. Neutralization. For example, parasites such as *Plasmodium* spp. spread to new cells by specific receptor attachment; blocking the merozoite binding site with antibody prevents attachment to the receptors on the erythrocyte surface and hence further multiplication. 3. Enhancement of phagocytosis. Complement C3b deposited on parasite membrane opsonizes it for phagocytosis by cells with C3b receptors (e.g. macrophages). Macrophages also have Fc receptors. 4. Eosinophils, neutrophils, platelets and macrophages may be cytotoxic for some parasites when they recognize the parasite via specific antibody (ADCC). The reaction is enhanced by complement.

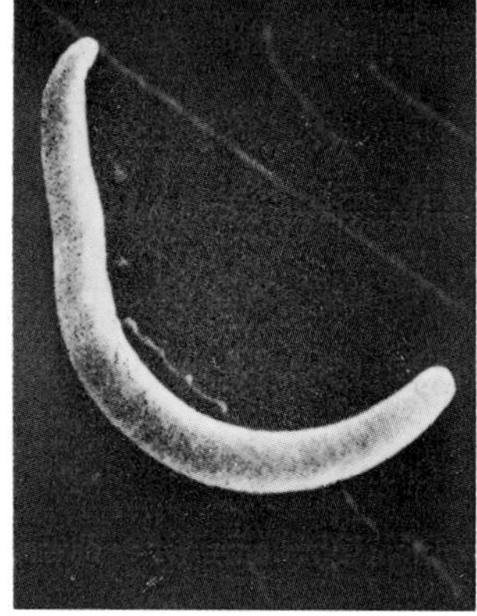

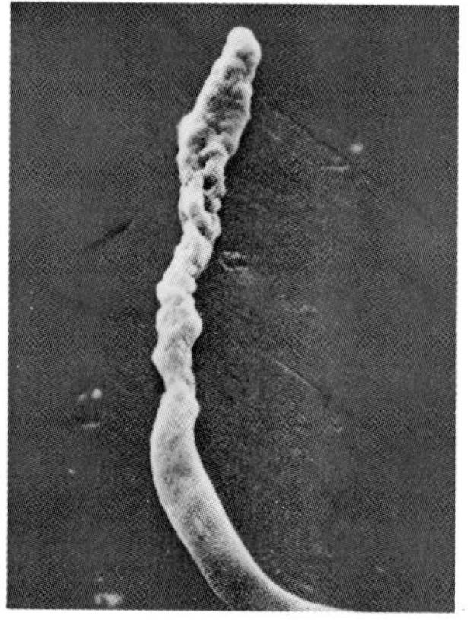

Fig. 17.13 Direct effect of specific antibody on sporozoites of malarial parasites. These scanning electron micrographs show a sporozoite of *Plasmodium berghei*, which causes malaria in rodents, before (left) and after incubation in immune serum (right). The surface of the parasite is damaged. Specific antibody protects against infection with *Plasmodium* spp. at several of the extracellular stages of the life cycle and the antibody is stage-specific in each case. Specific antibody perturbs the outer membrane of the sporozoite, causing leakage of fluid. (Courtesy of Dr R. Nussenzweig.)

In many infections it is difficult to distinguish between cell-mediated and antibody-mediated responses since both act in concert against the parasite. This is illustrated in Fig. 17.19 which summarizes the immune reactions which may occur against schistosomes.

NON-SPECIFIC EFFECTOR MECHANISMS

A variety of non-specific effector mechanisms act in parasitic infections. The blood phagocytes, both monocytes and granulocytes, and tissue macrophages all have some intrinsic anti-parasite activity although this is greatly enhanced by interaction with the different parts of the adaptive immune system, particularly antibody. It has also been postulated that NK cells may be active in some infections though this is still unproven.

Of the serum-soluble factors, complement has already been mentioned for its interaction with specific antibody via the classical pathway. Several parasites, including adult worms and infective larvae of *T. spiralis* and schistosomules of *S. mansoni*, activate the alternative pathway directly. This function is dependent on the nature of the molecules in their surface coats. The activation of the alternative pathway varies according to both the species of host and the species of parasite.

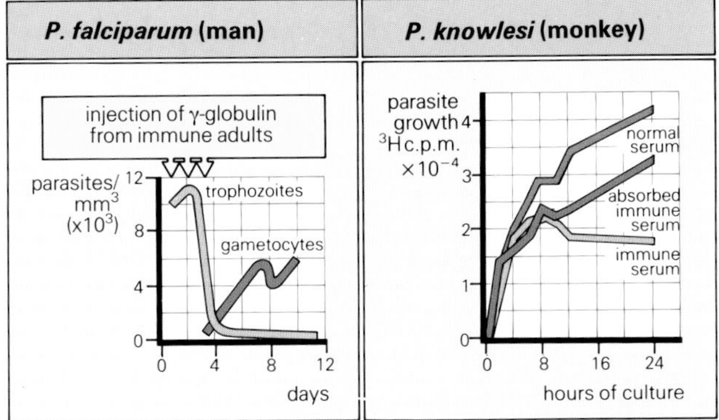

Fig. 17.14 Effect of antibody on malarial parasites. *Plasmodium falciparum.* In man, transfer of γ-globulin from immune adults to a child infected with *P. falciparum* caused a sharp drop in parasitaemia. Specific antibody acts at the merozoite stage in the life of the parasite and prevents the initiation of further cycles of multiplication in the blood. The development of gametocytes from existing intracellular forms is unaffected.
P. knowlesi. In culture, the presence of immune serum blocks the continued increase in number of *P. knowlesi* (a malarial parasite of monkeys), as measured by incorporation of ^{3}H-leucine. It stops multiplication at the stage after schizont rupture by preventing the released merozoites invading fresh red blood cells. The inhibitory activity of the immune serum can be reduced by absorbing the specific antibody with free schizonts.

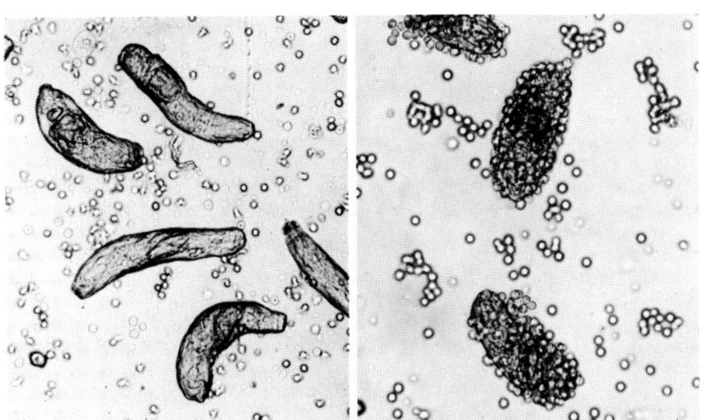

Fig. 17.15 Antibody-dependent cytotoxicity against schistosomes mediated by neutrophils. These photographs show schistosomules of *Schistosoma mansoni* incubated with neutrophils in the presence of normal rat serum (left) and in the presence of fresh immune serum containing active complement (right). The adherence of neutrophils to the surface of the larva, mediated by antibody and complement is demonstrated, and is the first step in the killing of the parasite. The worm is probably killed by hydrogen peroxide and other oxygen metabolites released from the neutrophil during the respiratory burst that follows the membrane perturbation resulting from contact between parasite and neutrophil. Neutrophils from patients with chronic granulomatous disease that are incapable of generating hydrogen peroxide are markedly impaired in their ability to kill schistosomules. (Courtesy of Dr D. McLaren.)

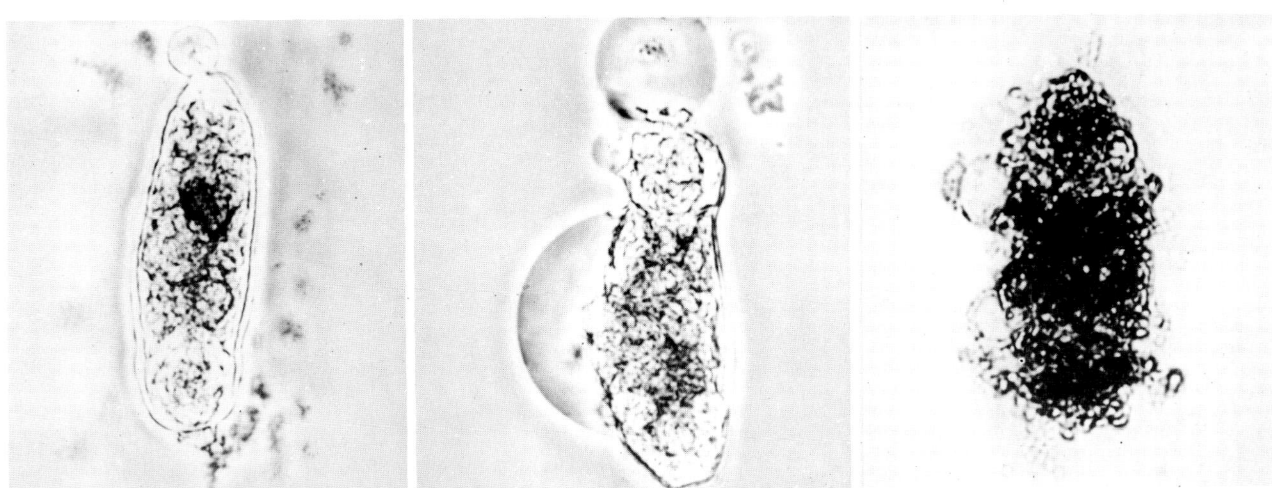

Fig. 17.16 Effect of basic protein of eosinophils on schistosomule larva. Killing of schistosomules by eosinophils can be associated with the major basic protein of the granules. These pictures show progressive surface damage and disruption of a larva caused by incubation in this cell product: intact worm (left), initial stage of damage to the tegument and worm surface (middle), total destruction of the worm (right). (Courtesy of Dr D. McLaren.)

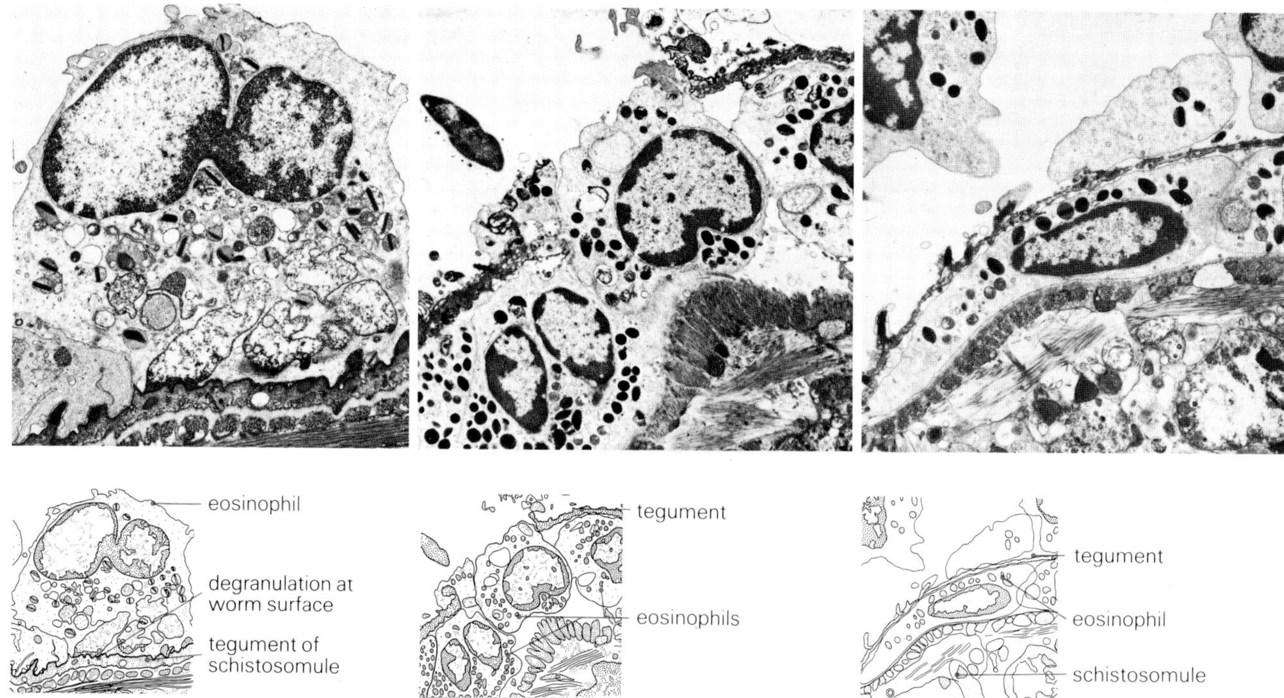

Fig. 17.17 Killing of schistosome larvae by eosinophils. Eosinophils can adhere to schistosomules and kill them. The damage is associated with degranulation of the eosinophils and the release of the contents of the granules onto the surface of the worm. This series of electronmicrographs shows adherence of the eosinophil and degranulation onto the surface of the worm larva (left), and stages in the formation of lesions in the worm tegument and migration of eosinophils through the lesions (middle, right). (Courtesy of Dr D. McLaren).

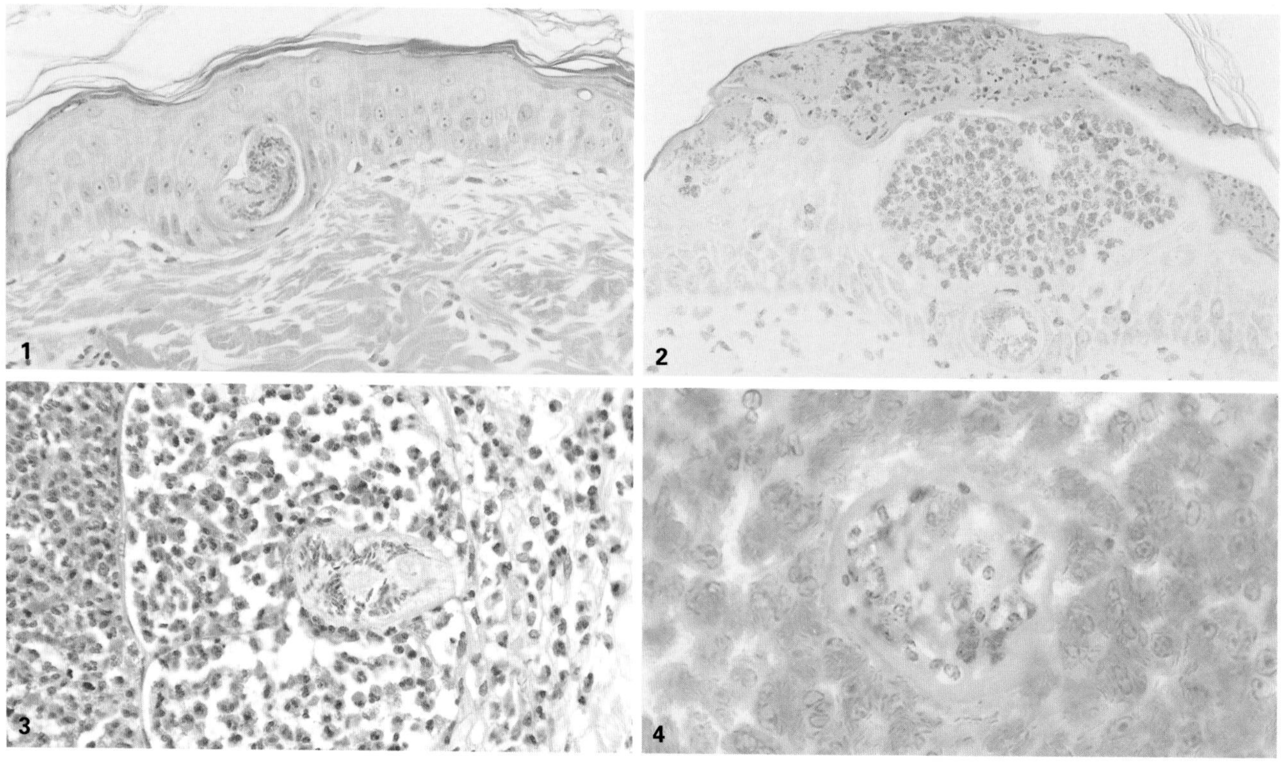

Fig. 17.18 Immunity to *Schistosoma mansoni in vivo.* Normal or previously infected baboons were infected percutaneously with 1000 cercariae of *S. mansoni*.
1. In control animals at 72 hours after challenge, there is no inflammatory or immune reaction and the schistosomes lie just above the basement membrane (H&E, x 160).
2. In animals infected 2 years previously, an inflammatory infiltration surrounds the schistosome by 24 hours after the challenge, and is predominantly eosinophilic (Giemsa, x 160).
3. In the immune animal 24 hours after challenge the schistosomule is trapped in an abscess of adherent eosinophils (Giesma, x 250).
4. The same animal as (3) showing a killed parasite in which the eosinophils have invaded its interior. (x 640).
(Courtesy of Dr B.J. Cottrell and Dr H.M. Seitz.)

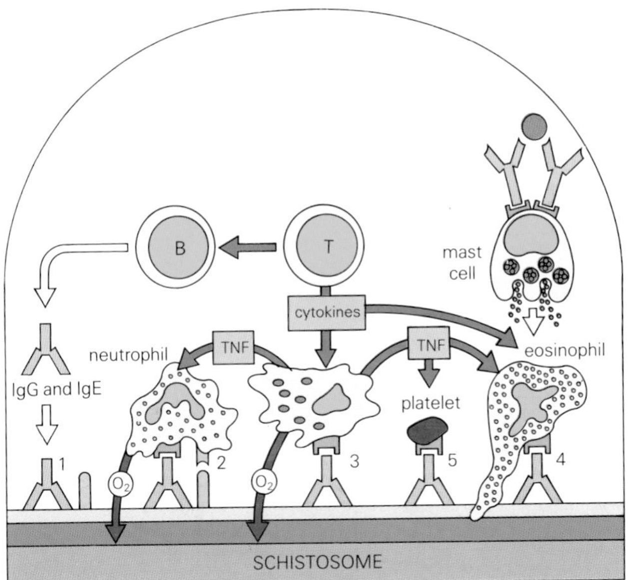

Fig. 17.19 Coordinated response to schistosomules. This diagram illustrates the various effector mechanisms that have been shown to damage schistosomes *in vitro*. Antibody and complement at high levels damage worms (1), and at lower levels antibody sensitizes neutrophils (2), macrophages (3), eosinophils (4) and platelets (5) for antibody-dependent cytotoxicity. Neutrophils and macrophages probably act by releasing toxic oxygen products, whereas eosinophils damage the worm tegument by release of major basic protein. The response is potentiated by cytokines (e.g. TNF) and IgE antibody is important both in sensitizing eosinophils and in sensitizing local mast cells, which release a variety of mediators, including mediators which activate the eosinophils.

ESCAPE MECHANISMS

It is a characteristic of all successful parasite infections that they can, in different ways, evade the full effects of the host's immune responses.

INTRINSIC RESISTANCE

Many parasites are protected from the host's defences by their anatomical inaccessibility. For example, those that have an intracellular habitat avoid the effects of antibody (for example *T. cruzi, Leishmania* spp. and the intracellular stages of *Plasmodium* spp.). Other parasites are protected by cysts (for example *T. spiralis, Entamoeba histolytica*) or live in the gut (intestinal nematodes). Those that live inside macrophages have evolved different ways of avoiding killing by oxygen metabolites and lysosomal enzymes (Figs 17.20 and 17.21).

Some parasites, for example *T. gondii*, avoid triggering the oxidative burst while others break down its products. These escape mechanisms are of more limited efficiency in the immune host. The ability to resist destruction by complement, for instance, may correlate with virulence. Thus *L. tropica* is easily killed by complement and causes a localized self-healing infection in the skin whereas *L. donovani* which is ten times more resistant to complement becomes disseminated throughout the viscera, causing a disease which is often fatal.

AVOIDANCE OF RECOGNITION

Parasites that may be exposed to antibody have evolved different methods of evading its effects. African trypanosomes, by antigenic variation, change the antigens of

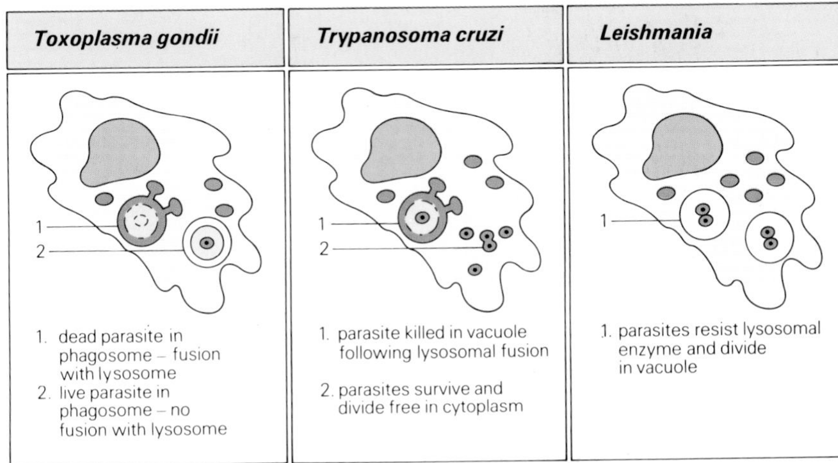

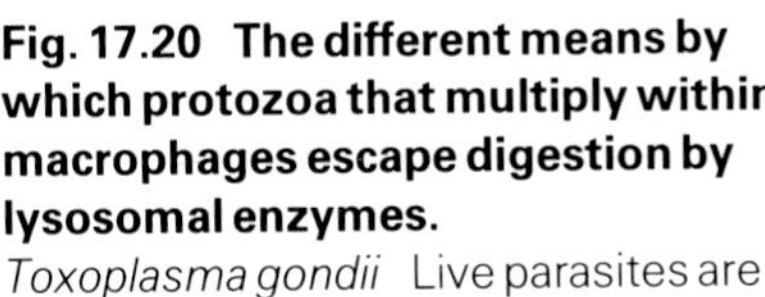

Fig. 17.20 The different means by which protozoa that multiply within macrophages escape digestion by lysosomal enzymes.
Toxoplasma gondii Live parasites are not exposed to the enzymes because fusion of secondary lysosomes with the phagosomal vacuole within which the parasites live is inhibited. Dead parasites – or those coated with antibody – lose the capacity to block fusion and are destroyed.
Trypanosoma cruzi Survival of these parasites depends upon their stage of development; trypomastigotes escape from the vacuole and divide in the cytoplasm whereas epimastigotes do not escape and are killed and digested. The proportion of parasites found in the cytoplasm is decreased if the macrophages are activated.
Leishmania spp. These parasites multiply in the phagocytic vacuole where they resist digestion. If the macrophages are first activated by treatment with lymphokines, the number of parasites entering the cell and the number that replicate diminish.

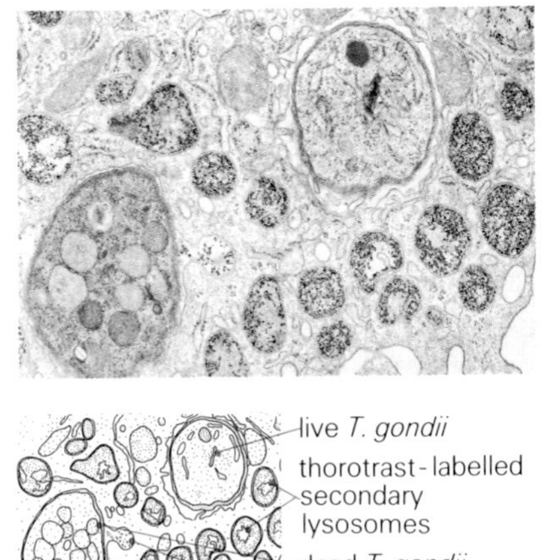

Fig. 17.21 Electronmicrograph showing a macrophage infected with *Toxoplasma gondii*. Following infection the macrophages are treated with thorotrast to make the contents of secondary lysosomes electron dense. The live parasite has inhibited fusion of the secondary lysosome with the phagosome. A dead parasite lies in a vacuole that contains thorotrast; it can be seen that a lysosome has just fused with the vacuole and emptied its contents into it. x 14,000 (Courtesy of Professor T. C. Jones.)

their surface coat (Fig. 17.22). Each variant possesses an antigenically distinct glycoprotein which forms its surface coat. The immunological uniqueness of these glycoproteins reflects diversity in amino acid sequence. Glycoproteins are identified on the organism by immunofluorescence or by radioimmunoassay of extracts. The surface coat presumably protects the underlying surface membrane from the host's defence mechanisms. Malarial parasites also show antigenic variation. Other parasites acquire a surface layer of host antigens so that the host does not distinguish them from 'self' (for example *Schistosoma* spp., Fig. 17.23). Schistosomules cultured *in vitro* in medium containing human serum and red blood cells can acquire surface molecules con-

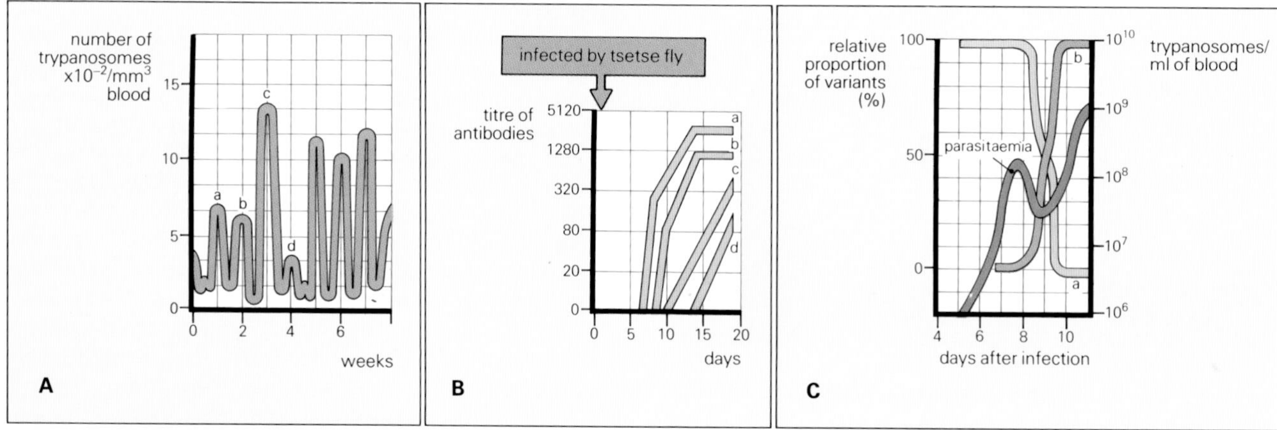

Fig. 17.22 Antigenic variation in African trypanosomes. Trypanosome infections, which can be initiated by a single parasite, may run for several months giving rise to successive waves of parasitaemia. Graph A shows a chart of the fluctuations in parasitaemia in a patient with sleeping sickness. Each wave is caused by an immunologically distinct population of parasites (a, b, c, d); protection is not afforded by antibody against preceding variants. There is a strong tendency for new variants to appear in the same order in different hosts. Variation does not occur in immunologically compromised animals, that is, treated in order to deprive the animal of some aspect of its immune function). Graph B shows the time course of production of antibody against four variants in a rabbit bitten by a tsetse fly carrying *Trypanosoma brucei*. Antibody to successive variants appears shortly after the appearance of the variant and rises to a plateau. The appearance of antibody drives the parasite towards another variant type. Graph C shows the kinetics of one cycle of antigenic variation in a rat infected with a homogeneous population of one variant (a) of *T. brucei*. The new wave of parasitaemia develops as the new variant (b) emerges and predominates.

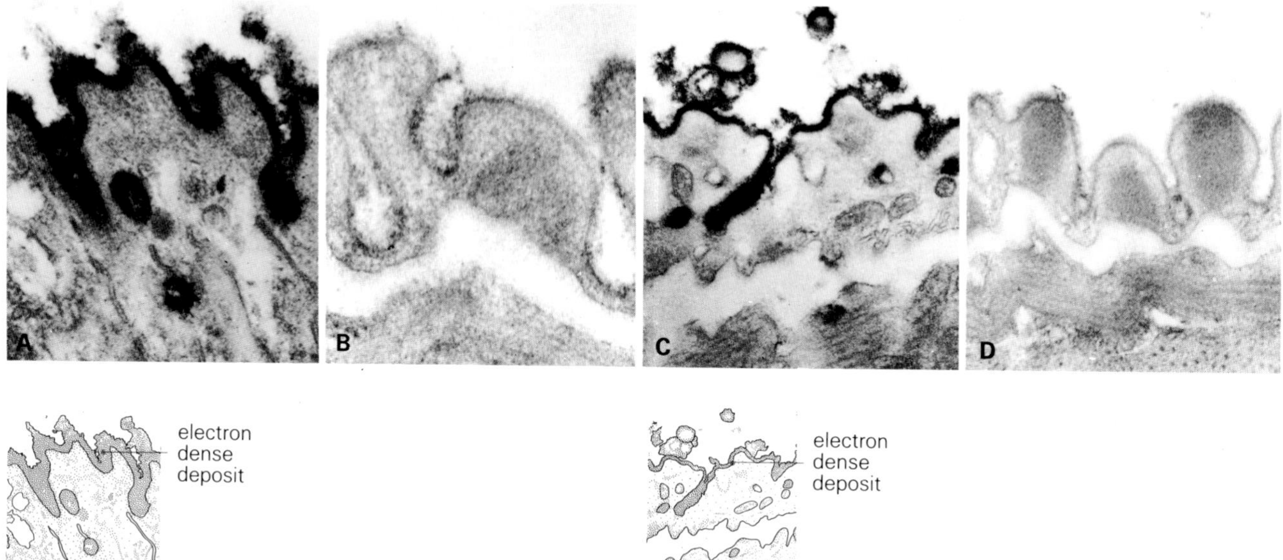

Fig. 17.23 Acquisition of host antigens by schistosomes. These electronmicrographs show sections of the surface of schistosomes that have been incubated with labelled antibody against schistosome antigens or against mouse red blood cells. Presence of each antigen is shown by the layer of electron-dense deposit of labelled antibody. Young 3-hour schistosomules bind specific antibody *in vitro* (A) but not after 4 days in a mouse host (B). Antibody against mouse antigens binds to the 4-day-old lung stage parasite (C) but not to the newly transformed schistosomules (D). Thus, older worms express the species-specific antigens of their host but not their own antigens. Lung stage worms are immune to attack by complement and antibody-mediated effectors *in vitro*. Worms transferred from one species to another die within 24 hours. They are only susceptible to attack by specific antibody *in vitro* if they are not coated with host protective antigens, whereas antibody to host red cell antigens causes severe damage to the worm surface. (Courtesy of Dr D. McLaren.)

taining A, B and H specific blood group determinants. They can also acquire antigens of the MHC. Acquisition of host molecules may protect the parasite from damage by antibody while within that host. Schistosomules maintained in medium devoid of host molecules, however, also become refractory to attack by antibody and complement so that changes in the parasite tegument occur that are independent of the adsorption of host antigens. Thus, the relative importance of this antigen masking in protection from recognition is hard to assess.

SUPPRESSION OF THE HOST'S IMMUNE RESPONSE

Parasites can cause disruption of lymphoid cells or tissue directly. For example, newborn larvae of *T. spiralis*

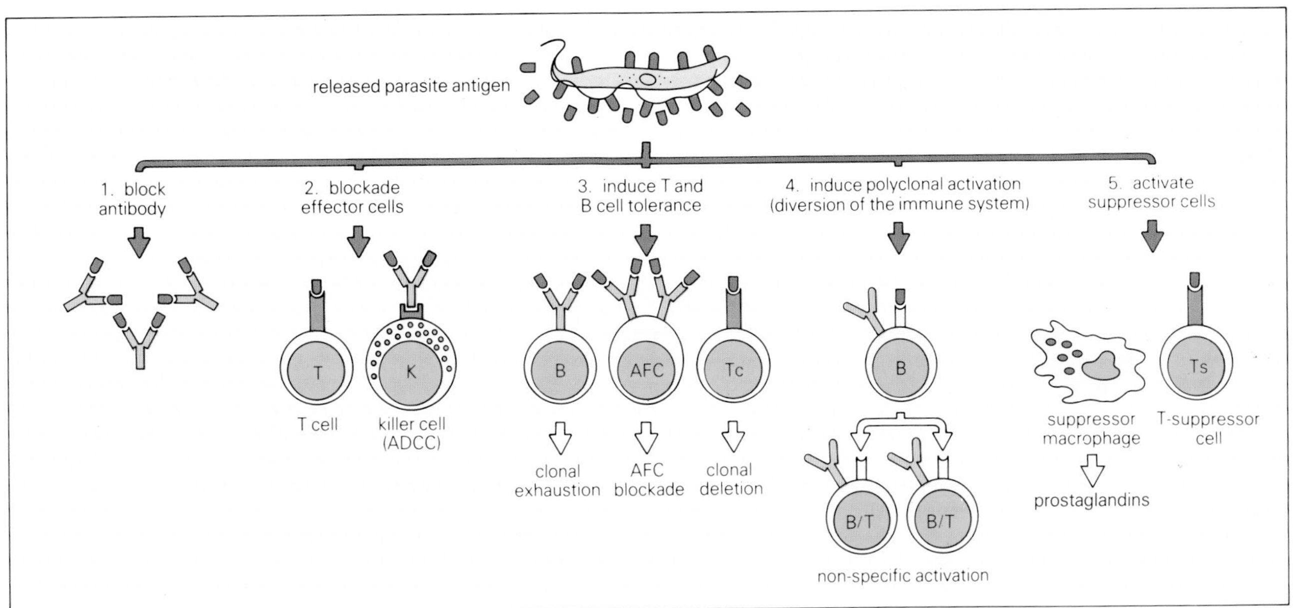

Fig. 17.24 Interference with host's immune response by antigens released from the parasite.
1. By combining with antibody and diverting it from the parasite.
2. By blockading effector cells, either directly or as immune complexes formed by combination with antibody. Circulating complexes for example, are able to inhibit the action of cytotoxic cells active against *Schistosoma mansoni.*
3. By inducing T or B cell tolerance, presumably by blockade of antibody-forming cells (AFC) or by depletion of the mature antigen-specific lymphocytes (i.e. clonal exhaustion).
4. By polyclonal activation. Many parasite products are mitogenic to B or T lymphocytes, and the high serum concentrations of non-specific IgM (and IgG) commonly found in parasitic infections probably result from this polyclonal stimulation. Its continuation is believed to lead to impairment of B cell function, the progressive depletion of antigen-reactive B lymphocytes and thus immunosuppression.
5. By activating suppressor cells, which may be T cells or macrophages or both.

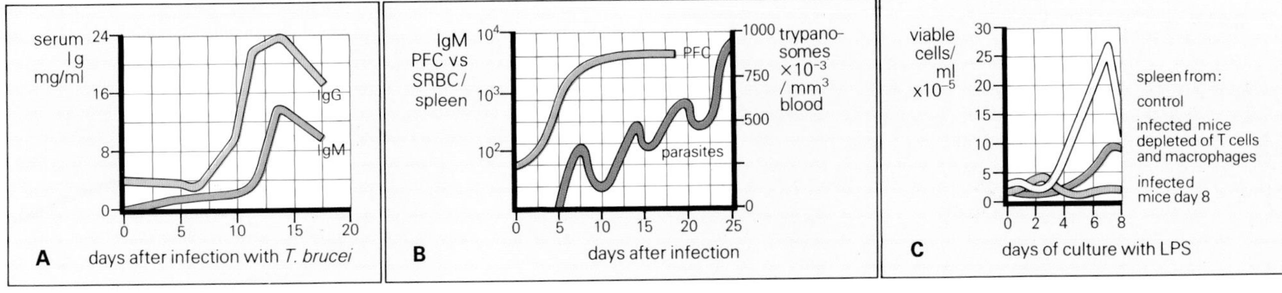

Fig. 17.25 Polyclonal activation by African trypanosomes. Graph A shows increasing concentrations of serum immunoglobulins observed in mice infected with *Trypanosoma brucei*. These levels are only consistent with polyclonal activation and not specific antibody alone. Graph B shows the increase in number of IgM-secreting cells forming plaques with sheep red blood cells (SRBC) that occurs spontaneously during infection, that is, without injection of SRBC. The number increases with the parasitaemia to reach a plateau of 20–30 times normal. Cells secreting antibody against other antigens, increase similarly. Soluble fractions derived from parasites have been shown to be mitogenic, their activity being enhanced by macrophages. Trypanosomes (and other parasites) thus cause proliferation of B lymphocytes and this may lead to the progressive depletion of antigen-reactive B cells. Graph C shows the failure of spleen lymphocytes taken from infected mice (at day 8) to proliferate in response to stimulation by lipopolysaccharide *in vitro*. Removal of T cells and macrophages from spleens taken soon after infection partly restores the response, but not later on when the B cell potential appears to become exhausted. Macrophages collected early in infection depress the ability of normal spleen cells to respond to LPS. Thus, the clonal exhaustion of B lymphocytes that have been stimulated directly to proliferate by parasites is partly mediated by the generation of suppressive macrophages and T cells.

release a soluble lymphocytotoxic factor. Similarly, schistosomes can cleave a peptide from IgG that inhibits many cellular immune responses. Soluble parasite antigens which can occur in enormous quantities may reduce the effectiveness of the host's response by a process termed immune distraction. Non-specific immunosuppression is a universal feature of parasite infection (Figs 17.24 and 17.25) and has been demonstrated for both antibody (Fig. 17.26) and cell-mediated responses. Much of the suppression of immune responses may be due to macrophage dysfunction associated with antigen overload. For example in mice infected with African trypanosomes, IL-1 production and antigen-presenting capacity are reduced. Macrophages also release prostaglandins which suppress some inflammatory reactions.

Specific suppression may also occur, as has been demonstrated in leishmaniasis (Fig. 17.27). In this case immunosuppression of T cell reactivity is harmful to the host because protection depends on cell-mediated immunity. Experiments have demonstrated that elimination of the suppressor cells allows mice to recover from the infection. However, immunosuppression may benefit both the host and parasite, as is seen in schistosomiasis. Many immune responses are depressed in this infection. The activity of T-helper cells is suppressed, as shown by decreased antibody responses to sheep red blood cells or to tetanus toxoid, and specific delayed hypersensitivity is suppressed, as shown by diminished foot pad responses to challenge by soluble worm egg antigen. Lymphocyte proliferation in response to mitogens such as a phytohaemagglutinin or concanavalin A is depressed. A factor produced by the worm inhibits lymphocyte proliferation directly and the existence of both suppressor T cells and suppressive macrophages has been demonstrated. Liver granulomata caused by schistosome eggs diminish in size with time

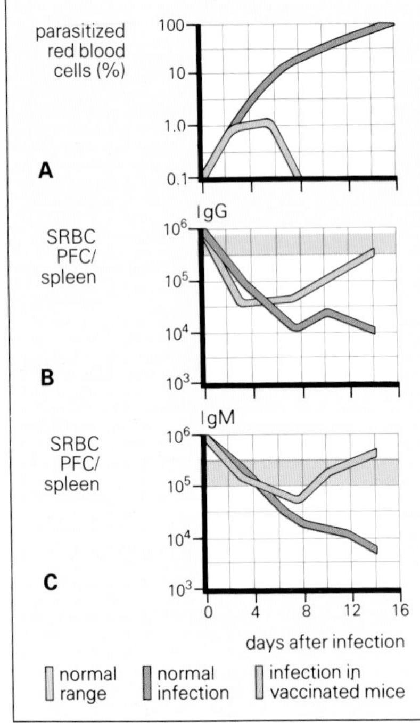

Fig. 17.26 Depression of non-specific antibody production in mice with malaria. Graph A (above) shows the course of parasitaemia in unvaccinated and vaccinated mice infected with a lethal variant of *Plasmodium yoelii;* unvaccinated mice die about 16 days later, vaccinated mice survive and all parasites disappear from the blood by 8 days. The time course of parasitaemia correlates with the immunosuppression. Graphs B and C show numbers of IgM- and IgG-plaque forming cells (PFC)/spleen obtained 5 days after infection of sheep red blood cells (SRBC) into two groups of mice. Antibody-producing cells decrease during infection and in vaccinated mice they return to normal as the mice recover. The depression of PFC, appears to reflect parasite load. Its mechanism is unknown.

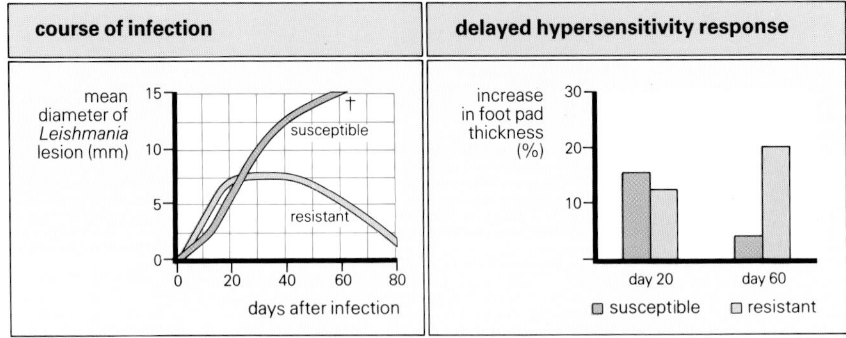

Fig. 17.27 Depression of specific delayed hypersensitivity in mice infected with *Leishmania*. The course of infection of *L. tropica*, as determined by the size of infection, is plotted for a susceptible strain and a resistant strain of mouse. Mice of the susceptible strain die about 70 days after infection. Delayed hypersensitivity to specific antigen injected into the footpad is illustrated as the percentage increase in footpad thickness. In resistant mice the response increases as the mice recover, whereas it is significantly depressed in the susceptible mice. The depression is antigen-specific and is mediated by cells which inhibit delayed hypersensitivity, but not antibody production. Recovery from this infection is associated with cell-mediated immunity.

parasite	habitat	effector	method of avoidance
African trypanosome	bloodstream	antibody + complement	antigenic variation
Plasmodium spp.	liver (hepatocytes) blood cell	cytokines antibody	intracellular habitat, antigenic variation
Toxoplasma gondii	macrophage	O_2 metabolites lysosomal enzymes	failure to trigger, inhibits fusion of lysosomes
Trypanosoma cruzi	macrophage	O_2 metabolites lysosomal enzymes	unknown escapes into cytoplasm avoids digestion
Leishmania	macrophage	O_2 metabolites lysosomal enzymes	O_2 burst impaired avoids digestion
Trichinella spiralis	gut, blood muscles	myeloid cells antibody+complement	encystment in muscle
Schistosoma mansoni	skin, blood, lungs portal vein	myeloid cells antibody+complement	acquisition of host antigens, blockade by soluble antigen and immune complexes

Fig. 17.28 Examples of ways evolved by parasites to avoid host defences.

and it is thought that diminishing local production of cytokines and eosinophil stimulation promoter may explain the decrease in size of the granulomata. This immunosuppression is to the benefit of both host and parasite because although extensive granulomata damage the host's liver, some macrophage accumulation is helpful in protecting the tissue against the toxic secretions of the egg. Some of the escape mechanisms discussed above are summarized in Fig. 17.28.

IMMUNOPATHOLOGICAL CONSEQUENCES OF PARASITE INFECTIONS

Apart from the directly destructive effects of some parasites and their products on host tissues, many immune responses themselves have pathological effects.

The IgE of worm infections can have severe effects on the host through the release of mast cell mediators; anaphylactic shock may occur when a hydatid cyst ruptures, and asthma-like reactions occur in *Toxicara canis* infections and in tropical eosinophilia when filarial worms migrate through the lungs.

The formation of immune complexes is common; they may be deposited in the kidney, as in the nephrotic syndrome of quartan malaria, and may give rise to many other pathological changes. For example, tissue-bound immunoglobulins have been found in the muscles of mice infected with African trypanosomes and in the choroid plexus of mice with malaria.

Autoantibodies, which probably arise as a result of polyclonal activation, have been detected against red blood cells, lymphocytes and DNA (for example in trypanosomiasis and in malaria). Antibodies against the parasite may cross-react with host tissues. For example, the cardiomyopathy, enlarged oesophagus and megacolon that occur in Chagas' disease are thought to result from the autoimmune effects on nerve ganglia of antibody or of cytotoxic T cells that cross-react with *T. cruzi.*

The splenomegaly and hepatomegaly of malaria, sleeping sickness and visceral leishmaniasis are all associated with increases in the numbers and activity of macrophages and lymphocytes in the liver and spleen. The enlarged liver and its fibrosis in schistosomiasis are a consequence of granulomata formation around the worm eggs, resembling a delayed hypersensitivity reaction (Fig. 17.6)

Excess production of some cytokines may contribute to some of the manifestations of disease. Thus the fever, anaemia, diarrhoea and pulmonary changes of acute malaria closely resemble the symptoms of endotoxaemia and are probably caused by tumour necrosis factor (TNF). Furthermore the development of cerebral malaria in mice has been shown to be inhibited by antibody to TNF. The severe wasting of cattle with trypanosomiasis also appears to be TNF-mediated. Many of the immunological mechanisms may be combined in their pathological effects, as is likely in the case of the anaemia of malaria (Fig. 17.29).

Lastly, the non-specific immunosuppression that is so universal, probably explains why people with parasite infections are especially susceptible to bacterial infections and to viral infections (for example measles) and it may account for the association of Burkitt's lymphoma with malaria.

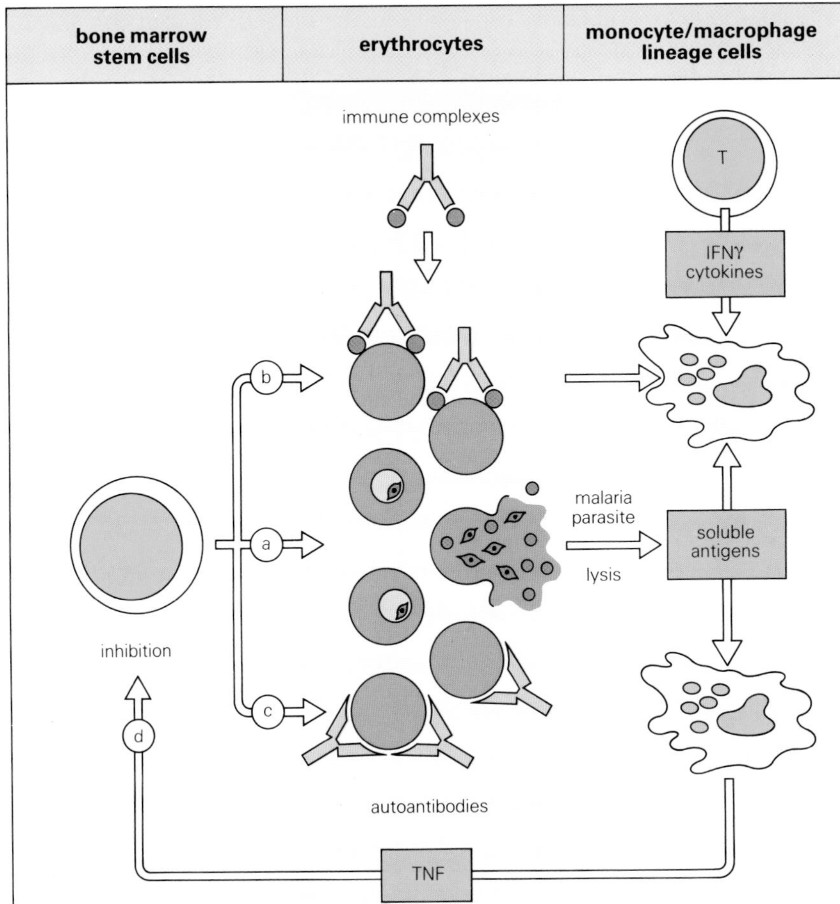

Fig. 17.29 Development of anaemia in malaria. In addition to the direct damage of erythrocytes by the malaria parasite (a), other immunopathological mechanisms contribute to the anaemia. Immune complexes containing parasite antigens may bind to unparasitized cells and accelerate their clearance by cells of the macrophage/monocyte lineage in spleen and liver (b). There is also some autoantibody produced to red cells which again accelerates their sequestration and breakdown (c). Tumour necrosis factor (TNF) released in response to infection inhibits red cell development from bone marrow stem cells (d).

VACCINES

Some vaccines composed of attenuated living parasites have proved successful in veterinary practice but now, as a result of recent exciting advances in the field of molecular biology, much effort is being directed towards the development of subunit vaccines against the important parasitic diseases of man.

Since protection in many cases depends upon both humoral and cell-mediated responses, a vaccine must induce a long-lived response from both T and B cells to be effective, and since determinants that are recognized by T cells often show a marked genetic restriction, it must also react with T cells of most MHC haplotypes, preferably without inducing suppression. Antigens that may induce the wrong kind of immune response must be avoided. In some circumstances protective antigens can induce antibodies that may cause dissemination of parasites; in addition, cell - mediated responses may cause pathology as well as induce protection.

STRATEGIES IN VACCINE DESIGN

The usual strategy is to identify protective antigens and then the key immunogenic portion of the molecule, which is likely to be separate from that causing suppression.

Isolation of protective antigens may be especially difficult in those diseases in which protection depends upon the development of good cell-mediated immunity since antigens are usually identified by reaction with antibody. Furthermore, humoral responses are likely to be strongest against surface antigens, so that antibody prepared from immune individuals may be selective for those antigens, whereas better protection may be obtained against antigens which are within the body of the parasite, such as the myosin of schistosomal worms.

Another approach under consideration is the development of vaccines which do not block initial infection but prevent the clinical manifestations of disease. In diseases like schistosomiasis, for instance, the objectives of such a vaccine might be to block the production of eggs, since they cause the characteristic granulomata in the liver which lead to pathology. Again, in malaria, since immune individuals can live with parasites in their blood without displaying any other effects of infection, the aim would be to vaccinate against these antigens which induce the secretion of tumour necrosis factor. Excess production of tumour necrosis factor is thought to be responsible for many of the symptoms of the disease.

Preparation of Antigens Once promising antigens have been identified there are then three usual approaches to their preparation and purification.

1. Genes coding for synthesis of the antigens may be cloned and transferred to bacterial or yeast cells which will secrete the recombinant antigens. This has the disadvantage that recombinant molecules may differ from natural peptides because translational processes in such cells are different from those of mammalian cells: recombinant samples of glycoproteins, for instance, remain unglycosylated.
2. The peptides may be sequenced and synthesized in the laboratory.
3. The antigens may be used to produce idiotypic vaccines which mimic the peptides. Idiotypic vaccines have the advantage that they can be made against carbohydrate moieties of antigens and they avoid the need to use the antigen itself.

Surface Antigens To date, recombinant DNA technology has been used to purify an antigen from the circumsporozoite protein of *P. falciparum* which coats the surface of the sporozoite, and a small peptide has been synthesized which is homologous to a part of the molecule. It is composed of a repeating sequence of a group of 4 amino acid residues, which in nature may be repeated up to 40 times in tandem in the whole molecule, depending upon the strain of parasite from which it was derived. Both cloned antigens and synthetic peptides induce the development of neutralizing antibodies against sporozoites. However, protection appears to require more than that. Unfortunately, responses to sporozoites show a clear genetic restriction, which in mice has been shown to be related to the MHC haplotype.

Several antigens from blood stage malarial parasites have also been cloned and sequenced, and synthetic peptides have been prepared that are similar to selected portions of various molecules. Again, these molecules have many repeated sequences that are immunodominant and induce antibody production. It is possible, however, that antigens inducing the necessary cell-mediated immunity may lie outside these regions of repeats, within variable regions of the molecules. The existence of this antigenic variation among parasites makes for poor prospects for the development of useful vaccines, especially in the case of African trypanosomiasis.

Enzyme Antigens Enzymes of parasites may be useful targets for immunological attack. Promastigotes of *Leishmania,* for instance, bear a molecule on their surface which acts as a protease. Antibody against the purified enzyme is not protective, but when the enzyme was used to vaccinate mice it induced strong cell-mediated responses and protection. Recently a gene without repeated sequences that codes for a polypeptide which functions as an enzyme, an aldolase, has been cloned from blood stage malarial parasites. It shares some homology with the mammalian aldolase but when it was used to vaccinate monkeys it conferred partial protection. Similarly, an antigen which is present on the surface of larvae of *S. mansoni* and below the tegument of the adult worm has been purified and found to share some homology with mammalian glutathione transferase. Antibody against this protein transferred protection. If, however, parasite enzymes give rise to cross-reactions with host enzymes, there is the possibility that such vaccines would induce autoimmune reactions.

Finally, experimental idiotypic vaccines have been made that induced protection against *S. mansoni* and *T. rhodesiense* and one has been described that induced the formation of parasite-binding antibodies against *T. cruzi.*

Ultimately, it seems likely that vaccines comprised of combinations of antigens made in various ways will be the most successful, given with an adjuvant and by a route that have yet to be determined.

EXAMPLES OF MAJOR HUMAN PARASITES

In the text above, a number of parasites infecting man are referred to. Their life cycles, geographical distributions and, in some cases, clinical and pathological presentation are illustrated in Figs 17.30–17.35.

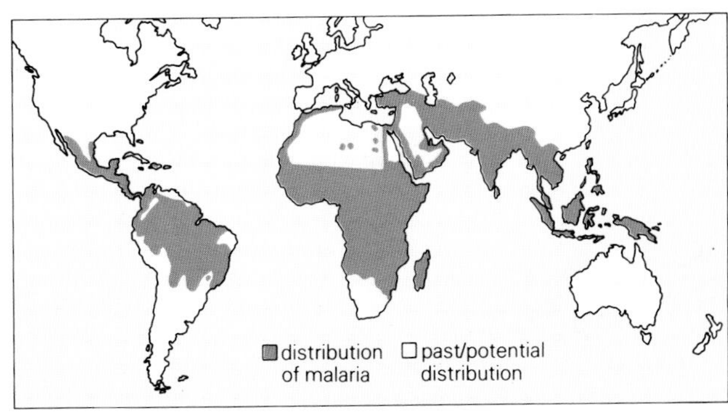

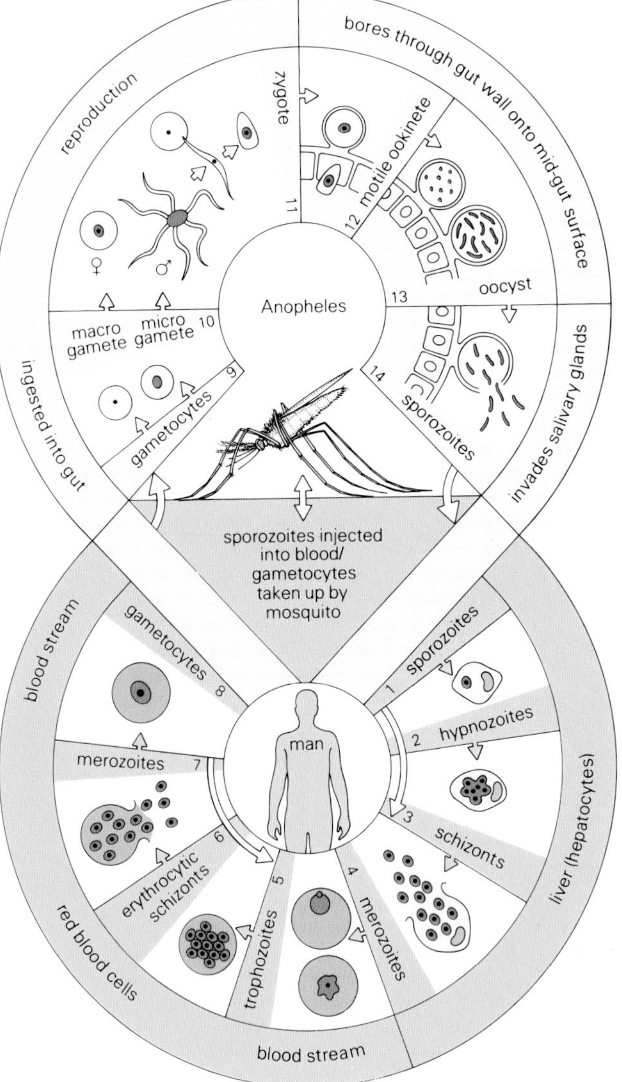

Fig. 17.30 Life cycle of *Plasmodium vivax* and the geographical distribution of malaria. The geographical distribution of malaria is shown for 1981. The life cycle of *Plasmodium vivax* is associated with a relapsing form of human malaria. In man the infection begins when sporozoites are injected into the blood by a mosquito of the genus *Anopheles* (1) (infective stage). The sporozoites migrate to the liver where they enter hepatocytes (2) and develop into schizonts (3) which give rise to the invasive form, the merozoites (4), some of which enter red blood cells. Some sporozoites may remain dormant in the liver as hypnozoites. They may later, after an interval of several months, develop into schizonts and then merozoites which enter the blood. In red blood cells, parasites become first trophozoites (5) and then erythrocytic schizonts (6), from each of which 12–24 merozoites are released to invade further cells (7). Some merozoites become gametocytes (8) and are ingested by a mosquito (9) in which they develop into microgametes and macrogametes (10) that fuse to form a zygote (11). This becomes a motile ookinete (12) which bores through the gut wall and forms an oocyst (13) from which large numbers of sporozoites are released (14). These invade the salivary glands from which they are injected into the human host when the mosquito feeds (1).

Bouts of fever are associated with the rupture of the schizonts which occurs every 48 hours with *P. falciparum, P. vivax* and *P. ovale* (tertian fever) and every 72 hours with *P. malariae* (quartan fever). The liver and spleen are grossly enlarged and haemolytic anaemia may be severe. The three photographs illustrate blood films showing ring forms of *P. falciparum* (left) and trophozoites of *P. vivax* in human erythrocytes (middle) (both courtesy of Dept of Protozoology, London School of Hygiene and Tropical Medicine) and placental blood showing schizonts of *P. falciparum* in erythrocytes (right). (Courtesy of Professor G. A. T. Targett.)

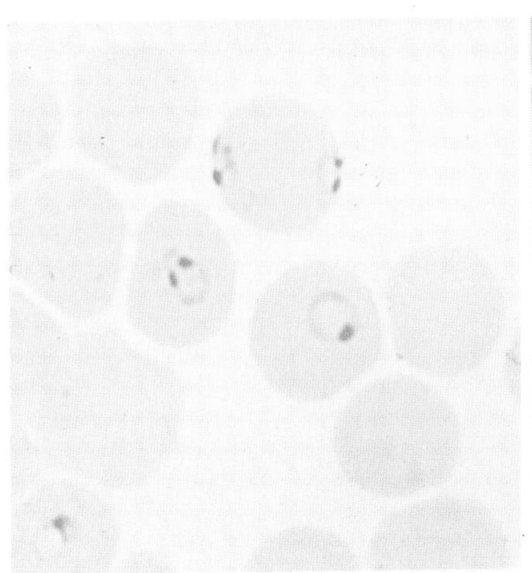

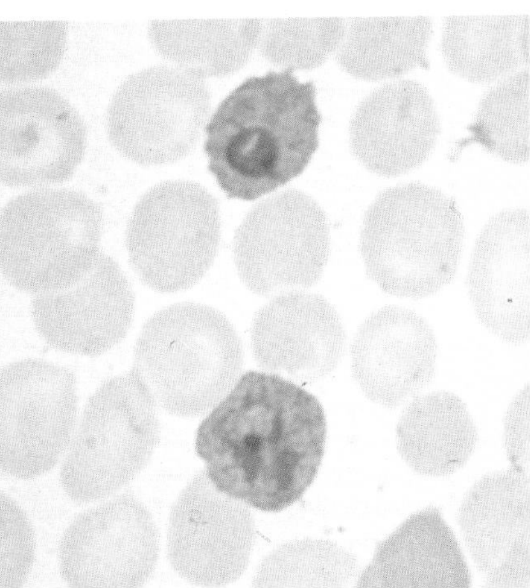

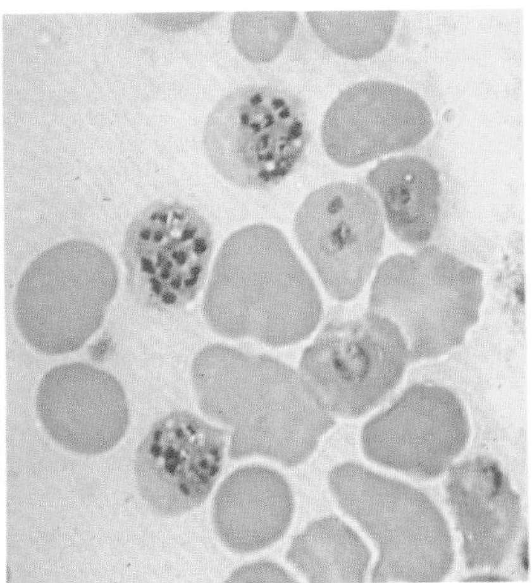

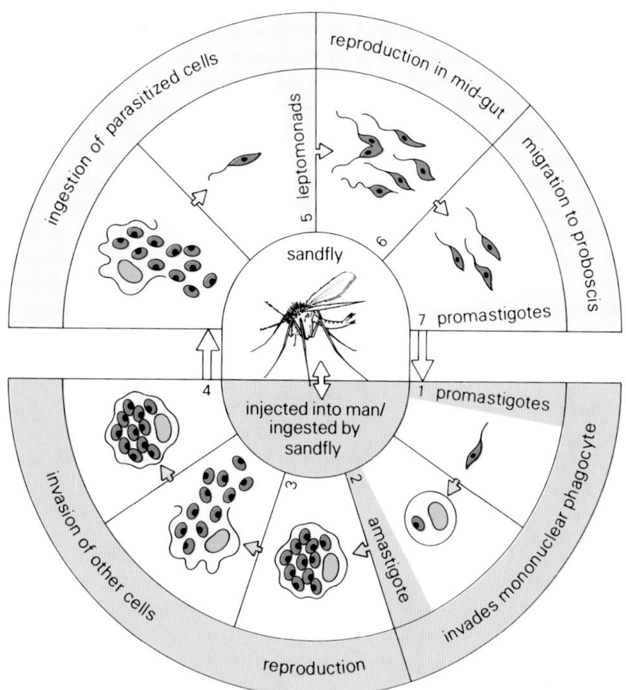

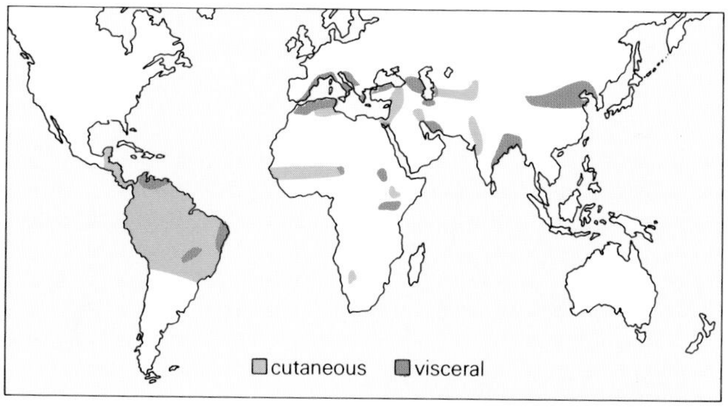

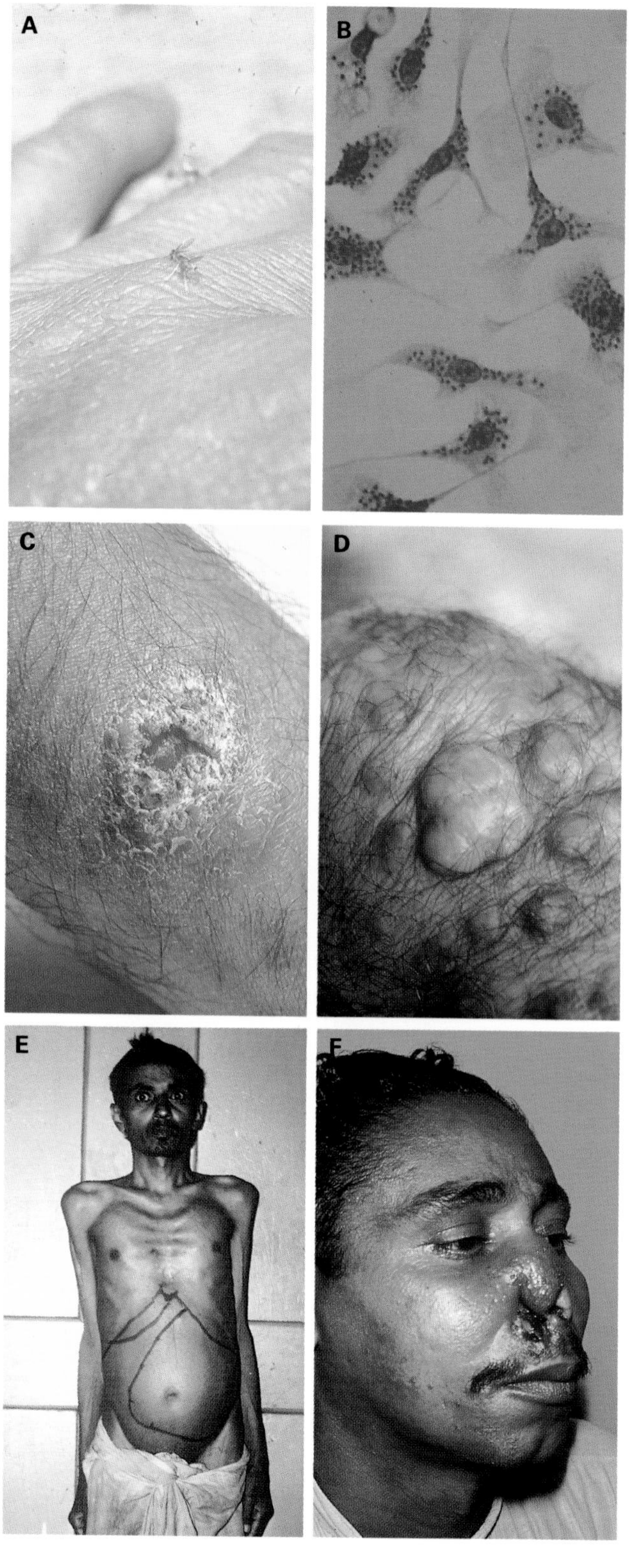

Fig. 17.31 Life cycle of *Leishmania* and the geographical distribution of leishmaniasis. The geographical distributions in 1981 of *Leishmania tropica*, the parasite which causes cutaneous leishmaniasis (involving skin) and *L. donovani*, which causes visceral leishmaniasis (kala-azar) involving internal organs are shown. Both the cutaneous and visceral forms are transmitted to man by certain species of *Phlebotomus* (sandflies). In India and some parts of Africa the parasite may be transmitted from man to man; in other areas dogs, rodents and some small mammals form a reservoir.

A generalized life cycle is shown. In man, infection begins when the promastigote is injected into the skin (1). It then enters mononuclear phagocytes (2) where it becomes an amastigote and multiplies (3). Further amastigotes are released which infect other cells (4). While in passage in the blood the infected cells may be picked up by the vector during feeding. After transformation into the leptomonad form (5), reproduction takes place in the mid-gut of the insect (6). From there the leptomonads migrate to the proboscis (7) to complete their maturation into promastigotes. *L. tropica* is restricted to macrophages of the liver, spleen and bone marrow. *L. tropica* causes the self-healing ulcer of oriental sore; *L. donovani* causes a systemic and often fatal disease.

A sandfly of the species *Lutzomyia longipalpis* seen in Lapinha, Brazil (A). (Courtesy of Professor W. Peters.) Resident peritoneal macrophages of CBA/Ca mouse strain infected with amastigotes 72 hours previously (B). Giemsa stain. (Courtesy of Dr J. Blackwell.) Tropical ulcer, caused by *L. major*, on the arm of an individual in Saudi Arabia (C). (Courtesy of Professor W. Peters.)

Diffuse cutaneous leishmaniasis caused by *L. mexicana amazoniensis,* in the knee of an individual from Belem, in the Amazon region in Brazil (D). Nodules indicate spread of the disease that occurs in the absence of cell-mediated immunity. (Courtesy of Professor W. Peters.) Visceral leishmaniasis (kala-azar), caused by *L. donovani* in a patient from Bihar, India (E). (Courtesy of Professor W. Peters.) Mucocutaneous leishmaniasis (espundia), caused by *L. braziliensis braziliensis*, showing severe destruction of nasopharyngeal tissues in a patient from Belo Horizonte, Brazil (F). (Courtesy of Professor W. Peters.)

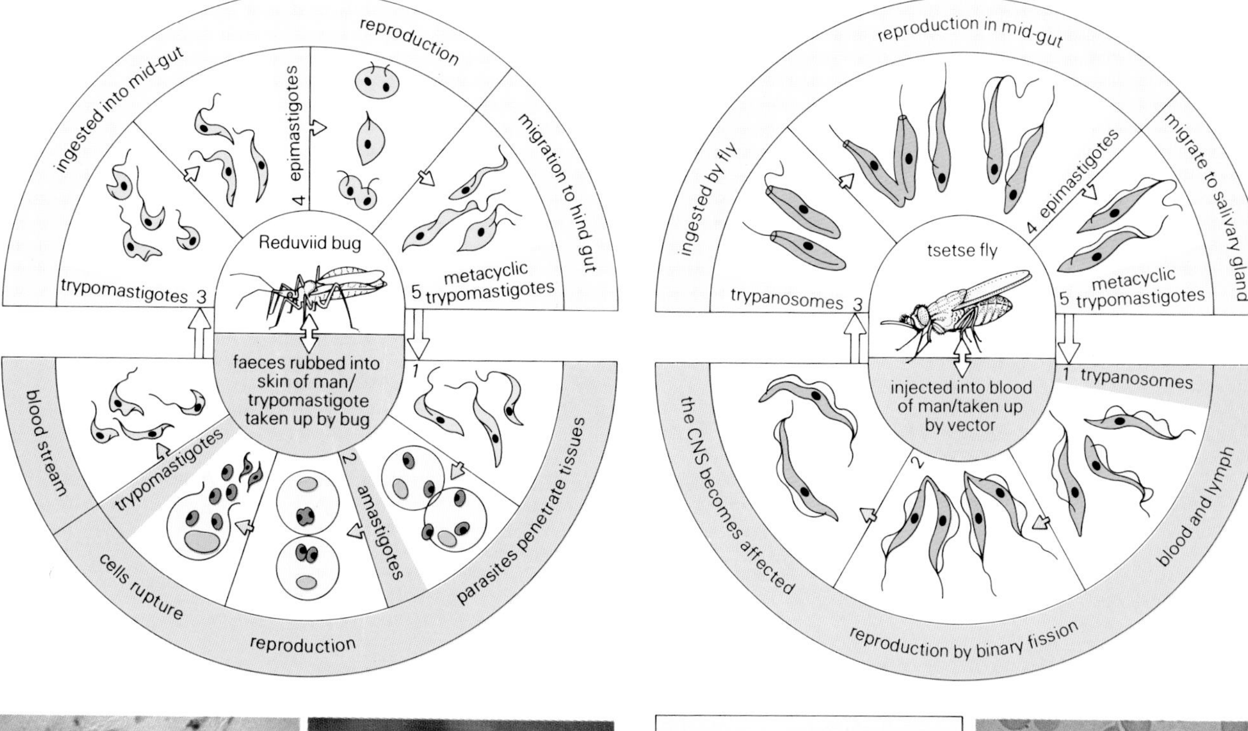

Fig. 17.32 Life cycle of *Trypanosoma cruzi*. *T. cruzi* causes Chagas' disease which is widespread in South America. These parasites exist in wild mammals such as armadillos and possums as well as in domestic animals. They are transmitted to man by the bite of Reduviid bugs, called 'kissing' or 'assassin' bugs, particularly of the genera *Triatoma, Rhodnius* and *Panstrongylus.* The vectors live in cracks in the walls of mud huts and bite at night. They transmit *T. cruzi* while feeding, not by inoculation but by faecal contamination. They defaecate and the victim then rubs the faeces into the skin when scratching.

After an initial trypomastigote parasitaemia (1), associated with fever in the acute stage of the disease, the parasites penetrate the tissues, for example cardiac muscle and smooth muscle of the gut, where they transform into amastigotes (2). There is a long chronic stage of infection, during which the heart may become enlarged and destruction of various ganglionic plexuses may occur, or various segments of the alimentary tract may become enlarged and denervated, causing conditions such as megacolon. Sudden death may result from heart block. The life cycle is completed when a feeding bug picks up blood trypomastigotes (3). The trypanosomes become epimastigotes (4) in the mid-gut, multiply and migrate to the hindgut where they become metacyclic trypomastigotes (5), the form which is the infective stage for man. Morphological appearance of amastigotes of *T.cruzi* in heart muscle (left). (Courtesy of the Wellcome Museum.) The Reduviid bug (right). (Courtesy of Dr W. Petana.)

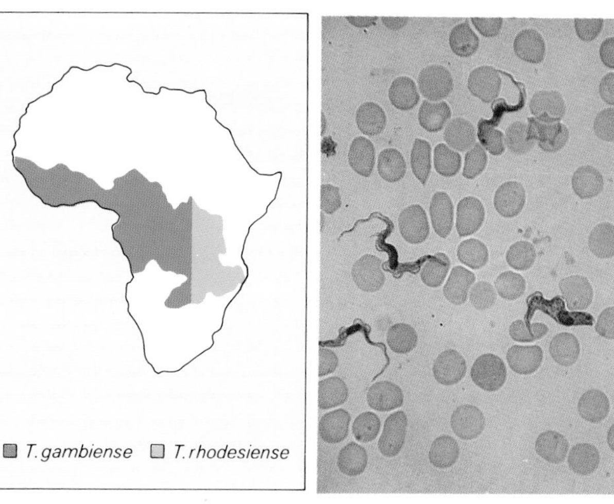

Fig. 17.33 Life cycle and geographical distribution of the African trypanosomes. African trypanosomiasis is confined to equatorial Africa. In man, the disease (sleeping sickness) is caused by two species of trypanosome, *Trypanosoma gambiense,* which is widespread in West and Central Africa and *T. rhodesiense,* which occurs in the East and east central areas. Trypanosomes are parasites of wild and domestic animals and are transmitted from host to host by the tsetse fly genus *Glossina.* Trypanosomiasis is a chronic and serious disease of domestic cattle, causing great economic loss.

Trypanosomes at the metacyclic stage are injected from the salivary gland of the tsetse fly during feeding (1). The entire life cycle in man occurs in the blood and lymph. The parasites are extracellular and divide by binary fission (2). As the CNS becomes affected the patient becomes progressively more wasted and finally comatose. The parasites are picked up by the vector during feeding (3); they divide and mature in the mid gut of the fly (epimastigote stage, 4), then return as a metacyclic trypanomastigote to the fly's salivary gland (5). Morphological appearance of the parasite in the blood (right); it is extracellular and motile, using its long free flagellum to propel itself. (Courtesy of Professor W. Peters.)

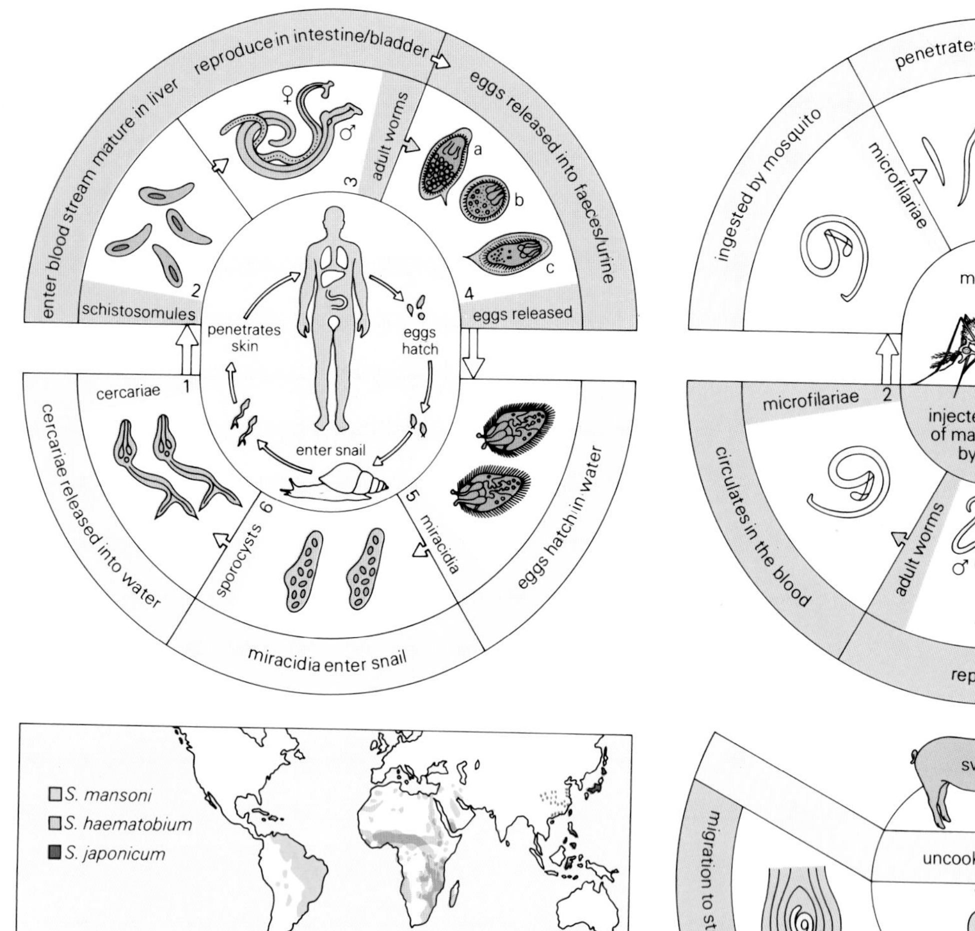

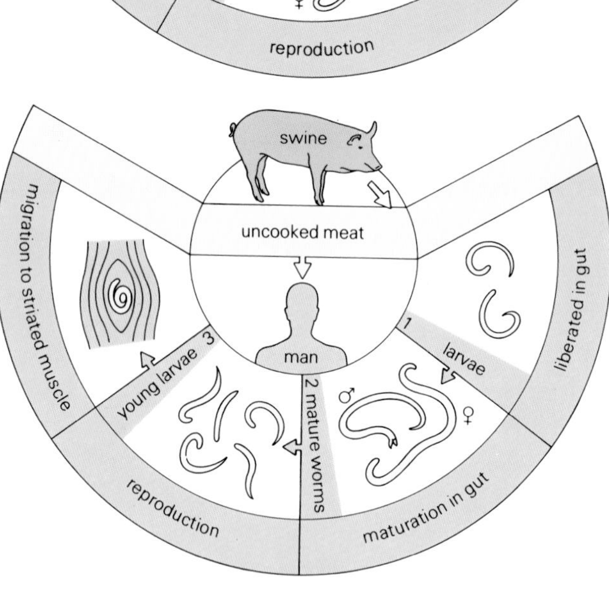

Fig. 17.34 Life cycle and geographical distribution of *Schistosoma mansoni, S. haematobium* and *S. japonicum*. Man becomes infected from water in which there are free swimming cercariae (larval form) which can penetrate the skin (1). The tail is shed and the worms (schistosomule stage) migrate through the circulation to the lungs and then to the liver, where they mature (2). They then enter the blood vessels of the gut or, in the case of *S. haematobium*, the bladder. The adult worms remain closely entwined in the portal vein (or blood vessels of the bladder) and the eggs released work their way out of the vessels into the tissues of the wall of the gut or bladder (3) and from there they escape into the faeces or urine (4). The three common species of schistosome infecting man can be distinguished by their eggs. Some eggs are carried to the lungs or liver, where granulomata develop around them. In water, the eggs hatch to become ciliated miracidia (5) which must enter a snail of a suitable species within 24 hours or die (6).

Fig. 17.35 The life cycles of two representative nematodes (roundworms). One is spread by an insect vector (*Wuchereria bancrofti*, upper right), and one (*Trichinella spiralis*, lower right) by direct transmission. *W. bancrofti*, a typical filarial worm, lives in the lymphatic vessels of man (adult stage) (1) and produces a prelarval form, the microfilaria, which circulates in the blood (2). The parasite is transmitted by mosquitoes, in which the microfilariae pass through three stages of development to reach the infective stage (3). The arthropod host is necessary for cyclical development; microfilariae circulating in transfused blood are unable to cause infection. *T. spiralis* develops through adult and larval stages within a single mammalian host, which may be carnivorous or omnivorous. The cycle in man is initiated by the ingestion of meat, usually undercooked pork, containing encysted larvae. The larvae liberated in the gut (1) mature rapidly (2) and the fertilized females then deposit further young larvae (3) which migrate to the tissues (4) by way of the lymphatics and the blood. They usually develop only in striated muscle, where they become encysted. The muscle biopsy of thigh muscle from a child in Kenya shows encysted larvae of *T. spiralis*. (Courtesy of Professor G. Nelson.)

FURTHER READING

GENERAL

Cohen, S. & Warren, K.S. (eds) (1982) *Immunology of Parasitic Infections*. 2nd edition. Oxford: Blackwell Scientific Publications.

Damian, R. (1987) Molecular mimicry revisited. *Parasitology Today*, **3**, 263.

Mitchell, G.F. (1987) Injection versus infection: the cellular immunology of parasitism. *Parasitology Today*, **3**, 106.

Parkhouse, R.M.E. (ed.) Parasite antigens in protection, diagnosis and escape. *Current Topics in Microbiology and Immunity*, **120**, Springer Verlag.

PROTOZOA

Clark, I.A. (1987) Cell-mediated immunity in protection & pathology of malaria. *Parasitology Today*, **3**, 300.

Den Hollander, N., Riley, D. & Beyfus, D. (1988) Immunology of Giardiasis. *Parasitology Today*, **4**, 124.

Greenwood, B.M. (1987) Asymptomatic malaria infections – do they matter? *Parasitology Today*, **3**, 206.

Hommel, M. (1985) Antigenic variation in malaria parasites. *Immunology Today*, **6**, 28.

Hudson, L. (1985) Autoimmune phenomena in chronic chagasic cardiopathy. *Parasitology Today*, **1**, 6.

Hughes, H.P.A. (1985) Toxoplasmosis – a neglected disease. *Parasitology Today*, **1**, 41.

Kierszenbaum, F. (1985) Is there autoimmunity in Chaga's disease? *Parasitology Today*, **1**, 4.

Steinert, M. & Pays, E. (1986) Selective expression of surface antigen genes in African trypanosomiasis. *Parasitology Today*, **2**, 15.

Stevenson, M.M. (ed.) *"Malaria: host responses to infection"*. CRC Press. In press.

HELMINTHS

Butterworth, A.E. & Hagan, P. (1987) Immunity in human schistosomiasis. *Parasitology Today*, **3**, 11.

Capron, M. & Capron, A. (1986) Rats, mice and men – models for immune effector mechanisms against schistosomiasis. *Parasitology Today*, **2**, 69.

Lee, T.D.G., Swieter, M. & Befus, A.D. (1986) Mast cell responses to helminth infection. *Parasitology Today*, **2**, 186.

Phillips, S.M. & Lammie, P.J. (1986) Immunopathology of granuloma formation and fibrosis in schistosomiasis. *Parasitology Today*, **2**, 296.

Filariasis. Ciba Foundation Symposium (1987), **127**.John Wiley & Sons.

VACCINES

Bordier, C. (1987) The promastigote surface protease of *Leishmania*. *Parasitology Today*, **3**, 151.

Greenblatt, C.L. (1988) Cutaneous leishmaniasis: the prospects for a killed vaccine. *Parasitology Today*, **4**, 53.

James, S.L. & Sher, A. (1986) Prospects for a non-living vaccine against schistosomiasis. *Parasitology Today*, **2**, 134.

Miller, L.H., Howard, R.J., Carter, R., Good, M.F., Nussenzweig, V. & Nussenzweig, R.S. (1986) Research toward malaria vaccines. *Science*, **234**, 1349.

Taylor, M.G. & Bickle, Q.D. (1986) Irradiated schistosome vaccines. *Parasitology Today*, **2**, 132.

Sadoff, J.C., Ballou, W.R., Baron, L.S., Majarian, W.R., Brey, R.N., Hockmeyer, W.T., Young, J.F., Cryz, S.J., Ou, J., Lowell, G.H. & Chulay, J.D. (1988) Oral *Salmonella typhimurium* vaccine expressing circumsporozoite protein protects against malaria. *Science*, **240**, 336.

18 Tumour Immunology

It has long been thought that the immune system could play a role in recognizing and reacting against tumours. Theoretically, immune reactions could either be important in preventing the initial appearance of tumours (the idea of immunosurveillance) or could occur following tumour initiation, and be involved in limiting their development. Even if neither of these mechanisms operates it might be possible to induce beneficial immune responses to some tumours therapeutically.

The concept of immunosurveillance, as proposed by Burnet, suggested that a major role of T cell-mediated immunity is to eliminate tumour cells as they arise and that this occurs because tumour cells express new epitopes whereby they are recognized as foreign. Several lines of evidence were seen to support immunosurveillance, for example, the frequency of occurrence of malignant tumours, which shows peaks in childhood and in old age, when it could be argued that the immune system is not fully functional. The rapidly expanding transplantation programme in the 1960s and the consequent use of powerful immunosuppressive drugs, provided evidence that the incidence of malignancy, albeit restricted to a few types of tumours, was indeed higher in immunosuppressed patients. More recently, the increased incidence of pathological immunosuppression associated with infection by the human immunodeficiency virus (HIV) has also suggested a relationship between immunosuppression and the development of certain kinds of malignant disease. Central to the concept of immunosurveillance is the hypothesis that malignant cells express novel antigens (sometimes referred to as tumour-associated or tumour-specific). There is evidence to suggest, at least in defined animal systems, that this may be so, although the definition of new antigens has to be extended to include re-expression or acquisition of embryonic or differentiation antigens, as well as simple quantitative differences in expression of 'normal' antigens.

HISTOLOGY OF TUMOURS

Some evidence for a role for the immune system in antitumour immunity can be gleaned from histological studies of tumours. Solid human tumours removed at surgery are frequently characterized by a marked mononuclear infiltrate unrelated to tumour necrosis, which is suggestive of host resistance of an immunological nature. Such infiltrates are heterogeneous and often comprise mononuclear phagocytes, lymphocytes of different subtypes and minority populations of other cells such as plasma cells and mast cells. In man, the opportunity to monitor the *in situ* immune responses usually arises only once – at surgery for the removal of the primary lesion; this reflects the situation of an isolated, often very late, point in the pathogenesis of the tumour. Although for some rare tumours, mononuclear infiltration is a good indicator of prognosis (for example in medullary carcinoma of the breast) and may even contribute to conventional anti-cancer therapy (for example in seminoma of the testis), there is no simple relationship between infiltration and prognosis and/or survival. The view that mononuclear infiltration has a defensive connotation is therefore an assumption. Infiltration may vary from the florid (Fig. 18.1) to none at all, and, with the exception of the neoplasms mentioned above, it rarely follows a consistent or predictable pattern. The *in situ* function of these cells is starting to be determined by studies on cells isolated from disaggregated tumours. Many experimentally-induced neoplasms are also characterized by mononuclear cell infiltrates. For some, such as Moloney virus-induced sarcomas, host cell infiltration is clearly associated with the frequent spontaneous regression of this tumour. This neoplasm is probably unique in this respect and its biological behaviour has little relevance for human neoplasia. For most tumours, the relationship is much more complex.

Since its proposal in 1970, the theory of immunosurveillance has undergone significant modification; for example, antitumour responses are no longer seen to be confined to cells of the adaptive immune system. It may be that immunosurveillance only applies to a restricted range of tumours or that its role is to limit the growth of established tumours or to prevent metastasis rather than to prevent tumour development.

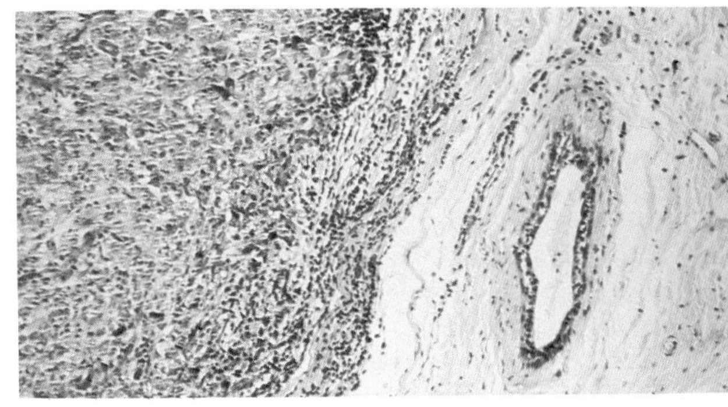

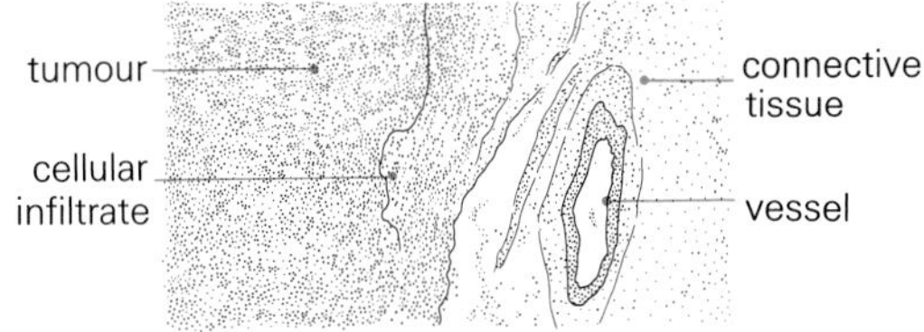

Fig. 18.1 Immunological reaction to a mammary carcinoma. The section shows a mammary carcinoma heavily infiltrated with mononuclear cells, suggesting that carcinomas may be recognized by cells of the immune system which are potentially active in limiting or eliminating the tumour cells. H&E stain, × 50.

IMMUNE RECOGNITION OF TUMOURS

Tumours may be induced experimentally in laboratory animals by treatment with carcinogens or by exposure to oncogenic viruses. Alternatively, tumours may arise spontaneously, usually in older animals. Spontaneously arising human tumours are often related to exposure to carcinogens such as benz-α-pyrene in tobacco smoke, to radiation or to viruses. There is increasing identification of tumours having viral aetiology such that it has been estimated that 20% of female and 8% of male human tumours may result from viral infection (Fig. 18.2). With some viruses such as hepatitis B virus (HBV), the association is direct whereas with others it is indirect, for example HIV and Kaposi's sarcoma in AIDS patients; the pathological immunodeficiency caused by the virus probably permits the reactivation of a latent cytomegalovirus (CMV) infection.

virus	cancer
hepatitis B virus (HBV)	hepatocellular carcinoma
Epstein-Barr virus (EBV)	non-Hodgkin's lymphoma nasopharyngeal carcinoma Burkitt's lymphoma
cytomegalovirus (CMV) [+HIV]	Kaposi's sarcoma
human T cell lymphotropic virus (HTLV-1)	T cell leukaemia
human papillomaviruses 16 and 18 (HPV16, HPV18)	cervical carcinoma

Fig. 18.2 Viruses associated with cancer. Burkitt's lymphoma is seen in Africa and nasopharyngeal carcinoma in South China.

TUMOUR-SPECIFIC ANTIGENS

Central to the theory of immunosurveillance lies the concept that tumour cells express antigens not found on normal tissue counterparts. Malignant transformation may be accompanied by phenotypic changes in the involved cells including the loss of normal cell surface antigenic components, the gain of neoantigens (antigens not detectable in the corresponding normal tissue) and other membrane changes which influence cell–cell interactions in the host. Whether 'public' (expressed on cells other than the tumour) or 'private' (expressed exclusively on the tumour) some of these neoantigens are capable of evoking an adaptive immune response (Fig. 18.3). In some systems the immune response to these antigens may be as strong as an allogeneic reaction whereas tumours which show minimal antigenic changes might be expected to elicit little or no adaptive immune response (spontaneous tumours of experimental animals are the major group in this category). Between these two extremes lies the theoretical possibility that tumours express neoantigens which evoke no response at all, or generate a response which is successfully evaded, a condition known as 'immunological escape' (see below).

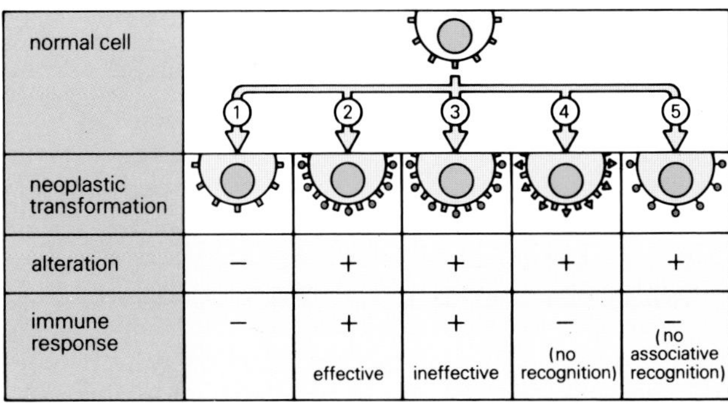

Fig. 18.3 Host recognition of tumours and adaptive immune responses. Cells which undergo neoplastic transformation do not necessarily change their surface phenotype, in which case no adaptive immune response can result (1). If the neoplastic cells do change their surface phenotype, immune responses may develop and are either effective (2) or ineffective (3), a condition referred to as 'immunological escape'. Some changed neoplastic cells do not induce immune responses, either because there is a failure to recognize the new antigens (4) or because other surface antigens (such as MHC products) are changed and there is no associative recognition of the neoplastic cell with its new antigens (5).

While neoantigens appear to be a stable, heritable property of some selected experimental tumours, the majority of cancers should properly be regarded as heterogeneous. Human tumours in particular are known to be heterogeneous with respect to such diverse properties as growth characteristics, drug resistance, metastatic potential, karyotype, tumour antigen expression. This heterogeneity reflects the presence within the tumour of several distinct clones of neoplastic cells resulting from genetic instability of the original transformed cell. Tumour heterogeneity has important consequences for tumour therapy since a secondary tumour arising after successful therapy of the primary is frequently drug resistant. This heterogeneity must also be borne in mind when developing immunotoxins. Selective destruction of antigenic tumour cells may result in the outgrowth of non-antigenic tumour variants present in the original tumours.

In addition to changes in the antigenic phenotype of malignant cells, tumour cell membranes apparently acquire an altered 'structure' which renders them susceptible to natural killer (NK) cells, although the molecular nature of this change is not known.

Antibodies against Tumour - Specific Antigens (TSAs) may be detected by use of (usually) xenogeneic antisera, exhaustively absorbed with normal cells of the appropriate histological origin. Monoclonal antibodies do not require such absorption. Nonetheless there are inherent difficulties in defining TSAs regardless of the type of antibodies used.

First, a tumour may anomalously express antigens which are not found on the normal cell from which it is derived, but which are produced by other normal cell types. This may result from the ability of tumours to make products inappropriate to their normal state of differentiation. Second, because most tumours arise from the clonal expansion of single cells they often express differentiation antigens normally only seen at particular phases of differentiation of a cell type. This is exemplified by the four major phenotypes of acute leukaemia which can be distinguished by membrane and enzyme markers. The antigenic profile of the leukaemic cell is qualitatively similar to the characteristics of the corresponding normal haemopoietic cells. Clonally expanded normal antigens may masquerade as tumour specific especially if the normal cell which undergoes transformation is present only as a small proportion of the normal cells of the tissue from which the tumour arises. For example, another type of antigen appears when tumours inappropriately express particular alloantigens such as blood group determinants. Some blood groups are determined by carbohydrate chains present on the cell surface. These chains may be lost or gained, resulting in inappropriate blood group expression. In isolated cases, illegitimate blood group antigens, that is, normal blood group antigens different from those present on normal tissue of the host, may appear.

Antigens of Solid Tumours Antigens associated with solid tumours may be classified serologically as follows.

1. Those which show an absolute restriction to a single tumour and are not found on any other normal or malignant cells.
2. Those which are shared by tumour cells in different individuals. These antigens may also be found on a restricted range of normal cells and should therefore be classified as *autoantigenic differentiation antigens*. One of the best known TSAs in this group is the TL antigen found on leukaemic cells in mice. TL antigens are structurally similar to MHC class I molecules and are normally found only on thymocytes of animals belonging to the TL^+ strain. The antigen is, however, expressed on the surface of leukaemic cells from mice belonging to the TL^- strain.
3. Those antigens which are pervasive and expressed on a wide variety of normal and malignant cells of human and animal origin. In the experimentally observed immune response to a patient's own tumour these antigens are observed more often than the antigens described in 1 and 2. In order to observe autologous reaction against the different classes it is necessary to absorb out reactivity against other classes using appropriate normal or tumour tissue.

Tumour-Associated Transplantation Antigens TSAs, which are defined by their ability to evoke rejection of a tumour in pre-immunized syngeneic hosts are known as tumour-associated transplantation antigens (TATAs) (Fig. 18.4). Expression of these functionally defined antigens is a feature of many, if not all, experimental neoplasms.

Where detectable, the major TATAs of chemically-induced tumours are unique (private) for each tumour, even within two tumours induced at the same time in an individual animal by the same chemical (Fig. 18.5). Cloning of a chemically-induced tumour may reveal subclones with private TATAs although the number of individual TATAs within a single tumour may be limited. The reason for the degree of polymorphism among TATAs probably reflects the multiplicity of genomic changes coding for cell surface antigens induced by carcinogen/DNA interaction. Private specificities on cells within such a tumour probably reflect individual transforming events induced by powerful carcinogens, rather than heterogeneity induced by genetic instability. In contrast, TATAs induced by the same oncogenic viruses cross-react regardless of the cell type from which the tumours are derived but not with tumours induced by other viruses (Fig. 18.6). In the case of the DNA viruses (for example, polyoma and SV40) the TATA is encoded by the viral DNA integrated into the cellular genome. These determinants are probably glycoproteins. In addition to

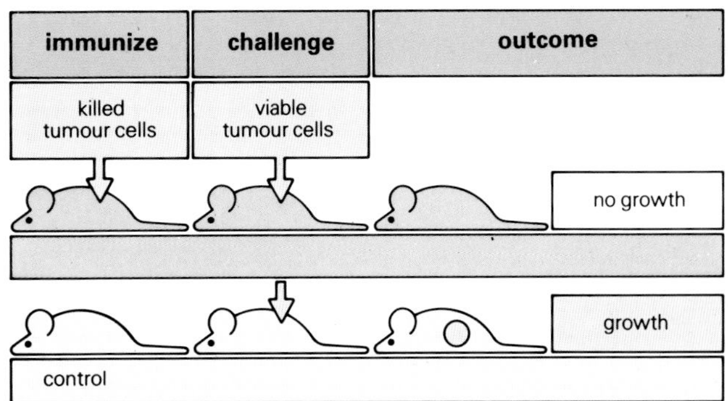

Fig. 18.4 Demonstration of tumour-associated transplantation antigens (TATAs). The presence of TATAs on transplantable tumours can be demonstrated by taking tumour cells from an animal and inactivating them chemically (e.g. with mitomycin C) or by irradiation. Animals which have been inoculated with inactivated tumour failed to produce a tumour when injected with viable tumour cells, whereas the control, uninoculated animals permitted tumour growth.

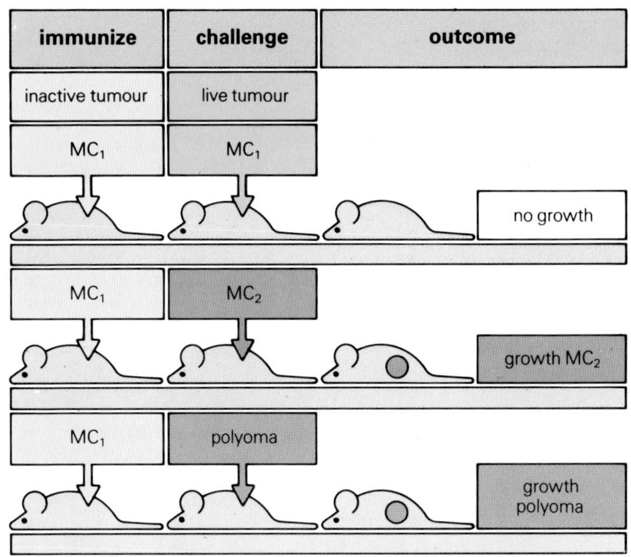

Fig. 18.5 Absence of common antigens on chemically-induced tumours. Three groups of animals were immunized to a methylcholanthrene-induced sarcoma (MC_1) by repeated implantation of inactivated tumour. (Methylcholanthrene is a chemical carcinogen.) Subsequently the groups were challenged with MC_1 or another methylcholanthrene-induced tumour (MC_2) or a virally-induced tumour (polyoma). Immunization was effective only for the specific tumour, MC_1 indicating that tumours induced by the same chemical do not share antigens nor do they share antigens with virally-induced tumours.

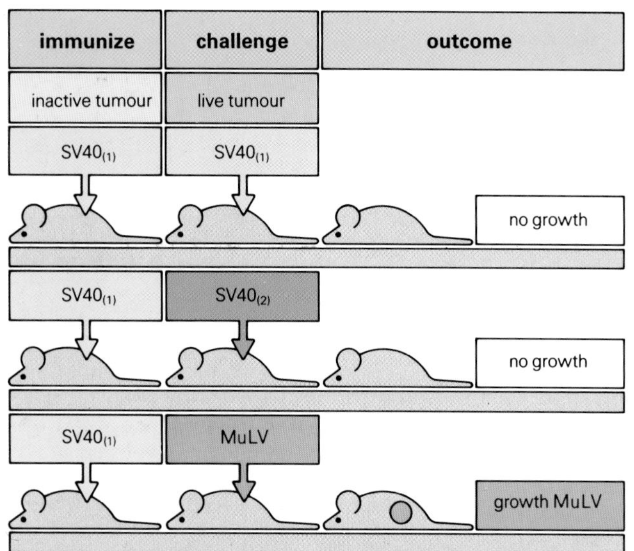

Fig. 18.6 Common antigens on virally-induced tumours. Three groups of animals were immunized to an SV40 virus-induced tumour ($SV40_{(1)}$) by repeated implantation of inactivated tumour. Subsequently the groups were challenged with live $SV40_{(1)}$ tumour or another similarly induced tumour, $SV40_{(2)}$, or with a tumour induced by murine leukaemia virus, MuLV. Immunization to $SV40_{(1)}$ protected against $SV40_{(1)}$ and $SV40_{(2)}$ but not against MuLV-induced tumours indicating that tumours induced by the same virus may have common antigens.

cell surface TATAs, other antigens may be concomitantly expressed, for example the T and U antigens located in the nucleus. These are both specified by the viral genome but are not part of the virus particle. In the case of RNA tumour viruses, for example, Rous sarcoma viruses, or feline leukaemia virus, cellular antigens are distinguishable serologically from the structural components of the virus including the envelope glycoproteins which enter the cell as part of the budding process. Viral envelope antigens are capable of inducing resistance, the major component being a glycoprotein with a molecular weight of 70 kD.

Malignant transformation in laboratory animals is sometimes accompanied by activation of latent oncogenic RNA viruses. For example, the antigens expressed by radiation-induced murine leukaemias are those of the murine leukaemia virus (MuLV) complex. Similar concomitant expression of virus-induced tumour antigens can occur during chemical carcinogenesis. 'Spontaneous' animal tumours where the aetiological agent is unknown, have very weak TATAs.

Oncofetal Antigens Certain tumours express antigens, or synthesize proteins normally expressed only by fetal tissue, a phenomenon known as retrogenetic expression. Most of these oncofetal antigens (OFA) are not strictly tumour associated and with the use of sensitive assays they have also been detected in small amounts in non-malignant adult cells. The best characterized of these antigens are alphafetoprotein (AFP) and carcinoembryonic antigen (CEA).

AFP, a glycoprotein (70 kD) is the first α globulin present in the serum of mammals during development and can reach concentrations of 2–3 mg/ml in humans. It is synthesized first by the yolk sac and later by endoderm and fetal liver. After birth, synthesis of AFP ceases and is replaced by albumin so that adult levels in healthy, non-pregnant adults are less than 5 ng/ml of human blood. Elevated levels of AFP in adults are associated significantly with primary hepatoma and with certain germ line tumours although it is also produced by regenerating liver.

Carcinoembryonic Antigen (CEA) is a heterogeneous cell surface glycoprotein (180,000 kD) produced by cells of fetal colon. Originally described as an antigen associated with carcinoma of the colon, elevated levels were subsequently found in the blood of patients with a variety

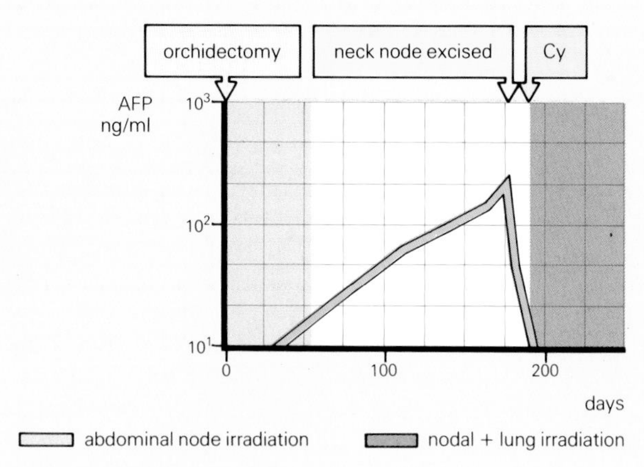

Fig. 18.7 Relationship of serum alphafetoprotein (AFP) levels to clinical course in a patient with teratoma of the testis. The progressive rise in AFP precedes relapse in the neck and lungs by about 150 days. After further therapy and treatment with cyclophosphamide (Cy) and irradiation, the AFP level returns to normal. (Courtesy of Professor T.J. McElwain.)

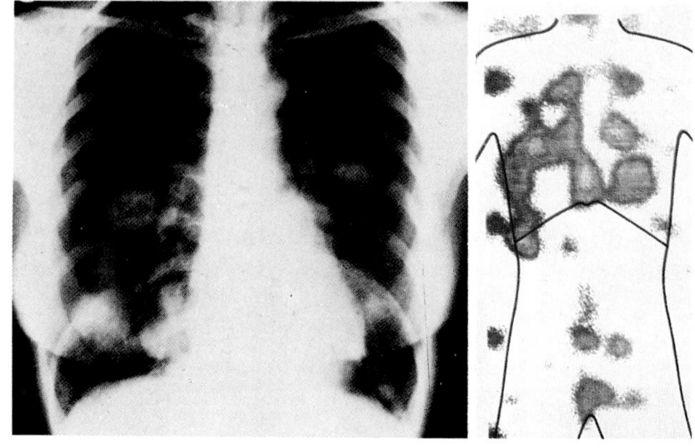

Fig. 18.8 Chest radiograph and immunoscintigraphy scan of a patient with carcinoma of the colon who has lung and liver metastases. The monoclonal antibody YPC2/12.1, raised against human colorectal cancer, binds to carcinoembryonic antigen and reacts with a glycoprotein of 180 kD. The antibody was radiolabelled with ^{131}I, administered intravenously and scintigrams obtained at 48 hours. The image is that obtained after a subtraction procedure to eliminate background blood-borne antibody. (Courtesy of Professor K. Sikora.)

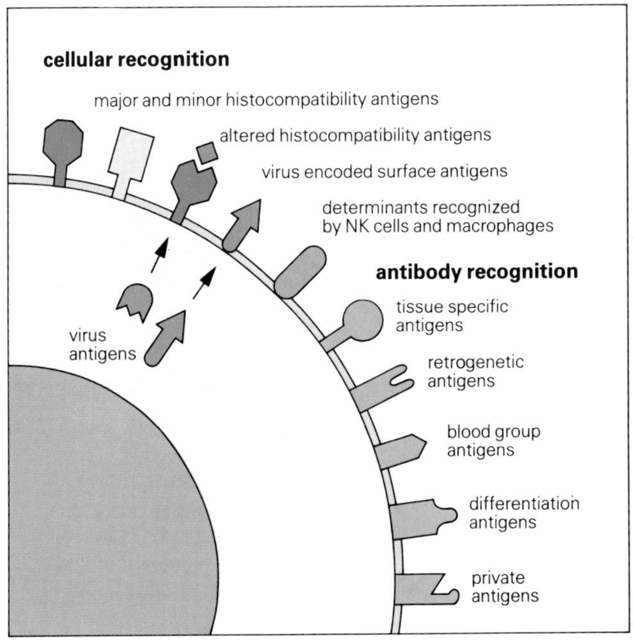

Fig. 18.9 Summary of tumour-specific antigens. Antigens on the upper segment are primarily recognized by immune effector cells, and those on the lower segment by antibodies.

of tumours of ectodermal origin – intestinal, pulmonary, pancreatic, gastric and mammary adenocarcinomas. Elevated levels are also associated with inflammatory disease of the bowel, lung and pancreas and heavy smoking, and low levels are found on normal adult colon. It is likely that different organs produce CEA molecules with public and private specificities and monoclonal antibodies have been produced which appear to be more specific to tumour-associated CEA than are polyclonal antibodies. Both AFP and CEA are readily measured by radioimmunoassay. While they are of no use in screening for cancer they do have a limited use in monitoring patients with certain types of cancer following tumour removal (Fig. 18.7). Blood levels of these antigens are directly related to the tumour burden such that increases are indicative of recurrence and/or metastasis. They have also been used for *in vivo* localization of metastatic disease with radiolabelled antibody (Fig. 18.8).

A composite scheme of tumour cell surface antigens based on *in vivo* studies and serology is given in Fig. 18.9. While not all of these may be immunogenic in the original host, they may still be of practical interest in immunodiagnosis and immunotherapy.

IMMUNE RESPONSES TO TUMOURS

IN SITU CELLULAR RESPONSES

Studies of the *in situ* host immune response were alluded to above where a mammary carcinoma was presented. With the advent of monoclonal antibodies to leucocytes and their subpopulations, the cellular nature of the inflammatory infiltrates can now be definitively analysed (Fig. 18.10). Ideally, the immunohistological examination of tumours should be followed by functional analysis of the recovered, purified cell populations. In man however this combined approach often presents

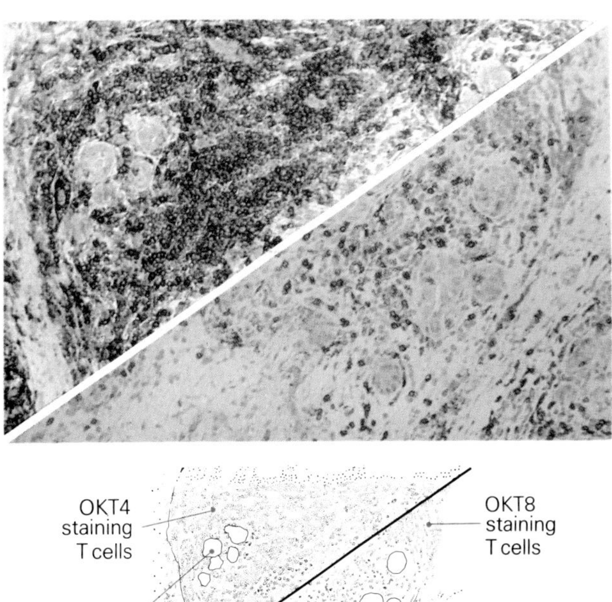

Fig. 18.10 $CD4^+$ and $CD8^+$ T lymphocyte subsets in carcinoma of the breast. Numerous dark staining $CD4^+$ cells (stained with monoclonal OKT4) are present throughout the tumour, whereas the fewer $CD8^+$ cells (stained with OKT8) tend to cluster round the periphery. Indirect immunoperoxidase technique, counterstained with haematoxylin.

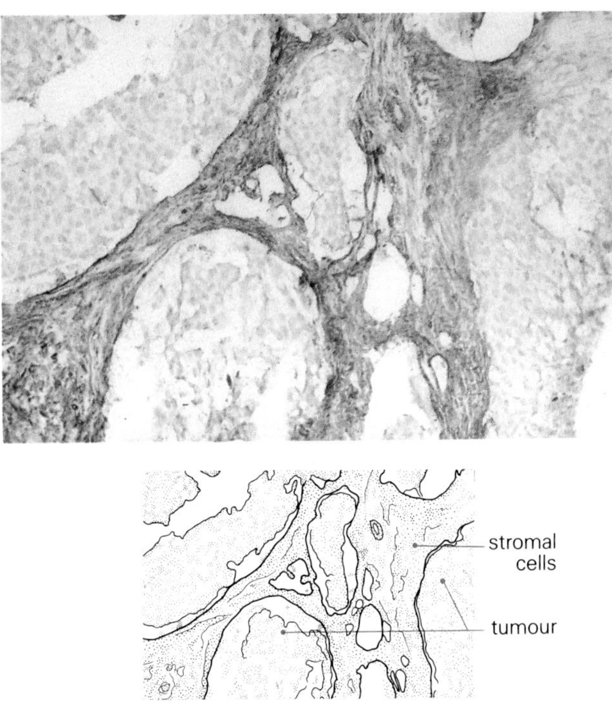

Fig. 18.11 Breast cancer tissue reactive with monoclonal antibody (2A1) to the monomorphic determinant of HLA class I antigens. Only the stromal cells are stained indicating that malignant epithelial cells fail to express MHC class I antigens. Some 50% of primary human breast cancers fall into this category. Aberrant class II expression may also occur on some tumours. Indirect immunoperoxidase technique, counterstained with haematoxylin.

insurmountable logistical problems. Monoclonal antibodies to T cell subsets, monocyte/macrophages and NK cells can determine the preponderance of a given subpopulation at the tumour site and its microanatomical distribution. The efficacy of this technique is exemplified in Fig. 18.10 for carcinoma of the breast. Much additional information can be obtained using monoclonal antibodies to MHC antigens. On the one hand, some tumours fail to express class I antigens (Fig. 18.11) while others express class II antigens. These have important implications particularly for cell-mediated immune reactions in that tumour cells lacking class I antigens may not be killed by cytotoxic T cells, whereas those expressing class I could possibly present self-antigen to helper T cells.

CELL-MEDIATED IMMUNITY TO TUMOURS

The adaptive immunity induced to tumour antigens is essentially similar to that evoked against T cell-dependent transplantation and other cell surface glycoprotein antigens (Fig. 18.12). T cell activation includes the generation of helper (TH) and suppressor (Ts) subsets as well as cytotoxic T lymphocytes (Tc). Tc cells recognize tumour antigen in association with class I MHC products. Activation also leads to the production of lymphokines by TH cells which are important in the recruitment and activation of macrophages, natural killer (NK) and lymphokine activated killer (LAK) cells (Fig. 18.13). The important lymphokines in this respect are as follows.

1. Interleukin-2 (IL-2); this lymphokine is essential for T cell division and the differentiation of B cells into plasma cells. It is also important in the amplification of NK cells and in the generation of LAK cells from precursors (see below). Whereas NK cells show restricted cytotoxicity against a limited range of tumour cell types *in vitro*, LAK cells are capable of destroying cells from a wide range of tumours. NK cells can also lyse virus-infected cells which may have implications for tumours of viral origin where viral products are expressed on cells.

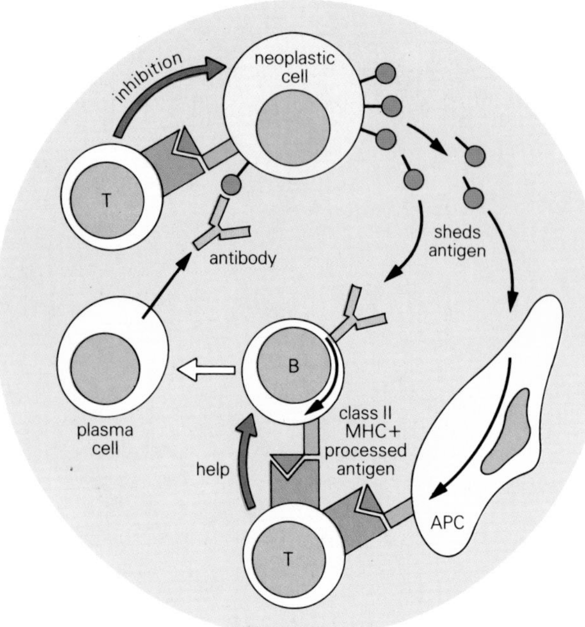

Fig. 18.12 Adaptive immunity to tumours. Antigens shed from neoplastic cells bind to antigen-presenting cells and in association with MHC class II antigens stimulate specific T and B cells. The activated lymphocytes cooperate in the production of tumour-specific antibody and activated T cells may also have cytostatic or cytolytic activity. (Memory cells are generated during the response.)

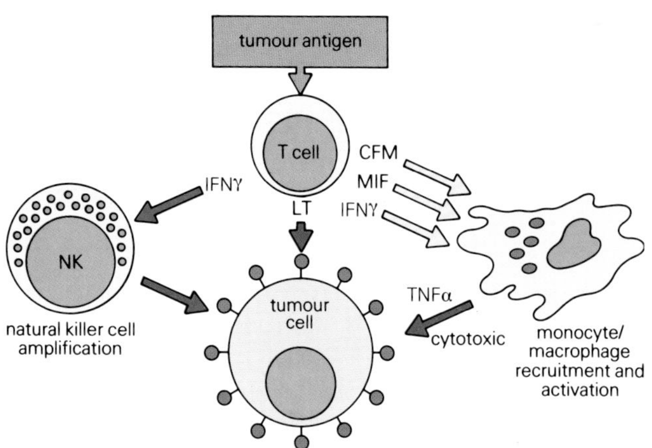

Fig. 18.13 The role of lymphokines in tumour killing. T cells activated by tumour antigen: (1) release interferon-ϒ (IFNϒ) to amplify the lytic action of natural killer (NK) cells and macrophages, (2) release lymphotoxin (LT) which acts directly, and (3) release chemotactic factors (CFM) and migration inhibition factor (MIF), all of which attract and activate macrophages. Macrophages have a cytotoxic effect on the tumour and prevent multiplication.

2. Migration inhibition factor (MIF); this binds to receptors on the macrophage surface, and increases the level of intracellular cyclic AMP, resulting in increased polymerization of microtubules and decreased migration. Its function is probably to arrest macrophages at the (antigenic) tumour site.
3. Macrophage activating factor (IFNϒ); macrophages cultured with IFNϒ develop some of the properties of activated macrophages, for example, increased tumoricidal activity.
4. Lymphotoxin (LT); this lymphokine can lyse some tumour cells *in vitro* and is also directly cytotoxic when injected into a tumour *in situ*. The significance of LT *in vivo* is not known. Whilst it is not wholly responsible for the killing capacity of Tc cells it may amplify T cell-mediated killing by other mechanisms.
5. Interferons (IFNs); antiviral and immunomodulatory properties of the different types of IFN overlap, though IFNϒ is consistently the most efficient immunomodulator. IFNs increase the cytotoxicity of NK cells as well as inducing MHC class I and II molecules on bystander cells with the possible consequences mentioned previously. Interferons also cause activation of macrophages rendering them more tumoricidal.
6. Chemotactic factors; separate chemotactic factors for macrophages and for granulocytes recruit phagocytic cells to the tumour site.
7. Mitogenic factors (MFs); these comprise a family of molecules generated by antigen or lectin stimulation of lymphocytes. A lymphocyte mitogenic factor (LMF) is probably identical to IL-2.

DETECTION OF T CELL-MEDIATED IMMUNITY

The methodology for the detection of tumour antigens on both human and experimental neoplasms which

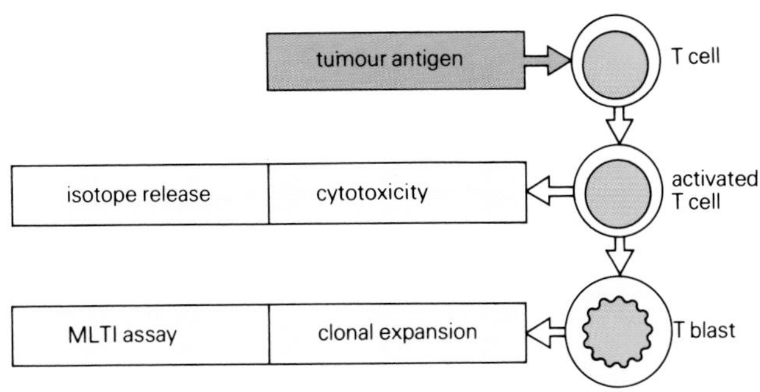

Fig. 18.14 Demonstration of T cell-mediated immunity to tumours *in vitro*. Cell-mediated immunity is measured in two assays. Following antigenic stimulation of specific T cells, the cells develop anti-tumour cytotoxic activity measured in an isotope release assay. Clonal expansion and proliferation of the cells is measured in the mixed lymphocyte/target cell interaction (MLTI) assay.

evoke adaptive immune responses relies upon T cell activation and the concomitant elaboration of lymphokines following exposure of T cells to tumour (target) cells. Tests have direct implications for the tumour–host relationship only if conducted, in animals, in strictly syngeneic systems, with target and effector cells from the same inbred strain, or, for human tumours, in autologous combinations, with target cells and T cells from the same donor. The tests fall into two major categories comprising assays of either T cell proliferation or effector function (Fig. 18.14).

T Cell Proliferation Specific T cell proliferation is measured by incorporation of ^{3}H-thymidine into autologous or syngeneic responder lymphocytes after 6 days' co-cultivation with irradiated tumour cells. Proliferating T cells may be CD4^{+} or CD8^{+}. Tc cells may be assayed by cytotoxicity assays (see below), TH cells by their capacity to undergo restimulation with appropriate antigen (primed lymphocyte test, PLT), and Ts cells by their capacity to inhibit primary lymphocyte transformation

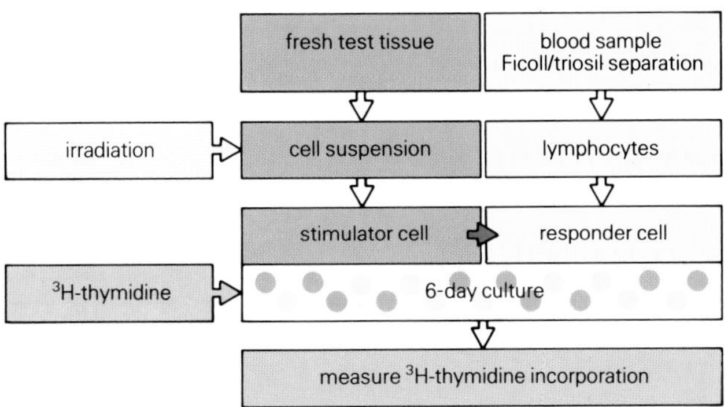

Fig. 18.15 Mixed lymphocyte/target cell interaction (MLTI) test. A cell suspension (target cells) is prepared from normal or tumour tissue. The cells are then irradiated which prevents them from dividing but does not alter their antigenicity. Meanwhile lymphocytes are prepared on a Ficoll/triosil gradient from a fresh heparinized blood sample and the lymphocytes and target cells co-cultivated for 6 days. Any antigen-specific lymphocytes are stimulated to divide as measured by pulsing the culture with tritiated thymidine and measuring the amount incorporated into the responder cells.

by lectins. Alternatively, immunohistological staining using monoclonal antibodies to CD4 and CD8 will distinguish between cells belonging to different subsets. T cells for proliferation assays may be obtained from peripheral blood or from the tumour infiltrate (tumour infiltrating lymphocytes, TIL) after enzymic disaggregation of the tumour, followed by separation of tumour cells and lymphocytes on Ficoll/triosil or Percoll gradients (Fig. 18.15).

T Cell Effector Function T cell effector function is commonly monitored in short-term cytotoxicity assays such as the release of ^{51}Cr from pre-labelled tumour targets. Since unfractionated or only partially purified T cells are generally used in such assays, it is important to distinguish T cell effector function from that of NK cells (see below) by using an NK-sensitive target as a control (Fig. 18.16).

Approximately one third of all cancer patients who undergo surgery exhibit peripheral blood or lymph node lymphocyte cytotoxicity which is directed against fresh autologous tumour cells. If the effector cells are first preincubated *in vitro* with inactivated tumour targets, as in the MLTI assay, and subsequently assayed against cryopreserved autologous targets on day 6 the incidence of cytotoxicity increases to approximately two thirds. This suggests that the frequency of Tc activity in the majority of operable patients is too low for detection without clonal amplification. Increased cytotoxicity can also be achieved if effector lymphocytes are cultured for short periods in exogenous IL-2 or under conditions in which IL-2 is generated endogenously. In patients in

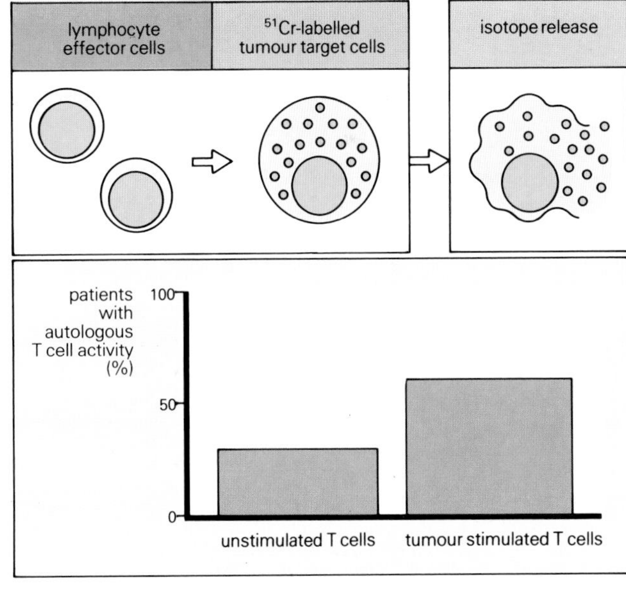

Fig. 18.16 Isotope release assay. Autologous T cell cytotoxicity (ATC) can be measured in an isotope release assay. Lymphocytes from peripheral blood or lymph node are incubated with autologous radiolabelled tumour cells (above). The lytic action of these effectors is measured by assaying released isotope. Approximately 30% of patients operated on to remove tumours display ATC against the tumour. If their lymphocytes are stimulated in an MLTI assay for 6 days prior to the isotope release assay up to 60% display ATC, implying that antigen-specific lymphocytes are present in the majority of patients but they may need stimulation, as in an MLTI, to become actively cytotoxic for the tumour (below).

whom autologous lymphocyte cytotoxicity is demonstrable in peripheral blood or draining lymph nodes, the activity of TIL is significantly depressed. This observation suggests *in situ* modulation of T cell function by tumour related products or accumulation of suppressor cells, either Ts or suppressor macrophages.

T Cell Clones The development of techniques for long-term culture of T cells in IL-2, has enabled cloning techniques to be applied to the T cells of tumour-bearing patients. T cells, obtained either from peripheral blood or as TIL, are clonally expanded in IL-2, using irradiated feeder cells. They can then be tested against cryopreserved tumour cells in either the MLTI or the cytotoxicity assays. Moreover the clones can be phenotyped using a panel of monoclonal antibodies against lymphocyte differentiation antigens. Where positive reactions occur, several patterns may emerge namely:

1. apparent specificity towards the autologous tumour
2. reactivity towards the autologous and some allogeneic tumours
3. a broad reactivity towards several tumour targets and towards NK-sensitive target cells. (This bears some resemblance to the activity of anomalous killer cells often generated in mixed lymphocyte cultures (MLC) and may represent the activity of LAK cells, which require several days incubation in IL-2 for their generation).

B CELL RESPONSES

That antibodies are produced against antigen expressed on the tumour cells may be demonstrated by a variety of techniques including immunofluorescence and cytotoxicity assays using isotope labelled tumour cells and exogenous complement (Fig. 18.17). Although cell-mediated reactions are probably of greatest significance, antibodies against tumour antigens which are detectable in autologous sera recruit cells carrying Fc receptors, for example, K cells and macrophages. Complement-dependent cytotoxic antibody is readily demonstrable in animals bearing lymphoid tumours if the tumour burden is not large, but is rarely demonstrated in the sera of humans bearing tumours. Antibody-dependent cellular cytotoxicity (ADCC) is demonstrable in some sera from patients with tumours. Antibodies forming soluble immune complexes with tumour antigens may subvert cellular responses (see below). Monoclonal antibodies and conventional polyclonal antibodies have been used to determine the complicated antigenic profile expressed by different tumours and are also being used for the immunolocalization of tumours *in vivo* (immunoscintigraphy). Monoclonal antibodies also have great potential for anti-tumour therapy by immunotargetting cytotoxic drugs and toxins.

IMMUNE COMPLEXES

The body fluids of cancer patients frequently contain immune complexes. To this extent they differ little from the sera of patients with non-malignant inflammatory or degenerative conditions of the same tissue or organ (Fig. 18.18). Theoretically, circulating immune complexes detectable in the sera of cancer patients and of patients with other pathological disorders may consist of several disparate antigens, including, in the case of cancer patients, some which are tumour-associated. In some malignant diseases, for example breast cancer, levels of circulating immune complexes have a tendency to rise in

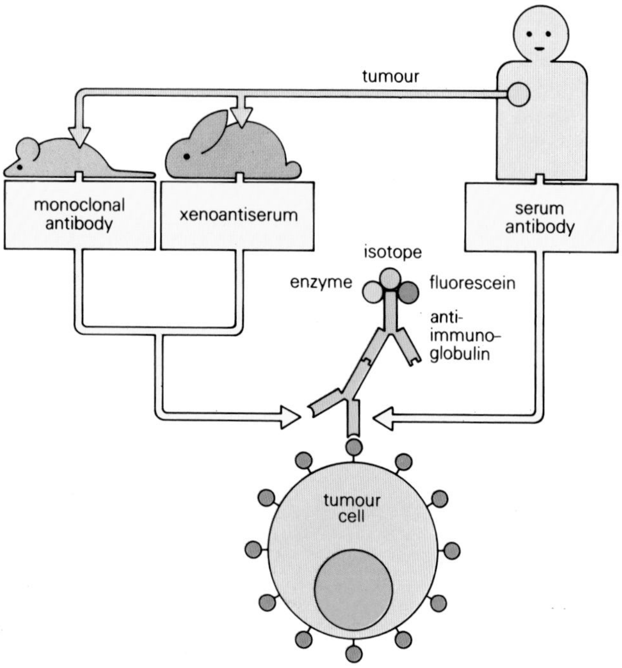

Fig. 18.17 Detection of tumour antigens by particular antibodies. The antibodies may occur in the patient's serum or they may be raised in experimental animals by immunization with the tumour. If this is done in mice, monoclonal antibodies can be produced. Binding of the antibody to the tumour is detected by a second layer of antibody specific for the first antibody and conjugated to an enzyme, an isotope or a fluorochrome.

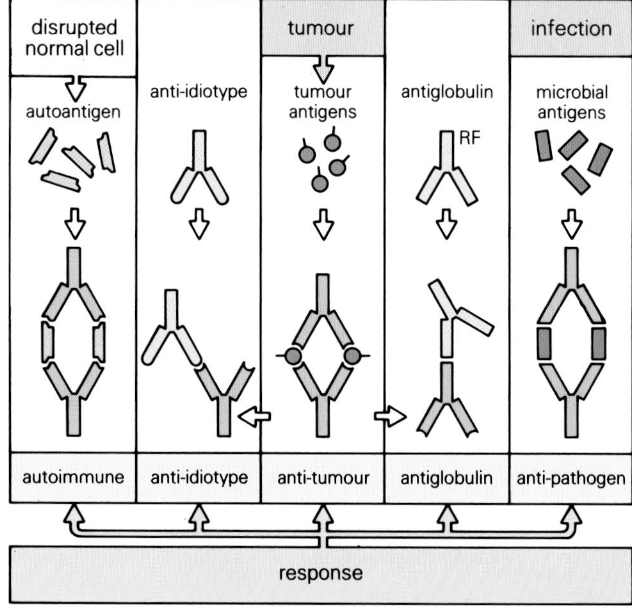

Fig. 18.18 Possible origin of circulating immune complexes in neoplasia. Immune complexes are detected in the body fluids of many patients with tumours. They may be due to antibodies reacting with autoantigens of damaged tissue or with microbial antigens. Intercurrent infections are seen more frequently in cancer patients who may be immunosuppressed by the action of the tumour or by cytotoxic drug therapy. They may also be due to anti-tumour antibodies forming complexes with tumour antigens, antiglobulin rheumatoid factor (RF) or specific anti-idiotypes.

patients who suffer relapse and to fall in patients who remain free of the disease. However, the nature of immune complexes in the sera of cancer patients is largely unknown.

NATURAL IMMUNITY

Natural immunity is effected by cells capable of lysing tumours spontaneously, that is, without prior sensitization. Strictly speaking, the effectors of natural immunity include mononuclear phagocytes and polymorphonuclear phagocytes as well as NK cells (Fig. 18.19). The original description of NK cells was based upon their apparent predilection for tumour cells adapted to tissue culture, against which cytotoxicity can be monitored in isotope release assays. Even so, NK cells and macrophages call for separate discussion. Unlike cytotoxic T cells, NK cells appear to lack both immunological memory and MHC restriction and are characterized by an ability to lyse a wide variety of targets including those which are syngeneic, allogeneic and xenogeneic to the NK donor. Virus infected targets are also highly sensitive as are normal cells of thymic and bone marrow origin. This has led to the hypothesis that the capacity to regulate tumours is an extension of the normal regulatory role of NK cells which is to combat virus-infected cells and regulate cellular differentiation in the thymus and bone marrow. LAK cells result from the incubation of peripheral blood lymphocytes in IL-2 for a minimum period of 48 hours. Although the percursors apparently lack the surface markers of NK cells, LAK cells may represent a further activation state of these cells.

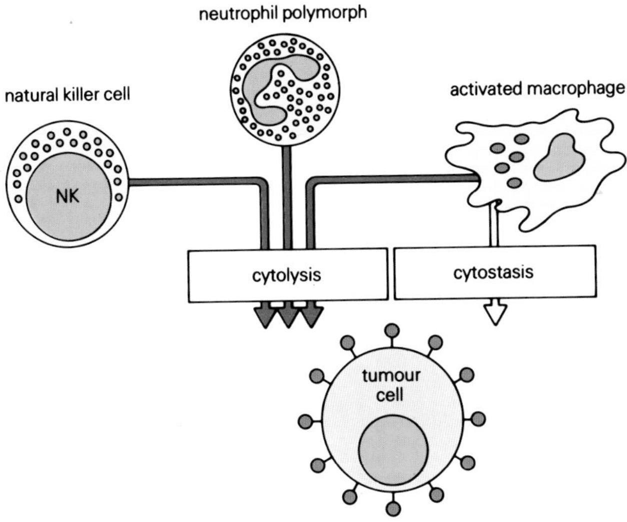

Fig. 18.19 Natural immunity to tumours. Natural immunity to tumours is mediated by activated macrophages, neutrophils and NK cells. Their action may be cytolytic, causing tumour cell lysis, or cytostatic, inhibiting growth. This type of immunity does not require antibody and displays no antigen specificity – the cells attack all tumour cells of a particular type, the origin of the cell donor being irrelevant.

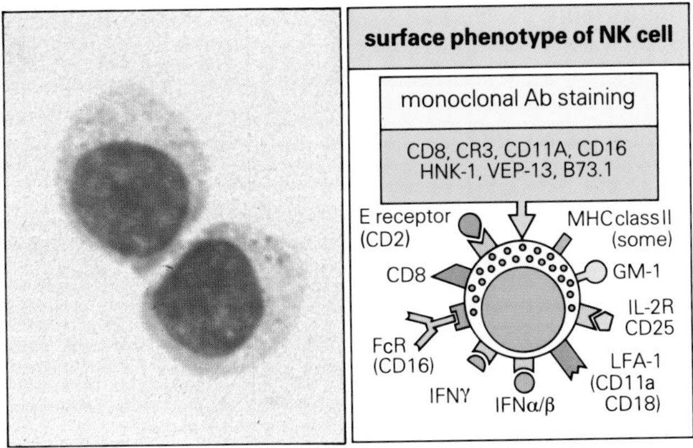

Fig. 18.20 The NK cell. NK cells are a heterogeneous group of cells, but a major proportion of them are large granular lymphocytes, here seen stained with Jenner-Giemsa (left). The surface phenotype (right) has been delineated with the help of the monoclonal antibodies listed.

NK and LAK Cells In man, the principal NK cell is the large granular lymphocyte (LGL), so called because of its intracytoplasmic azurophilic granules and high cytoplasmic : nuclear ratio (Fig. 18.20), which comprise 2–5% of peripheral blood lymphocytes. However, cytolysis experiments performed at the single cell level indicate that not all LGLs are NK cells and not all lytic cells are LGLs. LGLs display a number of phenotypic and functional markers, but studies on NK cell clones indicate considerable heterogeneity within this population not only in respect of cell surface phenotype but also regarding the target cell recognized. NK activity is demonstrable in peripheral blood and in the spleen, and to a much lesser extent in lymph nodes, bone marrow, thoracic duct and thymus. The target structures recognized by NK cells have not been defined but it appears from experiments using NK clones that some determinants are ubiquitous while others have a more restricted distribution. The determinants recognized by NK cells are more prevalent on tumours adapted to tissue culture. An alternative suggestion is that NK susceptibility depends on the absence of normal cell surface antigens such as MHC molecules and this theory has been supported by an observed increase in resistance to NK cell killing following incubation of the target in agents which induce MHC antigens on cell surfaces (such as interferon). Nevertheless, the first stage in NK cell lysis involves a readily demonstrable binding event which is essential for the triggering of lysis and which can be inhibited with cytochalasin-B which inhibits microfilaments. Such binding must involve a cell surface structure. Target susceptibility to lysis by the NK cell also depends on its differentiation status and its capacity to repair membrane damage.

There is virtual overlap of the NK population with the population which mediates ADCC (K cells). The Fc receptor of the NK cell is, however, not involved in the lytic process. There are also other mechanistic differences and K cell activity is less consistently augmented by interferon and other immunomodulators.

NK activity is subject to both positive and negative regulation both *in vivo* and *in vitro*. Peripheral blood NK cells show increased cytotoxicity after several hours incubation in either IFNγ or IL-2 (Fig. 18.21). The action of these agents is probably two-fold – transforming non-cytolytic NK precursors into a lytic state and enhancing the cytolytic capacity of already active cells. NK cells themselves produce IFNα (detectable by anti-IFNα) on binding to their targets and also respond to IL-2 by producing both IL-2 and IFNα. Production of IFNα on stimulation with IL-2 does not, however, account for all the increase in cytotoxicity which is still shown in the presence of antibodies to IFNα.

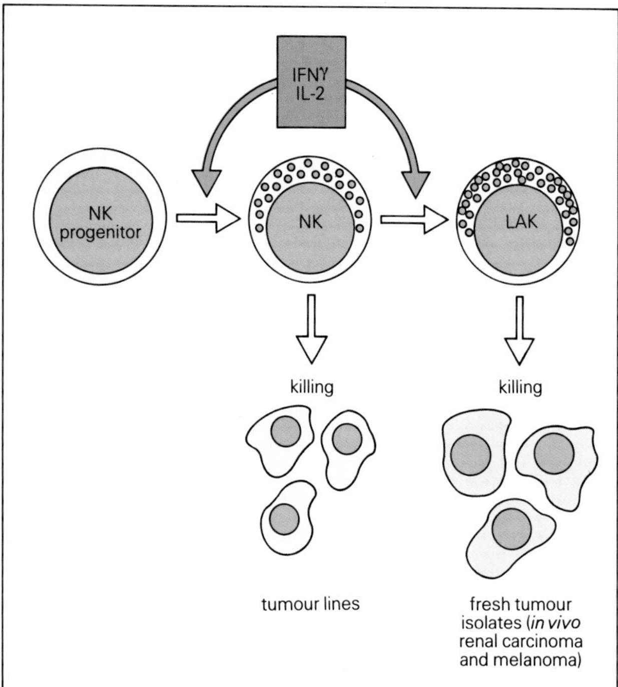

Fig. 18.21 Development of natural killer (NK) and lymphokine-activated killer (LAK) cells. NK cells develop from progenitors under the influence of interferon-ϒ (IFNϒ) and interleukin-2 (IL-2) and are capable of killing tumour lines, particularly those adapted to tissue culture. LAK cells are thought to develop from NK cells following further activation by cytokines. These cells are capable of killing freshly isolated tumours.

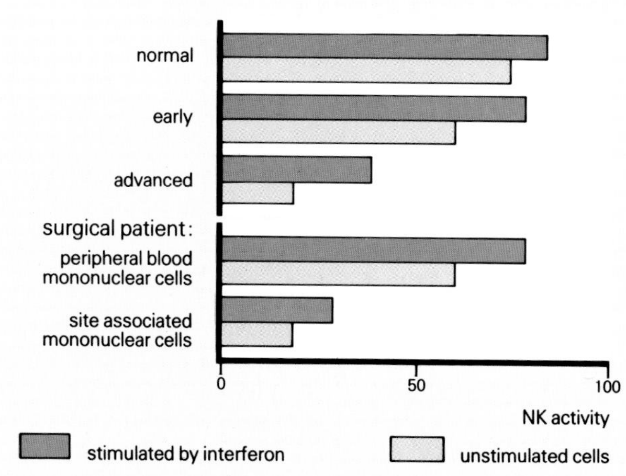

Fig. 18.22 Natural killer (NK) cell activity in disease. The activity of NK cells (defined as the percentage of maximum possible lysis of target cells) declines as the tumour progresses (upper chart). Activity is slightly reduced in the mononuclear cell population of patients with early cancer but is much reduced in those with advanced cancer. NK activity can be enhanced in all groups by interferon-ϒ (red) by comparison with unstimulated cells (grey). Mononuclear cells derived from the tumours of surgical patients with early cancer have less NK activity than their peripheral blood mononuclear cells (lower chart).

The biological role of NK cells is uncertain. There is circumstantial evidence from experimental systems that they participate in the rejection of transplanted tumour cells, in the prevention of metastases and in bone marrow graft rejection. However they have no impact on established cancers where their numbers are few and their functional ability greatly depressed. Anti-tumour effects are likely to be in the nature of a 'first line of defence' against a tumour nidus before the development of adaptive immune responses. Peripheral blood NK activity tends to wane with progressive disease (as indeed do many other aspects of the immune system) and is undetectable in some malignant proliferative disorders (Fig. 18.22).

More recently, attention has been focused on LAK cells, produced by incubation of PBL in IL-2 for more prolonged periods of time. Two of the interesting features of these cells are the broader specificity they apparently show towards a variety of freshly isolated solid tumours which are notoriously refractory to NK activity, and their relative lack of cytotoxicity towards normal tissue cells.

The precursors of LAK cells can be isolated from blood, spleen and lymph nodes and are found in the low density population which also includes the NK cells, but they lack some of the markers characteristic of the NK cell. It may be that LAK cells do in fact represent a further activation state of the NK cell but whatever their lineage, they hold out the prospect of a new form of therapy of tumours currently undergoing clinical trials, which is discussed later.

Macrophages In common with NK cells, macrophages can properly be regarded as effector cells of natural immunity, though this represents only one of several central roles in cellular immunity. Macrophages have also been implicated in the surveillance system against the development of tumours since the administration of macrophage 'poisons' significantly reduces the latent period for the development of ultraviolet light-induced skin tumours in mice. Conversely, administration of macrophage stimulants lengthens the latent period in the same system. Macrophages have also been implicated in the control of metastasis in experimental animal systems although the degree of infiltration of a tumour by macrophages rarely correlates with the spread of the tumour. In laboratory animals the macrophage content of tumours is frequently a constant characteristic of each individual neoplasm. Entry of macrophages into a tumour may be inhibited by certain tumour products, particularly retroviral protein. Conversely, some human and murine tumours produce factors with chemotactic activity for macrophages, the amount of which correlates with the number of macrophages in the infiltrate. As effectors, macrophages generally express little cytotoxicity unless activated, a process which is characterized by several morphological, biochemical and functional changes resulting in increased tumoricidal and bactericidal activity. Macrophages can be activated by a number of agents *in vitro* including endotoxin, immune complexes, aggregated IgG, muramyl dipeptide and lymphokines (see Chapter 9). The nature of the 'target' structure on tumours recognized by macrophages is unknown. They appear to display a remarkable ability to distinguish tumour cells from 'normal' cells and attempts to isolate tumour clones resistant to the tumoricidal activity of macrophages have generally been frustrated.

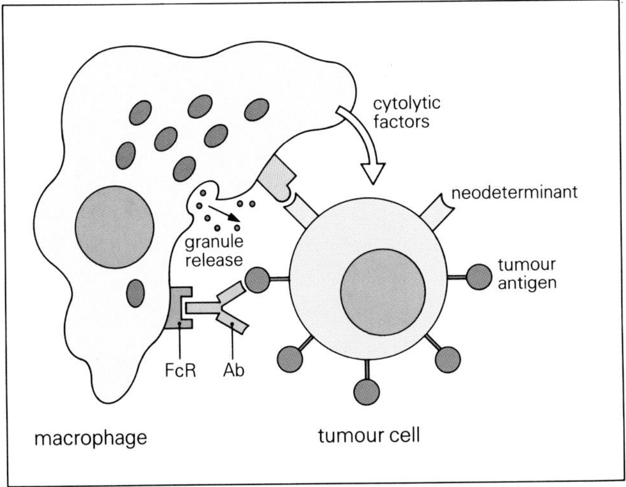

Fig. 18.23 Macrophage action against tumours. Macrophages recognize tumours either via their Fc receptors binding to antibody on the tumour surface or via neodeterminants which become expressed on cells which lose their contact inhibition. Macrophages damage their targets by the release of cytolytic factors including some cytokines, or by release of enzymes and oxygen metabolites.

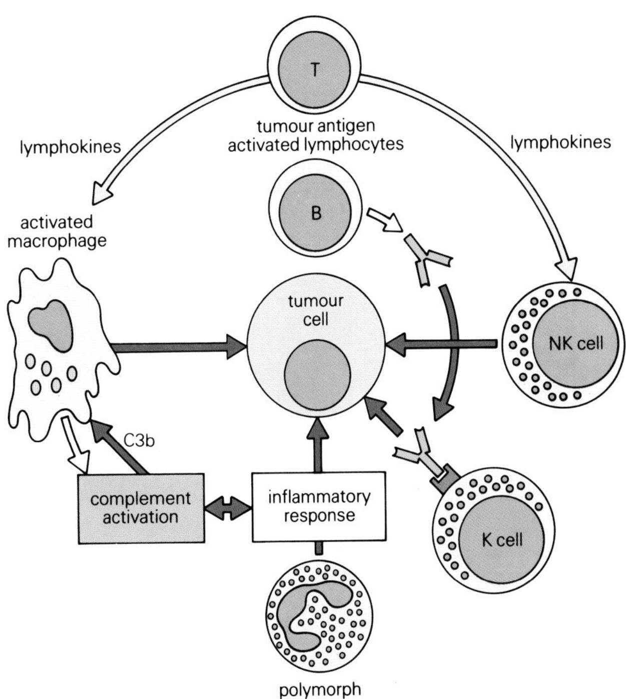

Fig. 18.24 Summary of the interactions between natural and adaptive immunity. Lymphokines activate macrophages and NK cells. Activated macrophages produce complement components locally which are involved in the development of the inflammatory response. C5a is chemotactic for neutrophils while C3b induces macrophage enzyme release. K cells are armed by antibody from tumour-specific B cells. This scheme should be interpreted bearing in mind that amplifying mechanisms only are shown.

Lack of contact inhibition displayed by tumour cell lines has been implicated but this is only one of numerous differences between tumour and 'normal' cells in culture. The cytotoxic process includes both cytolytic and cytostatic components. Tumour destruction results from a contact-mediated, non-phagocytic event and a later step may involve the secretion of lysosomal enzymes resulting in destabilization of the target cell membrane. Other macrophage secretions may also be implicated in tumour cell lysis and these include serine proteases, hydrogen peroxide, and tumour necrosis factor (TNF) produced in murine systems following stimulation of macrophages with endotoxins and bearing some similarities to lymphotoxin. Macrophages may also function as effectors in ADCC reactions against tumours although this is dependent on the amount of uncomplexed IgG (Fig. 18.23). Macrophages derived from tumour infiltrates frequently possess the characteristics of activated macrophages.

Macrophages can also mediate negative or inhibitory effects on various immune functions. This suppressive activity does not represent an abnormal state but a normal regulatory mechanism that may be intensified by the presence of a tumour or by certain treatments. Suppressor macrophages inhibit lymphoproliferative responses to allo- and tumour-associated antigens and this can be reversed by indomethacin which prevents prostaglandin E_2 (PGE_2) production. The fact that this reversal is rarely complete suggests that macrophages may be able to suppress via mechanisms not related to PGE_2. The primary effect of suppressor macrophages is not necessarily confined to the proliferation of lymphocytes. For example, suppressor macrophages interfere with the production of MIF, MAF and other lymphokines. In some cases an increase in macrophage content indicates a worsening prognosis and it has been suggested that they might secrete growth factors which encourage growth of the tumour. Like NK cells, macrophages may be involved in the regulation of their own activity.

A hypothetical scheme, based on data derived from *in vitro* studies, for the interaction of natural and adaptive immunity *in vivo* is shown in Fig. 18.24.

IMMUNOSURVEILLANCE

The original concept of immunosurveillance envisaged that control was exerted over oncogenesis, that is the development of tumours, so that the immune response was targetted towards small tumour cell foci. Thus, the development of large tumour burdens was due to immunological escape, possibly because the immune system was not functioning normally or because of some inherent property of the tumour itself with concomitant selective advantages. However, immunosurveillance could also occur after cancer has developed and this may perhaps manifest itself in the spontaneous regression of tumours (a rare event) or in demonstrable autologous anti-tumour responses of one kind or another using standard techniques *in vitro*. It is important to stress that immunosurveillance is only one form of host surveillance against tumour development. Other local and systemic mechanisms are concerned with the orderly maintenance of cells within tissues and the constant anatomical relationship between tissues of different kinds in controlling growth and development and in repair and regeneration after injury. Furthermore, immunosurveillance of all categories of neoplasm by a

cause	incidence of tumour		anti-tumour immune mechanisms
	nude	control	
spontaneous tumours	+	+	
chemical carcinogens	+	+	NK cells natural antibodies
oncornaviruses (RNA tumour virus)	+	+	
DNA tumour viruses	++	+	NK cells T cells antibodies

Fig. 18.25 Evidence for and against the role of T cells in immunosurveillance. The incidence of tumours (+) caused by different agents or spontaneously occurring in T cell-deficient (nude) and control (littermate heterozygote) mice is given. Only tumours caused by DNA viruses have a higher incidence in nudes than controls. This implies that if immunosurveillance is important for most types of tumour the function is performed by NK cells and other natural immune mechanisms. Only in the case of DNA virus-induced tumours is there evidence for T cell-mediated surveillance.

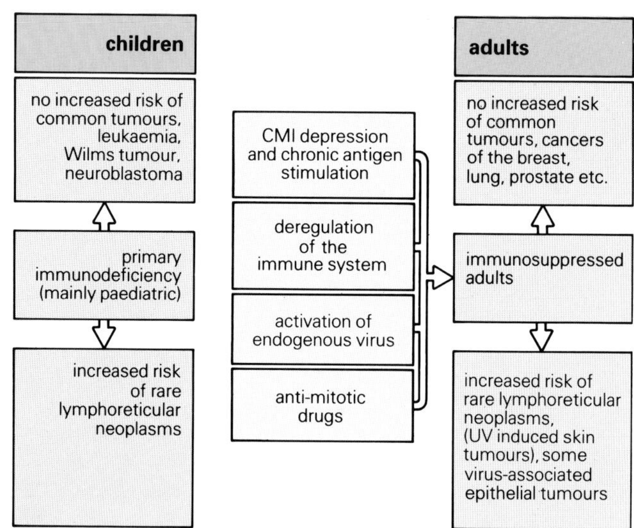

Fig. 18.26 A diagrammatic scheme relating to immunosurveillance in humans. Certain groups of tumours in children and adults can be related to impaired immune functions. It would be anticipated if immunosurveillance is operative that defects in the immune system would result in increased tumour incidence. In fact there is no increase in common tumours in primarily immunodeficient children or in immunosuppressed adults (usually transplant recipients), but there is an increase in the rarer tumours listed.

single mechanism, for example by T cells, is highly unlikely. Viewed in this context it may be seen that immunosurveillance, if it occurs, is a last line of defence against oncogenesis.

The most convincing evidence for T cell-mediated surveillance during oncogenesis is provided by tumours induced by the murine DNA viruses (for example, polyoma and SV40) (Fig. 18.25). Here the frequency of neoplasms in T cell-deficient mice is unequivocally greater than that in normal immunocompetent siblings. For other oncogenic agents (oncornaviruses, carcinogens), the frequency of neoplasms in T cell-deficient hosts is broadly comparable with that of their normal counterparts. In these circumstances T cell surveillance does not occur to any measurable extent and the fact that many of the emergent tumours express strong TATAs is not necessarily at variance with this (see 'Immunological Escape' below).

TUMOURS AND IMMUNODEFICIENCY

One big stumbling block to the theory of immunosurveillance has always been its failure to explain the lack of increase in the most common tumours (carcinomas of the breast, colon, lung etc.) in patients who are immunodeficient (Fig. 18.26). A consequence of immunosuppression in these patients is likely to be the release of ubiquitous viruses with oncogenic capability from immunological control by the host. Several human viruses are oncogenic and their evasion of control may result from abrogation of the T cell response to virus-infected and transformed cells. Alternatively, NK cells, known to kill virus-infected cells *in vitro*, may be implicated in this respect. Generalized immunosuppression could result in the loss of T-cell produced lymphokines which regulate NK activity (such as IL-2 and IFNγ). Provisional evidence for a role for NK cells in immunosurveillance comes from a study of the 'beige' mouse, in which a mutant gene confers some impairment of NK activity *in vitro* but which is neither selective nor absolute. In comparison to normal heterozygous littermates, these mice are marginally more susceptible to primary tumour development by carcinogens. Whether this relates to control of oncogenic viruses, however, is not certain.

Virus Surveillance Recent examples of the failure of immunosurveillance in human populations could be the unusual occurrence of Burkitt-like lymphoma (of Epstein-Barr virus association) and Kaposi's sarcoma (of cytomegalovirus association) in homosexual males with AIDS. Thus, the evidence in humans whereby there is an increased incidence of virally-induced tumours in immunodeficient patients, points to surveillance against the virus as opposed to the tumour, although the immune response could then destroy tumour cells as a consequence of viral antigens expressed thereon. It is conceivable that the immune system may have a role in preventing the occurrence of metastasis, where tumour foci are initially small, and immune suppression sometimes leads to increased metastasis in animal systems. Moreover, in such systems, small inocula of tumour cells can be rejected at a site distal from a progressively growing tumour in the same animal, a phenomenon known as concomitant immunity.

Escape Immunological escape does not necessarily invalidate immunosurveillance, since many tumours may be eliminated before their presence is detected. In other words, the tumours have been selected for their ability to evade an immune response. The relative inefficiency of therapy to date neither disproves immunosurveillance nor excludes the possibility that it may be made more effective. If immunosurveillance exists, its effectiveness is likely to depend on a balance between mechanisms minimizing tumour viability, immunological escape or immunodepression.

IMMUNOLOGICAL ESCAPE

Mechanisms of immunological escape address the central paradox of tumour immunology which is why neoplasms which are demonstrably immunogenic elude the effector arm of the immune response. Immunological escape may occur when the balance between factors favouring tumour growth and destruction is tilted in favour of the tumour. Some escape mechanisms are so potent that they could circumvent immunological therapy as well as the normal autologous response. The factors that may contribute to immunological escape include tumour kinetics, antigenic modulation, antigen masking, blocking factors, tolerance, genetic factors, tumour products, and growth factors (Fig. 18.27).

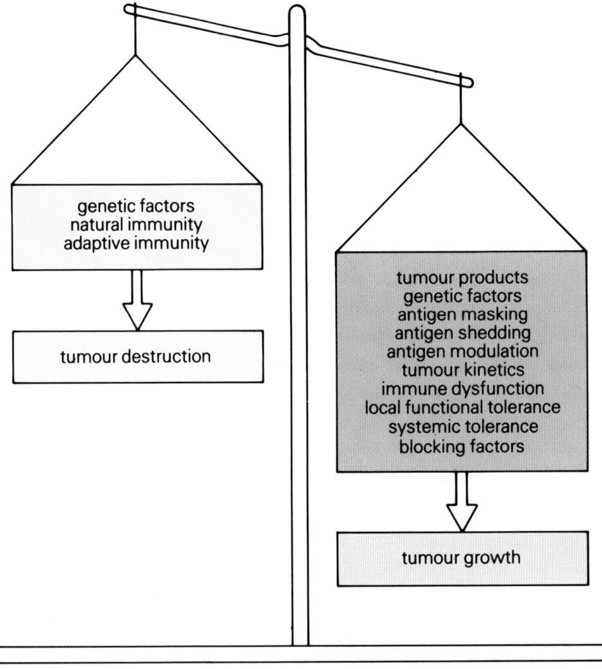

Fig. 18.27 Immunological escape. The ability of a tumour to escape from immunological control may depend on a balance between the effectiveness of the immune system and a variety of factors promoting escape.

Tumour Kinetics ('Sneaking Through') In immunized animals, tumour cells administered in sufficiently low doses develop into cancers when greater doses are rejected. Therefore, under conditions theoretically optimized for rejection, tumour cells may 'sneak through' and not be recognized until growth is established and beyond recall. This mechanism could account for many failures of immunosurveillance in both clinical and experimental situations.

Antigenic Modulation In the presence of antibody, some antigens are modulated off the cell surface. This involves antigen shedding, endocytosis and redistribution within the membrane without a complete loss of the determinant from the cell surface; it is a process distinct from capping. Antigenic modulation facilitates escape by removing the target antigens that the immune system's effector cells would recognize, and is known to occur in some instances when administering xenogeneic antibodies for immunotherapy. To some extent this is ameliorated by using monovalent antibodies.

Antigen Masking Facilitation of tumour escape from effector cells may occur because certain molecules such as sialomucin, which are frequently bound to the surfaces of tumour cells, mask tumour antigens and prevent adhesion of attacking lymphocytes. Masking can be overcome by treatment which degrades sialomucin, for example with *Vibrio cholerae* neuraminidase.

Blocking Factors Circulating soluble tumour antigens have been demonstrated in the sera of tumour-bearing animals and patients, where they have the capability to compromise the expression of T cell immunity by saturation of antigen-binding sites, particularly in the tumour microenvironment where the concentration of shed antigen is likely to be the highest. Similarly, when tumour antigens are shed they may form complexes with the host's specific antibody. Evidence exists from animal and human systems that these complexes can block the cytotoxicity of host T lymphocytes although the mechanism is uncertain. When the phenomenon was first described in the 1970s it was thought to be related to TH and Tc cells, but now it is thought to be more probably due to blocking of Fc receptors on LAK cells.

Tolerance Specific inhibition of the normal immune response to tumour antigens is exemplified by another murine tumour–host system, the mammary tumour virus (MTV). The virus is transmitted through the milk. Fostered mice are not infected and do not develop tumours. Transplantation experiments show that mammary tumours are far more antigenic in mice that lack the virus than those that acquire it at birth. Those mice which are infected congenitally become immunologically tolerant to certain antigens common to the virus and resulting tumours.

Genetic Factors Failure to induce an effector T cell response to a tumour could be a function of the MHC haplotype of the host in an analogous fashion to the T cell responses seen to virally infected cells. It has been shown with several viruses in mice and with influenza in humans that certain haplotypes are associated with poor induction of a cytotoxic T cell response, probably on account of the inability of the MHC products to form a suitable associated complex with the foreign antigen. Alternatively, inherent susceptibility to disease associated with particular haplotypes, may be explained in other ways; for example, the MHC antigen may act as the receptor for the known or putative infectious agent. In man, very few malignancies are associated with HLA but the ones where an association has been shown to be statistically significant include acute lymphoblastic leukaemia (HLA–A2, with a relative risk (RR) of 1.39), Hodgkin's disease (HLA–A1; RR=1.37), nasopharyngeal carcinoma in South China (HLA–A2, Bw46; RR=2.31), and carcinoma of the breast (Bw35; RR=1.35). Although the relative risks are generally small the association of HLA and malignancy could be important not just in susceptibility but also in the resistance to an established tumour. Indeed, some neoplasms fail to express class I antigens. Genetically determined unresponsiveness to tumour antigens need not deter immunological approaches to tumour therapy because it may be overcome by appropriate modification or presentation of the relevant antigen.

Tumour Products The subversion of immune responses by products of tumours other than antigens can also be envisaged. Prostaglandins which negatively regulate NK and K cell functions constitute one example. Similarly other humoral factors act non-specifically to impair inflammatory responses, chemotaxis, the complement cascade or to augment the formation of a blood supply within solid tumours.

Growth Factors Amplification of T cell responses is critically dependent on the availability of interleukins. Any perturbation in production of IL-1 by macrophages or in the degree of cooperation between the T cell subsets or in the availability of IL-2 could conceivably limit the overall response to a tumour.

POTENTIAL FOR THERAPY

The potential for therapy via the immune system lies on several fronts as follows.

1. Active intervention, whereby attempts have been made to stimulate by various means those components of the immune system most likely to be responsible for anti-tumour immunity.
2. Adoptive immunotherapy, with the transfer of immunocompetence from one individual to another.
3. Passive immunotherapy via the administration of monoclonal antibodies to tumour-specific antigens to localize within the tumour and to target a variety of cytotoxic agents within the tumour.
4. Where bone marrow transplants are given to leukaemic patients who have been irradiated, monoclonal antibodies may be administered to deplete the bone marrow either of tumour cells if autologous, or of T cells if allogeneic.

It is important to stress that, with few exceptions, no immunotherapy schedule is presently more efficient than conventional treatments. At best immunotherapy may facilitate the removal of tumour foci inaccessible to conventional treatment or may be exploited to enhance specific or non-specific anti-tumour activity (Fig. 18.28). The complexity of the immune response to tumours necessitates a multilateral approach to the problem of immunotherapy. Ideally, this should attempt to enhance specific and non-specific host resistance at the same time as minimizing the prospects of escape from immunological control by the induction of other potentially deleterious changes in immune regulation.

ACTIVE INTERVENTION

Attempts to vaccinate animals in order to induce tumour resistance have met with very limited success in animal systems and, in some circumstances, for example with some chemically-induced transplantable tumours, immunization with irradiated tumour cells prior to transplantation of the tumour can result in enhanced tumour growth possibly by stimulating the production of blocking antibodies. The increasing realization of the involvement of viruses in the development of tumours in man offers great hope for the prevention of certain tumours.

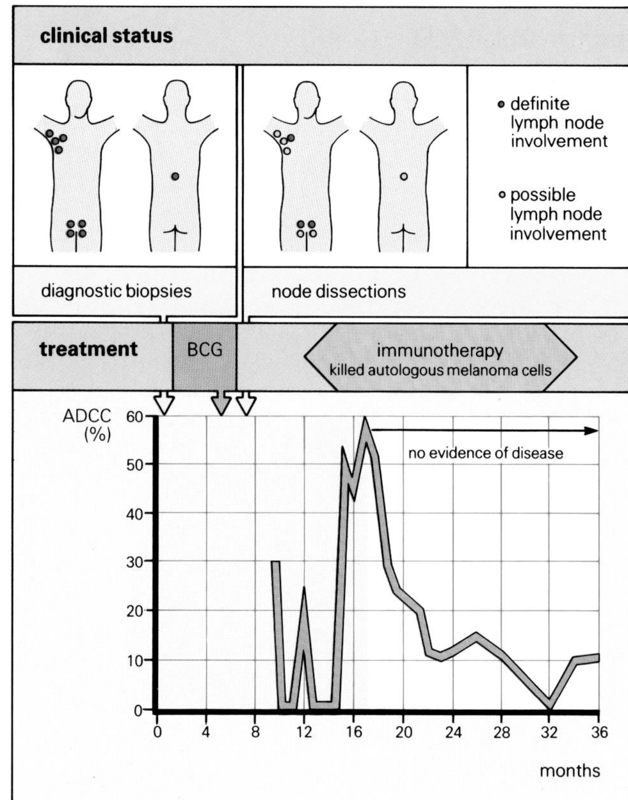

Fig. 18.28 Potential for immunotherapy of cancer. A patient with malignant melanoma was immunized with BCG (the key component of Complete Freund's Adjuvant) and separately with killed autologous melanoma cells and tested for the incidence of antibody-dependent cellular cytotoxicity (ADCC) (K cell activity) to the melanoma expressed as the percentage killing of the melanoma target cells. The patient's lymph nodes were examined for metastasis during the treatment. The clinical incidence of the tumour was inversely related to the activity of the effector cells. (Data from Dr L.J. Old and colleagues.)

For example, there is little doubt that the successful vaccine against hepatitis B virus will reduce the incidence of primary hepatoma. Similarly, where other strong associations exist, as with human papillomavirus 16 and 18 and cervical carcinoma, there is also the potential for vaccination of women at high risk, although in this case the immunity must be stimulated at mucosal surfaces. Modified cancer vaccines may offer a means whereby the immunogenicity of the tumour cells may be artificially enhanced for use in active immunization protocols (Fig. 18.29); these comprise the following.

1. Infection with certain viruses. In mice, homogenates prepared from virus-infected tumours are more effective immunogens than comparable preparations of non-infected tumour cells for the induction of transplantation immunity. In mice, myxoviruses are the viruses of choice, and vesicular stomatitis virus (VSV) infected melanoma cells are under study in man.
2. Chemical attachment of foreign determinants. Augmentation of the immunogenicity of tumour cells by chemical or enzymatic means has been achieved with chemically-induced murine sarcomas. PPD bound to tumour cell surfaces can augment the response if the host is immune to BCG.

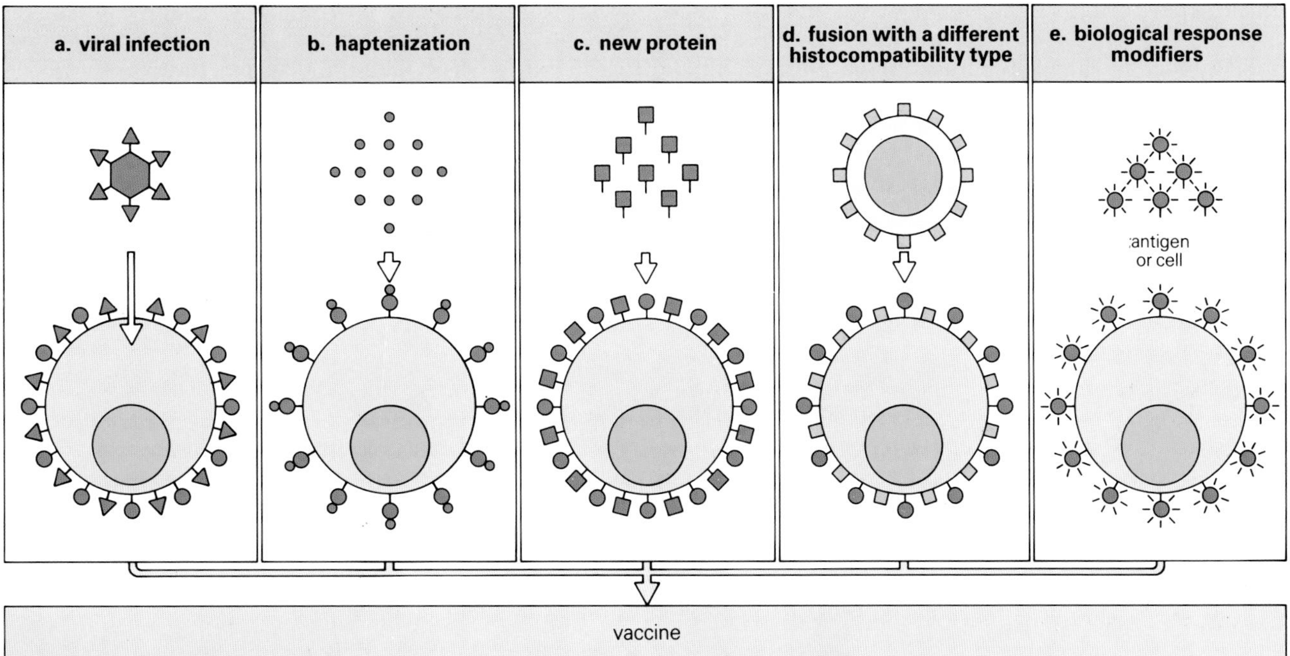

Fig. 18.29 Augmentation of host response. Vaccination against tumours is aimed at increasing the host response to tumour by: a. infecting the tumour with virus, b. coupling haptens to the tumour surface antigens, c. coupling protein antigens to the tumour surface, d. fusing the tumour with cells of a different histocompatibility type, e. increasing the immune response with adjuvants and other biological response modifiers.

3. Introduction of foreign determinants by somatic cell hybridization. Cell hybridization may provide another means of introducing foreign determinants onto the tumour cell surface.
4. Isolation and purification of tumour-specific antigens. Vaccines produced from purified tumour-specific antigens may be more effective than whole tumour cells where the relevant tumour antigens may be of low density and consequently 'swamped' by other determinants.

NON-SPECIFIC ACTIVE IMMUNIZATION

Non-specific active immunization employs a diversity of reagents which affect the immune response and are called biological response modifiers (BRM). Of these, the most extensively tested have been BCG, interferon, and IL-2 (Fig. 18.30). One of the continuing problems of the use of BRMs has been to ensure that the cells which are stimulated are the correct population, that is, it is essential that the treatment does not stimulate cells with suppressive activity.

type of BRM	examples	major effect
bacterial products	BCG, *C. parvum* muramyl dipeptide trehalase dimycolate	macrophage and NK activation
synthetic molecules	pyran copolymer MVE, poly I:C pyrimidines	interferon induction
cytokines	IFNα, IFNβ, IFNY IL-2, TNF	macrophage and NK activation
hormones	thymosin, thymulin thymopoietin	modulate T cell function

Fig. 18.30 Examples of biological response modifiers. Biological response modifiers (BRMs) are used to enhance immune responses and fall into four major groups. Broadly speaking, bacterial products have adjuvant effects on macrophages; a variety of synthetic polymers, nucleotides and polynucleotides induce interferon production and release; the cytokines administered directly act on macrophages and NK cells, and a variety of hormones including the thymic hormones, can be used to enhance T cell function. (MVE=maleic anhydride divinyl ether.)

BCG BCG has been widely used on the basis of its known stimulatory effect on macrophages, and has been reported to prolong the survival of children with acute lymphatic leukaemia and of adults with acute myelogenous leukaemia. Very little benefit has been found from its use on patients with various solid tumours, but intralesional BCG can cause regression of melanoma lesions. BCG exerts an adjuvant effect primarily through components in the cell wall of the bacillus.

Interferon Interferons α and ß probably exert antitumour activity principally by the inhibition of cell growth and division. All three classes of interferons have immunomodulatory properties (see Chapters 8 and 9). The results of interferon treatment of tumours have on the whole been most disappointing, and it has little or no effect on the course of the common tumours. Success has been achieved with its use against hairy cell leukaemia, a tumour which was previously refractory to conventional chemotherapy and radiotherapy.

IL-2 Administration of IL-2 for prolonged periods to patients with large tumour burdens has had very little measurable effect on the tumours. However, administration of IL-2 with LAK cells (produced by *in vitro* stimulation of autologous lymphocytes) has had some limited success in producing measurable regression of solid tumours including renal carcinoma and melanoma. Such treatments require multiple administration of IL-2 and LAK cells, a regimen which is both extremely expensive and logistically difficult.

ADOPTIVE IMMUNOTHERAPY

Adoptive immunotherapy involves the transfer of immunity from one individual to another, usually with leucocytes. The most likely prospect for adoptive immunotherapy in man depends upon the successful preparation of T cell clones with tumour-directed helper or cytotoxic activity. Animal models exist in which the adoptive transfer of tumour 'immune' lymphocytes is shown to mediate anti-tumour effects on established tumours. In man this would require the culture of large numbers of specific T cells *in vitro* using IL-2. Specific T cells may be obtained initially from a tumour infiltrate or from the blood of the patient. Alternatively there is the possibility of *in vitro* stimulation of lymphocytes with isolated and purified tumour-specific antigens. It has already been shown that allogeneic T cell clones able to lyse several kinds of fresh human tumours, but not untransformed human cells *in vitro*, are capable of inducing remission of malignant disease when administered to cancer patients. Since IL-2 was found to synergize with these clones in causing remission, it may well be that the clones were LAK cells possessing some T cell phenotypic markers.

PASSIVE IMMUNOTHERAPY

Passive immunotherapy using monoclonal antibodies entails the transfer of anti-tumour antibodies to cancer patients in order to cause tumour regression or prevent tumour recurrence. Several problems relate to the killing of tumour cells in this way. First, the specificity of the antibody and the distribution of the 'tumour' antigen is of paramount importance. Although monoclonal antibodies are uniquely specific for a given epitope, it is very rare for such an epitope to appear solely on cells of a single type. Thus, there is often a poor uptake of antibody and the ratio of the uptake by the tumour to that taken up by normal tissues is low. Second, even if the target antigen is tumour specific, a low surface density of the antigen will again lead to problems of low uptake. The affinity of the antibody is also important, although this can to some extent be controlled when selecting the hybridoma in the first instance. Since the blood supply to a given tumour represents a very small fraction of the total cardiac output, the binding of intravenously-injected antibody to tumour will be slow even in the presence of high affinity antibodies.

Assuming that antibody has successfully localized into the tumour, it is very unlikely that it will cause widespread regression of the tumour unless the tumour is well vascularized so that all parts of the tumour are reached. Should killing occur, complement dependent cytotoxicity may be involved, although ADCC is likely to be the significant factor. A number of clinical trials with anti-tumour monoclonal antibodies have been performed with little success but the greatest potential for this sort of therapy lies in the possibility of targetting cytotoxic agents to the tumour by way of tumour-specific monoclonal antibodies. Although uptake of antibody by the tumour remains an important factor, the cytotoxic effects of a low amount of antibody can be amplified if the antibody has attached to it either a cytotoxic drug such as chlorambucil, a toxin such as ricin, or a radioisotope such as ^{123}iodine.

Radioisotopes Radioisotopes are better suited to localize the tumour (immunoscintigraphy) rather than to destroy it since, in the latter case, the type of isotopes used could harm surrounding normal tissues. One advantage of radioisotopes not found with drugs or toxins is that radioactivity emitted from the surface of a tumour cell may kill bystander tumour cells which have failed to bind antibody.

Cytotoxic Drugs Initial attempts at immunotargetting used chlorambucil attached to a polyclonal anti-melanoma antibody. This technique was shown to cause some regression of the melanoma lesion. One advantage of using cytotoxic drugs is that much is already known about toxicity and pharmacokinetics following their extensive use in conventional cancer chemotherapy. They do, however, present a number of problems in that relatively high concentrations have to be taken up by the cell in order to kill it and this in turn necessitates high antigen density on the tumour cell surface.

Toxins Toxins are highly toxic proteins whose cytotoxic potential is invested in their ability to inhibit cell growth by enzymatic means. A cell may be killed by the entry of very few (possibly even one) molecules of the toxin so that only a few molecules of toxin need be attached to a single antibody molecule and a high antigen density at the target cell surface is not so essential. Toxins commonly employed include ricin and abrin from plants or diphtheria toxin. Immunotoxins employing a variety of antibody–toxin conjugates have been tested in animal systems for anti-tumour activity. The major predictive feature of activity appears to be the specificity and binding characteristics of the antibody but several other factors are also important for efficacy *in vivo* and these include the rate of clearance of the immunotoxin by cells of the mononuclear phagocytic system, the rate at which immunotoxin enters the tissue fluid from the vasculature, and the size of the tumour. While tumours of small size are consistently more susceptible to immunotoxin therapy, the destruction of large tumours depends on good vascularity within the tumour. The conjugates have been used against human tumours growing in nude mice with variable degrees of success but usually with a demonstrable prolongation of survival. Several trials have either just begun or are being planned using the conjugates in cancer patients and one study in melanoma patients using a ricin conjugate has produced partial success without toxicity to normal tissue.

IMMUNODEPLETIVE THERAPY

The major application of immunodepletion occurs in the field of bone marrow transplantation to irradiated leukaemic patients. Conventional chemotherapy has a long history in the treatment of leukaemia and is a well-documented method for inducing remissions. However, cytotoxic drugs rarely manage to kill all the tumour cells and the surviving cells may be drug-resistant. Whole body irradiation with or without chemotherapy provides a more reliable method for destroying all leukaemic cells particularly in the bone marrow. Such irradiated patients however require a bone marrow transplant from healthy donors to replace normal haemopoietic functions and such transplants often generate graft versus host (GVH) reactions. Immunotoxins, in which the monoclonal antibody is against a T cell-specific antigen (such as CD3) can be used, in the presence of exogenous complement, to purge the donor bone marrow of all T cells (and thus the potential GVH effector cells) prior to transplantation of the marrow. An alternative method, is to remove some autologous bone marrow prior to irradiation and to purge that bone marrow of tumour cells before giving it back to the irradiated patient. These techniques, however, require a tumour-specific antigen by which the tumours can be both identified and destroyed, and the monoclonal antibody must fix complement. Encouraging results have come from a number of trials in the reduction of GVH reactions with allogeneic bone marrow transplants although occasional rejection of the graft or relapse of the tumour points to incomplete destruction of tumour or the patients own T cells prior to transplant. Purging of autologous bone marrow has been used in patients with T cell leukaemia and lymphoma where the more frequent relapse rate (nearly 70% in one trial) may again be due to incomplete treatment of the patient rather than incomplete removal of tumour cells from the bone marrow.

SUMMARY OF POTENTIAL OF IMMUNOLOGICAL THERAPY

The potential for immunological intervention is summarized in Fig. 18.31. There is potential for cancer therapy using immunological methods, based on the observation that leucocytes expressing anti-tumour reactivity are found in cancer patients. However, since their activity is insufficient to control developed tumours, it is necessary to enhance the activity of tumour reactive leucocytes. This in turn requires the identification of antigens or other structures on the tumour surface which can stimulate the immune system and through which the immunological attack can be directed. It is not certain that these target antigens exist for every tumour, but if immunological surveillance does occur those tumours which do arise in immunocompromised patients may be potentially immunogenic and so susceptible to immunological destruction. On the other hand, tumours which arise in normals may be insufficiently immunogenic. Thus, there is evidence to offer hope of useful immunological intervention in some tumours. In particular, the development of monoclonal antibodies against tumour-associated antigens and of related conjugates holds out an exciting prospect for future therapy as well as for cancer diagnosis and monitoring.

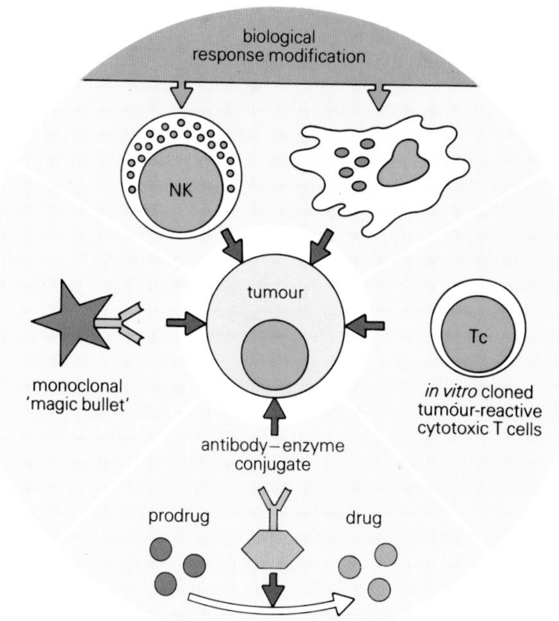

Fig. 18.31 Prospects for immunological intervention. Biological response modifiers could be used to activate NK cells and macrophages. Monoclonal antibodies directed to tumour antigens and coupled to cytotoxic drugs or toxins provide a possible 'magic bullet' against the tumour. Alternatively antibody–enzyme conjugates located at the tumour site could act on systemically administered pro drugs to release toxic drugs selectively at the critical site. Cloning of Tc cells of appropriate specificity might also be possible.

FURTHER READING

Bock, G. & Marsh, J. (eds) (1987) *Tumour Necrosis Factor and Related Cytokines. Ciba Foundation Symposium*, **131**. Chichester: Wiley & Sons.

Bolognesi, D. (ed.) (1988) *Human Retroviruses, Cancer and AIDS. Approaches to Prevention and Therapy.* New York: Alan R. Liss Inc.

Borrow, L.G. & Norton, A.J. (1987) Immunohistology in the identification of tumour types. *Cancer Surveys*, **6**, 209.

Franks, L.M. & Teich, N. (eds) (1986) *Introduction to the Cellular and Molecular Biology of Cancer.* Oxford: Oxford Science Publications.

Herlyn, M. & Koprowski, H. (1988) Melanoma antigens: immunological and biological characterisation and clinical significance. *Annual Review of Immunology*, **6**, 283.

Ruddon, R.W. (1987) *Cancer Biology.* 2nd edition. Oxford: Oxford University Press.

Strander, H. (ed.) (1986) Interferon treatment of human neoplasia. *Advances in Cancer Research*, 46.

Schreiber, H., Ward, P.L., Rowley, D.A. & Strauss, H.J. (1988) Unique tumour-specific antigens. *Annual Review of Immunology*, **6**, 465.

Tannock, I.F. & Hill, R.P. (eds) (1987) *The Basic Science of Oncology.* Oxford: Pergamon Press.

Tonaka, K., Yoshioka, T., Bieberich, C. & Jay, G. (1988) Role of the major histocompatibility complex class I antigens in tumour growth and metastasis. *Annual Review of Immunology*, **6**, 359.

Truitt, R.L., Gale, R.T. & Bortin, M.M. (eds) (1987) *Cellular Immunotherapy of Cancer.* New York: Alan R. Liss Inc.

Vogel, C.W. (ed.) (1987) Immunoconjugates. *Antibody Conjugates in Radioimaging and Therapy of Cancer.* Oxford: Oxford University Press.

Wright Jr, G.L. & Cox, A.D. (1987) Monoclonal antibodies to human tumour antigens. *Current Topics in Pathology*, **77**, 1.

19 Hypersensitivity–Type I

TYPES OF HYPERSENSITIVITY

When an adaptive immune response occurs in an exaggerated or inappropriate form causing tissue damage, the term hypersensitivity is applied. Hypersensitivity is a characteristic of the individual and is manifested on second contact with the particular antigen evoking hypersensitivity. Coombs and Gell have described four types of hypersensitivity reaction (Types I, II, III and IV), but in practice these types do not necessarily occur in isolation from each other. These reactions are no more than expressions of the beneficial immune responses acting inappropriately, and sometimes causing inflammatory reactions and tissue damage. The first three types are antibody-mediated; the fourth is mediated primarily by T cells and macrophages.

Type I, or immediate hypersensitivity, occurs when an IgE response is directed against innocuous antigens, such as pollen; the resulting release of pharmacological mediators, for example histamine, by IgE-sensitized mast cells produces an acute inflammatory reaction with symptoms such as asthma or rhinitis. Type II, or antibody-dependent cytotoxic hypersensitivity, occurs when antibody binds to antigen on cells, and leads to phagocytosis, killer cell activity or complement-mediated lysis. Type III, or immune complex-mediated hypersensitivity, develops when complexes are formed in large quantities, or cannot be cleared adequately by the reticuloendothelial system, leading to serum sickness type reactions. Finally, Type IV or delayed type hypersensitivity (DTH), is most seriously manifested when antigen, for example tubercle bacilli, trapped in a macrophage, cannot be cleared. T lymphocytes are then stimulated to elaborate lymphokines which mediate a range of inflammatory responses. Other aspects of DTH reactions are seen in graft rejection and allergic contact dermatitis. These four types of hypersensitivity reaction are summarized diagrammatically in Fig. 19.1.

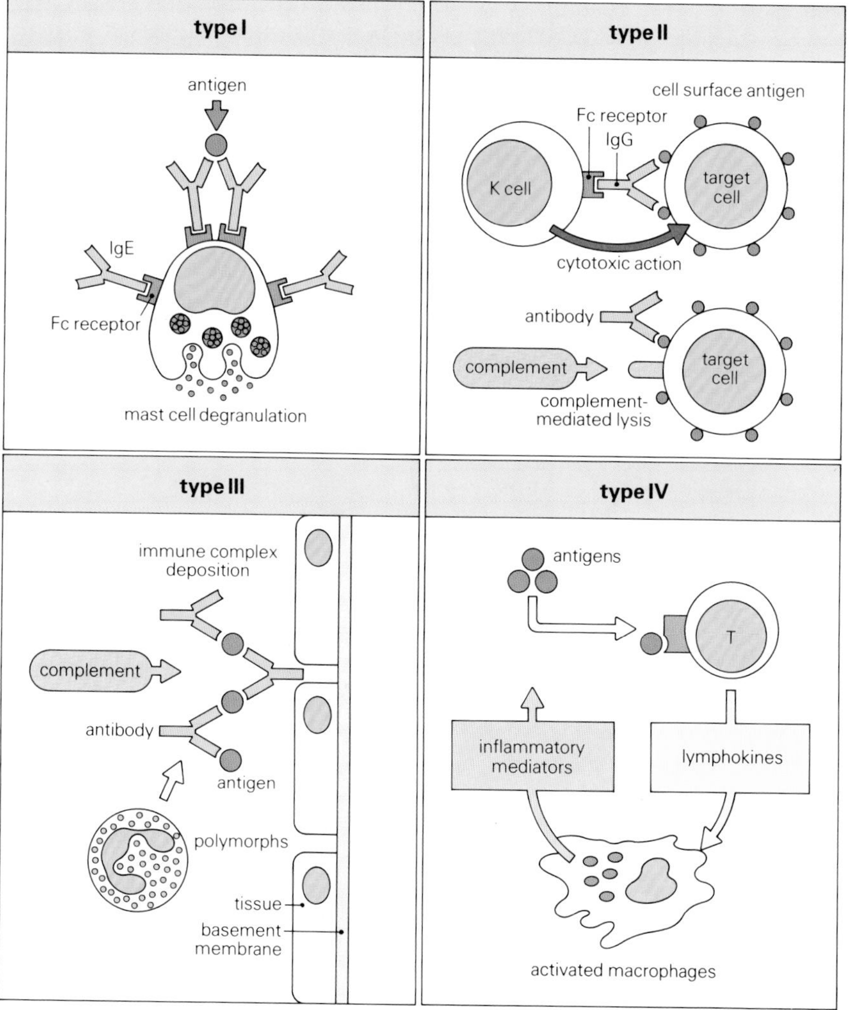

Fig. 19.1 Summary diagram of the four types of hypersensitivity reaction.
Type I Mast cells bind IgE via their Fc receptors. On encountering antigen the IgE becomes cross-linked, inducing degranulation and release of mediators.
Type II Antibody is directed against antigens on an individual's own cells (target cell). This may lead to cytotoxic action by K cells or complement-mediated lysis.
Type III Immune complexes are deposited in the tissue. Complement is activated and polymorphs are attracted to the site of deposition, causing local damage.
Type IV Antigen-sensitized T cells release lymphokines following a secondary contact with the same antigen. Lymphokines induce inflammatory reactions and activate and attract macrophages which release mediators.

TYPE 1 – IMMEDIATE HYPERSENSITIVITY

DEFINITION

Type I hypersensitivity is characterized by an allergic reaction immediately following contact with the antigen, which is referred to as the allergen (Fig.19.2). The term 'allergy', meaning 'changed reactivity' of the host when meeting an 'agent' on a second or subsequent occasion, was originally coined in 1906 by von Pirquet. He made no strictures as to the type of immunological response made by the host. It is only in recent years that 'allergy' has become synonymous with Type I hypersensitivity. These reactions are dependent on the specific triggering of IgE-sensitized mast cells by antigen resulting in the release of pharmacological mediators of inflammation (Fig. 19.3).

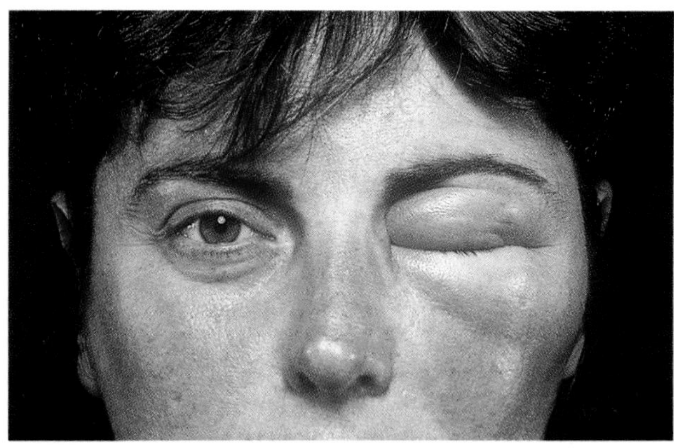

Fig. 19.2 The anaphylactic response to bee venom. This patient has been stung on her face by a bee. The immediate hypersensitivity to bee venom is a clear cut example of Type I hypersensitivity due to the release of pharmacological mediators, including histamine, from mast cells. The reaction can produce generalized anaphylaxis and even death since the allergen is injected into the patient rather than being inhaled. The reaction can be aggravated by mellitin in the venom which can trigger mast cells non-immunologically.

ATOPY

Originally described by Coca and Cooke (1923), the term atopy describes the clinical features of Type I hypersensitivity, which include asthma, eczema, hay fever and urticaria, in subjects with a family history of these or similar conditions and showing positive immediate wheal and flare skin reactions to common inhalant allergens.

It had already been suggested that anaphylaxis in animals, discovered by Portier and Richet (1902), was related to hay fever or asthma in humans, but whereas 90% of animals developed precipitating antibodies to injected heterologous proteins or toxins, only 5–10% of the human population exposed to an airborne allergen became sensitized to it. Furthermore, human allergy shows strong hereditary linkages which were not then appreciated in the animal model. Thus, Coca and Cooke considered that human allergic diseases were different from animal anaphylaxis and called them 'atopic diseases'. There is still some advantage in keeping the term atopy as it is a convenient umbrella term for a number of diseases, which share some common features, such as asthma, eczema, and hay fever.

The first description of the mechanism of the allergic reaction was by Prausnitz and Küstner (1921), who showed that a serum factor (termed reagin) could mediate the reaction on passive transfer to the skin of a normal subject. Some 45 years later, Ishizaka and colleagues showed that this 'atopic reagin' was a new class of immunoglobulin – immunoglobulin E (IgE).

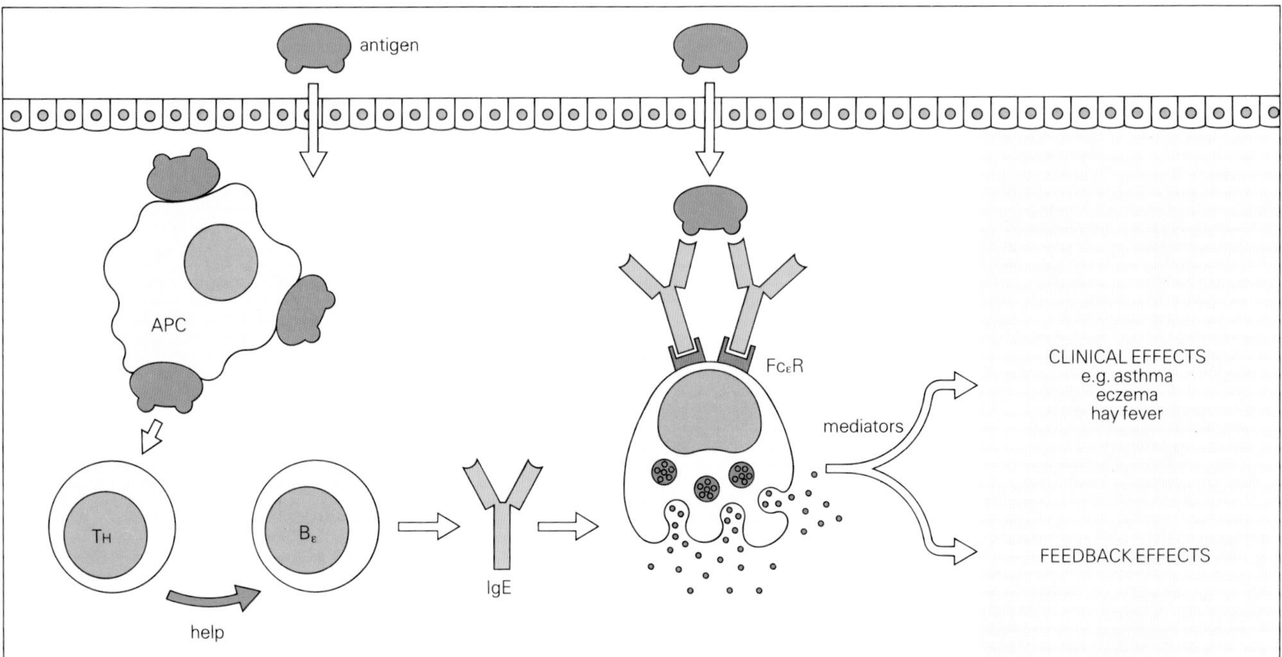

Fig. 19.3 Overall scheme for Type I hypersensitivity. Antigen stimulates B_ε cells to produce specific IgE with T cell help. This antigen-specific IgE binds to mast cells via Fc_ε receptors ($Fc_\varepsilon R$) thus sensitizing them. When antigen subsequently reaches the sensitized mast cell, it cross-links surface bound IgE and the cell degranulates, releasing mediators which cause the symptoms associated with Type I hypersensitivity.

IMMUNOGLOBULIN E

Following the initial contact of allergen with the mucosa there is a complex series of events before IgE is produced and before allergic symptoms result after a second contact with the same allergen. The IgE response is a local event occurring at the site of the allergen's entry into the body, that is, at mucosal surfaces and/or at local lymph nodes. IgE production by B cells involves antigen presentation via antigen-presenting cells, T cell help and the stimulation of B cells to produce IgE. Locally produced IgE will first sensitize local mast cells, and 'spill-over' IgE enters the circulation and binds to receptors on both circulating basophils and tissue-fixed mast cells throughout the body.

The structure of IgE is compared with that of IgG in Fig. 19.4. As with other immunoglobulins, IgE is comprised of two heavy and two light chains but the IgE heavy chain has five domains.

The major characteristics of IgE include its heat lability and its ability to bind to mast cells and basophils. It is notable that although the serum half-life of IgE is only 2½ days, mast cells may remain sensitized for up to 12 weeks following passive sensitization with atopic serum containing IgE. As has been mentioned above, the original description of the passive transfer of allergy by a serum component was by Prausnitz and Küstner. Küstner was allergic to fish and injection of his serum into the skin of Prausnitz, who was allergic to pollen, led to an immediate wheal and flare reaction when fish antigen was subsequently injected into the sensitized site. Interestingly, Küstner was allergic to cooked but not fresh fish. This test is similar to the passive cutaneous anaphylaxis (PCA) test which is used for the assay of IgE production in experimental animals.

The skin-sensitizing capacity of IgE resides in the Fc portion of the molecule and by heating the immunoglobulin at 56°C for half an hour the skin-sensitizing capacity is destroyed: the antigen-binding capacity, which resides in the Fab portion, is preserved. Thus, PCA tests before and after heating the serum will distinguish IgE from other antibodies which may sensitize mast cells, for example IgG1 in the guinea-pig.

IgE LEVELS IN DISEASE

IgE levels are often raised in allergic disease and grossly elevated in parasitic infestations. When assessing children or adults for the presence of atopic disease, a raised level of IgE aids the diagnosis although a normal IgE level does not exclude atopy (Fig. 19.5). The determination of IgE alone will not predict an allergic state as there are genetic and environmental factors which play an important part in the production of clinical symptoms. When skin tests are performed on a large number of subjects, many more give positive skin tests than complain of symptoms. A recent survey has shown that up to 30% of a random group of 5000 subjects had a positive wheal and flare reaction to one or more common allergens. Thus, these subjects can produce specific IgE but lack some factor (factor X, see Fig. 19.38), which precipitates the symptoms of atopy.

binds to FcεR

	IgE	IgG1
heavy chain domains	5	4
molecular weight	188,000	146,000
carbohydrate	12%	2–3%
half-life (serum)	2½ days	21 days

Fig. 19.4 IgE structure compared with IgG1. IgE is a trace protein in serum (<0.001% of total serum immunoglobulin). It has five domains in the heavy chain and varies from the basic IgG structure as shown. A part of the Fc region of IgE (C_H3 and C_H4) is involved in binding to Fc_ε receptors (FcR) on mast cells and basophils. This Fc binding is heat labile and activity is destroyed by heating at 56°C for 30 minutes. Antigen binding to the Fab portion is not heat labile. IgE serum levels are raised in parasitic infections and atopy.

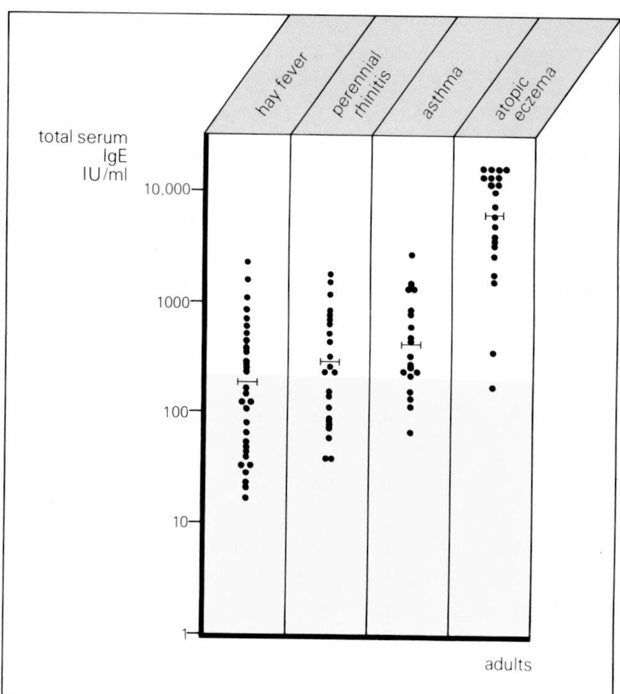

Fig. 19.5 IgE levels in allergic patients. Each point in this chart represents the serum IgE level of a patient. IgE levels vary over a wide range, but the levels in atopic patients are generally elevated above the levels in normal subjects of the same age. For many atopic individuals with less severe disease, the serum IgE level falls within the normal range. IgE titres are usually expressed in international units/ml, by reference to standard sera, where 1IU = 2.4 ng. The normal range of IgE in non-atopic subjects is shaded yellow.

CONTROL OF IgE PRODUCTION

Cellular Control – Early Studies The early studies by Tada and colleagues in the early 1970s using rats clearly demonstrated the T cell control of IgE production. Animals immunized with the antigen DNP-*Ascaris,* with *Bordetella pertussis* as adjuvant, showed a rise in IgE titres which peaked between 5 and 10 days and returned to normal over the next 6 weeks. If these animals were thymectomized or irradiated as adults, the IgE response was enhanced and prolonged. If during this phase of enhanced IgE production the animal was passively given thymocytes or spleen cells from *Ascaris*-primed animals, IgE production was suppressed (Fig. 19.6). The suppression of the IgE response was due to T-suppressor cells in the transferred cell population suggesting that thymectomy or irradiation treatment reduces suppressor activity. The IgG and IgM levels were unchanged by the cell transfer, showing that the IgE responses are particularly sensitive to the effects of T-suppressor cells. However, neonatal thymectomy completely abolishes the capacity to produce IgE to DNP-*Ascaris,* showing the need for T-helper cells in the IgE response. In several clinical conditions there is an association between low T-suppressor cell numbers and high levels of IgE, thus supporting the hypothesis for T cell control of IgE production in man.

Molecular Control – Recent Studies In the last five years, the complex interactions which regulate IgE production have been studied at the cellular and molecular levels, in experimental animals and man. Much of the work was performed by Ishizaka and his colleagues and the results of these studies are summarized in Fig. 19.7.

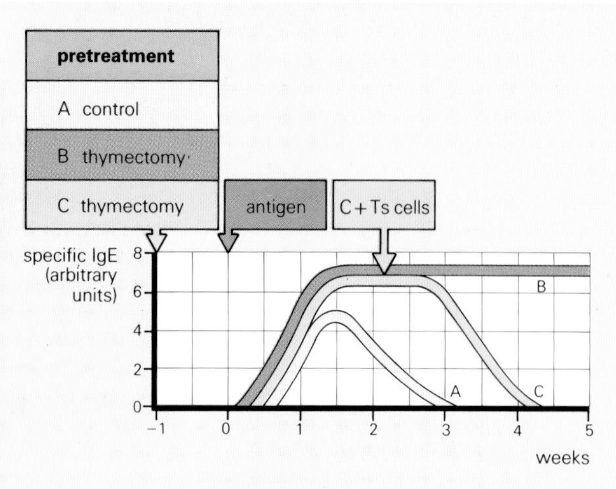

Fig. 19.6 T cell control of the IgE response. The IgE response is under both T-helper (TH) and T-suppressor (Ts) cell control. This experiment uses three groups of rats – a control group (A) receiving no pretreatment 1 week before antigen challenge, and two groups which are first thymectomized (B, C). Following antigen challenge the IgE response is measured regularly. On immunization with antigen there is a transient rise in antigen-specific IgE (A, control). Thymectomy (or irradiation) causes a prolonged response (B) which can be curtailed by the addition of antigen-stimulated spleen cells containing Ts cells (C). (If neonatally thymectomized rats are immunized no IgE response is seen, indicating the requirement for TH cells in the IgE response.)

The central T-helper cell bearing Fc_ε receptors ($Fc_\varepsilon R$) in this system makes IgE binding factors (IgE-BF), in response to factors derived from antigen-specific T-helper cells activated by antigen-presenting cells and antigen. Two types of IgE-BF can be made; these are IgE potentiating factor (IgE-PF) and IgE suppressor factor (IgE-SF). It has been demonstrated that a single gene codes for both these molecules and the difference between them is in the post-translational glycosylation (addition of carbohydrate to proteins). The relative amounts of IgE-PF and IgE-SF produced are controlled by factors derived from other antigen-specific T cells. These factors either enhance (glycosylation enhancing factor, GEF) or inhibit (glycosylation inhibiting factor, GIF) glycosylation of IgE-BF. GIF is produced by a T-suppressor cell, whereas GEF is produced by an $Fc_\varepsilon R^+$ T-helper cell. The levels of these factors control the production of IgE-PF and IgE-SF by the central T-helper cell, and ultimately whether or not an IgE response will be made.

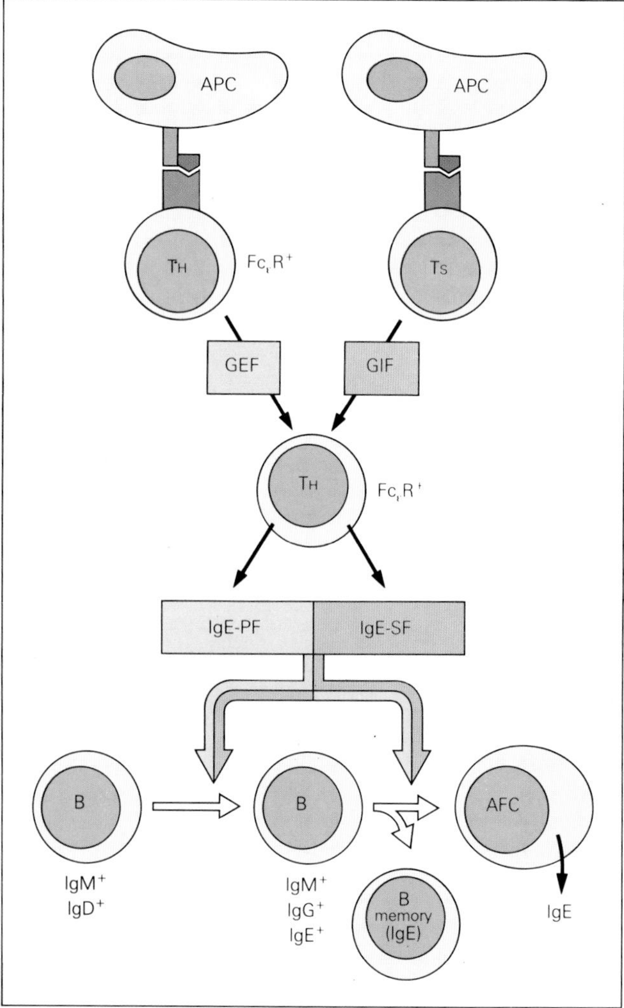

Fig. 19.7 Molecular control of IgE. There is a central role for the $Fc_\varepsilon R^+$ T-helper (TH) cell which, under the influence of other TH and T-suppressor (Ts) cells makes binding factor (IgE-BF) which potentiates (IgE-PF) or suppresses (IgE-SF) IgE production by B cells. A single gene codes for both these factors, the difference being in the post-translational glycosylation. The proportion of these factors is governed by other factors from antigen-specific TH and Ts cells, namely glycosylation inhibiting factor (GIF) and glycosylation enhancing factor (GEF).

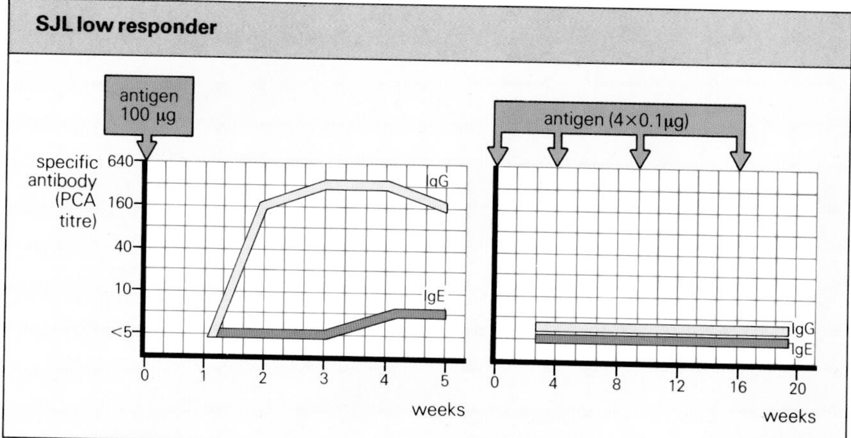

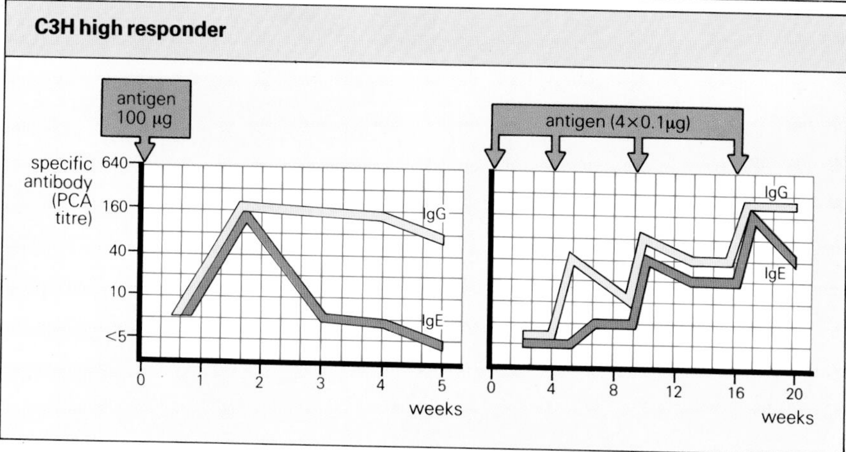

Fig. 19.8 Dependence of the IgE response on the antigen dose and the genetic constitution of the animal. A 'low responder' SJL mouse (top) makes predominantly IgG to a single large dose (100 μg) of antigen (left), but makes little or no specific IgG or IgE in response to repeated small doses (0.1μg). By contrast a C3H 'high responder' mouse (bottom) makes a transient large IgE response to a single high antigen dose which decays over 3–4 weeks, whilst repeated low dose antigen stimulation produces rising titres of both IgE and IgG with each injection.

IgE-BFs probably interact with surface IgE (sIgE) positive B cells and either stimulate (IgE-PF) or inhibit (IgE-SF) IgE production by these cells. The mechanisms involved are not yet fully understood but may include regulation of B_ε cell proliferation and/or maturation. It is likely that complexes of IgE plus antigen, or IgE plus IgE-BF, are formed during an IgE response and the binding of such complexes to $Fc_\varepsilon R^+$ B and T cells may also play a role in regulating the production of IgE-BF, memory B_ε cells and IgE antibody itself. Such feedback mechanisms are very important and typical of many physiological systems, since they result in the self-controlled production of the end-product which, in this case, is IgE.

The presence of $sIgE^+$ B cells is crucial in the above scheme, but as yet it is not known what mechanism(s) or factor(s) induce the switch from $sIgM^+$, $sIgD^+$ B cells to $sIgM^+$, $sIgE^+$ cells. Interestingly, interleukin-4 (IL-4) preferentially induces IgE production by mitogen activated B cells, and increases $Fc_\varepsilon R$ expression and release of IgE-BF by murine B cells. Furthermore, neutralizing antibodies against IL-4 can suppress IgE responses in experimental animals. Since IL-4 also has mast cell growth factor activity, the development of drugs which inhibit the action of IL-4 may have important therapeutic potential for controlling IgE responses and allergy.

Genetic Control of IgE in Mice The finding that different strains of animal vary in their ability to produce IgE suggests that IgE production is also under direct genetic control. Low responder strains of mice such as SJL do not produce high titres of IgE even when subjected to an optimum injection schedule for its production. In these studies, both the dose of antigen and the mode of its administration is critical (Fig. 19.8). It must be emphasized that although many animal model systems are available for studying IgE production, these are not models of allergy; there are no strains of laboratory mouse that develop hay fever spontaneously, although some dogs do. Clinically, however, man is sensitized with multiple low dose exposures to allergen, such as pollen during the summer, and the route of sensitization is by mucosal surfaces and not by intraperitoneal injection! The production of IgE in response to allergen, which is under genetic control, is just one factor in the development of atopy as discussed below.

GENETICS OF THE ALLERGIC RESPONSE IN MAN

Early studies in the 1920s showed that allergic parents tended to have a higher proportion of allergic children than parents who were not allergic. When large numbers of families are examined the figures show that with two allergic parents there is a greater than 50% chance of the children having allergy. Even with one allergic parent the chances are still almost 30%. Thus, both genetic background and elevated serum IgE levels are risk factors (Fig. 19.9).

It has been calculated that the annual challenge of individuals by airborne pollens is in the order of 1 μg, which is clearly a low-dose challenge. It is perhaps surprising that some 15% of the population respond to this exceptionally low-dose challenge. A variety of non-genetic factors also play an important role, such as the

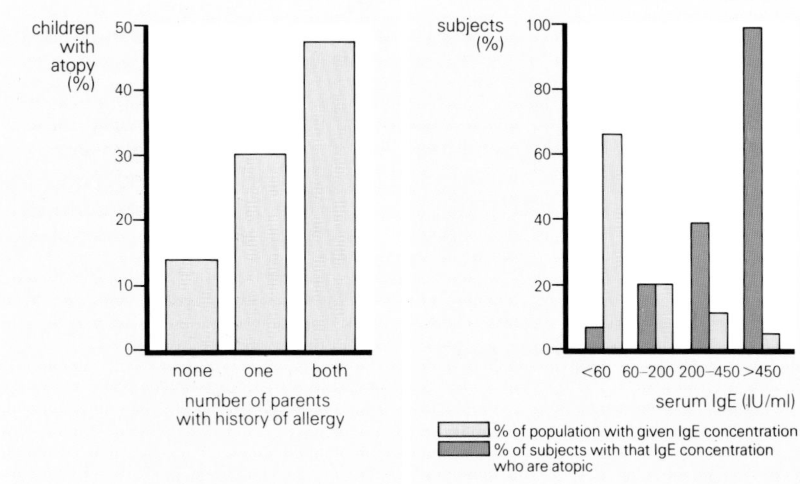

Fig. 19.9 Risk of allergy: family history and IgE levels. The left hand bar diagram shows the percentage of atopic children born to parents where none, one or both of the parents have a history of allergy. The greater the parental or family history of allergy, the greater is the risk of atopy in the child. The right hand diagram shows that the majority of the population has low levels of IgE. However, the higher the level of total serum IgE, the greater the likelihood of atopy.

systematic name	old name	mol.wt (daltons)	primary association	*p* value
Ambrosia (ragweed) spp.				
Amb a I	AgE	37,800	none	–
Amb a III	Ra3	12,300	A2	0.01
Amb a VI	Ra6	11,500	DR5	$<10^{-7}$
Amb a V	Ra5	5000	DR2/Dw2	$<10^{-9}$
Amb t V	Ra5G	4400	DR2/Dw2	$<10^{-3}$
Lolium (ryegrass) spp.				
Lol p I	Rye I	27,000	DR3/Dw3	$<10^{-3}$
Lol p II	Rye II	11,000	DR3/Dw3	$<10^{-3}$
Lol p III	Rye III	11,000	DR3/Dw3	$<10^{-4}$

Fig. 19.10 HLA associations of IgE responses to allergens from ragweed and ryegrass. (Courtesy of Dr D. Marsh.)

quantity of the exposure, the nutritional status of the individual and the presence of chronic underlying infections or acute viral illnesses (see Fig. 19.39).

There are three main genetic mechanisms regulating the allergic response; these mechanisms affect the total IgE levels, the antigen-specific response and general hyperresponsiveness, and are discussed in more detail below.

1 Total IgE levels Studies of families in which at least one member has high IgE levels have confirmed the hypothesis that a low IgE level is associated with a dominant gene.

2 HLA linked allergen-specific response The association between HLA and a specific response to allergens is most striking when ultrapure (>99.5% pure) preparations are used. It is more pronounced for very low-dose allergen exposure and especially for low molecular weight minor determinants, for example the ragweed allergen, Ra5, 5000 daltons, than for abundant high molecular weight allergens, for example AgE, 38000 daltons. With Ra5, more than 90% of IgE responders are HLA–Dw2, whereas with AgE there is as yet no HLA association (Fig. 19.10).

The association is greater with IgE antibody and immediate hypersensitivity skin tests than with IgG antibody. However, following hyposensitization to ragweed it is only the HLA–Dw2, Ra5$^+$ subjects who make a good IgG response showing that the immune response to Ra5 is not restricted to IgE, but includes other immunoglobulin classes.

Lastly, there is a higher association with HLA linkage when the subject has a low total IgE. For example, of patients who are allergic to ragweed, only 1 in 6 respond to Ra3, which is a minor determinant. Of the Ra3$^+$ patients with low levels of total IgE, 9 out of 10 subjects carry HLA–A2 (Fig. 19.11). With increasing total IgE levels, the number of determinants which are recognized is less restricted and the HLA association disappears.

3 General hyperresponsiveness The concept of hyperresponsiveness to a broad range of antigens has been tested in patients attending an allergy clinic who were divided solely on the basis of having positive or negative skin tests (Fig. 19.12). The results showed that HLA–B8 and HLA–Dw3, but not HLA–A1, are present at a significantly higher frequency in the allergic group. This hyperresponsiveness can also be seen in those already making anti-ragweed IgE antibodies, where those with HLA–B8 have higher titres of antibody and also high levels of total IgE.

HLA–B8 is also strongly associated with other forms of immune 'hyperactivity', for example autoimmune diseases. This raises the possibility that HLA–B8 is linked to T-suppressor cell control of immune responses, since depressed T-suppressor cell activity is thought to be involved in the development of both autoimmune and IgE responses.

The main features of the three genetically controlled parameters which predispose to allergy are summarized in Fig. 19.13. There is also a fourth possible mechanism; this is an HLA-linked association with immunosuppressive genes.

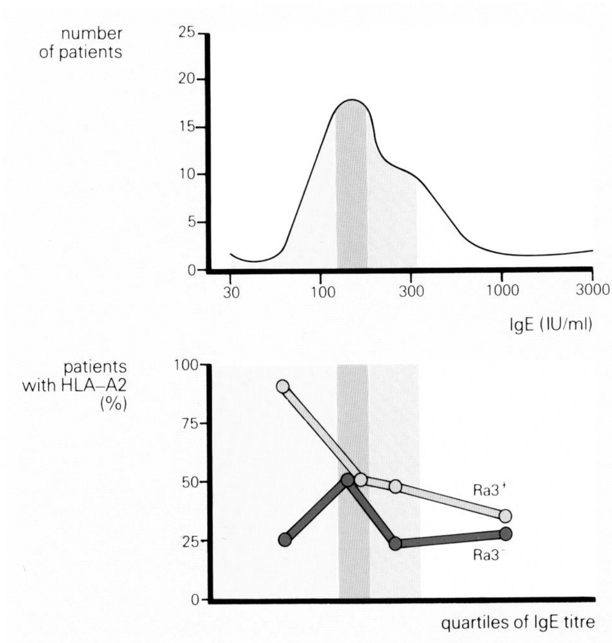

Fig. 19.11 Atopy: IgE levels and tissue type. The upper chart shows the number of ragweed allergic patients ($Ra3^+$) with given levels of total IgE; quartiles of the range are indicated in different shades. The lower chart shows the percentage of patients in the four quartiles possessing HLA–A2 for $Ra3^+$ and $Ra3^-$ individuals. It appears that a person is more likely to be sensitive to Ra3 if he possesses HLA–A2. This association is most marked where the IgE level is low. HLA–A2 is present in 47% of the population.

HLA	skin test		*p*
	positive (%)	negative (%)	
A1	28.7	24.1	0.4
B8	22.3	11.5	0.01
Dw3	25.2	11.7	0.002

Fig. 19.12 IgE response: genetic association. In atopic subjects who have positive skin tests to a number of common environmental allergens (e.g. pollens, housedust mite), there is a significant association between HLA–B8 and HLA–Dw3 and skin test positivity, compared with skin test negative non-allergic controls. The IgE response to antigens is clearly genetically linked, both in terms of the ability to respond to a given antigen and the general 'atopic ability' to produce an IgE antibody response to any antigen.

antigen non-specific		antigen-specific
basal IgE levels	**general hyperresponsiveness**	**HLA-linked antigen-specific response**
dominant for low levels not HLA-linked IgE class-specific	HLA-linked not IgE class-specific	HLA-linked Ir genes not IgE class-specific

Fig. 19.13 Summary of the three genetically controlled parameters predisposing to allergy.

MAST CELLS

It has long been recognized that there is a species difference in mast cell morphology. These morphological differences may be seen not only in the staining properties of the cells and the outer structure of their granules, but also in the detailed mechanism of the degranulation process. This last point can be clearly demonstrated and is illustrated in Figs 19.14 and 19.15; in man, the membranes surrounding the mast cell granules fuse before exocytosis, whereas in rats the granules are expelled singly.

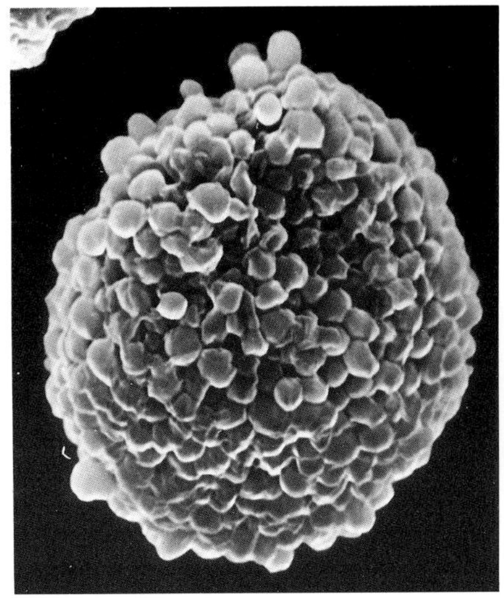

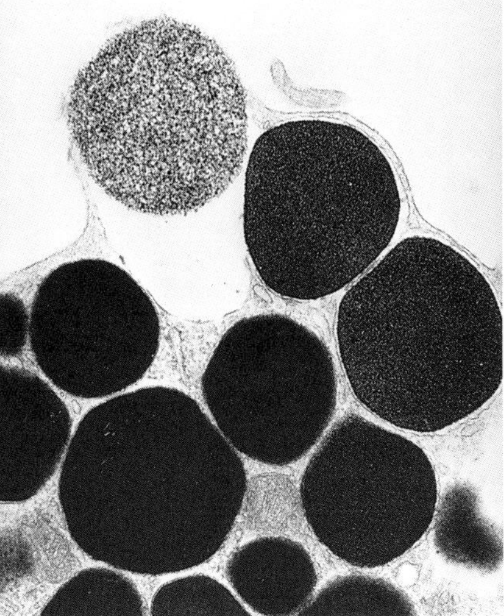

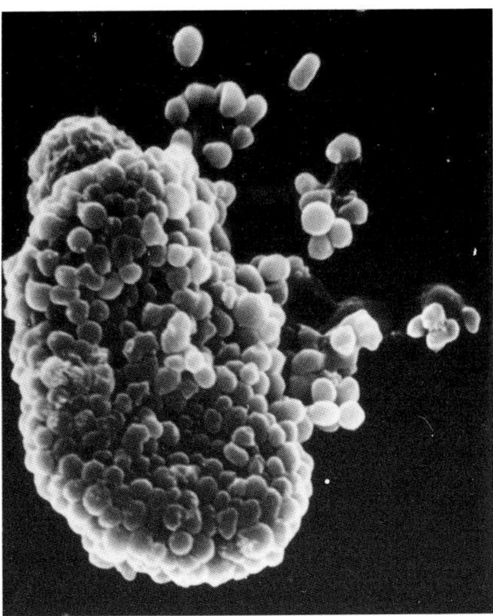

Fig. 19.14 Electronmicrograph study of mast cells – I. On the left is an intact rat peritoneal mast cell with the cell membrane shrunk on to the granules (scanning electronmicrograph; x1500). The middle transmission electronmicrograph (x15,000) shows a granule in exocytosis. On the right, a rat peritoneal mast cell is degranulating following incubation with anti-IgE for 30 seconds (scanning electronmicrograph, x1500). (Courtesy of Dr T. S. C. Orr.)

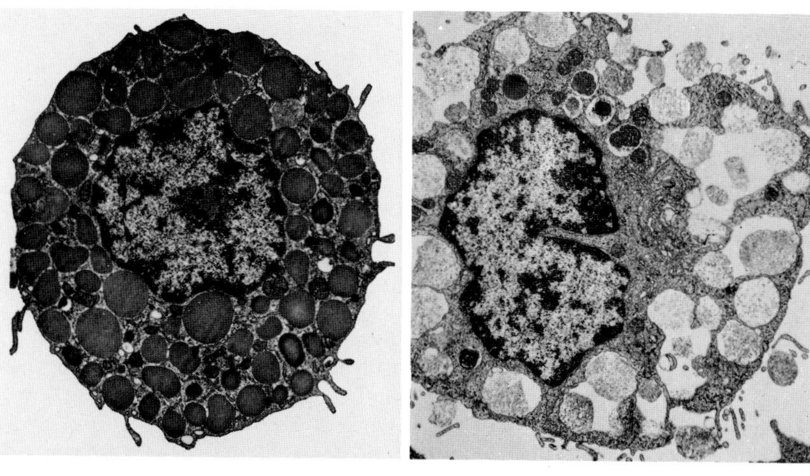

Fig. 19.15 Electronmicrograph study of mast cells – 2. These transmission electronmicrographs of rat peritoneal mast cells show election-dense granules (left), and following incubation with anti-IgE (right), vacuolation with exocytosis of the granule contents has occurred. x2700. (Courtesy of Dr D. Lawson).

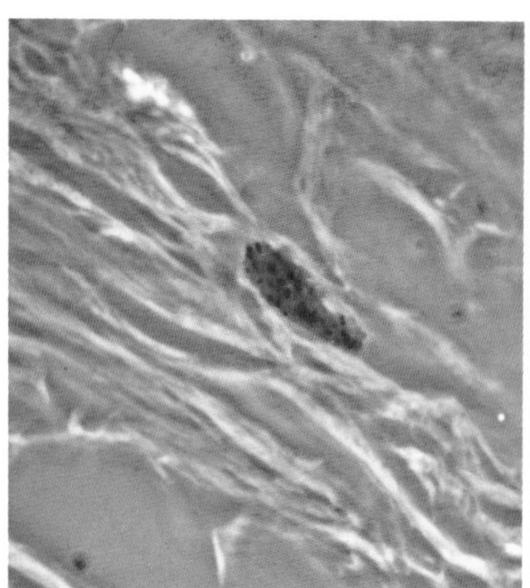

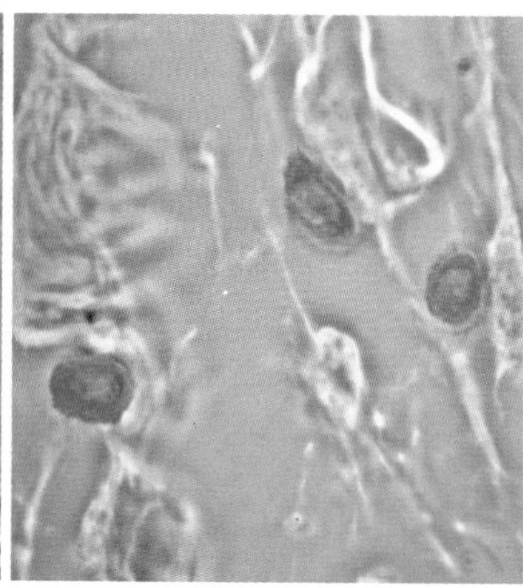

Fig. 19.16 Histological appearances of rat ileum mast cells. Connective tissue mast cell showing both blue and brown granules (left) and three mucosal mast cells with only blue granules (right). The tissue was fixed in formol saline and stained with alcian blue and safranin. x600. (Courtesy of Dr B. Greenwood.)

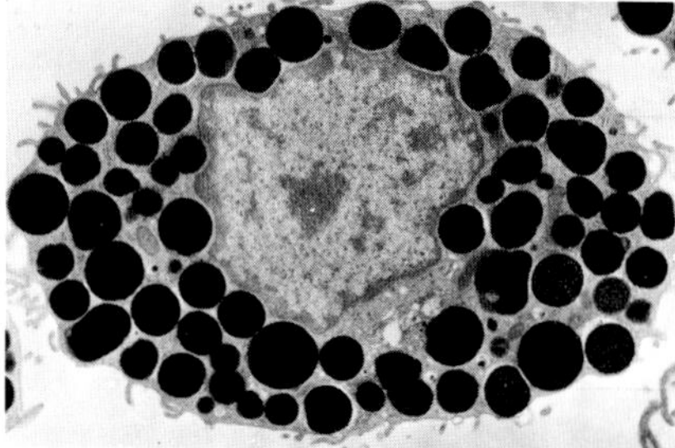

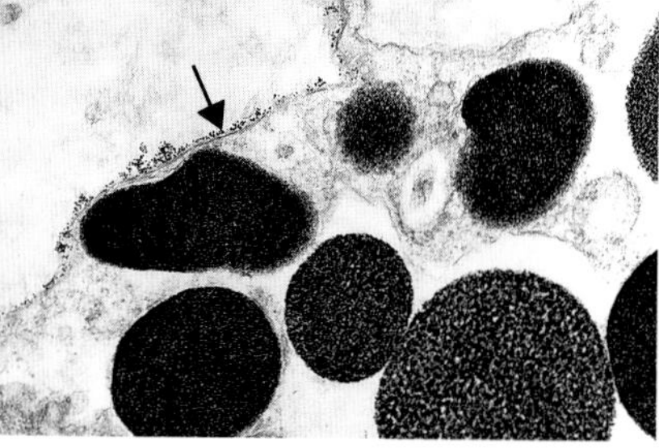

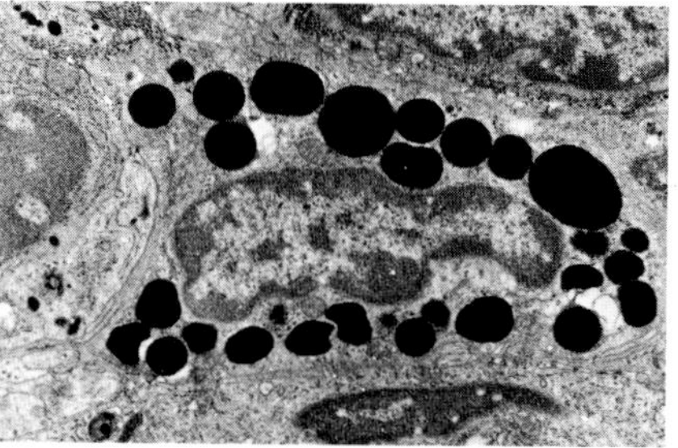

Fig. 19.17 Electronmicrographs of rat mast cells. On the left, the connective tissue mast cell (CTMC) has electron-dense granules characteristic of the rat. On the right, the mucosal mast cell of an ileal villus has fewer granules, with considerable diversity of size. In the centre, at far higher magnification, is a rat CTMC on which membrane bound IgE has been marked with colloidal gold particles. (Courtesy of H. Coleman.)

In addition to the morphological differences there are also functional differences between species and between mast cells derived from different sites within the same animal. The functional differences are seen in response to secretagogues (histamine liberators) and to drugs which block or enhance histamine release.

It used to be thought that mast cells comprised a homogeneous population of cells, the morphology being similar to that which is now recognized as the connective tissue mast cell (CTMC). The staining technique used to demonstrate CTMCs involves formalin fixation of sections and toluidine blue staining. It is now realized that these stains do not adequately show up the mucosal mast cell (MMC) which is only shown with special fixatives and stains (Figs 19.16 and 19.17).

DISTRIBUTION OF MAST CELLS

CTMCs are found around blood vessels in most tissues. Although CTMCs from different sites may have similar properties, the gross morphology of CTMCs from the peritoneum and the skin for example, may be quite different in terms of the number and size of the granules, the density of staining and their pharmacological properties. MMCs have a different distribution to that of CTMCs; in man the highest concentration is found in the mucosa of the midgut and the lung. During parasitic infections there is a marked increase in MMCs in the gut. This increase is also seen in Crohn's disease and ulcerative colitis, and in the synovium of patients with rheumatoid arthritis. In rats infected with *Nippostrongylus brasiliensis* there is an increase in MMCs in the gut mucosa. It has been suggested that the precursors of the cells arise in the mesenteric lymph nodes which drain the gut and then migrate via the thoracic duct back to the intestine. It is clear that MMC proliferation after such infection is dependent on T cell derived lymphokines including IL-3 and IL-4. CTMC clones arise in culture from fibroblast layers, independent of T cells or T cell factors, and are found in normal numbers in nude mice.

Recent evidence suggests that MMCs and CTMCs are derived from the same precursor cell, with the end-cell phenotype depending on factors found in the local microenvironment.

Clinical Studies A number of recent clinical studies have demonstrated the presence of MMCs infiltrating the nasal epithelium in patients with hay fever during, but not before, the pollen season. Similarly, increased numbers of mast cells (the identity of which is not clear) are found in the bronchoalveolar lavage fluid of asthmatics. Since the mucosal surface is the first site of contact for inhaled allergen, the interaction of superficial mast cells and allergen will lead to the release of mediators from mast cells and result in increased permeability of the mucosa to allergen; this results in further mediator release by submucosal mast cells, thereby amplifying the clinical symptoms.

A better understanding of the nature of these superficial, bronchoalveolar mast cells and their responsiveness to anti-allergic drugs will have important therapeutic implications for the future. For instance, in experimental rats infected with the nematode parasite *Nippostrongylus brasiliensis,* the accumulation of MMCs in the gut is rapidly and dramatically suppressed by corticosteroids. Interestingly, local corticosteroids also suppress the increase in nasal mast cell numbers seen in patients during the pollen season. The mechanism of this suppression is not clear, but it is known that corticosteroids inhibit T-helper cell lymphokine production, including IL-3, which has mast cell growth factor activity.

	mucosal mast cell	connective tissue mast cell
location *in vivo*	gut and lung	ubiquitous
life span	<40 days (?)	>40 days (?)
T cell-dependent	+	–
number of Fc_ε receptors	2×10^5	3×10^4
histamine content	+	++
cytoplasmic IgE	+	–
major AA metabolite LTC_4:PGD_2 ratio	25:1	1:40
DSCG/theophylline inhibits histamine release	–	+
major proteoglycan	chondroitin sulphate	heparin

Fig. 19.18 Differences between mast cell populations. There are at least two subpopulations of mast cells, the mucosal mast cell (MMC) and the connective tissue mast cell (CTMC). The differences in their morphology and pharmacology suggest different functional roles *in vivo*. MMCs are associated with parasitic worm infections and possibly allergic reactions. In contrast to the CTMC, the MMC is smaller, shorter lived, T cell dependent, has more surface Fc_ε receptors and contains intracytoplasmic IgE. Both cells contain histamine and serotonin in their granules; the higher histamine content of the CTMC may be accounted for by the greater number of granules. Major arachidonic acid metabolites (prostaglandins and leukotrienes), are produced by both mast cell types, but in different amounts. For example, the ratios of production of the leukotriene LTC_4 to the prostaglandin PGD_2 are 25:1 in the MMC and 1:40 in the CTMC. The effect of drugs on degranulation is different between the two cell types. Sodium cromoglycate (DSCG) and theophylline both inhibit histamine release from the CTMC but not from the MMC and this may have important implications in the treatment of asthma. Much of the data comes from rodent studies and may not apply to man.

Effect of Drugs Crucial from the functional and clinical points of view is the effect of drugs on mast cell degranulation. In the rat, sodium cromoglycate and theophylline both inhibit histamine release from CTMCs but not from MMCs. Because of mast cell heterogeneity and species differences, the development of 'pure' human mast cell lines may be of great use in the development of drugs for the management of the allergic patient. Features of MMCs and CTMCs are compared in Fig.19.18.

STRUCTURE AND FUNCTION OF Fc RECEPTORS FOR IgE

THE HIGH AFFINITY RECEPTOR – $Fc_\varepsilon RI$

Analysis of the $Fc_\varepsilon RI$ receptor was initiated in the mid-1970s and it is now known to have the structure shown in Fig. 19.19.

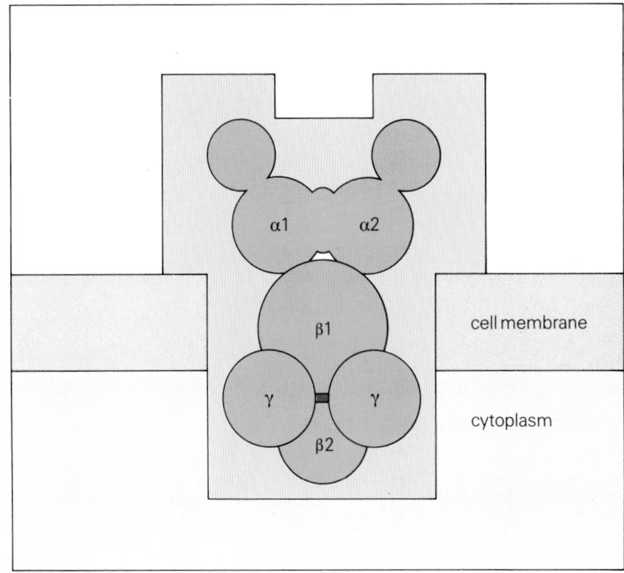

Fig. 19.19 The high affinity Fc_ε receptor. The receptor is composed of six sub-units illustrated as spheres, whose size is in proportion to their molecular weight. A disulphide bond (red) links the γ chains. (Based on data of Dr H. Metzger.)

The two subunits of the α chain polypeptide (molecular weight 55kD) are glycosylated and exposed on the surface, and it has been shown that antibodies against the α chain can block IgE binding to the receptor and trigger histamine release from rat basophil leukaemia cells. The role of carbohydrate is probably protection of the α chain from serum protease activity, as is the case with many cell surface proteins. It is unlikely that carbohydrate plays a role in IgE binding and IgE-mediated histamine release *per se*. However, as shown later (Fig. 19.21), carbohydrate binding lectins can trigger histamine release although this may not be of importance under physiological conditions.

The single ß chain (molecular weight 33kD) and the two disulphide-linked γ chains (molecular weight 9kD) are not exposed on the outer cell surface, but are essential components of the $\alpha_2\beta_2\gamma_2$ receptor unit, perhaps playing a role in signal transduction.

The receptor interacts with the distal portion of the IgE heavy chain, that is, the regions of the CH2 and/or CH3 domains. The interaction is highly specific and the binding constant for IgE is also very high (approximately 10^{10} M^{-1}). The interaction of monovalent IgE with the receptor complex does not appear to activate mast cells or basophils since no histamine release occurs and, as discussed later, it is the cross-linking of surface bound IgE by antigen and other molecules which stimulates degranulation. It is also worthy of note that the carbohydrate associated with IgE itself does not seem to be of importance in its interaction with $Fc_\varepsilon RI$. Its role seems to be in the secretion of IgE from B cells.

THE LOW AFFINITY RECEPTOR – Fc_εR II

The exact molecular structure of the Fc_εRII receptor has not yet been described. The human lymphocyte Fc_εRII however, has already been cloned and the cDNA predicts a 321 amino acid polypeptide with an approximate molecular weight of 36 kD. It shows the characteristics of a membrane bound molecule; that is, a cytoplasmic amino-terminal domain with 23 hydrophilic residues, a hydrophobic membrane spanning region (residue 24–44) and the extracellular domain from residue 45 to the carboxy-terminal end at residue 321.

Interestingly, it has been shown by immunoprecipitation with monoclonal antibody that Fc_εRII shares several antigenic determinants with the IgE-Bf obtained from B cell supernatants and peptide mapping has shown several identical fragments after digestion of Fc_εRII and IgE-Bf with trypsin, chymotrypsin or papain. This may indicate that IgE-Bf represents a breakdown product of the Fc_εRII. It has also been shown that Fc_εRII shares antigenic determinants with CD 23, which is a B cell-specific marker that is thought to be involved in B cell differentiation.

OTHER Fc_εR-BEARING CELLS

Mast cells and basophils express the high affinity Fc receptor for IgE (Fc_εRI), whereas many other cells of the immune system express a low affinity IgE receptor (Fc_εRII, Fig. 19.20). It is notable that Fc_εRII positive T cells and IgE levels rise during the pollen season. The levels of monocytes possessing Fc_εRII are increased in the circulation in some atopics, particularly in those who have severe atopic eczema. These cells, when armed with IgE, may have a local cytotoxic potential. Alveolar macrophages may also be sensitized with IgE and release enzymes when they are challenged by allergen, and this could play an important role in allergen-induced lung disease.

Fc_εR I	comment
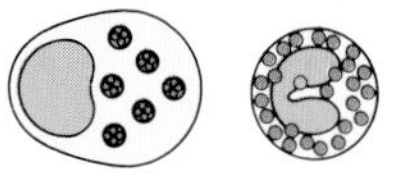 mast cell and basophil	main effectors of IgE-mediated reactions
Fc_εR II	**comment**
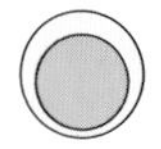 T cell and B cell	T cells: about 1% $Fc_\varepsilon RII^+$ increase in atopics during pollen season B cells: about 30% $Fc_\varepsilon RII^+$ increasing as above
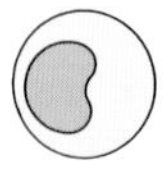 monocyte	about 2% $Fc_\varepsilon RII^+$ increasing up to 20% in some allergic disorders
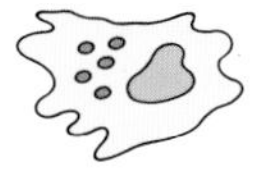 alveolar macrophage	receptors demonstrated by IgE-mediated enzyme release
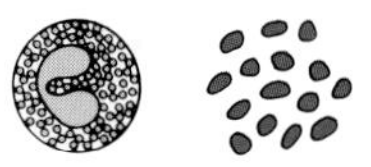 eosinophil and platelet	effectors of IgE-mediated damage to schistosomes

Fig. 19.20 Fc_ε receptor-bearing cells. Mast cells and basophils express high affinity (Kd≃10^{10}) Fc receptors. The Fc receptors on other cells (Fc_εRII) are of much lower affinity (Kd≃10^{6}) and their function on T and B lymphocytes and monocytes is not yet clear. IgE bound to alveolar macrophage Fc_ε receptors when reacted with antigen can stimulate lysosomal enzyme release and production of leukotrienes, which may be important in asthmatic reactions. Fc_ε receptor-bearing eosinophils and platelets have been shown to mediate the killing of IgE-sensitized schistosomes.

Both eosinophils and platelets have been shown to bear the low affinity Fc_ε receptors and when these cells are sensitized with IgE they are found to have a greatly enhanced capacity for cytotoxicity against some parasites including schistosomes. It may be that these cells perform important functions in patients with allergy when sensitized by circulating immune complexes containing IgE, since they both contain a variety of active pharmacological mediators which have the capability of accentuating (platelets) or controlling (eosinophils) allergic reactions.

MAST CELL TRIGGERING

Once IgE binds to the Fc_ε receptors on the mast cells and basophils, degranulation may be triggered by cross-linking the IgE, thereby cross-linking the Fc_ε receptors. Degranulation may also be effected by manoeuvres which directly cross-link the receptors (Fig. 19.21). Lectins, including PHA and ConA can also cross-link IgE by binding to carbohydrate residues on the Fc region, thus

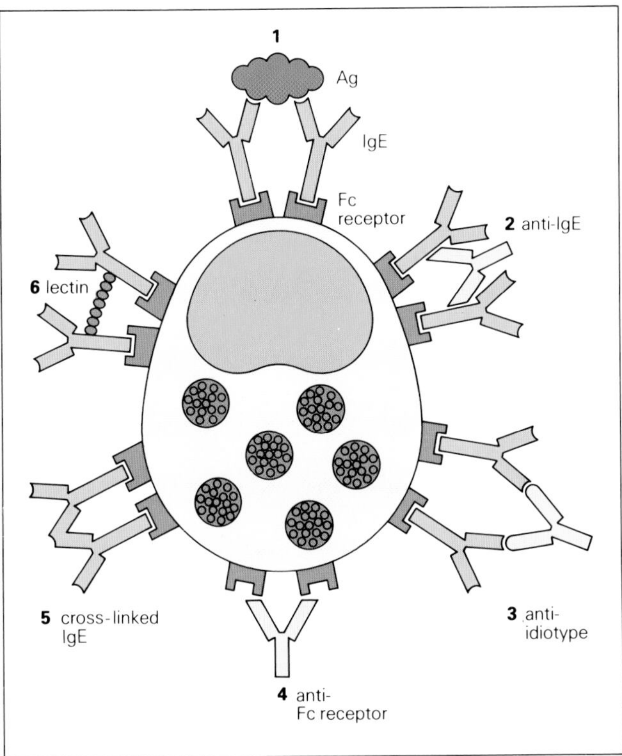

Fig. 19.21 Fc$_\varepsilon$ receptor-mediated mast cell triggering. Mast cells are triggered when their Fc$_\varepsilon$ receptors are cross-linked. This may occur when (1) surface bound antigen-specific IgE binds antigen (Ag); (2) by divalent antibody to the Fc region of IgE or (3) by anti-idiotype antibodies to the idiotopes of that IgE. The receptors may also be cross-linked by direct binding of anti-receptor antibody (4). Experimentally, covalently cross-linked IgE dimers can bridge the receptors (5), or lectins (carbohydrate binding glycoproteins) can link sugar residues on IgE and thus cause degranulation (6). It is the perturbation of the mast cell membrane which is caused by the cross-linking of the Fc$_\varepsilon$ receptors that is the first stage in mast cell activation. Thus, monovalent antigen or antibody will not cause mast cell activation, since cross-linking is not achieved.

causing degranulation. This might explain the urticaria induced in some individuals by strawberries which contain large amounts of lectin.

As well as the methods of bridging the Fc$_\varepsilon$ receptors that are described in Fig. 19.21, there are compounds which are extremely active in degranulating mast cells. Probably the most important of these *in vivo* are the breakdown products of complement activation, that is, the anaphylatoxins C3a and C5a. The anaphylatoxins also affect many other cells, including neutrophils, platelets and macrophages. There are also a number of compounds that can directly activate mast cells, for example calcium ionophore, mellitin and compound 48/80, as well as some drugs, such as synthetic ACTH, codeine and morphine (Fig. 19.22). All of these compounds lead to the activation of mast cells by causing an influx of calcium ions.

T CELLS AND MAST CELL TRIGGERING

The mucosal mast cell needs T cell factors (IL-3, IL-4) for maturation, but there also seems to be a more direct relationship between these cells in the induction of mediator release. Lymphokines from stimulated human lymphocytes can release histamine from basophils and this release is additional to that due to IgE and antigen. This histamine releasing factor may be involved in non-specifically amplifying delayed hypersensitivity and also in modulating Type I hypersensitivity reactions. In addition to this non-specific factor, an antigen-specific T cell factor can also arm mast cells to release mediators following contact with antigen. This factor, produced by TDTH cells, sensitizes mast cells for a few hours only, whereas IgE sensitizes them for months. The link between T cells and mast cells therefore extends beyond growth factors (that is, IL-3, IL-4) to the production of antigen-specific sensitizing factors – T cell factors and non-specific histamine releasing factors. These may be important in the early induction of delayed type hypersensitivity.

MEDIATOR RELEASE

The antigen-induced calcium ion influx into mast cells has two main results. Firstly, there is an exocytosis of granule contents with the release of preformed mediators, the major one being histamine. Secondly, there is the induction of synthesis of newly formed mediators from arachidonic acid which leads to the

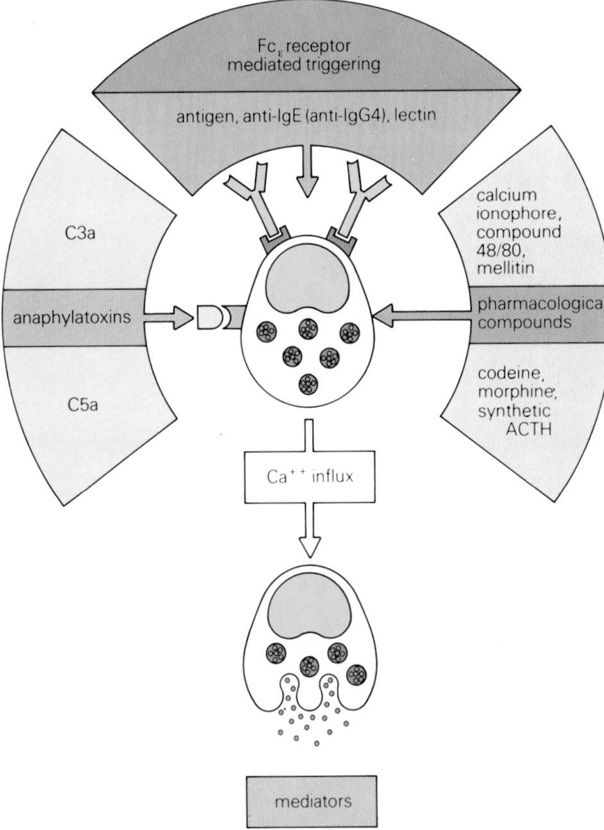

Fig. 19.22 Mast cell activation – I. Mast cell activation can be produced by immunological stimuli which cross-link Fc$_\varepsilon$ receptors and by other stimuli, such as anaphylatoxins and secretagogues (e.g. compound 48/80, mellitin and calcium ionophore A23187). Some other drugs such as codeine, morphine and synthetic ACTH have also been found to activate mast cells directly. The common feature in each case is the influx of Ca^{++} ions into the mast cell which initiates the biochemical processes leading to mast cell degranulation and mediator release.

production of prostaglandins and leukotrienes (Figs 19.23 and 19.24). These mediators have a direct effect on the local tissues and in the lung cause immediate bronchoconstriction, mucosal oedema and hypersecretion leading to asthma (Figs 19.25 and 19.26).

It is becoming clear that different newly formed mediators arise from the different populations of mast cells, thus the different clinical effects in different organs may be related to the differing population of mast cells in each.

Drugs may block the release of mediators either by increasing the intracellular levels of cAMP by stimulating ß-receptors, for example isoprenaline, or by preventing the breakdown of cAMP by phosphodiesterase, for example, theophylline. The mode of action of sodium cromoglycate in preventing histamine release is not clear, but it may involve inhibition of the initial antigen-induced calcium influx.

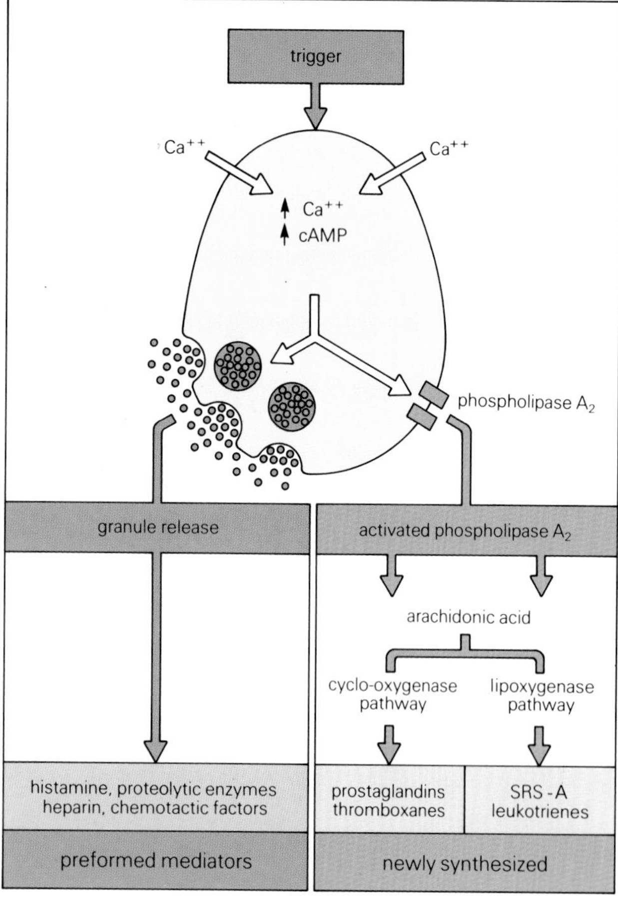

Fig. 19.23 Mast cell activation – II. Immunological triggers (e.g. antigen or anti-IgE) perturb the mast cell membrane, leading to calcium ion influx which is crucial for the degranulation. Microtubule formation and movement of the granules to the cell membrane lead to fusion of the granule and plasma membrane and the release of granule-associated mediators into the intercellular space. Changes in the plasma membrane associated with activation allow phospholipase A_2 to release arachidonic acid; this can then be metabolized by lipoxygenase or cyclo-oxygenase enzymes, depending on the mast cell type. The newly synthesized products include prostaglandin A_2 and thromboxane A_2 (cyclo-oxygenase pathway), and SRS-A (which is leukotriene LTC_4+LTD_4) and chemotactic LTB_4 (lipoxygenase pathway).

granule-associated preformed mediators		
histamine	mol.wt = 111	vasodilation, increased capillary permeability chemokinesis bronchoconstriction
heparin	mol.wt = 60,000	anticoagulant
enzymes	tryptase (mol.wt = 130,000) β-glucosaminidase (mol.wt = 150,000)	proteolytic C3 convertase cleaves glucosamine residues
chemotactic and activating factors	ECF-A (mol.wt = 380/2000) NCF (mol.wt > 750,000)	chemotaxis of eosinophils, neutrophils
newly formed mediators		
SRS-A(LTC_4+LTD_4) chemotactic leukotrienes (LTB_4)	lipoxygenase pathway products	vasoactive, broncho-constriction, chemotactic and/or chemokinetic
prostaglandins thromboxanes	cyclo-oxygenase products	bronchial muscle contraction, platelet aggregation, vasodilation
chemotactic and activating factors	PAF (mol.wt = 600)	platelet activation

Fig. 19.24 Human mast cell derived mediators. In man the major vasoactive amine is histamine, which leads to immediate inflammatory effects and is stored in mast cell granules in association with heparin. Granule-associated proteases, such as tryptase and chemotactic factors may lead to the inflammation associated with late phase reactions. Of the newly formed mediators, SRS-A (LTC_4 + LTD_4) is associated with early inflammation, although later than that induced by histamine. Prostaglandins, thomboxane and chemotactic factors such as ECF-A, NCF and LTB_4 may be involved in initiating the late phase reaction and inducing the cellular infiltrate which includes neutrophils, eosinophils, basophils and mononuclear cells.

CLINICAL TESTS FOR ALLERGY

The classical skin test in atopy is the Type I wheal and flare reaction in which antigen introduced into the skin leads to the release of preformed mediators, increased vascular permeability, local oedema and itching (Figs 19.27 and 19.28). A positive skin test usually correlates with a positive radioallergosorbent test (RAST, a laboratory test for antigen-specific IgE in serum) and a positive relevant provocation test, for example, nasal or bronchial provocation with the allergen.

The late response following skin testing is not often seen because it is rarely looked for and when it does occur it has the appearance of a lump in the skin which is painful rather than itchy. End-point titration of skin testing is useful for determining an approximate estimation of the patient's sensitivity to the allergen.

There is a small group of patients who give a clear-cut history of, for example, allergic rhinitis, but in whom skin tests and RAST are negative. These patients, however, do make a local mucosal antibody response as can be shown by a positive nasal provocation test and by

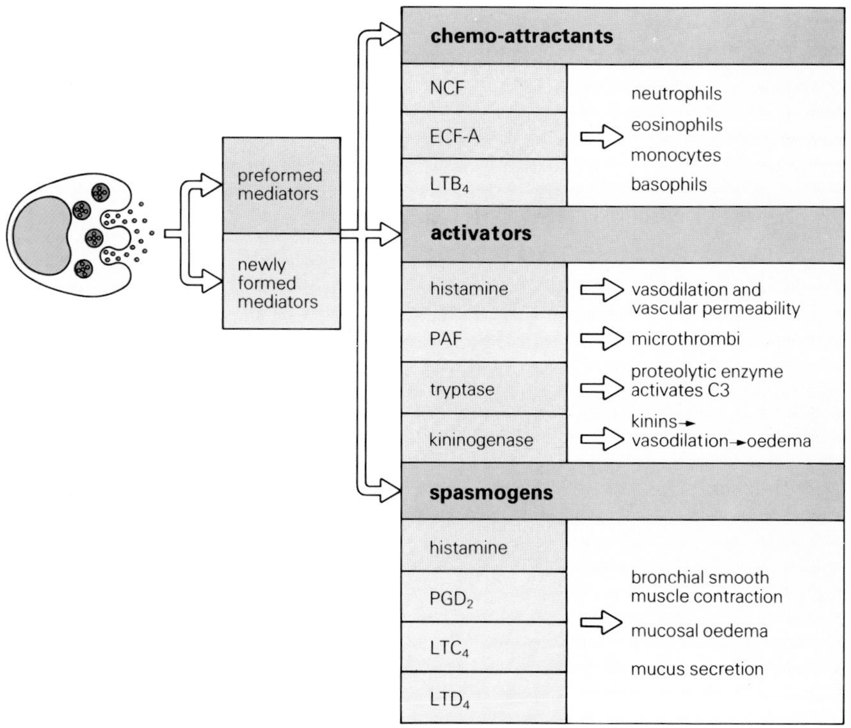

Fig. 19.25 Physiological effects of mast cell derived mediators. Both the pre-formed granule-associated and the newly formed mediators have three main areas of action.

As **chemotactic agents:** a variety of cells can be attracted to the site of mast cell activation, in particular eosinophils, neutrophils and mononuclear cells including lymphocytes. **Inflammatory activators** can lead to vasodilatation, oedema and, via platelet activating factor (PAF), to microthrombi – leading to local tissue damage. Tryptase, the major protein of human lung mast cells can activate C3 directly, this function being inhibited by heparin. Kininogenases are also released and these affect small blood vessels by generating kinins from tissue kininogens, again leading to inflammation. The **spasmogens** have a direct effect on bronchial smooth muscle but can also increase mucus secretion leading to bronchial plugging.

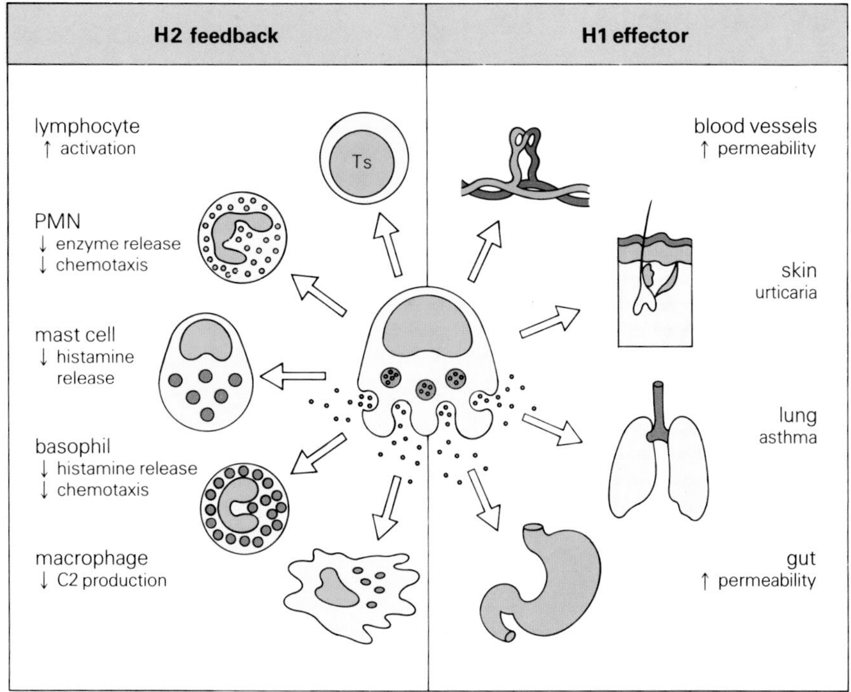

Fig. 19.26 Histamine has functions mediated by H1 and H2 receptors. The inflammatory effect of histamine is due to its pharmacological effects on blood vessels, smooth muscle and mucosal surfaces mediated by H1 receptors. The anti-inflammatory effects are mediated by H2 receptors and the second messenger cAMP· leading to the indicated effect on the target cells.

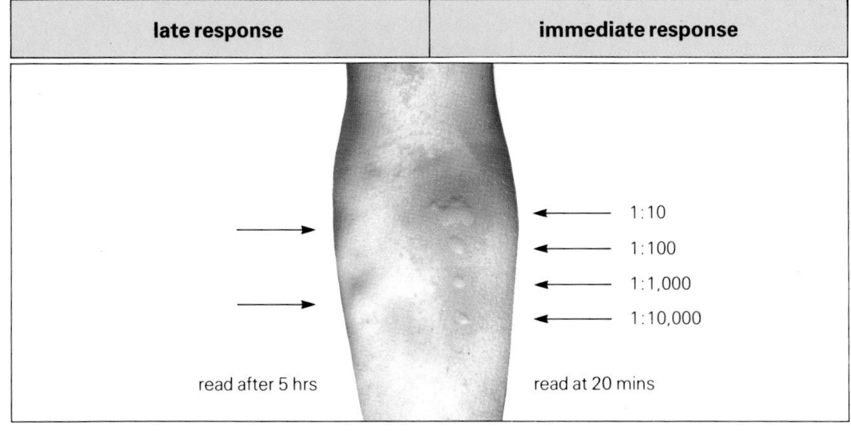

Fig. 19.27 Skin prick tests with grass pollen allergen in a patient with typical summer hay fever. Skin tests were performed 5 hours (left) and 20 minutes (right) before the photograph was taken. The tests on the right show a typical end-point titration of a Type I immediate wheal and flare reaction. The late phase skin reaction (left) can be clearly seen at 5 hours, especially where a large immediate response has preceded it. Figures for allergen dilution are given.

the presence of the relevant specific IgE in the nasal secretion.

Patients with a variety of atopic disorders show the classical immediate wheal and flare response following skin prick tests, demonstrating that IgE is bound to skin mast cells. If the lymphocytes of these patients are stimulated with allergen, lymphocyte transformation and lymphokine production result, indicating T cell reactivity to the allergen. This does not necessarily imply that delayed hypersensitivity is contributing directly to the disease process but indicates that T cells specific for allergen are present in these patients and may be providing 'help' in the IgE response.

In patients with atopic eczema (Fig. 19.29) who have IgE antibodies to the house dust mite, it has been shown that when mite allergen is applied to abraded non-affected skin, a positive patch test results (Fig. 19.30).

It is interesting that a proportion of patients with allergic rhinitis due to the house dust mite (Fig. 19.31) also show positive patch tests to the house dust mite with basophil infiltration, suggesting that the infiltration is an immune response to house dust mite antigen and is not specific for atopic eczema. The recruited basophils may be sensitized to many different allergens and could degranulate in response to allergens other than the one used to induce the lesion.

When the late phase skin reaction was originally described, it was thought that the mechanism might have been a Type III reaction (immune complex-mediated) due to a precipitating IgG antibody, as occurs in bronchopulmonary aspergillosis. However, precipitating antibodies have not been found to be associated with this late reaction and further research has confirmed that the late response is an IgE-dependent sequel to the immediate response.

Bronchial reactions to allergens also show an immediate and late phase response (Fig. 19.32). Sodium cromoglycate is a very effective treatment in allergic asthma and prevents both the immediate and late phase responses which follow bronchial provocation with allergen. This implies that the development of a late reaction in the lung is dependent on an initial

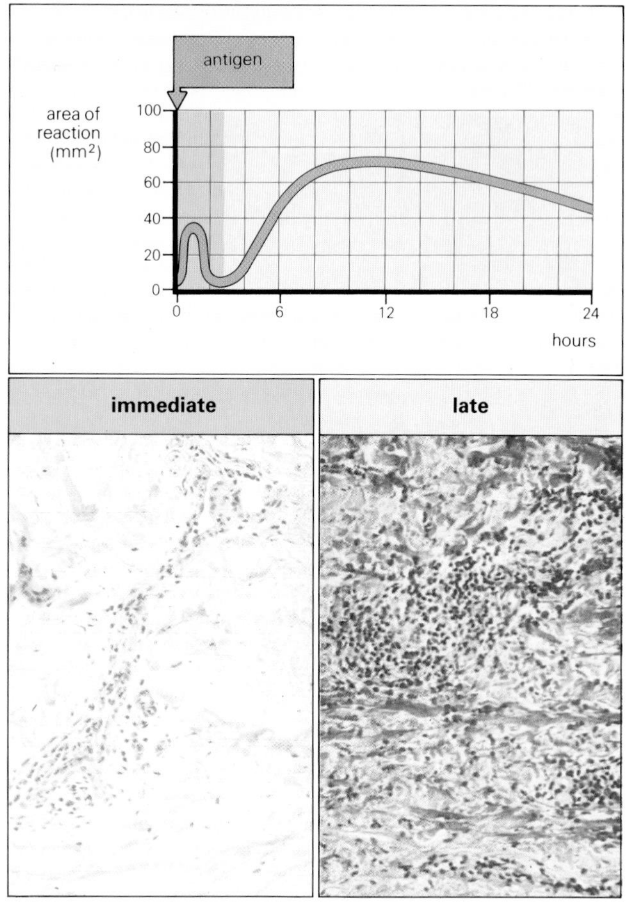

Fig. 19.28 Immediate and late skin reactions. Using the skin prick or intradermal method of skin testing, an immediate wheal and flare reaction is often followed by a late phase reaction. This phase may last 24 hours and the reaction is larger and generally more oedematous than the immediate response. The immediate type of reaction has a sparse cellular infiltrate around the dermal vessels consisting primarily of neutrophils; the late reaction has a dense infiltrate, with many basophils. The late phase reaction can be seen after challenge of the skin, nasal mucosa and bronchi and may be particularly important in chronic asthma. (Courtesy of Dr A.K. Black (left) and Dr G. Gleich (right).)

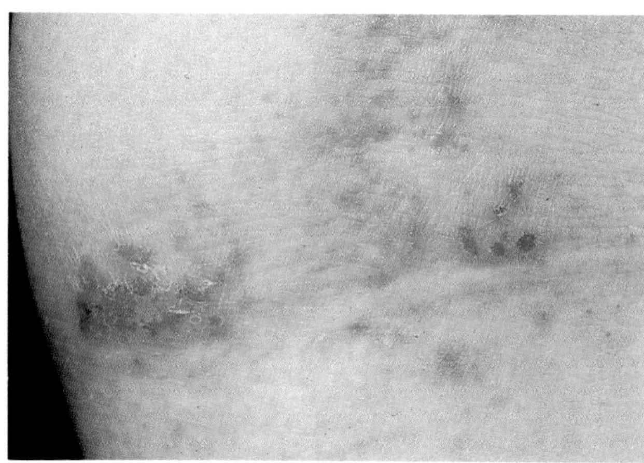

Fig. 19.29 The appearance of atopic eczema on the back of a knee in a child allergic to rice and eggs.

Fig. 19.30 Skin patch tests in a patient with atopic eczema using purified house dust mite *(Dermatophagoides pteronyssinus)* antigen. The surface keratin of an unaffected area is removed by gentle abrasion and the extract is placed on the skin (right) and occluded for 48 hours at which time the site is examined. The lesions are macroscopically eczematous and microscopically contain infiltrates of eosinophils and basophils. Saline control (left). (Courtesy of Dr E. B. Mitchell.)

allergen/IgE/mast cell interaction; preventing degranulation with sodium cromoglycate prevents all subsequent events. If patients are pretreated with corticosteroids or prostaglandin synthetase inhibitors, late reactions alone are abolished leaving the immediate response unchanged. This indicates a role for mast cell-derived arachidonic acid metabolites, such as prostaglandins and leukotrienes, in the late response (see Figs 19.23 and 19.25).

Most asthmatics with reversible airway obstruction benefit from treatment with corticosteroids. Although these drugs have little or no effect on the immediate IgE-mediated reaction, the late reaction is abolished by corticosteroids. This suggests that the late reaction is of major clinical importance in chronic asthma. The beneficial effect of corticosteroids in chronic asthma may be related to the reduction of cell infiltration in the bronchi (Fig. 19.33). Much evidence has been accumulated suggesting a central role for inflammatory cell infiltration during the late phase reaction. In particular, eosinophils, which are found in increased numbers in the bronchoalveolar lavage during the late phase but not during the early phase reaction of asthmatics, are thought to cause damage to the respiratory epithelium through the release of myelobasic protein and eosinophil cationic protein (ECP). This in turn may facilitate the access of inflammatory mediators to afferent nerve endings, causing bronchoconstriction through axon reflex pathways.

Associated with asthma is hyperreactivity of the bronchi to histamine and non-specific stimuli such as cold air and water vapour. Normal subjects become asthmatic following inhalation of 10 ng of histamine whereas asthmatics respond to amounts which are at least 20-fold less.

The fact that this hyperreactivity is a response to chronic antigen challenge is strongly supported by the data of Platts-Mills who removed asthmatics from their allergenic environment (house dust mite) for up to 3 months and showed that at the end of that time their sensitivity to histamine was greatly reduced and in some cases had returned to normal.

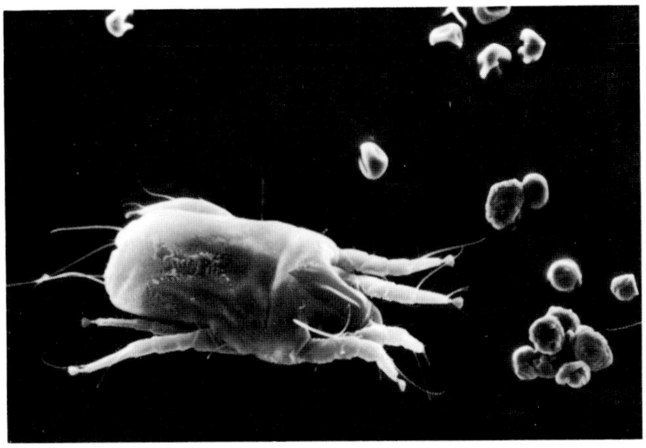

Fig. 19.31 House dust mite – a major allergen. Electronmicrograph showing the house dust mite, *Dermatophagoides pteronyssinus,* and faecal pellets (bottom right) which represent the major source of allergen. Biconcave pollen grains (top right) are shown for comparison of size showing that the faecal pellet and not the mite itself can become airborne and reach the lungs. (Courtesy of Dr E. Tovey.)

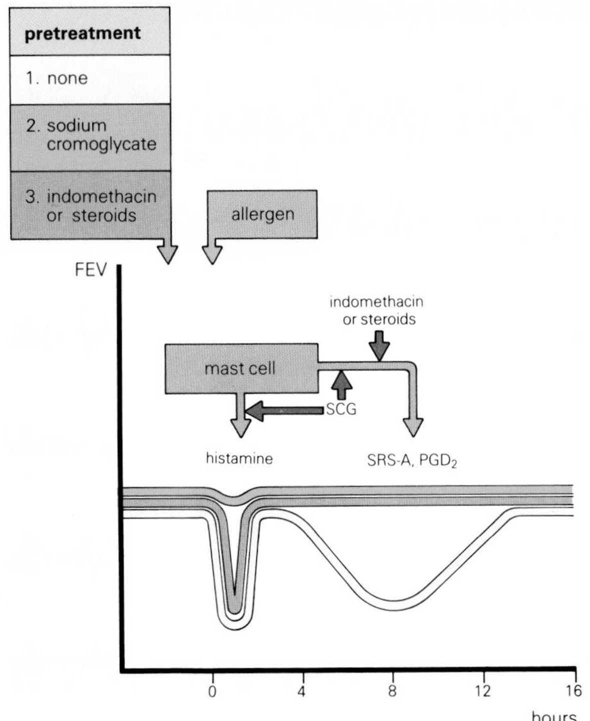

Fig. 19.32 Immediate and late phase bronchial reactions. This graph plots the forced expiratory volume (FEV) in three groups of individuals prior to and several hours after bronchial provocation with an allergen. Each group is pretreated differently. In the control group (1) there is a biphasic (initial and late) bronchial constriction. The initial reaction lasts for 1 hour and is followed by a late reaction lasting several hours. Histamine released from degranulating mast cells is thought to be the major mediator of the immediate reaction in man. Pretreatment with sodium cromoglycate (SCG) inhibits mast cell degranulation thus preventing both early and late reactions (2). Pretreatment with indomethacin and corticosteroids, which block arachidonic acid metabolic pathways, inhibit the late phase reaction but not the immediate reaction (3) thus implicating SRS-A and PGD_2 in the development of the late reaction.

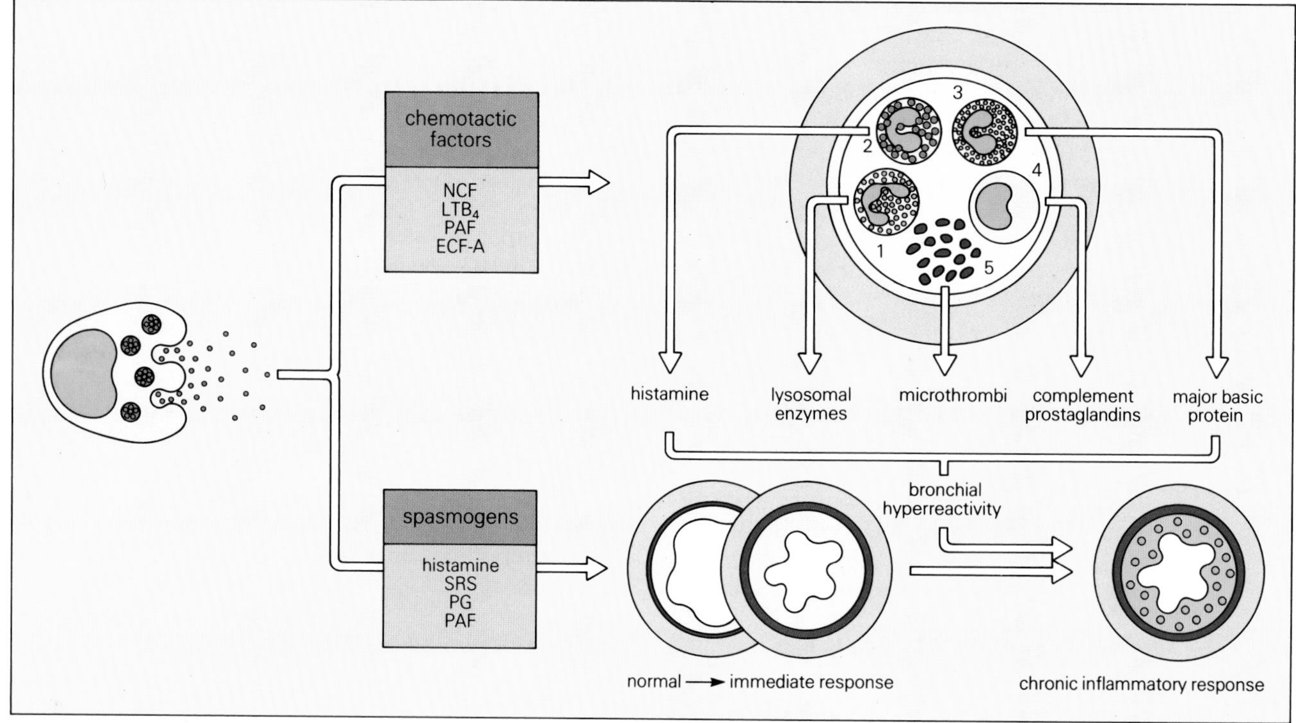

Fig. 19.33 The inflammatory response in the asthmatic lung. Mast cell mediators may be divided into chemotactic and direct acting (spasmogenic) factors. The **chemotactic factors** lead to active accumulation of granulocytes (1), basophils (2), eosinophils (3), macrophages (4) and platelets (5). Production of a further set of inflammatory molecules by these cells leads to the late phase response. **Spasmogenic mediators** produce the immediate response on bronchial provocation and also lead to increased small vessel permeability, oedema and cell emigration. All these factors, including hypersecretion of mucus, smooth muscle hypertrophy and cellular infiltration, with associated bronchial hyperreactivity lead to subacute or chronic inflammation.

FACTORS INVOLVED IN THE DEVELOPMENT OF ALLERGY

As well as the known genetic predisposition for developing allergy, it is now appreciated that other factors may also be important and these are discussed below.

T CELL DEFICIENCY

There is substantial evidence for a role for T cells in the IgE response (see Fig. 19.6). This has led to the suggestion that a defect in T cells and in particular, suppressor T cells, may be involved in the aetiology of atopy. There are reduced numbers of E-rosette forming cells and suppressor T cells in patients with severe atopic eczema, but this is not seen so clearly in patients with rhinitis and asthma (Fig. 19.34). In addition, T cell mitogen responses are reduced in severe atopics (those with eczema) (Fig. 19.35), and these reduced T cell responses *in vitro* correlate with reduced cell-mediated immunity, which is seen *in vivo* as depressed delayed hypersensitivity skin responses.

Until recently it was not clear whether this T cell defect was a cause or a consequence of the atopic disease. Interestingly, recent studies have provided some evidence for a causal relationship between the T cell defect in atopy and the type of feeding in infancy. Soothill and colleagues have shown that the incidence of eczema in children is reduced if they are breast fed, and work by

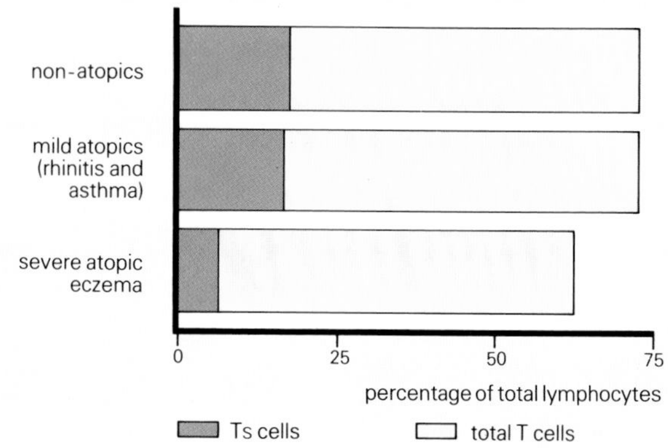

Fig. 19.34 Suppressor T cells in atopy. The total number of T cells was estimated by E-rosetting, and T-suppressor (Ts) cells by staining with an anti-Ts monoclonal antibody (OKT8). Patients with severe atopic eczema, but not patients with rhinitis or asthma, have a reduced total number of T cells, which is almost wholly accounted for by fewer OKT8 staining, Ts cells. Decreased numbers of circulating Ts cells are associated with the often grossly elevated serum IgE levels seen in atopic eczema.

other groups has shown a relationship between bottle feeding with cows' milk in infancy, IgE levels and T cell numbers (Fig. 19.36). The implication is that bottle feeding in infancy associated with reduced numbers of some subsets of regulatory T cells causes increased IgE levels, although it is not certain whether the bottle feeding itself affects T cell numbers.

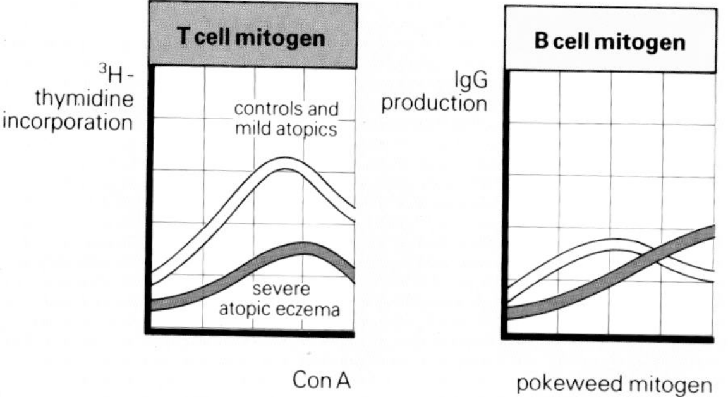

Fig. 19.35 Mitogen responses in atopy. *In vitro* studies show that the response of purified peripheral blood lymphocytes (PBLs) to the two mitogens, ConA and pokeweed mitogen, can be used as a measure of T cell and B cell activity respectively. Mitogens react with cell surface glycoproteins, stimulating cell transformation and proliferation, measured by ^{3}H-thymidine incorporation into cellular DNA. PBLs from mild atopics (those with rhinitis or asthma), and non-atopics respond similarly to the T cell mitogen (ConA), whilst the response of PBLs from patients with severe atopic eczema is generally depressed. In contrast, the response of atopic and non-atopic subjects to a B cell mitogen (pokeweed) is very similar when measured by either ^{3}H-thymidine incorporation or IgG antibody production.

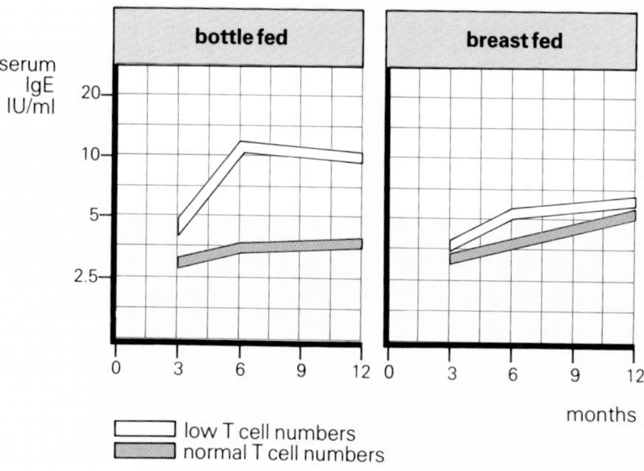

Fig. 19.36 Effect of early bottle feeding and T cell deficiency on serum IgE levels. In infants with low numbers of circulating T cells, IgE levels in the serum were found to be elevated when those children were bottle fed with cows' milk early in life. Other infants with low T cells, but breast fed, had similar IgE levels to those infants with normal levels of T cells who were breast or bottle fed. These data show that the type of feeding and T cell numbers affect IgE levels and suggest that a T cell defect in association with an environmental factor (feeding) may influence the development of the atopic state.

MEDIATOR FEEDBACK

Mast cell mediators such as histamine, prostaglandins and leukotrienes are generally thought to be pro-inflammatory. However, recent evidence suggests an anti-inflammatory role for these compounds on a variety of cells. Histamine, a major mast cell mediator has been particularly well studied in this respect and the major feedback effects are outlined in Fig. 19.26.

In contrast to the inflammatory effects of histamine mediated by H1 receptors, the anti-inflammatory effects are mediated by H2 receptors and cAMP. The original hypothesis of Szentivanyi that a defect of cAMP-mediated signalling was the basis of atopy is now not generally accepted. However, it has been shown that H2 receptor-mediated inhibition of lysosomal enzyme release and activation of suppressor T cells by histamine is defective in atopic subjects. Thus, the role of mediator feedback in atopy is a subject of current interest.

ENVIRONMENTAL FACTORS

Environmental pollutants such as SO_2, nitrogen oxides, diesel fumes and fly ash may increase mucosal permeability and therefore enhance antigen entry and IgE responsiveness. The effect of smoking seems to be biphasic, with an enhancement of IgE levels with low level cigarette consumption and suppression at high levels. Smoking also leads to a substantial reduction in the immune response to inhaled antigens. Diesel exhaust particulates (DEP) can act as a powerful adjuvant for IgE production (Fig. 19.37). They are less than 1 μm in diameter, are buoyant in the atmosphere of polluted districts and are inhaled. The concentration in urban air is approximately 2 $\mu g/m^3$ of air, but on main roads can reach 30 $\mu g/m^3$ and during times of peak traffic, levels of

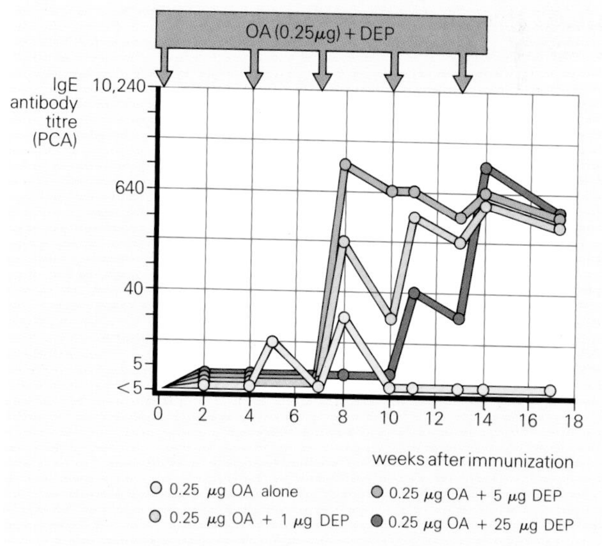

Fig. 19.37 The effect of pollutants (diesel exhaust particulates, DEP) on IgE anti-ovalbumin responses in mice. When mice are immunized intranasally with ovalbumin (OA), a small peak of IgE antibody is seen at weeks 5 and 8, and none thereafter. If DEP are added to the OA, there is a dose-related increase in IgE persisting after immunization ceases. Thus, DEP are good adjuvants for IgE production and may help to explain the increase in allergy in recent years. (Courtesy of Dr S. Takafuji; with permission from *Journal of Allergy and Clinical Immunology* 1987, **79**, 639–45.)

500 $\mu g/m^3$ have been recorded. DEP given intranasally with antigen produces a marked increase in antigen-specific IgE. This adjuvant effect can be seen with low dose antigen exposure of the order that might be experienced in natural conditions. The increase in allergic rhinitis and asthma in the last 3 decades parallels an increase in air pollution and diesel exhaust. Thus, environmental pollutants may be affecting IgE responses, thereby contributing to the increase in allergic disease.

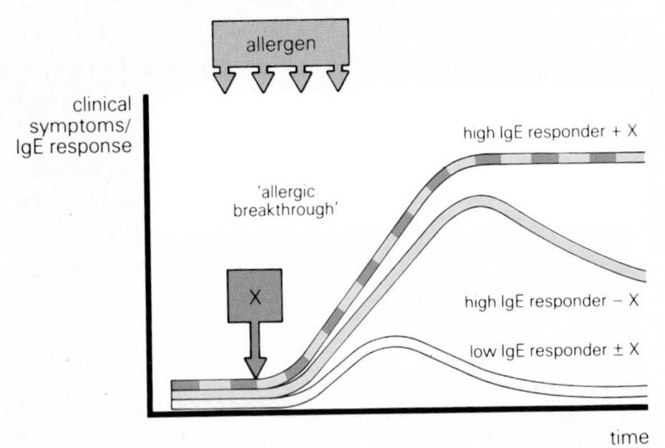

Fig. 19.38 Allergic breakthrough in man: hypothesis. On exposure to allergen an IgE response may develop transiently in low IgE responders before being controlled by normal T-suppressor cell activity. In high responders, the IgE response to allergen is much greater than in low responders, but the overt expression of clinical symptoms is only seen when allergic breakthrough is exceeded. This may depend on the presence of concomitant factors (X) such as viral infections of the upper respiratory tract, transient IgA deficiency or decreased T-suppressor cell activity, which will allow unrestrained IgE responses and clinical symptoms to develop. In the absence of factor X, the high responder subject may not show clinical symptoms after a short period of allergen exposure alone, but may be induced to express clinical symptoms of allergy by future exposure to allergen and factor X.

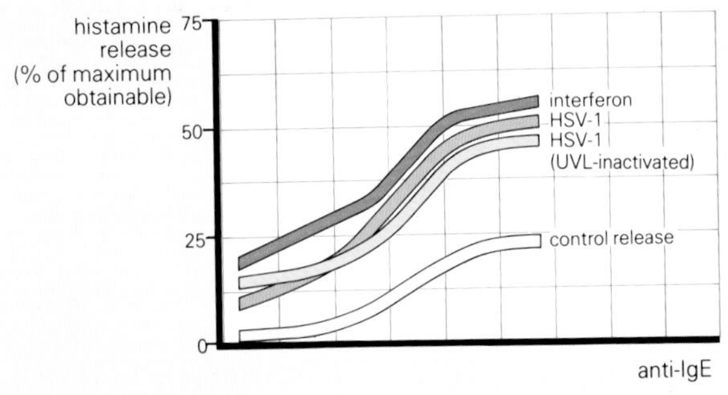

Fig. 19.39 Virus enhancement of IgE-mediated histamine release. Basophils can be induced to release histamine by anti-IgE which cross-links the Fc receptors (control). Histamine release is enhanced in the presence of live *Herpes simplex* virus (HSV-1) or ultraviolet light (UVL)-inactivated HSV. Interferon is thought to be responsible for this enhancement because it mimics the virus effect. This might explain the exacerbation of asthma seen in atopics following upper respiratory tract virus infections.

THE CONCEPT OF ALLERGIC BREAKTHROUGH

It is evident that a number of factors must contribute to allergy and this has led to the hypothesis of allergic breakthrough, where clinical symptoms of allergy are only seen when an arbitrary level of immunological activity (allergic breakthrough) is exceeded (Fig. 19.38). This will depend on a number of conditions, including exposure to allergen, genetic predisposition, the tendency to make IgE, and other factors, such as the presence of upper respiratory tract viral infections, decreased suppressor activity or transient IgA deficiency.

Viral infections may exacerbate allergic symptoms and this may be due to the fact that some viruses, for example *Herpes simplex*, enhance basophil histamine release (Fig. 19.39). Both live and ultraviolet light-inactivated viruses can enhance histamine release, and interferon has been shown to be the mediator of this effect. Additionally, viruses can also enhance allergen entry through damaged epithelial surfaces and the responsiveness of target organs to histamine. Thus the role of viruses in the development of allergy is an area of particular interest.

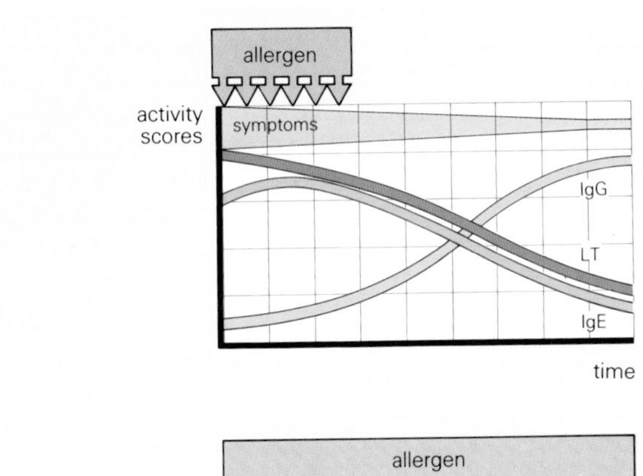

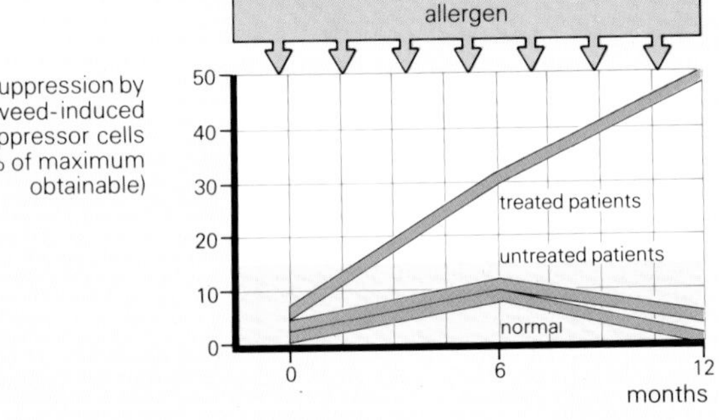

Fig. 19.40 Hyposensitization: a prospect for allergy treatment. Hyposensitization treatment involves repeated injection of increasing doses of allergen. There is an increase in antigen-specific IgG (upper graph) accompanied by a fall in antigen-specific IgE. This fall is thought to be due to an increase in activity of T-suppressor cells, which is reflected in reduced antigen-induced lymphocyte transformation (LT) *in vitro*. The lower graph shows evidence to support this concept. Following successful hyposensitization of ragweed-sensitive patients over 6 or 12 months there is an increase in antigen-specific T-suppressor activity compared to that of untreated patients or controls. This is measured by co-cultivating the patient's lymphocytes with autologous antigen-generated T-suppressor cells, and then measuring proliferation of the lymphocytes in response to allergen. The background level of suppression seen with an irrelevant antigen is the same in all groups.

HYPOSENSITIZATION

Hyposensitization therapy involves the injection of increasing doses of allergen. Although clinical benefit is often obtained, the exact mechanism by which it occurs is unknown. Following treatment there is an increase in serum levels of allergen-specific IgG and suppressor T cell activity whilst specific IgE levels tend to fall (Fig. 19.40, upper graph), but in most cases, there is no clear-cut correlation between any of these findings and clinical improvement in the patient. However, it has been shown that allergen-specific suppressor T cells develop in successfully hyposensitized ragweed allergic patients and this may have a number of effects such as suppression of the IgE response and may also lead to suppression of T cell-dependent mast cell recruitment (Fig. 19.40, lower graph). In the case of people allergic to bee venom where IgG produced by hyposensitization protects by neutralizing the injected venom antigen, there is an excellent correlation between specific IgG antibodies and clinical protection.

There is now good evidence in experimental animals for very long-lived, suppressor T cells and radiation resistant B_ε cells. In rats and mice repeated inhalation of antigen (ovalbumin) results in tolerance, especially of IgE responses. However, using high IgE responder animals, Holt's group have shown that B_ε memory and plasma cells are very resistant to the effects of ovalbumin specific T-suppressor cells and ongoing IgE responses are unaffected, although administration of such T-suppressor cells to unimmunized animals prevents subsequent IgE response to ovalbumin. These results are clearly relevant, since allergic humans are clinically diagnosed after sensitization and this may explain the relative lack of success of desensitization in many subjects. An understanding of the mechanism(s) by which these long-lived B_ε cells are maintained, for example, by continued presentation of antigen on dendritic cells or by the idiotypic network system, will undoubtedly be important in the future for control of IgE responses in man.

Interestingly, Holt's group also showed that inhalation of noxious substances (nitrous oxides or histamine) before inhalation of antigen can induce significant IgE responses in low responder animals, suggesting a role for environmental factors in promoting IgE responses as indicated above.

THE BENEFICIAL ROLE OF IgE

With so many disadvantages inherent in producing an IgE response to an allergen the question arises as to what useful function IgE actually has (Fig. 19.41). It has long been considered that IgE plays a major role in the

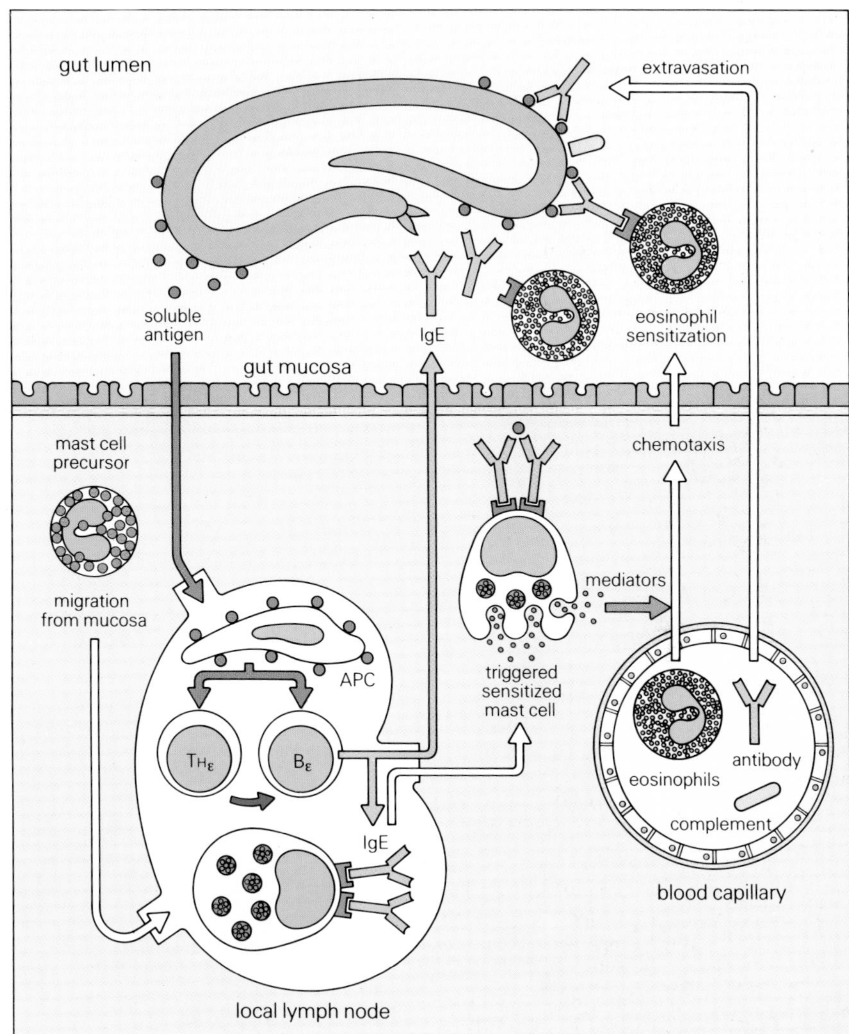

Fig. 19.41 The beneficial role of IgE in parasitic worm infections. During a parasitic worm infection soluble worm antigens diffuse across the gut mucosa into the body and are transported to the local lymph node where an IgE response occurs. Mast cell precursors migrate from the gut mucosa to the same local lymph nodes where they mature, and acquire worm-specific IgE on their surface and then migrate back to the gut mucosa via the thoracic duct and bloodstream. These mast cells degranulate following contact with worm antigen, releasing mediators which increase vascular permeability and attract inflammatory cells, including eosinophils, to the area. IgE from the lymph node also sensitizes the worm to attack by eosinophils which bear Fc receptors for IgE. Complement and worm-specific IgG also enter the site due to increased vascular permeability caused by mediators such as histamine. There is also an associated increase in mucus production by goblet cells in the mucosa. All of these mechanisms lead to worm damage and expulsion.

defence against parasitic worms and the mechanisms involved are illustrated. If IgA does not prevent the penetration of the gut mucosa by an organism or worm, contact with IgE-sensitized mast cells will lead to release of mediators which recruit serum factors (IgG and complement), whilst chemotactic factors will attract eosinophils and neutrophils needed for local defence. It is significant that IgA deficiency has been implicated in the aetiology of atopy thus drawing a parallel between the induction of an immune response to infectious agents and airborne allergens. It is worth noting that since approximately one-third of the world's population has parasitic worm infections this may have represented the evolutionary pressure which initiated development of the IgE class, allergies being an unfortunate by-product of this evolutionary step.

FURTHER READING

Brostoff, J. & Challacombe, S.J. (eds) (1987) *Food Allergy and Intolerance*. London: Ballière Tindall.

Bruynzeel-Koomen, C., Wichen, D., Toonstra, J., Berren, S.L. & Bruynzeel, P.L.B. (1986) The presence of IgE molecules on epidermal Langerhans' cells in patients with atopic dermatitis. *Archives of Dermatological Research*, **278**, 199–205.

Capron, A., Dessaint, J.P., Capron, M., Joseph, M., Ameisen, J.C. & Tonnel, A.B. (1986) From parasites to allergy: a second receptor for IgE. *Immunology Today*, **7**, 15–18.

Cooke, R.A. & Vander-Veer, A. (1916) Human sensitization. *Journal of Immunology*, **1**, 201.

Craig, S.S., Schechter, N.M. & Schwartz, L.B. (1988) Ultrastructural analysis of human T and Tc mast cells identified by immunoelectron microscopy. *Laboratory Investigation*, **58**, 682–691.

Gleich, G.J. (1988) Current understanding of eosinophil function. *Hospital Practice*, March 15, 97–120.

Ishizaka, K. (ed.) (1984) Mast cell activation and mediator release. *Progress in Allergy*, Vol.34. Basle: Karger

Iwata, M., Adachi, M. & Ishizaka, K. (1988) Antigen-specific T cells that form IgE-potentiating factor, IgG-potentiating factor, and antigen-specific glycosylation-enhancing factor on antigenic stimulation. *Journal of Immunology*, **140**, 2534–2542.

Joseph, M., Capron, A., Ameisen, J-C., Capron, M., Vorng, H., Pancre, V., Kusnierz, J-P. & Auriault, C. The receptor for IgE on blood platelets. *European Journal of Immunology*, **16**, 306–312.

Juto, P. (1980) Elevated serum immunoglobulin E in T cell deficient infants fed cow's milk. *Journal of Allergy and Clinical Immunology*, **66**, 402.

Kaliner, M.A. (1987) The late-phase reaction and its clinical implications. *Hospital Practice*, October 15, 73–83.

Metzger, H., Alcaraz, G., Hoffman, R., Kinet, J.P., Pribluda, V. & Quarto, R. (1986) The receptor with high affinity for immunoglobulin E. *Annual Review of Immunology*, **4**, 419–470.

Rocklin, R.E. (1983) Clinical and immunologic aspects of allergen specific immunotherapy in patients with seasonal allergic rhinitis and or allergic asthma. *Journal of Allergy and Clinical Immunology* **72**, 323.

Sedgwick, J.D. & Holt, P.G. (1986) Induction of IgE-secreting cells in the lymphatic drainage of the lungs of rats following passive antigen inhalation. *International Archives of Allergy and Applied Immunology*, **79**, 329–331.

Stanworth, D.R. (1973) *Immediate Hypersensitivity* Amsterdam: North Holland Publications.

Takafuji, S., Suzuki, S., Koizumi, K., Tadokoro, K., Miyamoto, T., Ikemori, R. & Muranaka, M. (1987) Diesel-exhaust particulates inoculated by the intranasal route have adjuvant activity for IgE production in mice. *Journal of Allergy and Clinical Immunology*, **79**, 639–645.

Vercelli, D., Jabara, H.H., Lee, B-W., Woodland, N., Geha, R-F. & Leung, D.Y.M. (1988) Human recombinant interleukin-4 induces Fc_{ε}RII/CD23 on normal human monocytes. *Journal of Experimental Medicine*, **167**, 1406–1416.

Wide, L., Bennich, H. & Johansson, S.G.O. (1967) Diagnosis of allergy by an *in vitro* test for allergen antibodies. *Lancet*, **ii**, 1105.

20 Hypersensitivity — Type II

The different forms of hypersensitivity were originally described in terms of the mechanisms involved in damage to tissues. Both type II and type III hypersensitivity are caused by IgG and IgM antibodies. The main distinction is that type II reactions involve antibodies directed to antigens on the surface of specific cells or tissues, whereas type III reactions are due to antibodies against widely distributed antigens, or soluble antigens in serum. Thus, damage caused by type II reactions is localized to a particular tissue or cell type, while damage caused by type III reactions affects those organs where antigen–antibody complexes are deposited.

These hypersensitivity reactions are related to normal immune responses seen against microorganisms and parasites; in the reactions against pathogens, exaggerated immune reactions may be as damaging to the host as the effects of the pathogen itself. In these cases the borderline between a normal, useful immune response and hypersensitivity is blurred. Hypersensitivity reactions may also occur in many other conditions involving immune reactions. Two areas where these types of reaction are particularly notable are autoimmunity and transplantation. The mechanisms of tissue damage which underlie autoimmune immunopathology and graft rejection are described in the chapters covering types II, III and IV hypersensitivity.

MECHANISMS OF DAMAGE

In type II hypersensitivity, antibody directed against cell surface or tissue antigens interacts with molecules of the complement system and a variety of effector cells to bring about damage to the target cells (Fig. 20.1). Antibodies interact with complement by activating C1 of the classical pathway; alternatively they may cross-link the antibody-sensitized tissue to effector cells via Fc receptors on the effectors. The complement system can act in two ways in these reactions (Fig. 20.2).

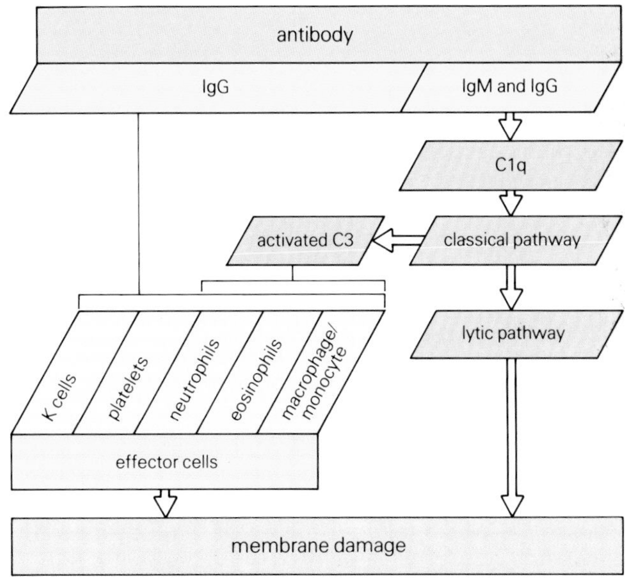

Fig. 20.1 Antibody-dependent cytotoxicity. The action of antibody occurs through Fc receptors. Platelets, neutrophils, eosinophils and cells of the mononuclear phagocyte series all have receptors for Fc, by which they can engage target tissues. K cells are functionally defined Fc receptor$^+$ cytotoxic cells. Clq is a soluble Fc receptor and the first molecule of the complement classical pathway. Activation of complement C3 can generate complement-mediated lytic damage to target cells directly, and also allows phagocytic cells with receptors for activated C3 to bind to the target.

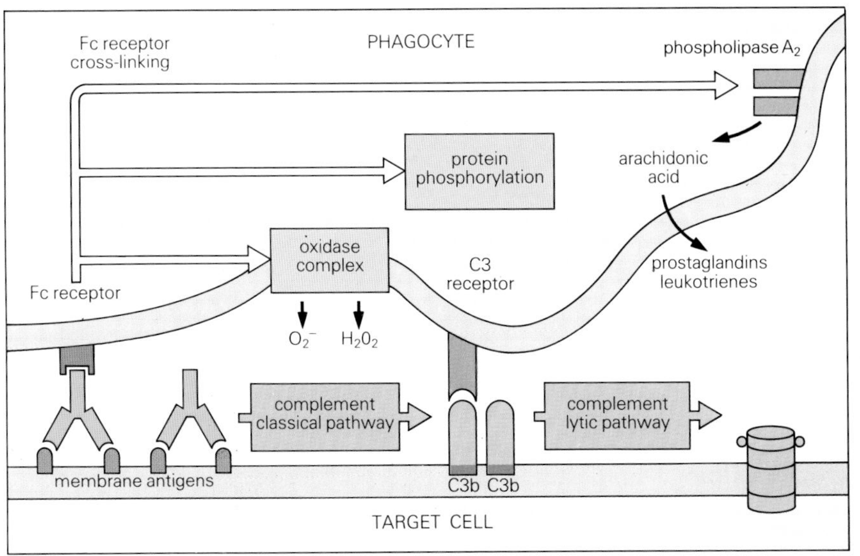

Fig. 20.2 Type II cytotoxic mechanisms. Antibody bound to membrane antigens on effector cells opsonizes them for phagocytes. Cross-linking of the Fc receptors activates a membrane oxidase complex to secrete oxygen radicals; it causes increased protein phosphorylation and hence cellular activation; it also causes increased arachidonic acid release from membrane phospholipids effected by phospholipase-A. Immune complexes induce complement C3b deposition which can also interact with opsonic adherence receptors on phagocytes. Activation of the lytic pathway causes the assembly of the membrane attack complex (MAC) by components C5–C9.

1. Antibody-sensitized cells can be lysed by activation of the classical and lytic pathways, resulting in the deposition of the C5b–9 membrane attack complex on the target cells.
2. C3b can be deposited onto target tissues by activation of the classical pathway and amplification loops. This sensitizes the targets for interaction with effector cells, such as macrophages and neutrophil polymorphs, which carry receptors for activated complement components (CR1, CR3).

C3b binds to targets by a covalent bond formed after the breaking of an internal thiolester linkage during C3 activation by C3 convertases. After inactivation of C3b by factor I and other serum enzymes, C3d remains covalently bound to the target. Both C3b and C3d can act as recognition structures for cells with complement receptors, as detailed in Chapter 13.

In addition to their ability to activate the complement classical pathway, antibodies can also interact with cells carrying Fc receptors. These include macrophages, neutrophils, eosinophils and K cells. The different antibody subclasses vary in their ability to interact with different effector cells and with C1q. This reflects the binding characteristics of the different kinds of Fc receptor. For example, C1q binds to a site in the Cγ2 domain of IgG1, whereas macrophages bind to a site which involves the Cγ2 and Cγ3 domains (Fig. 20.3). In fact many cells have several different Fc receptors, and these may vary in their ability to bind different subclasses. An example of this is mouse macrophages which have different receptors for the IgG2a and IgG2b subclasses.

Complement fragments and IgG present as opsonins on tissues and microorganisms also serve to activate phagocytes which take up the opsonized particles. By enhancing lysosomal activity of phagocytes and potentiating their capacity to produce reactive oxygen intermediates, the opsonins increase the phagocytes' capacity to destroy pathogens, but also increase their capacity to produce immunopathological damage in hypersensitivity reactions (Fig. 20.4). For example, neutrophils isolated from the synovial fluid of patients with rheumatoid arthritis produce more superoxide in response to suitable stimuli than blood neutrophils; this is thought to be related to their activation in the rheumatoid joint by mediators which include immune complexes and complement fragments.

Fc receptor of effector system	IgG subclass				IgG fragment		
	IgG1	IgG2	IgG3	IgG4	Cγ2	Cγ3	Fc
monocytes	+	±	+	–	–	–	+
neutrophils	+	+	+	some	–	–	+
K cells	+	+	+	some	–	–	+
C1q	+	±	+	–	+	–	+

Fig. 20.3 Human IgG subclass domains activating different effector systems. The ability to interact with Fc receptors on cells and Clq varies with the different IgG subclasses. Additionally the site recognized on the Fc region varies for the different cell types. For example, Clq binds to a site in Cγ2 whereas K cells bind to a site which requires the whole Fc region (Cγ2 and Cγ3).

neutrophil function	activator					
	IgG	C3	IgG+C3	C5a	C5b67	IgA
adherence	+	+++	+++	+	–	+
oxygen metabolism	+	±	++++	+++	++	+
lysosomal enzyme release	+	+	++++	+++	++	+
chemotaxis	+	–	+	+++	++	?
phagocytosis	+	±	++++	–	–	?

Fig. 20.4 Neutrophil activation. Neutrophils are activated by complexed IgG and activated complement components. Each mediator has a particular spectrum of activity. Note how activated C3 (including C3b, C3bi and C3d, depending on the maturity of the cells involved) and activation via IgG Fc receptors potentiate each other and present a particularly powerful signal to the cells when both are present.

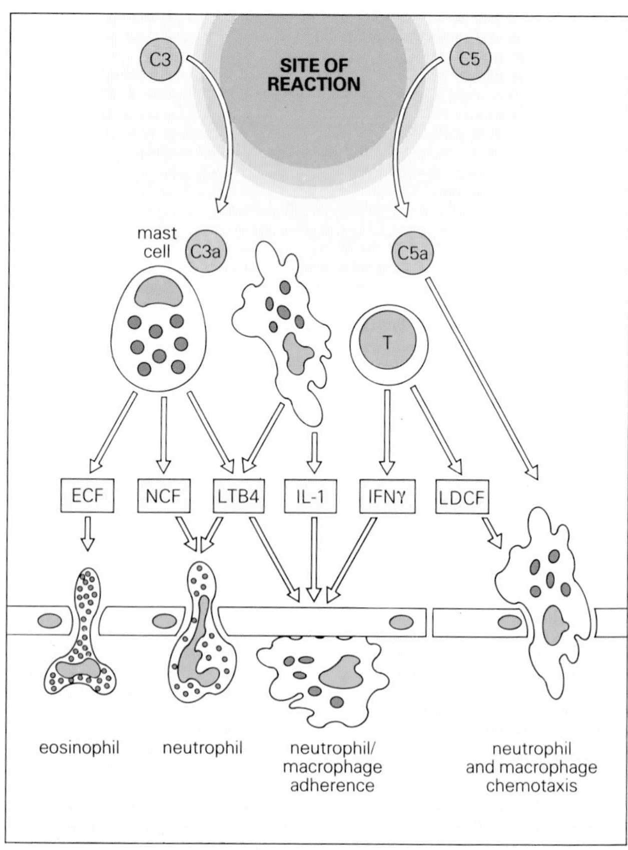

Fig. 20.5 Chemotactic factors in hypersensitivity reactions. Activated mast cells release eosinophil chemotactic factors (ECF) including active tetrapeptides and neutrophil chemotactic factor (NCF), and leukotriene B4 (LTB4). LTB4 is also produced by macrophages and is chemotactic for neutrophils and macrophages. LTB4, IL-1 and IFNϒ act on endothelium to increase neutrophil and monocyte adherence. C5a is a major chemoattractant for both neutrophils and macrophages. Activated T cells release both IFNϒ and a lymphocyte derived chemotactic factor (LDCF) which appears to be important in macrophage infiltration of delayed hypersensitivity reactions.

Additionally arachidonic acid release is stimulated, supplying the precursor for production of prostaglandins and leukotrienes, which are involved in the development of inflammation.

Other complement fragments, for example C5a, are involved in attracting phagocytic cells to the sites of hypersensitivity reactions. Fibrin peptides, leukotrienes (LTB4) and chemotactic polypeptides from mast cells and lymphocytes are also active in signalling to incoming effector cells. This again reflects their normal functions in the development of inflammatory reactions (Fig. 20.5).

The mechanisms by which Fc receptor-bearing effector cells damage their targets also reflect their normal physiological functions in dealing with infectious pathogens (Fig. 20.6). Most pathogens, unless they are resistant to phagocyte-mediated attack, are killed inside the phagolysosome by a combination of oxygen metabolites, radicals, ions, enzymes, altered pH and other factors which interfere with their metabolism. Phagocytes cannot adequately phagocytose large targets and so granule and lysosome contents are released in apposition to the sensitized target, thereby damaging host tissue (Fig. 20.7). The process of releasing cellular contents is referred to as exocytosis. In some reactions, such as the eosinophil reaction to schistosomes, exocytosis of granule contents is beneficial, but if the host tissue has been sensitized by antibody it will activate similar effector mechanisms and damage, rather than benefit, will occur.

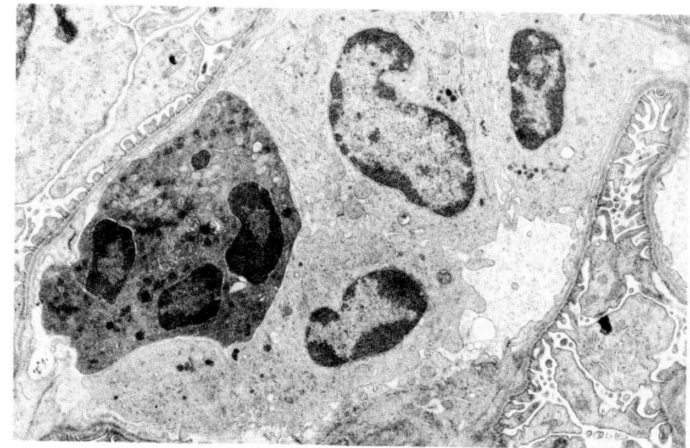

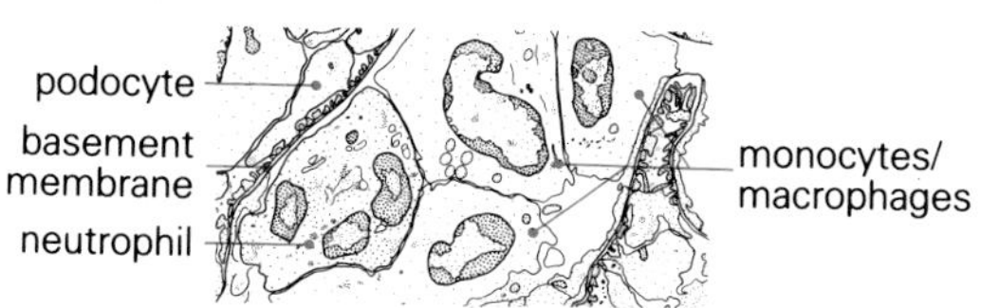

Fig. 20.7 Phagocytes attacking a basement membrane. This electronmicrograph shows a neutrophil and three monocytes binding to the capillary basement membrane in the kidney of a rabbit containing anti-basement membrane antibody. ×3500 (Courtesy of Professor G. A. Andres).

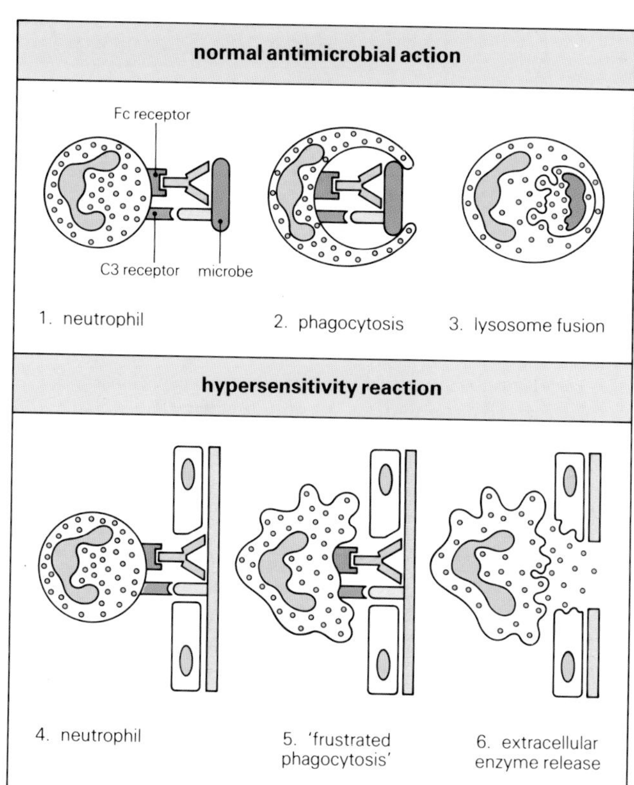

Fig. 20.6 Damage mechanisms. Neutrophil-mediated damage is a reflection of normal antibacterial action. Neutrophils engage microbes with their Fc and C3 receptors (1). The microbe is then phagocytosed (2) and destroyed as lysosomes fuse to form the phagolysosome (3). In hypersensitivity reactions, host cells coated with antibody are similarly phagocytosed, but where the target is large, for example a basement membrane (4), the neutrophils are frustrated in their attempt at phagocytosis (5) and release their lysosomal contents to the outside, causing damage to cells in the vicinity (6).

Antibodies also mediate hypersensitivity by cross-linking K cells to target tissues. K cells are mainly found in the population of large granular lymphocytes, and bind sensitizing antibody via their high-affinity Fc receptors. Cytotoxicity then appears to follow the same mechanisms as used by cytotoxic T cells. Although K cell activity may be demonstrated against a number of different cell types *in vitro*, it is difficult to assess the impact of K cells in hypersensitivity reactions. One problem is the varying susceptibility of different target cells to the actions of the various effector cells (Fig. 20.8). This is due

	target			
effector	nucleated mammalian cells	group A human erythrocytes	pyogenic micro-organisms	parasites
K cells	+++	–	±	?
mononuclear phagocytes	++	+++	+++	?
neutrophils	±	+++	++++	?
eosinophils	?	?	?	++
platelets	±	?	?	?

Fig. 20.8 The susceptibility of different targets to damage by effector cells. Susceptibility differs with the cell type. For example, K cells are inactive against pyogenic bacteria. Note that cytotoxic T cells and K cells both require extracellular Mg^{2+} and Ca^{2+} for optimum killing – neutrophil and macrophage activation by aggregated IgG does not.

to such factors as the amounts of particular antigens expressed on the target cell's surface and on the inherent ability of different target cells to sustain damage. For example, a red cell may be lysed by a single active C5 convertase site, whereas it takes many such sites to destroy most nucleated cells. Nucleated cells are particularly susceptible to K cell-mediated damage, and chick erythrocytes (nucleated red cells) are often used as a standard target to test for K cell activity.

The remainder of this chapter examines some of the instances where type II hypersensitivity reactions are thought to be of prime importance in causing target cell destruction or immunopathological damage.

REACTIONS AGAINST BLOOD CELLS AND PLATELETS

Some of the most clear-cut examples of type II reactions are seen in the responses to red blood cells. These may occur following incompatible blood transfusions, where the recipient becomes sensitized to antigens on the surface of allogeneic erythrocytes. Other important examples include autoimmune haemolytic anaemias and thrombocytopenias, where the patient becomes sensitized to his own erythrocytes or platelets, respectively.

TRANSFUSION REACTIONS

At least 20 blood groups have been recognized in man, with more than 200 allogeneic variants. Each system consists of a gene locus specifying antigens on the erythrocyte surface and, in some cases, on the surface of other cells too. An individual with a particular blood group can recognize red cells carrying allogeneic blood group antigens and produce antibodies to them. The antibodies may be produced naturally, without prior

system	gene loci	antigens	phenotype frequencies
ABO	1	A, B or O	A 42% B 8% AB 3% O 47%
Rhesus	3 closely linked loci: major antigen=RhD	C or c D or d E or e	RhD$^+$ 85% RhD$^-$ 15%
Kell	1	K or k	K 9% k 91%
Duffy	1	Fy^a, Fy^b or Fy	Fy^{a}Fy^b 46% Fy^a 20% Fy^b 34% Fy 0.1%
MN	1	M or N	MM 28% NN 50% MN 22%

Fig. 20.9 Five major blood group systems involved in transfusion reactions. Not all are equally antigenic in transfusion reactions: thus, RhD evokes a stronger reaction in an incompatible recipient than the other Rhesus antigens; and Fy^a is stronger then Fy^b. Frequencies stated are for Caucasian populations – other races have different gene frequencies.

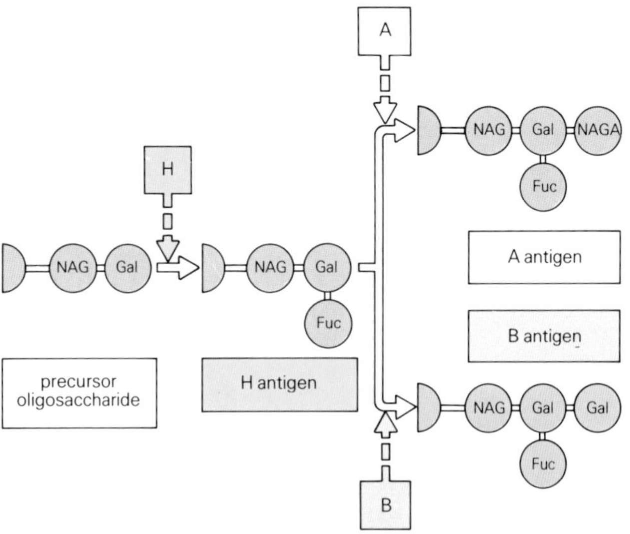

blood group (phenotype)	genotypes	antigens	antibodies to ABO in Serum
A	AA,AO	A	anti-B
B	BB,BO	B	anti-A
AB	AB	A and B	none
O	OO	H	anti-A and anti-B

Fig. 20.10 ABO blood group reactivities. The diagram presents a simple account of the way the ABO blood groups are constructed. The enzyme produced by the H gene attaches a fucose residue (Fuc) to the terminal galactose (Gal) of the precursor oligosaccharide. Individuals possessing the A gene now attach *N*-acetylgalactosamine (NAGA) to this galactose residue, while those with the B gene attach another galactose, producing A and B antigens, respectively. People with both genes make some of each. The table indicates the genotypes and antigens of the ABO system. Most people naturally make antibodies to the antigens they lack. (NAG = *N*-acetylglucosamine.)

immunization with foreign red cells, or only after contact with allogeneic cells. Some blood group antigens are stronger immunogens than others and are more likely to induce antibodies. It is important that donors and recipients are cross-matched for major blood groups before transfusion, otherwise transfusion reactions will occur. Some major human blood groups are listed in Fig. 20.9.

The ABO system is of primary importance. The antigens are expressed on carbohydrate units of glycoproteins. The structure of these carbohydrates and of those determining the related Lewis blood group system is determined by allelic genes which transfer terminal sugars to a carbohydrate backbone (Fig. 20.10). In the case of the ABO system, individuals develop antibodies to allogeneic specificities without prior sensitization with red cells. It is thought that most people become sensitized to ABO system antigens by encountering identical antigenic determinants which are coincidentally expressed on a variety of microorganisms. Since antibodies to the ABO system antigens occur naturally, it is particularly important to match donor blood to the recipient for this system.

The Rhesus system is also of great importance, since it is a major cause of haemolytic disease of the newborn. Rhesus antigens are lipid-dependent proteins which are sparsely distributed on the cell surface, and are generated by three closely linked genes, of which the Rhesus D locus is most important due to its high immunogenicity. The MN system antigens are expressed on the *N*-terminal glycosylated region of glycophorin A, present on the erythrocyte surface. Antigenicity is determined by polymorphisms at amino acids 1 and 5. The related Ss system antigens are carried on glycophorin B. It has recently been shown that the Kell antigen occurs on a membrane protein of 93kD. Transfusion reactions caused by the minor blood groups are less common, but the risks are greatly reduced by accurately cross-matching the donor blood to the recipient.

The principle of cross-matching is to ensure that the recipient does not have antibodies which react with the donor red cells. Antibodies to ABO blood groups antigens cause incompatible cells to agglutinate, but weaker reactions may only be detectable by an indirect Coombs' test (see below). If an individual is transfused with whole blood, it is also necessary to check that the donor serum does not react to the recipient erythrocytes. Transfusion of whole blood is unusual, however; most blood donations are separated into different cellular and serum fractions to be used individually.

Transfusion of blood cells into a recipient who has antibodies to those red cells produces an immediate transfusion reaction (Fig. 20.11). The severity of the reaction depends on the class and the amounts of the antibodies involved. Antibodies to ABO system antigens are usually IgM. They cause agglutination, complement activation and intravascular haemolysis. Other blood groups induce IgG antibodies, and these agglutinate the cells less well than IgM. Severe reactions may cause red cell destruction by complement activation, but more often the IgG-sensitized cells are taken up by Fc receptor-bearing cells in the liver and spleen. Red cell destruction may cause circulatory shock, and the released contents of the red cells can produce acute tubular necrosis of the kidneys. Transfusion reactions to incompatible blood may also develop over days or weeks in previously unsensitized individuals as antibodies to the foreign cells are produced, resulting in anaemia or jaundice.

fever

hypotension

lower back pain

feeling of chest compression

nausea and vomiting

Fig. 20.11 Clinical indications of transfusion reactions.

Transfusion reactions to other components of blood, including leucocytes and platelets, may also occur, though their consequences are not usually as severe as reactions to erythrocytes.

HAEMOLYTIC DISEASE OF THE NEWBORN

Haemolytic disease of the newborn (HDNB) appears in newborn infants where the mother has been sensitized to the blood group antigens on the infant's erythrocytes and makes IgG antibodies to these antigens. These antibodies cross the placenta and react with the fetal red cells, causing their destruction (Figs 20.12 and 20.13). Rhesus D (RhD) is the most commonly involved antigen

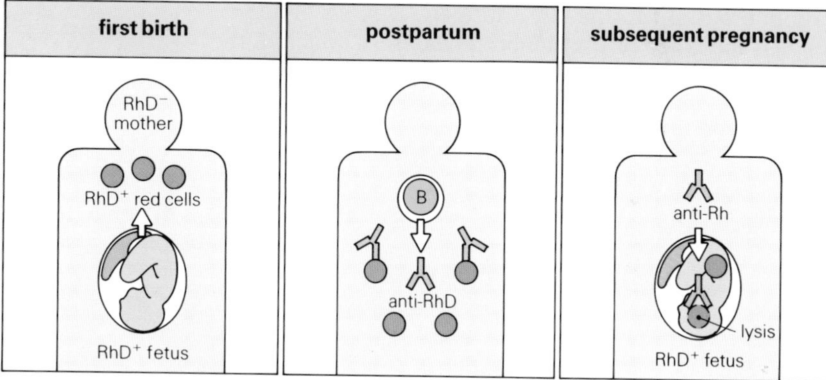

Fig. 20.12 Haemolytic disease of the newborn – I. Erythrocytes from a Rhesus$^+$ (RhD$^+$) fetus leak into the maternal circulation during a first incompatible pregnancy. This stimulates the production of anti-Rh antibody of the IgG class postpartum. During subsequent pregnancies, antibodies are transferred across the placenta into the fetal circulation (IgM antibodies cannot cross the placenta). If the fetus is again incompatible the antibodies cause red cell destruction.

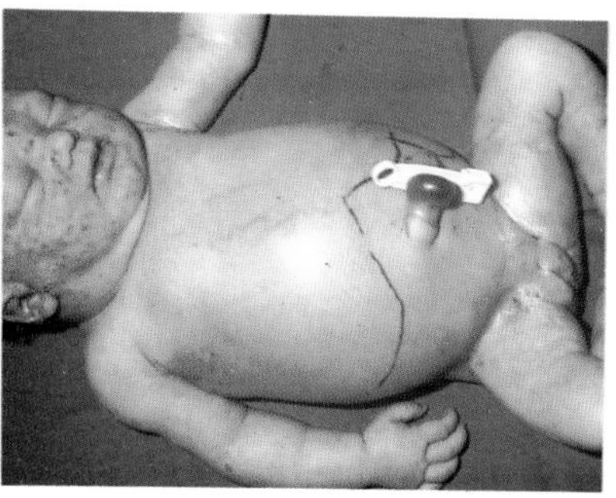

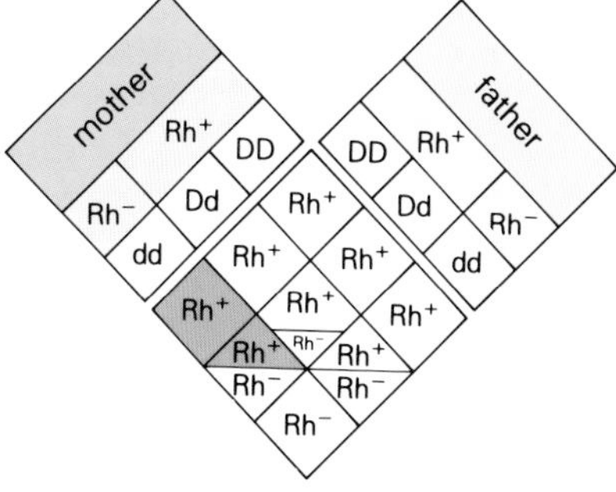

Fig. 20.13 Haemolytic disease of the newborn – II. The child is suffering from HDNB. There is considerable enlargement of the liver and spleen associated with red cell destruction caused by maternal anti-red cell antibody in the fetal circulation. The child had elevated bilirubin (breakdown product of haemoglobin) and the facial petechial haemorrhaging was due to impaired platelet function. (Courtesy of Dr K. Sloper.) The most commonly involved antigen is RhD. The table indicates the phenotypes of children from parents with different RhD phenotypes. The Rh+ individuals may be homozygous (DD) or heterozygous (Dd). Rh$^-$ individuals are always homozygous (dd). The danger of HDNB arises in Rh$^-$ mothers carrying Rh$^+$ children (red).

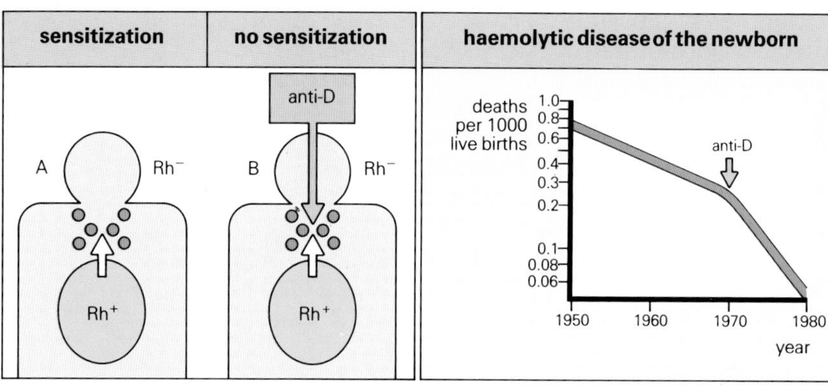

Fig. 20 14 Rhesus prophylaxis. Without prophylaxis Rh^+ red cells leak into the circulation of a Rh^- mother and sensitize her to the Rh antigen(s) (A). If anti-Rh antibody (anti-D) is injected immediately postpartum it eliminates the Rh^+ red cells and prevents sensitization (B). The incidence of deaths due to HDNB fell during the period 1950–1966 with improved patient care. The decline in the disease was accelerated by the general advent of Rhesus prophylaxis in 1969.

and a risk arises when a Rh^- mother carries a Rh^+ infant. Sensitization of the Rh^- mother to the Rh^+ red cells usually occurs during birth, when some fetal red cells leak back across the placenta into the maternal circulation to be recognized by the maternal immune system. For this reason the first incompatible child is usually unaffected, but the second and later children have an increasing risk of being affected as the mother is repeatedly immunized with successive pregnancies. Reactions to other blood groups may cause HDNB, the second most common being the Kell system K antigen. This is much less frequent than reactions due to RhD because of the relative infrequency of the K antigen (9%) and its weaker antigenicity.

It was noticed that in cases where haemolytic disease of the newborn due to Rhesus incompatibility was expected, there was a lower incidence of the condition if the father was of a different ABO group to the mother. This led to the idea that Rh^+ fetal cells would be destroyed in a Rh^- mother by the mother's natural antibodies if they were also ABO-incompatible. Consequently they would not be available to sensitize the maternal immune system to the RhD antigen. This observation formed the basis of Rhesus prophylaxis, in which anti-RhD antibodies were given to Rh^- mothers immediately after delivery of Rh^+ infants. This has led to a fall in the incidence of HDNB due to Rhesus incompatibility (Fig. 20.14). Although it is not certain, it is assumed that the prevention of sensitization is due to destruction of fetal red cells.

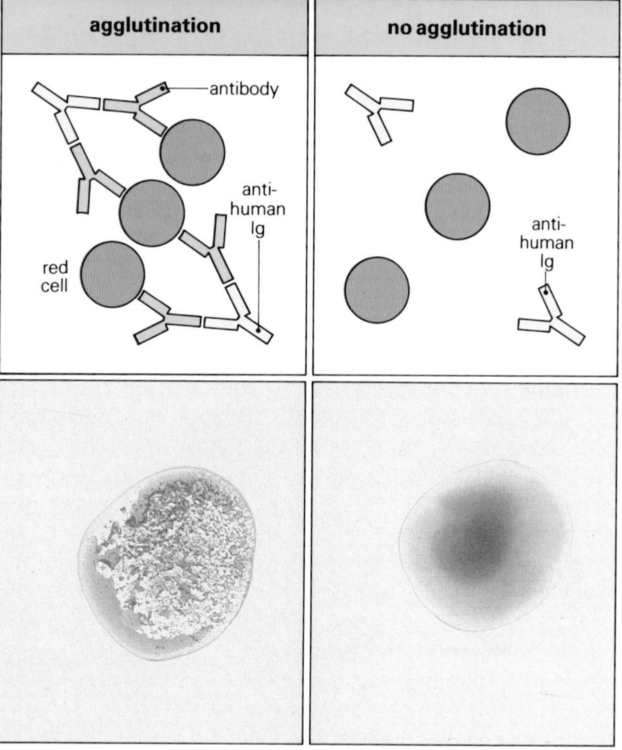

Fig. 20.15 Indirect Coombs' test. This test, also called the direct antiglobulin test, is used to detect antibody on a patient's erythrocytes. If antibody is present the erythrocytes can be agglutinated by anti-human immunoglobulin. If no antibody is present on the red cells they are not agglutinated by anti-human immunoglobulin.

AUTOIMMUNE HAEMOLYTIC ANAEMIAS

Reactions to blood group antigens also occur in the autoimmune haemolytic anaemias, in which patients produce antibodies to their own red cells. A diagnosis of autoimmune haemolytic anaemia would be suspected if a patient gave a positive Coombs' test (Fig. 20.15). This test identifies antibodies present on the patient's red cells, and is usually indicative of either antibodies directed towards erythrocyte antigens or immune complexes adsorbed onto the red cells' surface. The Coombs' test is also used to detect antibodies on red cells caused by mismatched transfusions and in haemolytic disease of the newborn. Autoimmune haemolytic anaemias can be divided into three types, depending upon whether they are due to:

1. warm-reactive autoantibodies which react with the antigen at 37°C
2. cold-reactive autoantibodies which only react with antigen below 37°C
3. antibodies provoked by allergic reactions to drugs.

Warm-reactive autoantibodies Warm-reactive autoantibodies are frequently found against Rhesus system antigens, including determinants of the RhC and RhE loci as well as RhD. The type of reactivity displayed by these autoantibodies is, however, not typical of the antibodies which develop in transfusion reactions to these antigens, in the sense that they appear to react with different epitopes on the Rh antigens than otherwise occurs. Occasionally autoantibodies to other blood group antigens are found. The cause of the majority of warm antibody haemolytic anaemias is unknown but some are associated with other autoimmune diseases. The anaemia seen in these patients appears to be caused by accelerated clearance of the sensitized red cells by spleen macrophages more often than by complement-mediated lysis.

Cold-reactive autoantibodies Cold-reactive autoantibodies are often present in higher titres than the warm-reactive autoantibodies. The antibodies are primarily IgM and fix complement strongly. In most cases they are specific for the Ii blood group system. These antigens are expressed on the precursor polysaccharides which also produce the ABO system antigens. Incomplete glycosylation of the core polysaccharide produces increased expression of the I and i antigens.

The reaction of the antibody with the red cells takes place in the peripheral circulation (particularly in winter) where the temperature in the capillary loops of exposed skin may fall below 30°C. This can cause peripheral necrosis in severe cases. Since organs such as the spleen and liver are at 37°C, and the antibodies do not bind at this temperature, anaemia is apparently caused not by Fc-mediated removal of sensitized red cells in the centre of the body but by complement-mediated destruction in the periphery. The severity of the anaemia is related to the complement fixing ability of the patient's serum.

Most cold antibody autoimmune haemolytic anaemias occur in older people; their cause is unknown, but it is notable that the autoantibodies produced are usually of very limited clonality. Other cases may follow infection with *Mycoplasma pneumoniae.* This is usually an acute onset disease of short duration and with polyclonal autoantibodies. Its occurrence is thought to be due to cross-reacting antigens on the bacteria and the red cells, producing bypass of normal tolerance mechanisms, as described in Chapter 23.

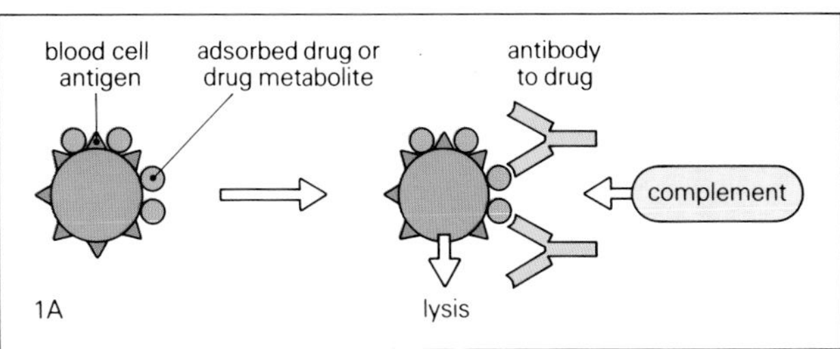

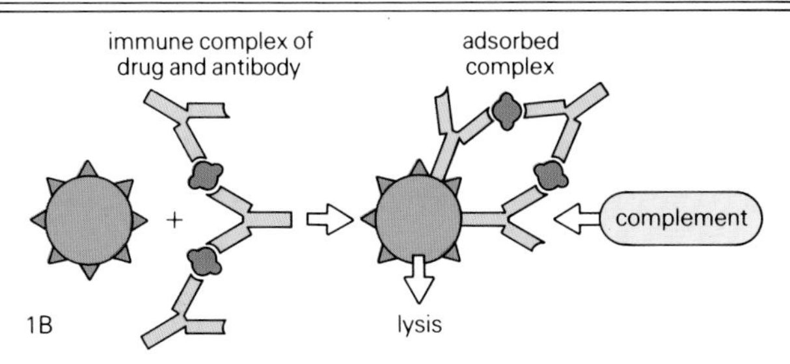

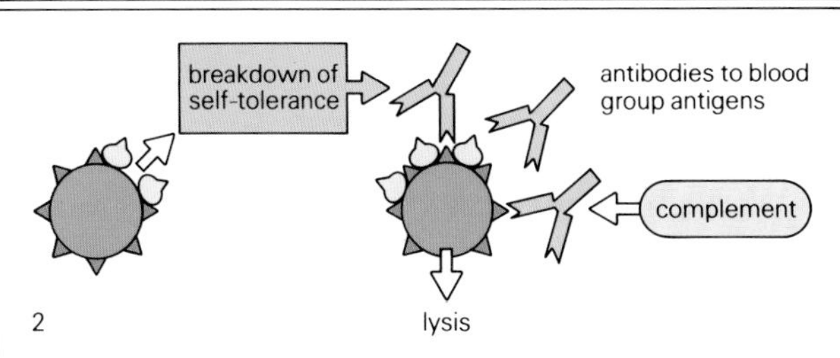

Fig. 20.16 Drug-induced reactions to blood cells: ways in which drug treatment may induce damage.
1A. Drugs (or metabolites) adsorb to cell membranes. If the patient makes antibodies to them they will bind to the cell and complement-mediated lysis will occur.
1B. Immune complexes of drugs and antibody become adsorbed to the red cell. This appears to be mediated by the immune adherence receptor (CR1) and/or the immunoglobulin Fc region. It is uncertain whether Fc-dependent binding is specific. Damage occurs by complement-mediated lysis.
2. Drugs, presumably adsorbed onto cell membranes, induce a breakdown of self-tolerance, possibly by stimulating T-helper (TH) cells. This leads to formation of antibodies to other blood group antigens on the cell surface. Note that in 1A and 1B the antibody is to the drug while in 2 it is to normal cell surface antigens, therefore in 2 the antibody can destroy cells whether they carry adsorbed drug or not.

DRUG-INDUCED REACTIONS TO BLOOD COMPONENTS

Drugs can provoke allergic and autoallergic reactions against blood cells, including erythrocytes and platelets. This can occur in three different ways (Fig. 20.16). Usually the reaction occurs to the drug or its metabolites, in which case it is necessary for both the drug and the antibody to be present to produce the reaction. The first observation of this type was made by Ackroyd, who observed thrombocytopenic purpura (destruction of platelets) following administration of the drug sedormid. Haemolytic anaemias have been reported following administration of a wide variety of drugs, including penicillin, quinine and sulphonamides. All these conditions are rare.

Occasionally drugs may induce allergic reactions where autoantibodies directed against the red cell antigens are produced, as is the case with 0.3% of patients given α-methyldopa. The antibodies produced are similar to those in patients with warm-reactive antibody but, unlike those diseases, the condition remits shortly after the cessation of drug treatment.

REACTIONS TO LEUCOCYTES AND PLATELETS

Autoantibodies to neutrophils (Fig. 20.17), and lymphocytes are sometimes reported. The autoantibodies to neutrophils are true tissue-specific antibodies, unlike antibodies to ABO system antigens. (ABO antigens are found on many tissues, for example, red cells, kidney,

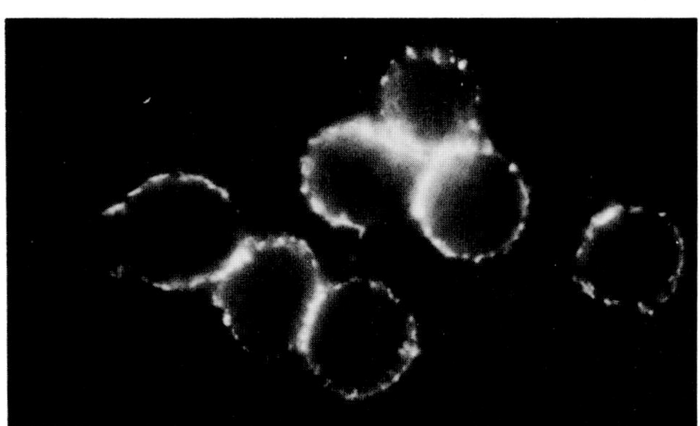

Fig. 20.17 Immunofluorescence of normal neutrophils incubated with SLE serum and goat anti-human F(ab')$_2$FITC. Antibodies to neutrophils occur in SLE, as demonstrated by immunofluorescence of normal neutrophils. Acute transfusion reactions to neutrophils may cause pyrexia, presumably due to pyrogens released from the damaged neutrophils. This indicates that anti-neutrophil antibodies can damage neutrophils, although their role in the pathogenesis of SLE is uncertain. (Reproduced from the *Journal of Clinical Investigation,* 1979, **64**, pp 902–912.)

salivary gland; the neutrophil-specific antigens are found only on PMNs.) Antibodies to both neutrophils and lymphocytes are observed in systemic lupus erythematosus (SLE), but their contribution to the pathogenesis of the disease appears to be relatively small, possibly because these cells remove bound antibodies from their surface quite rapidly.

Autoantibodies to platelets are seen in up to 70% of cases of idiopathic thrombocytopenic purpura, a disorder in which there is accelerated removal of platelets from the circulation, mediated primarily by splenic macrophages. The mechanism of removal is via the immune adherence receptors on these cells. The condition most often develops after bacterial or viral infections, but may also be associated with autoimmune diseases including SLE. In SLE, antibodies to cardiolipin, present on platelets, can sometimes be detected. Autoantibodies to phospholipids can inhibit blood clotting (lupus anticoagulant) and are associated, in some cases, with venous thrombosis and recurrent abortions. Thrombocytopenia may also be induced by drugs, by similar mechanisms to those outlined in Fig. 20.16.

HYPERACUTE GRAFT REJECTION

Hyperacute graft rejection occurs when a transplant recipient has preformed antibodies directed against the graft. The reaction occurs between a few minutes and 48 hours after completion of the transplantation; the recipient's antibodies react immediately against antigens exposed on the grafted cells. The most serious reactions of this type are due to ABO group antigens which are expressed on kidney, but since donors and recipients are now always cross-matched for these antigens, this is very rare. Preformed antibodies to other tissue antigens, including MHC class I molecules, may also cause this type of rejection. Such antibodies might arise after previous transfusions or failed engraftments. Hyperacute rejection is further minimized by cross-matching donor T cells with recipient sera, to ensure that the recipient lacks such antibodies.

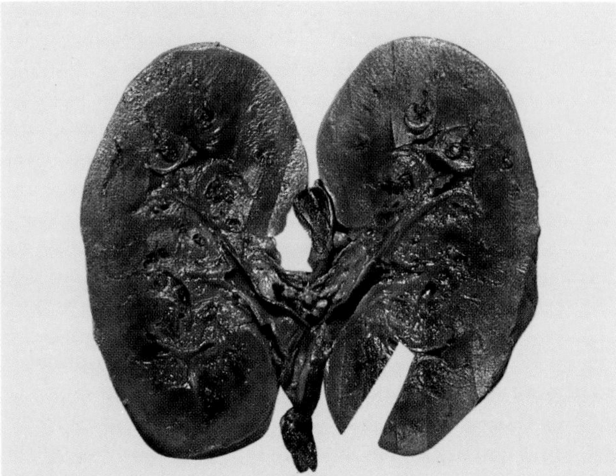

Fig. 20.18 Hyperacute graft rejection. This human kidney, removed 18 hours after transplantation, is thrombosed and haemorrhagic. The whole tissue is dark and necrotic. (Courtesy of Dr K. Welsh.)

The reaction is only seen in grafts which are revascularized directly after transplantation, such as kidney grafts. Within one hour of revascularization there is an extensive infiltration of neutrophils and this is followed by major damage to the glomerular capillaries and haemorrhage. Thrombi deposit in the arterioles and the graft is irreversibly destroyed (Fig. 20.18). The major effectors are the neutrophils and platelets, interacting with the sensitized cells via Fc, C3b and C3d receptors.

REACTIONS TO TISSUE ANTIGENS

A number of autoimmune conditions occur in which antibodies to tissue antigens cause immunopathological damage by activation of type II hypersensitivity mechanisms. The antigens may be expressed on extracellular structural proteins or, on the surface of cells. Examples of such diseases include Goodpasture's syndrome and myasthenia gravis. There are many other examples in which it is possible to demonstrate autoantibodies to particular cell types, but in these cases the importance of the type II mechanisms is less well established.

REACTIONS TO BASEMENT MEMBRANES

A number of patients with nephritis are found to have antibodies to a glycoprotein of the glomerular basement membrane (Fig. 20.19). The antibody is usually IgG and in at least 50% of patients it appears to fix complement.

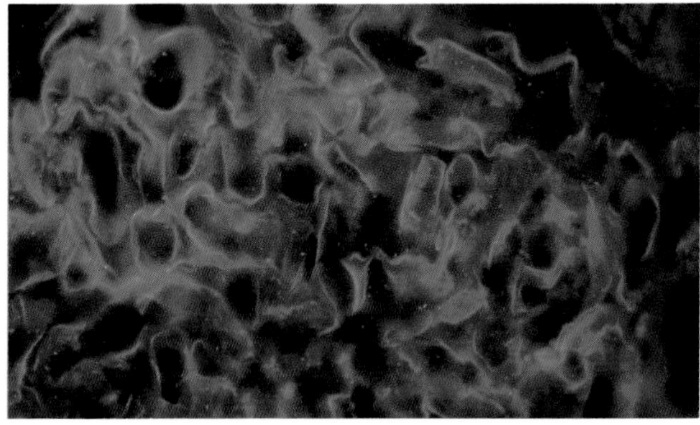

Fig. 20.19 Autoantibody to glomerular basement membrane in Goodpasture's syndrome. Antibody to a basement membrane antigen forms an evenly bound layer on the basement membrane. This is visualized with fluorescent anti-IgG. (Courtesy of Dr F. Hay.)

The condition usually results in severe necrosis of the glomerulus, with fibrin deposition. The association of this type of nephritis with lung haemorrhage was originally noticed by Goodpasture (hence Goodpasture's syndrome). Although the lung symptoms do not occur in all patients, the association of lung and kidney damage is due to cross-reactive autoantigens in the two tissues.

One animal model for Goodpasture's syndrome is nephrotoxic serum nephritis (Masugi glomerulonephritis). In this model heterologous antibodies to glomerular basement membrane are injected into rats or rabbits, resulting in acute nephritis. Antibody deposition occurs on the basement membranes, and there is further deposition of antibodies formed in the host animal to the heterologous immunoglobulin. Development of nephritis and proteinuria depends on the accumulation of polymorphs, which bind via complement-dependent and complement-independent mechanisms. Similar lesions can be induced by immunization with heterologous basement membrane (Stablay model). Another animal model (Heyman nephritis), caused by raising autoantibodies to a protein present in the brush border of glomerular epithelial cells, resembles human membranous glomerulonephritis. Interestingly the damage in this model is mostly complement-mediated; complement depletion of the animals alleviates the condition.

MYASTHENIA GRAVIS

It has recently been recognized that myasthenia gravis, a condition in which there is extreme muscular weakness, is associated with antibodies to the acetylcholine receptors present on the surface of muscle membranes. The acetylcholine receptors are located at the motor endplate where the neuron contacts the muscle. Transmission of impulses from the nerve to the muscle takes place by the release of acetylcholine from the nerve terminal and its diffusion across the gap to the muscle fibre.

It was noticed that immunization of experimental animals with purified acetylcholine receptors produced a condition of muscular weakness that closely resembled human myasthenia. This suggested a role for antibody to the acetylcholine receptor in the human disease. Analysis of the lesion in myasthenic muscles indicated that the disease was not due to an inability to synthesize acetylcholine, nor was there any problem in secreting it in response to a nerve impulse. It appeared that the released acetylcholine was less effective at triggering depolarization of the muscle (Fig. 20.20).

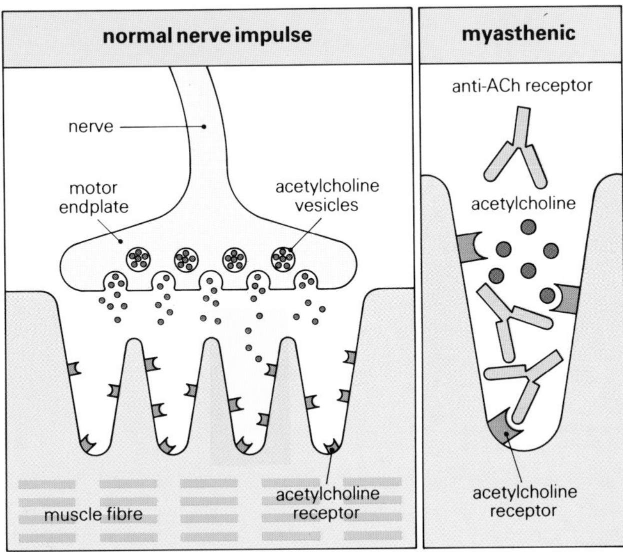

Fig. 20.20 Myasthenia gravis. Normally a nerve impulse passing down a neuron which arrives at a motor endplate causes fusion of acetylcholine-containing vesicles with the cell membrane and release of the acetylcholine (ACh). This diffuses across the neuromuscular junction and combines with ACh receptors on the muscle, causing opening of ion channels in the muscle membrane. In myasthenia gravis antibodies to the receptor block binding of the ACh transmitter and so the effect of each released vesicle is reduced. This is probably only one of the factors operating in the disease.

Examination of neuromuscular endplates by immunochemical techniques has demonstrated IgG, C3 and C9 on the postsynaptic folds of the muscle (Fig. 20.21). The IgG and complement are thought to act in two ways: by increasing the rate of turnover of the acetylcholine receptors and by some blockage of acetylcholine binding, with reduced ability to depolarize the muscle. Myasthenic serum injected into experimental animals reduces the size of the MEPPS (the amount of depolarization caused by a single vesicle quantum of acetylcholine). Cellular infiltration of myasthenic endplates is rarely seen, so it is assumed that damage does not involve effector cells. The transient muscle weakness in babies born to myasthenic mothers is further evidence for a pathogenetic role for IgG antibody, which can cross the placenta.

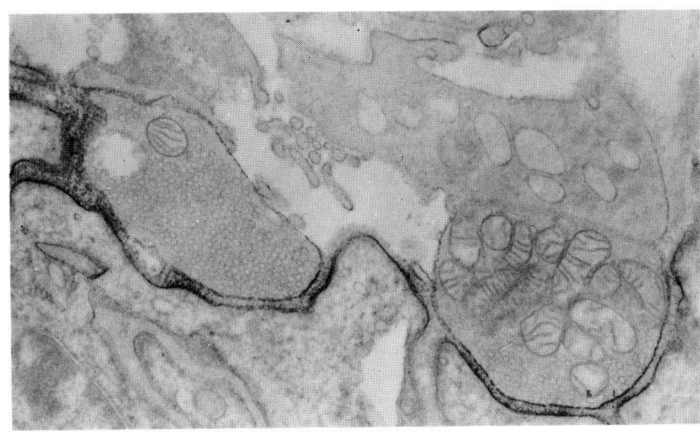

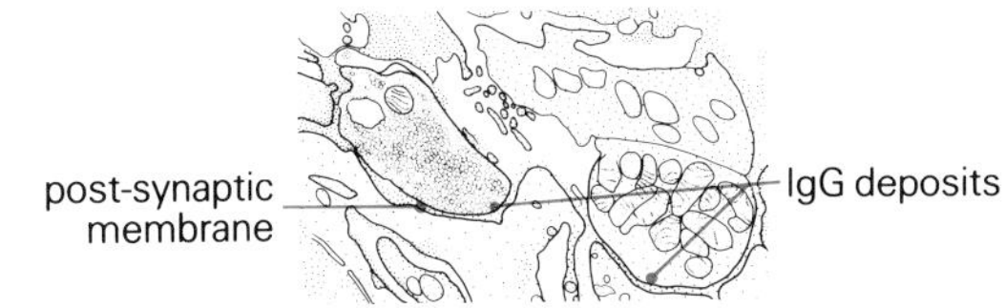

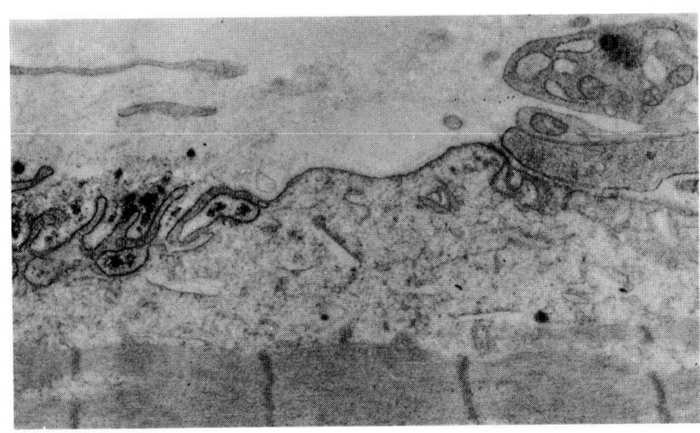

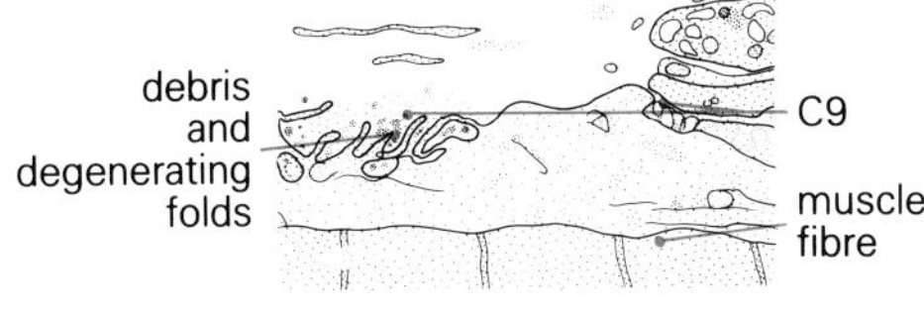

Fig. 20.21 Electronmicrographs showing IgG autoantibody (above) and complement C9 (below) localized at the motor endplate in myasthenia gravis. The upper micrograph shows IgG deposits in discrete patches on the postsynaptic membrane × 13,000. The micrograph illustrating C9 shows the postsynaptic region denuded of its nerve terminal: it consists of debris and degenerating folds. There is a strong reaction for C9 on this debris. ×9000. (Courtesy of Dr A. G. Engel.)

REACTIONS TO CELLULAR ANTIGENS

Although a great number of autoantibodies react with tissue antigens, their significance in causing tissue damage and pathology *in vivo* is uncertain. It is possible to demonstrate antibody-mediated cytotoxic reactions to thyroid cells using antibody to the thyroid microsomal-microvillous antigen (thyroid peroxidase), and cytotoxicity to pancreatic islet cells using sera from some diabetic patients *in vitro* (Fig. 20.22), but it is not certain whether this makes a major contribution to the immunopathological damage relative to that thought to be caused by autoreactive T cells. Alternatively the autoantibodies may be formed only after tissue breakdown and release of autoantigens has occurred. The autoantibodies to many of the cellular antigens detected in autoimmune diseases are directed towards intracellular molecules, present in the cytosol or organelles. Nevertheless, traces of these antigens can appear at the surface of the cell to act as potential targets for type II damage mechanisms. In some cases autoantibodies may actually stimulate receptors on cells, leading to disturbances in physiological regulation but not necessarily to cytotoxic damage (see Chapter 23).

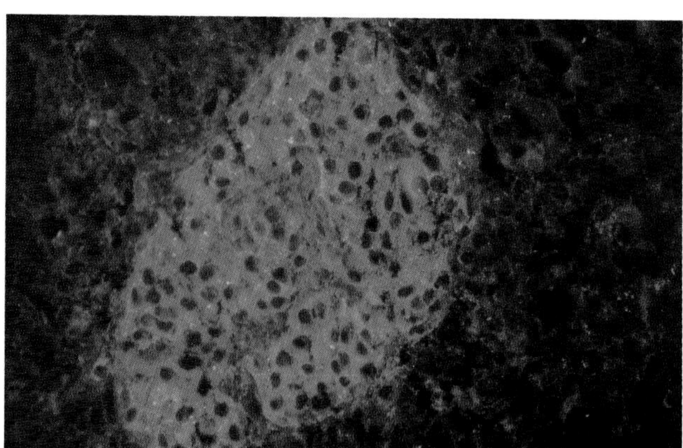

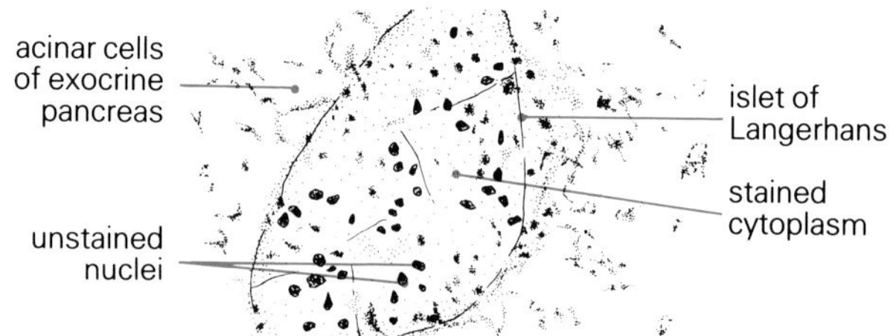

Fig. 20.22 Islet cell autoantibodies. Autoantibodies to the pancreas in diabetes mellitus may be demonstrated by immunofluorescence. The antibodies may be cytotoxic for islet cells *in vitro*, indicating a pathological role in disease. (Courtesy of Dr B. Dean.)

FURTHER READING

Bloy, C., Blanchard, D., Lambin, P., Goossens, D., Rouger, P., Salmon, C., Masoureclin, S. P. & Cartron, J-P. (1988) Characterization of the D, c, E and G antigens of the Rh blood group system with human monoclonal antibodies. *Molecular Immunology*, **25**, 925–930.

Burton, D. R. (1985) Immunoglobulin G: functional sites. *Molecular Immunology*, **22**, 161-206.

Druet, P. & Glotz, D. (1984) Experimental autoimmune nephropathies: induction and regulation. *Advances in Nephrology*, **13**, 115.

Fearon, D. T. (1984) Cellular receptors for the third component of complement. *Immunology Today*, **5**, 105–110.

Hughes-Jones, N. C. (1987) Monoclonal antibodies as potential blood typing reagents. *Immunology Today*, **9**, 68.

Lindstrom, J. (1985) Immunobiology of myasthenia gravis, experimental autoimmune myasthenia gravis and Lambert – Eaton syndrome. *Annual Review of Immunology*, **3**, 109-131.

Race, R. & Sanger, R. (1975) *Blood Groups in Man.* 6th edition. Oxford: Blackwell Scientific Publications.

Watkin, W. M. (1987) Biochemical genetics of the blood group antigens: retrospect and prospect. *Biochemical Society Transactions*, **15**, 614–624.

21 Hypersensitivity – Type III

TYPES OF IMMUNE COMPLEX DISEASE

Immune complexes are formed every time antibody meets antigen and generally they are removed effectively by the reticuloendothelial system, but occasionally their formation can lead to a hypersensitivity reaction. Diseases resulting from immune complex formation can be placed broadly into three groups (Fig. 21.1).

cause	antigen	sites of complex deposition
persistent infection	microbial antigen	infected organ(s), kidney
autoimmunity	self-antigen	kidney, joint, arteries, skin
extrinsic	environmental antigen	lung

Fig. 21.1 Three categories of immune complex disease. This table indicates the source of the antigen and the organs most frequently affected.

1. Where there is persistent infection such as occurs with α-haemolytic *Streptococcus viridans* or staphylococcal infective endocarditis, or with a parasite such as *Plasmodium vivax,* or in viral hepatitis, the combined effects of a low grade persistent infection together with a weak antibody response leads to chronic immune complex formation with the eventual deposition of complexes in the tissues (Fig. 21.2).
2. Immune complex disease is a frequent complication of autoimmune disease where the continued production of autoantibody to a self-antigen leads to prolonged immune complex formation, overload of the mononuclear phagocyte system (which is responsible for the removal of complexes) and tissue deposition of complexes, as occurs in systemic lupus erythematosus (SLE) (Fig. 21.3).
3. Immune complexes may be formed at body surfaces, for example in the lungs, following repeated inhalation of antigenic materials from moulds, plants or animals. This is exemplified in Farmer's lung disease and Pigeon Fancier's disease – examples of extrinsic allergic alveolitis – where there are circulating antibodies to actinomycete fungi following repeated exposure to mouldy hay or pigeon antigens. The antibodies induced by these antigens are primarily IgG, rather than IgE, which are produced in an immediate (Type I) hypersensitivity reaction. When antigen enters the body again by inhalation of

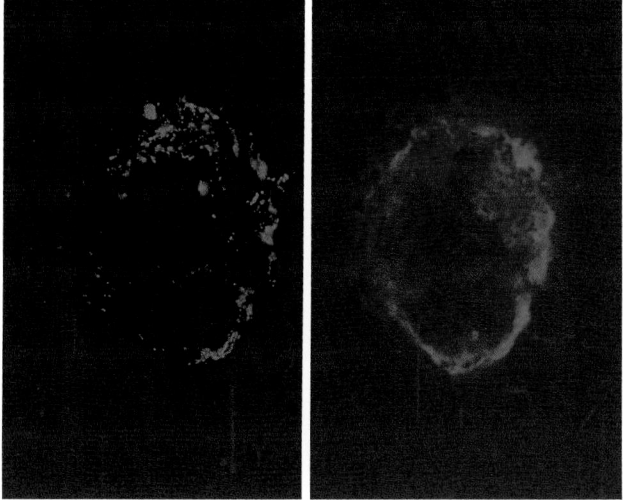

Fig. 21.2 Immunofluorescence study of immune complexes in infectious disease. These two serial sections of the renal artery of a patient with chronic hepatitis B infection are stained with fluoresceinated anti-hepatitis B antigen (left) and rhodaminated anti-IgM (right). The presence of both antigen and antibody in the intima and media of the arterial wall indicate the deposition of the complexes at this site. IgG and C3 deposits are also detectable with the same distribution. (Courtesy of Dr A. Nowoslawski.)

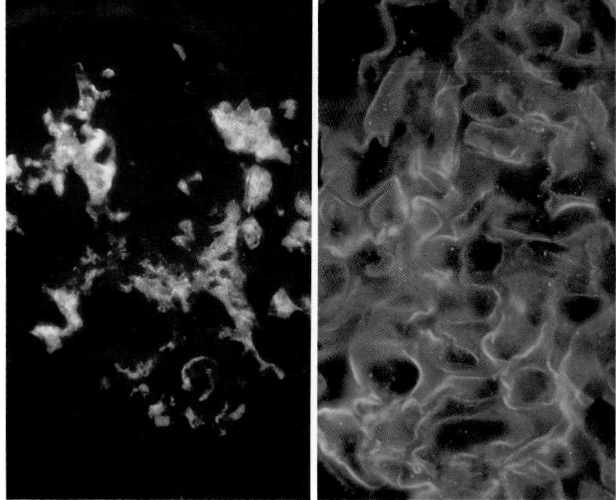

Fig. 21.3 Immunofluorescence study of immune complexes in autoimmune disease. In these renal sections from patients with systemic lupus erythematosus (SLE) and Goodpasture's syndrome the antibody is detected with fluorescent anti-IgG. Complexes deposited in the kidney form characteristic 'lumpy bumpy' deposits (left). The anti-basement membrane antibody in Goodpasture's syndrome (lung and kidney) in this Type II reaction (right) forms an even layer on the basement membrane.

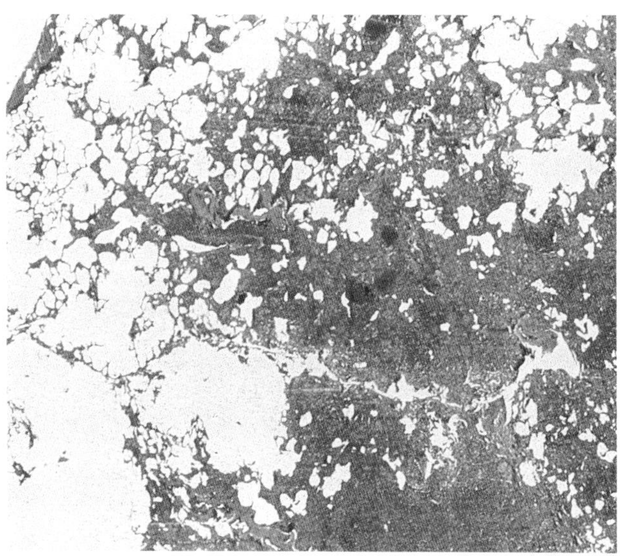

Fig. 21.4 Histological appearance of the lung in extrinsic allergic alveolitis (Pigeon Fancier's disease). There is considerable destruction of the alveoli with consolidated areas of darkly stained inflammation and fibrosis. H & E stain, x 150. (Courtesy of Dr G. Boyd.)

fungal spores, local immune complexes are formed in the alveoli leading to inflammation (Fig. 21.4). Precipitating antibodies to the inhaled antigens are found in the sera of 90% of patients with Farmer's lung, but since they are also found in some people with no disease and are absent from some sufferers, it seems that other factors are also involved, including Type IV hypersensitivity reactions.

Diseases in which immune complexes are important are summarized in Fig. 21.5. The sites of deposition of the complexes are partly determined by the localization of the antigen in the tissues and partly by how circulating complexes become deposited.

INFLAMMATORY MECHANISMS IN TYPE III HYPERSENSITIVITY

Immune complexes trigger a variety of inflammatory processes. They can interact with the complement system leading to the generation of C3a and C5a, which have anaphylatoxic and chemotactic properties. They also cause the release of vasoactive amines from mast cells and basophils, thus increasing vascular permeability and attracting polymorphs. Immune complexes can also interact with platelets through their Fc receptors leading to aggregation and microthrombus formation and hence a further increase in vascular permeability due to the release of vasoactive amines (Fig. 21.6).

The attracted polymorphs will attempt to phagocytose the complexes but in the case of tissue-trapped complexes this is difficult and the phagocytes are more likely to release their lysosomal enzymes to the exterior, causing tissue damage (Fig. 21.7). Simply released into the blood or tissue fluids these lysosomal enzymes are unlikely to cause much inflammation as they are rapidly neutralized by serum enzyme inhibitors, but if the phagocyte applies itself closely to the tissue-trapped complexes serum inhibitors are excluded and the enzymes then damage the underlying tissue.

EXPERIMENTAL MODELS OF IMMUNE COMPLEX DISEASE

Experimental models are available for each of the three main types of immune complex disease described above: serum sickness representing the presence of a persistent infection, the NZB/NZW mouse for autoimmunity and the Arthus reaction for local damage by extrinsic antigen. Care must be taken when interpreting animal experiments as rodents and lagomorphs (for

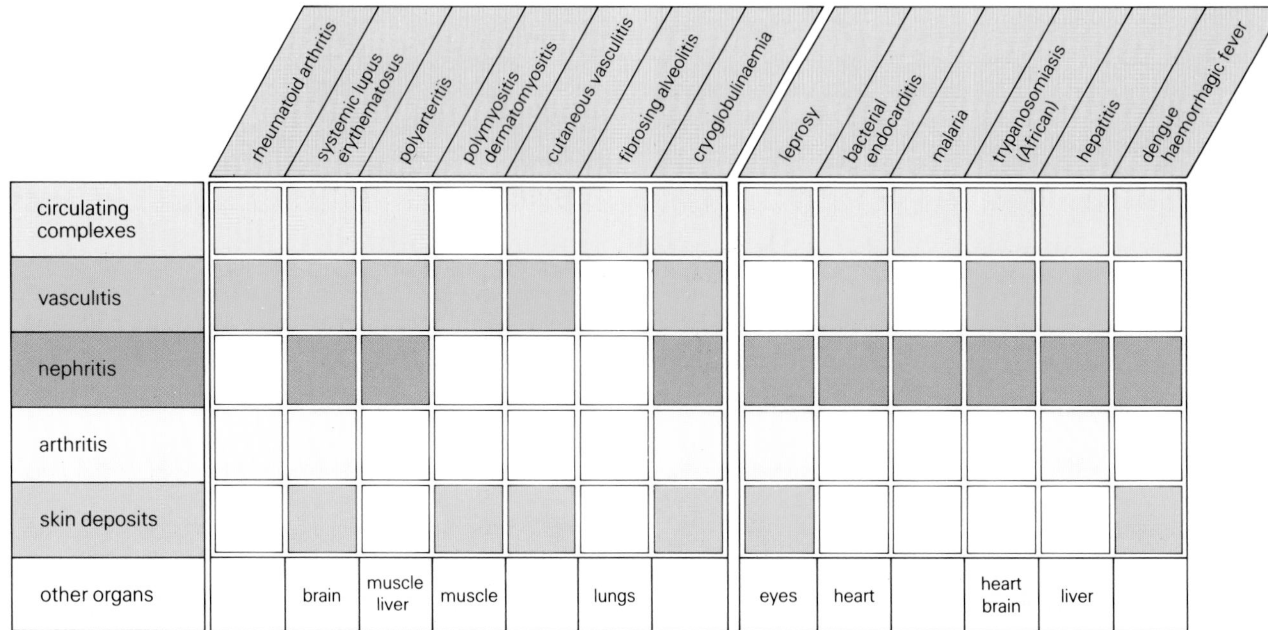

Fig. 21.5 Some of the main diseases in which immune complexes are implicated, indicating sites of deposition. Diseases on the left of the table are primarily autoimmune, those on the right are due to microbial antigens.

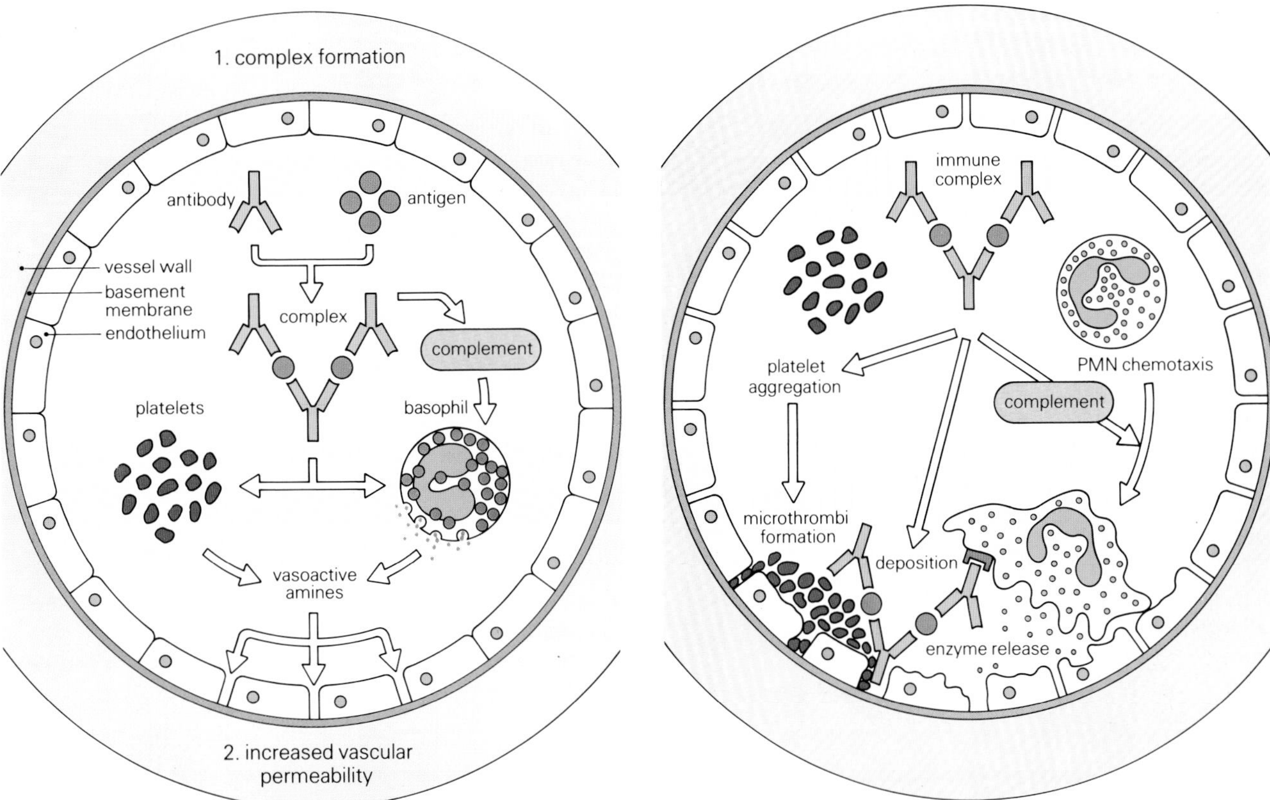

Fig. 21.6 Deposition of immune complexes in blood vessel walls – I. Antibody and antigen combine to form immune complexes (1). The complexes act on complement (to release C3a and C5a), which in turn acts on basophils to release vasoactive amines. The complexes also act directly on basophils and platelets (in humans) to produce vasoactive amine release. The amines released include histamine and 5-hydroxytryptamine, which cause endothelial cell retraction and thus increased vascular permeability (2).

Fig. 21.7 Deposition of immune complexes in blood vessel walls – II. With increased vascular permeability, immune complexes become deposited in the blood vessel wall. These complexes induce platelet aggregation and complement activation. The platelets aggregate to form microthrombi on the exposed collagen of the basement membrane of the endothelium. Polymorphs (PMNs) which are attracted to the site by chemotactic complement peptides cannot phagocytose the complexes and so release their lysosomal enzymes to the exterior of the cell, thus causing damage to the vessel wall.

example, rabbits) lack the receptor for complement fixing immune complexes (CR1) which is present on primate erythrocytes.

SERUM SICKNESS

In serum sickness circulating immune complexes deposit in the tissues when vascular permeability is increased, thus leading to inflammatory diseases such as glomerulonephritis and arthritis. In the pre-antibiotic era, serum sickness was a complication of serum therapy with massive doses of antibody for diseases such as diphtheria – horse anti-diphtheria serum was usually used and some individuals made antibodies against this foreign protein.

Serum sickness is now commonly studied in rabbits given an intravenous injection of a foreign soluble protein, such as bovine serum albumin. After about 1 week antibodies are formed which enter the circulation and complex with antigen in antigen excess (Fig. 21.8). These small complexes are only removed slowly by the mononuclear phagocyte system and persist in the circulation. With the formation of complexes there is an abrupt fall in total haemolytic complement and the clinical signs of serum sickness develop as granular deposits of antigen–antibody and C3 form along the glomerular basement membrane and in small vessels elsewhere. As the

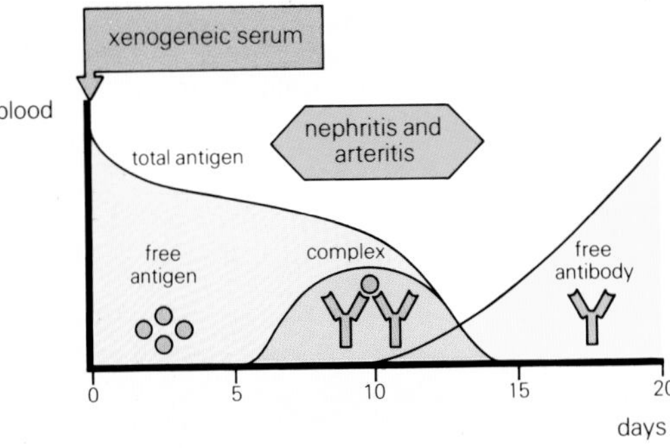

Fig. 21.8 Time course of experimental serum sickness. Following an injection of xenogeneic serum there is a lag period of approximately 5 days in which free antigen is detectable in serum. After this time, antibodies are produced to the foreign proteins and immune complexes are formed in serum, and it is during this period that the symptoms of nephritis and arteritis appear. As the antibody titres rise, the immune complexes are cleared and the syndrome resolves.

complexes are cleared the animals recover but the disease may be made chronic by the continued daily administration of antigen.

AUTOIMMUNE IMMUNE COMPLEX DISEASE

Autoimmune immune complex disease is demonstrated using the F1 hybrid NZB/NZW mouse which simulates various features of human SLE. These mice make a range of autoantibodies including anti-red cell, anti-nuclear, anti-DNA and anti-SM. The animals are born clinically normal but within 2–3 months show signs of haemolytic anaemia, and have positive Coombs' tests (for anti-red cell antibody), anti-nuclear antibodies, positive lupus cell tests and circulating immune complexes with deposits in the glomeruli and the choroid plexus.

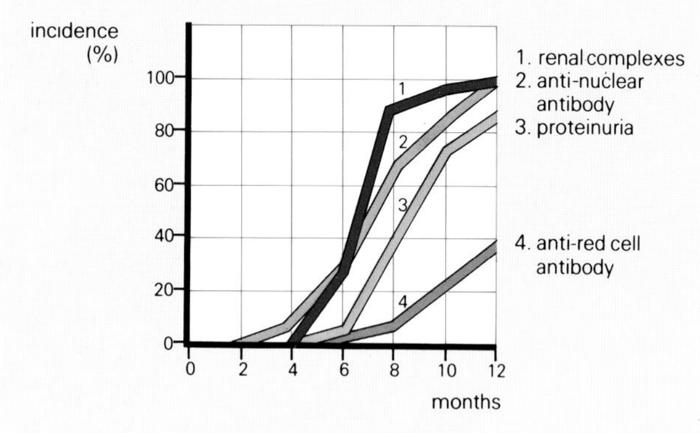

Fig. 21.9 Autoimmune disease in NZB/NZW mice. The graph shows the onset of autoimmune disease in female NZB/NZW mice with advancing age. Incidence refers to the percentage of mice with the features identified. Immune complexes were detected by immunofluorescent staining of kidney sections and anti-nuclear antibodies were detected in serum by indirect immunofluorescence. Proteinuria reflects kidney damage. Autoantibodies to red cells develop later in the disease and are therefore less likely to relate to kidney pathology. The onset of autoimmune disease is delayed in male mice by approximately 3 months.

The disease is much more marked in the females and these die within a few months of developing symptoms (Fig. 21.9).

THE ARTHUS REACTION

The Arthus reaction takes place at a local site in and around the walls of small blood vessels; it is most frequently demonstrated in the skin. Animals are immunized repeatedly until they have appreciable levels of precipitating, mainly IgG, antibody. On injecting antigen subcutaneously or intradermally a reaction develops which reaches peak intensity in 4–10 hours (Fig. 21.10). Depending on the amount of antigen injected, marked oedema and haemorrhage develop at the site of injection. The reaction then wanes and is usually markedly decreased by 48 hours.

Immunofluorescent studies have shown that initial deposition of antigen, antibody and complement in the vessel wall is followed by a polymorphonuclear neutrophil infiltration and intravascular clumping of platelets (Fig. 21.11) This platelet reaction can lead to vascular occlusion and necrosis in severe cases. After 24–48 hours the polymorphs are replaced by mononuclear cells and eventually some plasma cells appear.

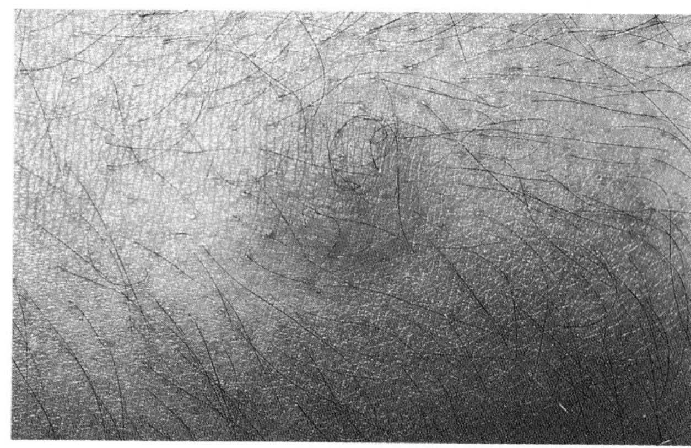

Fig. 21.10 The gross appearance of the Arthus reaction. The reaction is marked by a reddened area of inflammation which is maximal 5–6 hours after injection of antigen.

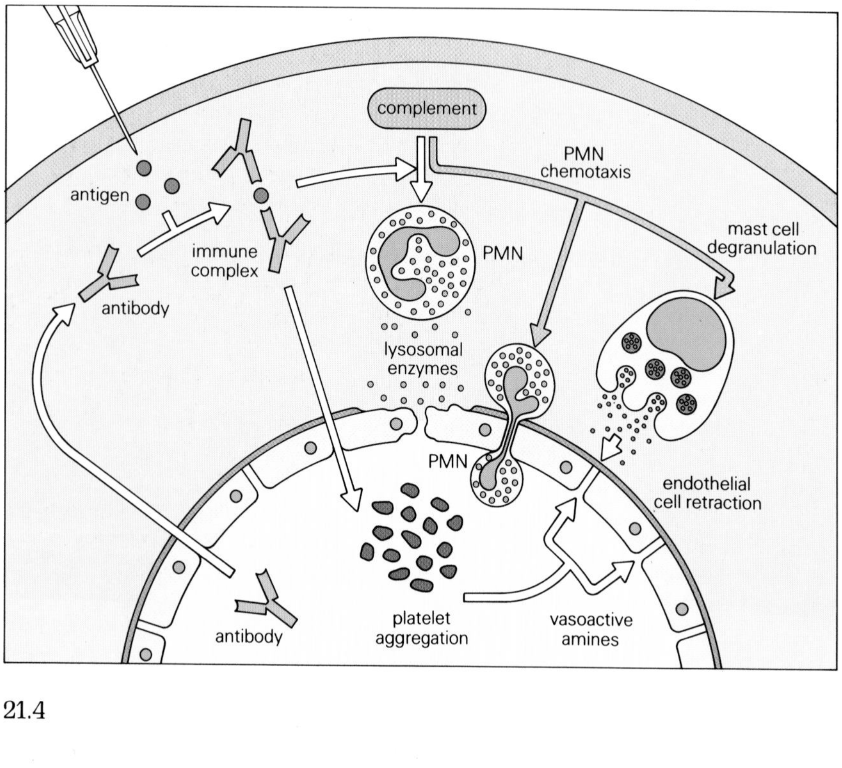

Fig. 21.11 The Arthus reaction. Antigen injected intradermally combines with specific antibody from the blood to form immune complexes. The complexes activate complement and act on platelets, which release vasoactive amines. Complement C3a and C5a fragments cause mast cell degranulation and polymorph chemotaxis into the tissues. Mast cell products, including histamine and leukotrienes, induce increased blood flow and capillary permeability. The inflammatory reaction is potentiated by lysosomal enzymes released from the polymorphs. Furthermore, C3b deposited on the complexes opsonizes them for phagocytes.

Complement activation via either the classical or alternative pathways is essential for the Arthus reaction to develop and only a mild oedema will occur in the absence of the polymorphs. The ratio of antibody to antigen is important for producing maximum reactivity. Generally, complexes formed in either antigen or antibody excess are much less toxic than those formed at equivalence.

WHY DO COMPLEXES PERSIST ?

Normally immune complexes are ultimately removed by the mononuclear phagocyte system, particularly in the liver, spleen and lungs. Some confusion has arisen owing to the separate immune complex removal system in primates in comparison with that in rodents and lagomorphs. Primate red cells have the CR1 receptor for C3b/C4b (see Chapter 13) whereas red cells in rodents and lagomorphs do not. The CR1 receptor readily binds immune complexes which have fixed complement. The complexes are then transported via the red cells to the liver, where they are removed by fixed tissue macrophages (Fig. 21.12). Complexes can also be released from red cells in the circulation by the action of Factor I. These complexes containing C3dg must then be removed by phagocytic cells bearing receptors for IgG Fc or C3d (Fig. 21.13).

The size of an immune complex is very important in regulating its clearance – in general, larger complexes are rapidly removed by the liver within a few minutes, while smaller complexes circulate for longer periods (Fig. 21.14). Larger complexes are more effective at fixing complement and thus bind better to red cells. Also larger complexes are released more slowly from the red cells by the action of Factor I. Factors which affect the size of complexes are therefore likely to influence clearance. It has been suggested that a genetic defect leading to the enhanced production of low affinity antibody could well lead to formation of smaller complexes, and so to immune complex disease. Generally when an individual forms antibodies to self-antigens, only a few epitopes

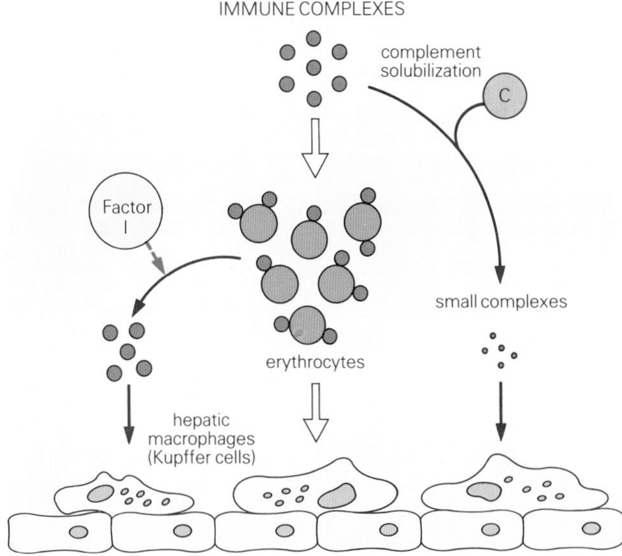

Fig. 21.13 Immune complex transport and removal. In man and primates, complexes may be taken up by the CR1 receptor on erythrocytes and transported to the liver where they are removed by hepatic macrophages. Complexes released from red cells by Factor I are taken up by Fc receptor and CR3 bearing cells. Complement solubilization of large complexes produces small soluble complexes which may be taken up directly by tissue macrophages.

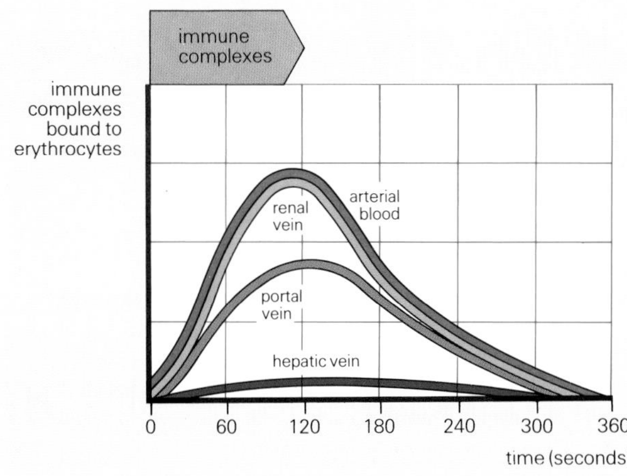

Fig. 21.12 Clearance of immune complexes in the liver. ^{125}I BSA/anti-BSA complexes were infused into a primate over a period of 120 seconds. Blood was sampled from renal, portal and hepatic veins, and the level of immune complexes bound to the red cells from each vessel was measured by counting radioactivity in the red cell fraction. The levels of complexes in the renal and portal veins were similar to that in arterial blood, but complexes were absent from hepatic venous blood, indicating that complexes bound to erythrocytes are removed during transit through the liver. (Based on data of Cornacoff and colleagues, 1983)

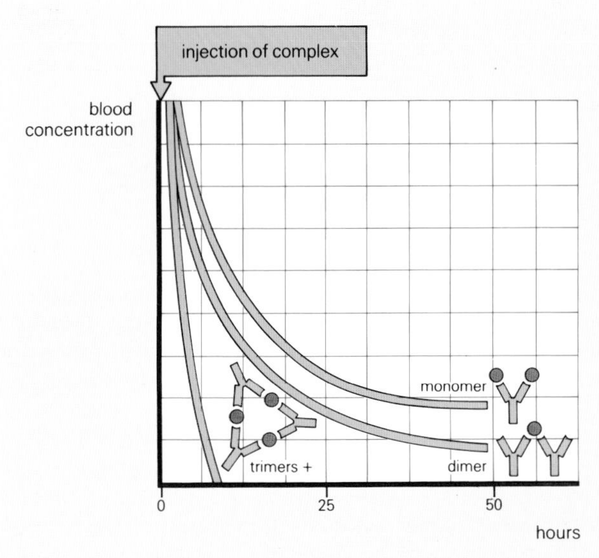

Fig. 21.14 Complex clearance by the reticuloendothelial system – I. Large immune complexes are cleared most quickly because they present an IgG–Fc lattice to reticuloendothelial cells with Fc receptors, permitting higher avidity binding to these cells. They also fix complement (C1q) better than small complexes.

are recognized and this favours the generation of small complexes since the formation of a cross-linked lattice is restricted. It is probable that many of these effects relating to size of complex are linked to the ability of complexes to fix complement. Interestingly, if complexes are infused into primates with a depleted complement system, they are removed from the circulation even more rapidly than in normal animals, but not to the usual sites for complex removal such as the liver. This obviously has relevance for patients with hypocomplementaemia. Striking differences have been observed in the clearance of complexes with different immunoglobulin classes. IgG complexes are bound by erythrocytes and are gradually removed from the circulation, whereas IgA complexes bind poorly to erythrocytes but are rapidly removed from the circulation, with increased deposition in the kidney, lung and brain.

When large amounts of complex are present the mononuclear phagocyte system may become overloaded. Certainly in experimental animals it is possible to block the mononuclear phagocyte system which then leads to prolonged circulation of immune complexes with some complex deposition in the glomerulus. There is evidence for a defective mononuclear phagocyte system in human immune complex disease but this may well be the result of overload rather than a primary defect.

Recently the carbohydrate groups on immunoglobulin molecules have been shown to be important for removal of immune complexes by phagocytic cells and there may be abnormalities of the immunoglobulin carbohydrates in certain immune complex diseases, particularly in rheumatoid arthritis and SLE. It is not certain, however, whether the abnormalities of carbohydrate are primary or are themselves caused by the disease.

Although immune complexes may persist in the circulation for prolonged periods, simple persistence is not usually harmful in itself; problems start to occur when they deposit in the tissues.

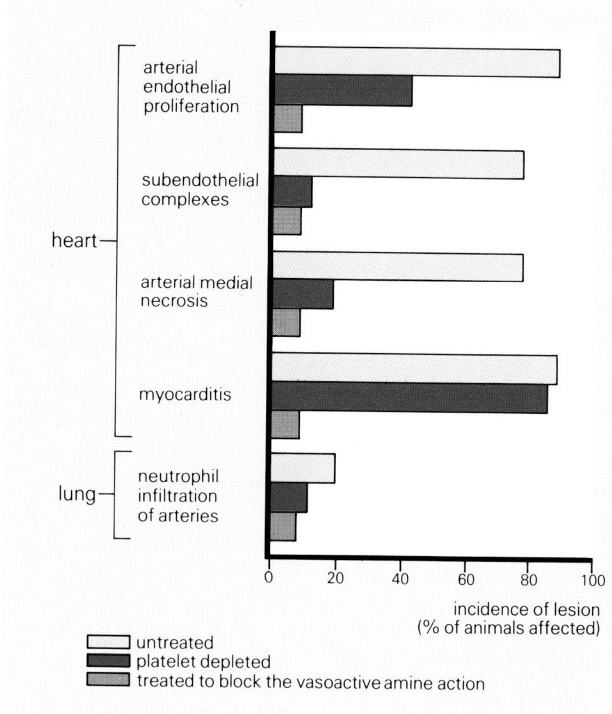

Fig. 21.15 Effect of vasoactive amine antagonists on immune complex disease. Serum sickness was induced in rabbits with a single injection of bovine serum albumin. The animals were either untreated (pink), platelet depleted (red) or treated with drugs to block vasoactive amine action (purple). The incidence of serum sickness lesions in the heart and lung was scored. Drug treatment considerably reduced the signs of disease by minimizing complex deposition.

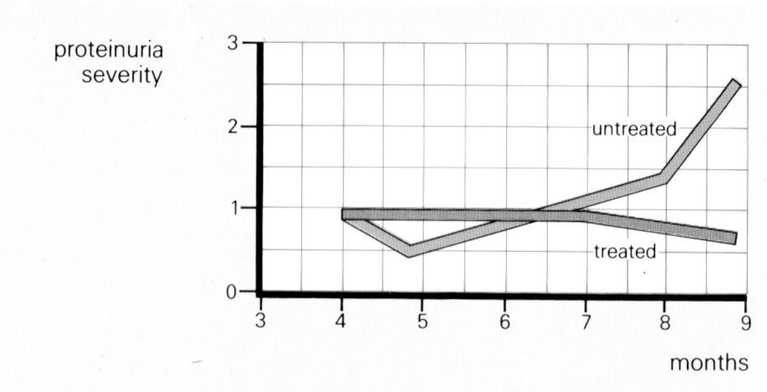

Fig. 21.16 Effect of the vasoactive amine antagonist methysergide on kidney damage. Kidney damage, assessed by proteinuria, was measured in NZB/NZW mice over a period of months. Untreated animals developed severe proteinuria, while methysergide-treated animals did not. Methysergide blocks formation of the vasoactive amine, 5-HT, and thus platelets are depleted of this.

WHY DO COMPLEXES DEPOSIT IN TISSUES?

Two questions are relevant to tissue deposition:

1. why do complexes deposit?
2. why do complexes show affinity for particular tissues in different diseases?

INCREASE IN VASCULAR PERMEABILITY

The most important trigger for tissue deposition of immune complexes is probably an increase in vascular permeability. This can be initiated by a range of mechanisms which may vary in importance in various diseases and in different species. This makes interpretation of some of the animal models difficult. Complement, mast cells, basophils and platelets must all be considered as potential contributors to the release of vasoactive amines. Inert substances, for example colloidal carbon, can be made to deposit in vessel walls if animals are given vasoactive substances such as histamine or serotonin. Similarly, circulating immune complexes may be caused to deposit by the infusion of agents which cause liberation of mast cell vasoactive amines. Pretreatment with antihistamines blocks this effect. In studies of experimental immune complex disease, long-term administration of vasoactive amine antagonists, such as chlorpheniramine or methysergide, considerably reduced complex deposition (Fig. 21.15). More importantly, young NZB/NZW mice treated with methysergide showed less renal pathology than controls (Fig. 21.16).

HAEMODYNAMIC PROCESSES

Immune complex deposition is most likely where there is high blood pressure and turbulence (Fig. 21.17). In the glomerular capillaries the blood pressure is approximately four times that of most other capillaries – many

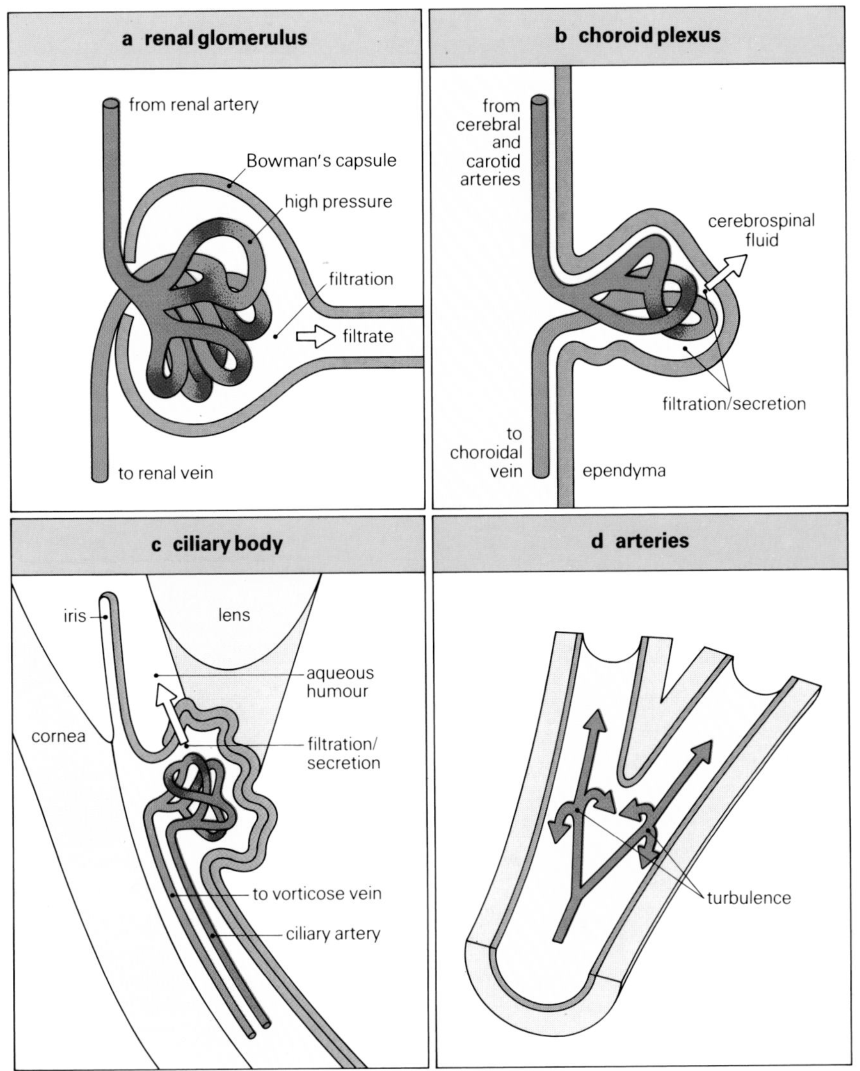

Fig. 21.17 Haemodynamic factors affecting complex deposition. Factors include filtration, which occurs in the formation of the glomerular ultrafiltrate (a), the formation of the cerebrospinal fluid by the choroid plexus, which lies along the ventricles of the brain (b), and in the formation of the aqueous humour by the epithelium of the ciliary body in the eye (c). High pressure in the renal glomerulus also favours deposition as does turbulence such as occurs at curves or bifurcations of arteries (d).

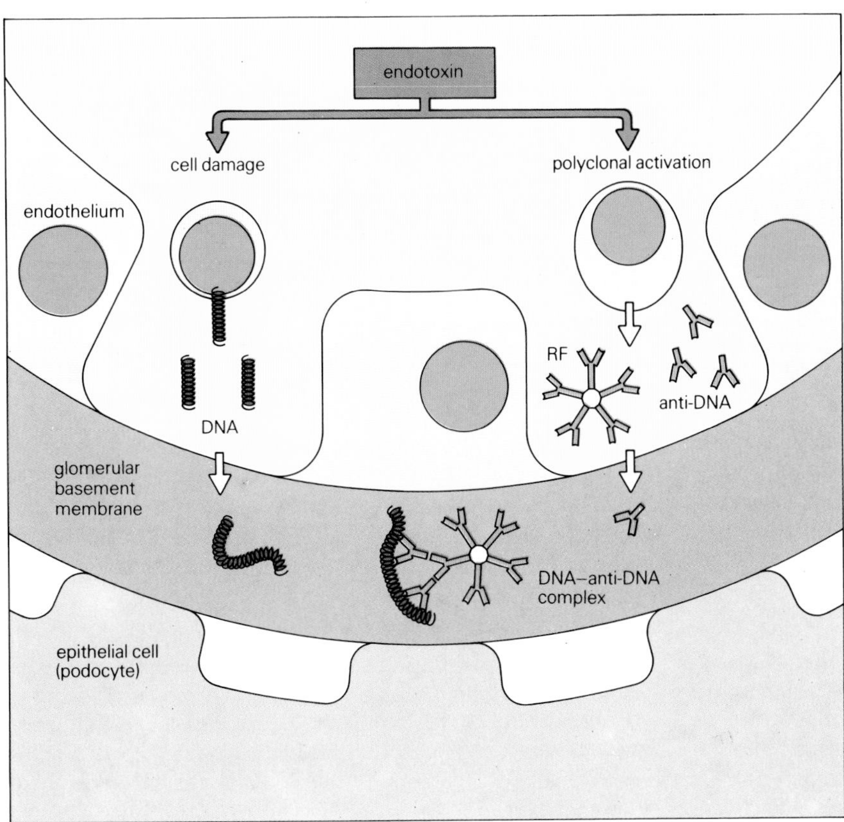

Fig. 21.18 A model for the formation and deposition of immune complexes in the kidney. Endotoxin induces cell damage with release of DNA which becomes deposited on the collagen of the glomerular basement membrane. Endotoxin also induces a polyclonal stimulation of B cells, some of which produce anti-DNA antibodies and auto-anti-IgG antibodies – these are termed rheumatoid factors (RFs). Anti-DNA binds to the deposited DNA, and RFs which have low affinity for monomeric IgG, bind to the assembled DNA–anti-DNA complex. Thus immune complex formation occurs *in situ*.

macromolecules favour a glomerular localization. If the pressure is reduced by partially constricting the renal artery, or ligating the ureter, deposition is reduced; experimentally induced hypertension enhances the development of the symptoms of acute serum sickness in the rabbit. Similarly at other sites, such as the walls of arteries, the most severe lesions occur at sites of turbulence, such as vessel bifurcations, or in filters such as the choroid plexus or the ciliary body of the eye.

ANTIGEN TISSUE BINDING

Although local high blood pressure explains a general tendency for certain organs to be particular sites for complex deposition, it does not explain why complexes home in on different organs in different diseases. For example, in SLE the kidney is a particular target whereas in rheumatoid arthritis, although circulating complexes are present, the kidney is usually spared and the joints are the principal target. It is possible that the antigen in the complex provides the organ specificity. It has been shown that DNA has a strong affinity for collagen in the basement membrane of the glomerulus and this could lead to the deposition of DNA–anti-DNA complexes in the kidney in SLE where anti-DNA antibodies are such a marked feature. A convincing model has been established where mice are given endotoxin, causing cell damage and release of DNA, which binds to the glomerular basement membrane. Anti-DNA is then produced by polyclonal activation of B cells and is bound by fixed DNA leading to local immune complex formation (Fig. 21.18). It is possible that in other diseases further antigens will be identified with affinity for other organs.

The charge of the antigen and antibody may be important in some systems; for example, positively charged (cationic) antigens and antibodies are more likely to deposit in the negatively charged basement membrane. In certain diseases the antibodies and antigens are both produced within the target organ. The extreme of this is reached in rheumatoid arthritis where the anti-human IgG is produced by plasma cells within the synovium; the antibodies combine with each other and self-associate so setting up an inflammatory reaction.

SIZE OF IMMUNE COMPLEXES

The exact localization of immune complexes is partly dependent on the size of the complex. This is exemplified in the kidney where small immune complexes are able to pass through the glomerular basement membrane so ending up on the epithelial side of the membrane, while large complexes are unable to cross the membrane and largely accumulate between the endothelium and the basement membrane or in the mesangium (Fig. 21.19). The size of immune complexes depends on the valency of the antigen, and the titre and affinity of the antibody.

IMMUNOGLOBULIN CLASS

The class of immunoglobulin in an immune complex can influence its deposition. With anti-DNA antibodies in SLE, there are marked age and sex-related variations in the class and subclass distribution. As the NZB/NZW mice age there is a class switch of these antibodies from predominantly IgM to IgG2a. This occurs earlier in

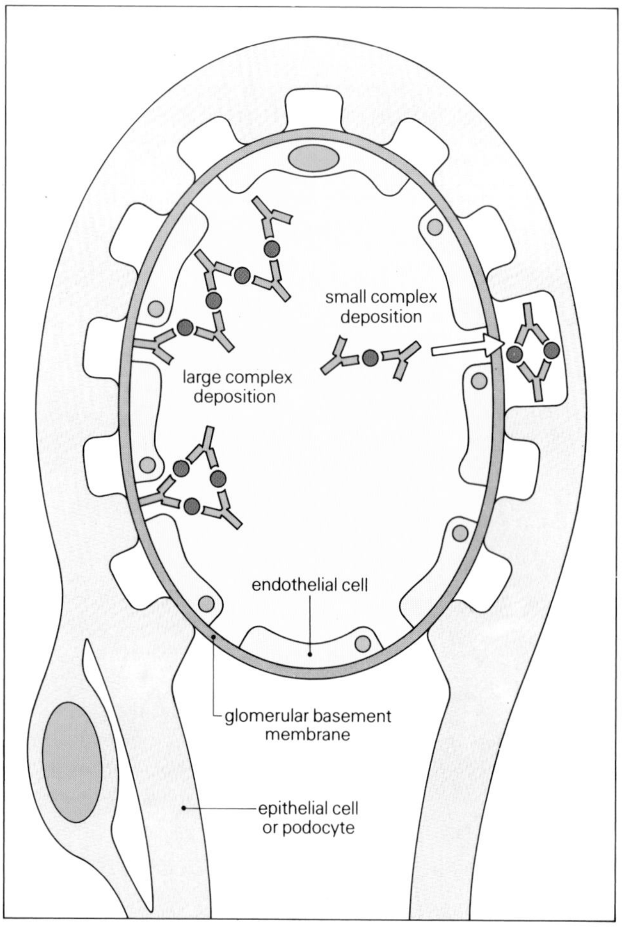

Fig. 21.19 The site of complex deposition in the kidney is dependent on the size of the complexes in the circulation. Large complexes become deposited on the glomerular basement membrane, while small complexes pass through the basement membrane and are seen on the epithelial side of the glomerulus.

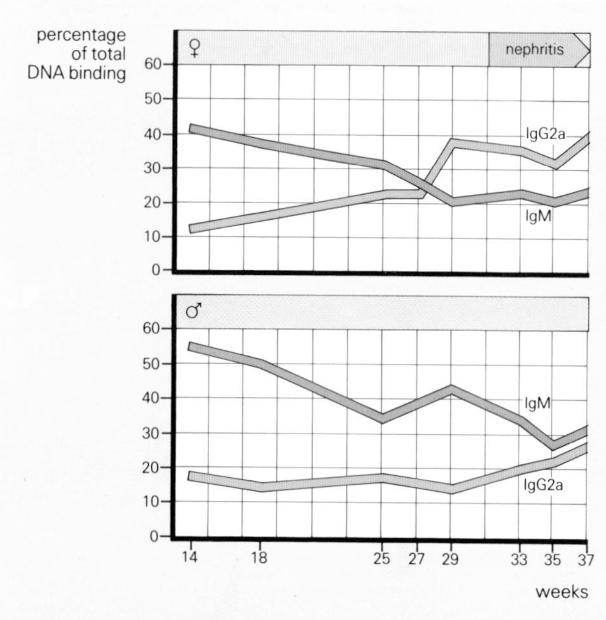

Fig. 21.20 Antibody classes in immune complex disease. Immune complex disease in the NZB/NZW mouse follows a class switch from IgM to IgG2a. The graphs show the titres of anti-DNA antibodies (IgM and IgG2a) in females (upper graph) and males (lower graph). The class switch and fatal renal disease occurs earlier in the female mice of this strain.

females than in males and coincides with the onset of renal disease preceding the time at which death occurs by 2–3 months, indicating the importance of antibody class in the tissue deposition of complexes (Fig. 21.20).

COMPLEMENT SOLUBILIZATION OF IMMUNE COMPLEXES

Once complexes have deposited in the tissues, a mechanism exists for making them soluble again; this mechanism is complement.

Complement can rapidly resolubilize precipitated complexes (Fig. 21.21). The solubilization appears to occur by the insertion of complement C3b and C3d fragments into the complex. It may be that complexes are continually being deposited in normal individuals, but are removed by solubilization. If this is the case, the process would be inadequate in hypocomplementaemic patients and lead to prolonged complex deposition. Solubilization defects have been observed in sera from patients with systemic immune complex disease, but whether the defect is primary or secondary is not known.

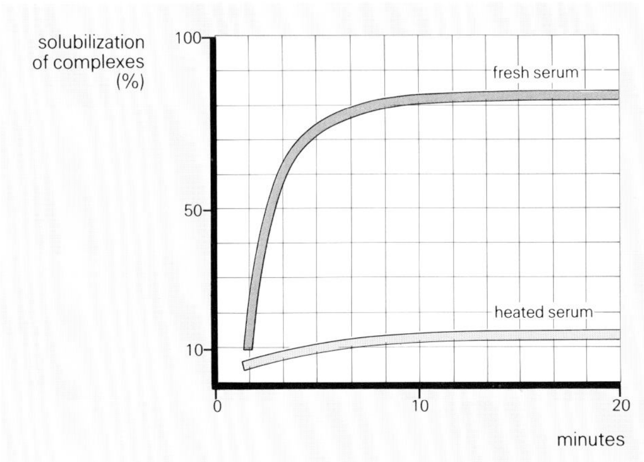

Fig. 21.21 Solubilization of immune complexes by complement. Complement can solubilize precipitable complexes *in vitro*. Addition of fresh serum containing active complement to insoluble complexes induces solubilization over about 15 minutes at 37°C. Some of the complexes resist resolubilization. Heated serum (56° for 30 minutes) lacks active complement and cannot resolubilize the complexes. It appears that intercalation of complement components C3b and C3d into the complex causes their solubilization.

DETECTION OF IMMUNE COMPLEXES

There are many techniques for detecting and quantitating immune complexes. The ideal place to look for the complexes is in the affected organ. Tissue samples may be examined by immunofluorescence for the presence of immunoglobulin and complement. The composition, pattern and particular area of tissue affected all provide useful information on the severity and prognosis of the disease. For example, the poor prognosis of the patient with continuous, granular, sub-epithelial deposits of IgG found in membranous glomerulonephritis can be contrasted with the relatively good prognosis of patients in whom the complexes are localized in the mesangium. Not all tissue-bound complexes give rise to an inflammatory response; for example in SLE, complexes are frequently found in skin biopsies from unaffected, as well as inflamed areas. Complexes may also be found in the circulation where they may be detected physically as high molecular weight immunoglobulin.

Circulating complexes are found in two separate compartments: bound to erythrocytes and free in plasma. Erythrocyte-bound complexes are potentially less pathogenic and therefore it is of more interest to determine the level of free complexes. For this reason care is required when collecting the sample as red cell-bound complexes may be easily released during clotting by the action of Factor I. It may be better to rapidly separate the red cells from the plasma to prevent complex release.

Precipitation of the immune complex with polyethylene glycol and estimation of the precipitated IgG is frequently used to identify high molecular weight IgG and forms the basis for one of the commercial assays (Fig. 21.22). Circulating complexes are often identified

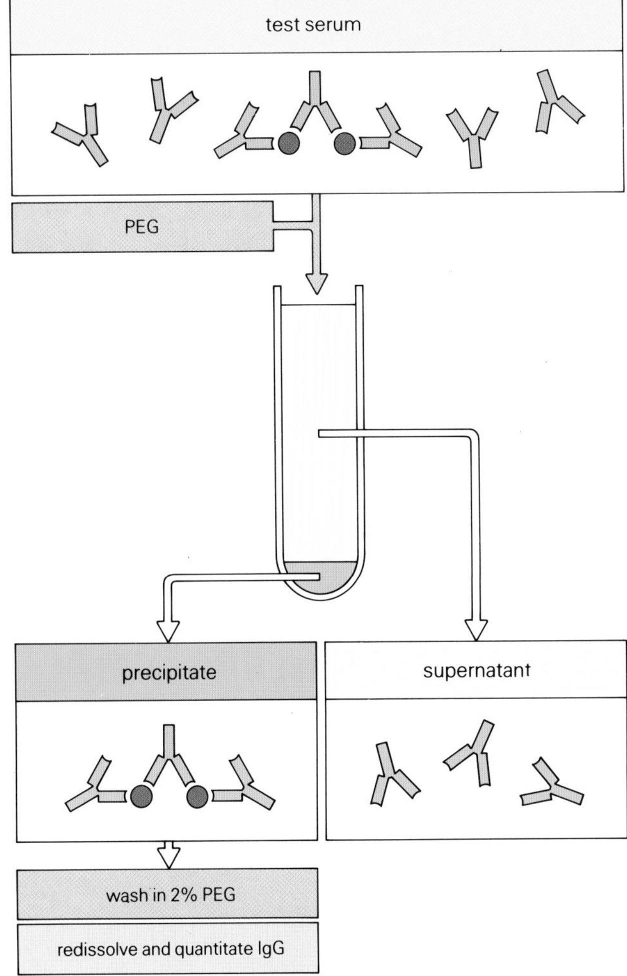

Fig. 21.22 An assay for immune complexes based on polyethylene glycol (PEG). PEG is added to the test serum containing complexes of IgG and IgG monomer, to produce a final concentration of 2% PEG. At 2% PEG, complexes are selectively precipitated and the supernatant contains free antibody. After washing, the precipitate is redissolved and complexed IgG can be quantitated (e.g. by single radial immunodiffusion, nephelometry, or radioimmunoassay).

by their affinity for complement, C1q, using either radiolabelled C1q or C1q linked to a solid support (solid phase C1q) (Fig. 21.23). Other receptors may be used such as the C3 receptor on RAJI (a B-cell tumour) cells or the Fc receptor on platelets. Even more care than that exercised over the interpretation of tissue complexes must be given to the evaluation of the importance of circulating complexes since many circulating complexes will not in themselves be harmful unless they deposit in the tissue.

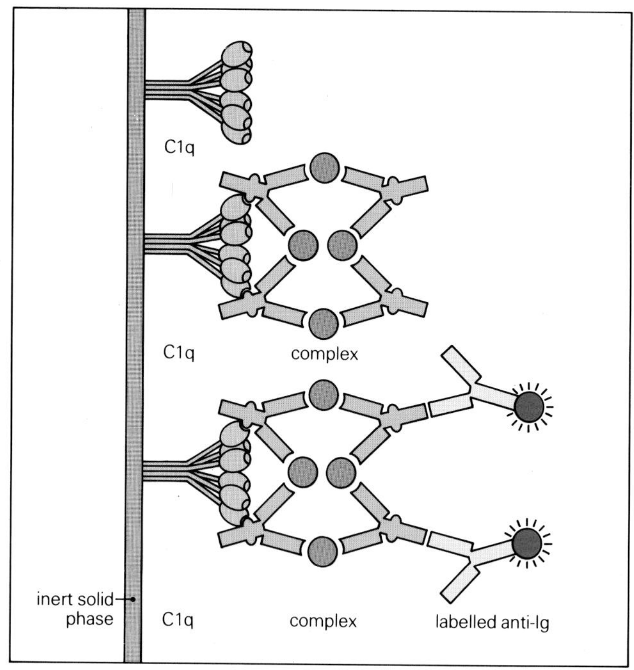

Fig. 21.23 A three layer radioimmunoassay for immune complexes based on the use of C1q.
1. C1q is linked to an inert solid phase support, usually a polystyrene tube or plate.
2. Serum containing complexes is added and the complexes bind to the solid phase C1q via the array of Fc regions presented to the C1q.
3. The amount of complex bound to the C1q is detected using a radiolabelled antibody to IgG and the radioactivity measured in a gamma counter.

FURTHER READING

Agnello, V. (1983) Immune complex assays in rheumatic diseases. *Human Pathology*, **14**, 343.

Arthus, M. (1903) Injections repete de serum de cheval chez le lapin. *Comptes Rendus des Seances de la Societé de Biologie et de ses Filiales*, **55**, 817.

Cornacoff, J.B., Hobart, L.A., Smead, W.L., Vanaman, M.E., Birmingham, D.J. & Waxman F.J. (1983) Primate erythrocyte immune complex clearing mechanism. *Journal of Clinical Investigation*, **71**, 236.

Czop, J. & Nussenweig, V. (1976) Studies on the mechanism of solubilisation of immune precipitates by serum. *Journal of Experimental Medicine*, **143**, 615.

Dixon, F.J., Feldman, J.D. & Vazquez, J.J. (1961) Experimental glomerulonephritis: the pathogenesis of a laboratory model resembling the spectrum of human glomerulonephritis. *Journal of Experimental Medicine*, **113**, 899.

Dixon, F.J., Vazquez, J.J., Weigle, W.O. & Cochrane, C.G. (1958) Pathogenesis of serum sickness. *Archives of Pathology*, **65**, 18.

Inman, R.D. (1982) Immune complexes in SLE. *Clin. Res. Dis.*, **8**, 49.

Kjilstra, H., Van Es, L.A. & Daha, M.R. (1979) The role of complement in the binding and degradation of immunoglobulin aggregates by macrophages. *Journal of Immunology*, **123**, 2488.

Sedlacek, H.H. & Seiler, F.R. (eds) (1979) Immune complexes. *Behring Institute Mitteilungen*, **64**.

Schifferli, J.A., Ng, Y.C. & Peters, D.K. (1986) The role of complement and its receptor in the elimination of immune complexes. *New England Journal of Medicine*, **315**, 488.

Takata, Y., Tamura, N. & Fujita, T. (1984) Interaction of C3 with antigen–antibody complexes in the process of solubilisation of immune precipitates. *Journal of Immunology*, **132**, 2531.

Theofilopoulos, A.N. & Dixon, F.J. (1979) The biology and detection of immune complexes. *Advances in Immunology*, **28**, 89.

Whaley, K. (1987) Complement and immune complex diseases. In *Complement in Health and Disease*. Edited by K. Whaley. Lancaster: MTP Press Ltd.

Williams, R.C. (1980) *Immune Complexes in Clinical and Experimental Medicine*. Massachusetts: Harvard University Press.

World Health Organisation Scientific Group. (1977) *Technical Report 606. The Role of Immune Complexes in Disease*. Geneva: WHO.

22 Hypersensitivity–Type IV

In the classification of hypersensitivity suggested by Coombs and Gell in 1963, delayed hypersensitivity (cell-mediated hypersensitivity or Type IV) was used as a general category to describe all those hypersensitivity reactions which took more than 12 hours to develop. At that time the mechanisms underlying the phenomena were not known, and they are still not well understood. It has become evident, however, that several different types of immune reaction can produce delayed hypersensitivity.

Unlike other forms of hypersensitivity it cannot be transferred from one animal to another by serum, but can be transferred by T lymphocytes bearing a variety of surface phenotypes, for example, in the mouse, L3T4 (CD4). It is obviously associated with T cell protective immunity but does not necessarily run parallel with it. The T cells necessary for producing the delayed response, T delayed hypersensitivity or TD cells, are cells which have become sensitized to the particular antigen by a previous encounter. But although sensitized T cells are instrumental in producing delayed hypersensitivity reactions, they frequently act by recruiting other cell types to the site of the reaction.

delayed reaction	maximal reaction time
Jones-Mote	24 hours
contact	48–72 hours
tuberculin	48–72 hours
granulomatous	at least 14 days

Fig. 22.1 The four types of delayed hypersensitivity. The Jones–Mote response is maximal at 24 hours. Contact and tuberculin-type hypersensitivities, which have a similar time course, are maximal at 48–72 hours. In certain circumstances, tuberculin-type reactions may develop at 21–28 days into a granulomatous hypersensitivity reaction which may continue for several weeks (e.g. skin testing in leprosy).

REACTIONS OF DELAYED HYPERSENSITIVITY

Four types of delayed hypersensitivity reaction are recognized and of these the first three, the Jones–Mote reaction, contact hypersensitivity and tuberculin-type hypersensitivity, all occur within 72 hours of antigen challenge. By contrast, the fourth type, granulomatous reactions, develop over a period of weeks. The position is complicated because these different types of reaction may overlap to some extent, or occur sequentially following a single antigenic challenge; therefore many of the hypersensitivity reactions seen in practice do not correspond to one category alone.

The four different types of delayed hypersensitivity were originally distinguished according to the reaction they produced when antigen was applied directly to the skin or injected intradermally. The degree of the reaction is assessed in animals by measuring thickening of the skin, which occurs at the site of antigen application and is accompanied by a variety of immune reactions.

The first type of reaction to appear is the Jones–Mote, which is maximal at 24 hours. Contact and tuberculin-type hypersensitivities both peak at 48–72 hours after antigen challenge. These may be followed by an even more delayed response, characterized histologically by the aggregation and proliferation of macrophages which form granulomas which may persist for weeks. The granulomatous hypersensitivity reaction is, in terms of its clinical consequences, by far the most serious type of delayed response.

The four types of reaction and times taken to produce maximal skin swelling, are listed in Fig. 22.1. In addition to the difference in timing and degree of skin swelling, the four types of delayed hypersensitivity are characterized in other ways which will now be described.

JONES–MOTE HYPERSENSITIVITY

Jones–Mote hypersensitivity is characterized by infiltration of the area immediately under the epidermis by basophils, and is frequently called cutaneous basophil hypersensitivity when induced in experimental animals such as the guinea-pig. It is induced by soluble antigen, is maximal seven to ten days after induction and tends to disappear when antibody appears. The skin swelling is maximal 24 hours after antigen challenge. A reaction with a similar time course may be induced in the guinea-pig by an intradermal injection of the antigen ovalbumin in Freund's Incomplete Adjuvant (FIA), a mild antigenic stimulus. If, however, a powerful antigenic stimulus is applied by injecting ovalbumin with Freund's Complete Adjuvant (adjuvant containing tubercle bacilli), a tuberculin-type response is seen. In the Jones–Mote reaction, studies of the cellular infiltrate reveal numerous basophils, but less basophils may be seen in guinea-pig tuberculin reactions. Interestingly, if ovalbumin in FIA is combined with cyclophosphamide before treatment, a skin response with a longer time course is seen which superficially resembles the tuberculin response but may not be identical.

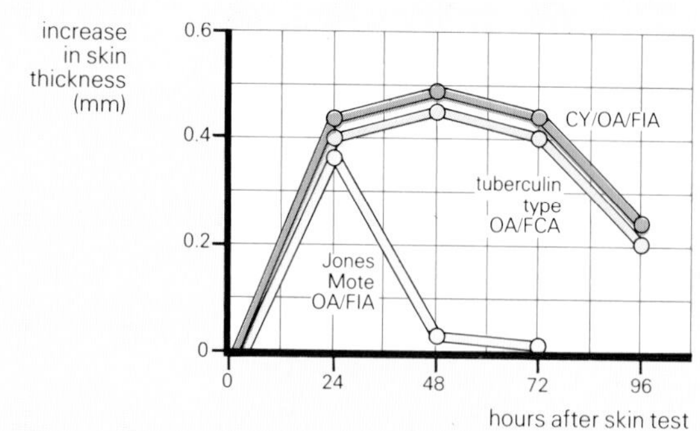

Fig. 22.2 The induction of Jones–Mote and tuberculin-type reactions in the guinea-pig using ovalbumin and Freund's Adjuvant. This graph plots the skin swelling induced when guinea-pigs are injected with different combinations of ovalbumin (OA), Freund's Adjuvant and cyclophosphamide. Intradermal injection of OA with Freund's Incomplete Adjuvant (FIA) induces skin swelling which is maximal at 24 hours; this is the Jones–Mote response. If OA and Freund's Complete Adjuvant (FCA) are injected, a swelling is induced, which is maximal at 48 hours – the tuberculin-type response (which may also show a basophil leucocyte infiltration). When the animal is pretreated with cyclophosphamide (CY) before injection of OA and FIA, a reaction is obtained which has a similar time course to the tuberculin-type reaction. However, B cells from Jones–Mote animals are able to suppress the skin response of Jones–Mote animals treated with CY but not those of animals immunized with FCA. This provides some evidence to suggest that the tuberculin-type response and the skin test of Jones–Mote animals treated with CY, although of similar time course, have different immunological effector mechanisms.

It is concluded that the Jones–Mote response is strongly regulated by cyclophosphamide-sensitive lymphocytes (suppressor lymphocytes; Fig. 22.2).

CONTACT HYPERSENSITIVITY

Contact hypersensitivity, characterized clinically by eczema (dermatitis) at the site of contact with the allergen, is usually maximal at 48 hours both in sensitized humans and experimental animals. In Europe the most common antigens are haptens, such as nickel, chromate, and chemicals found in rubber (Fig. 22.3); in the USA poison ivy and poison oak are the most important antigens. Contact dermatitis, although often irritant and not allergic, is a major cause of occupational disease.

The small haptens which induce contact hypersensitivity would not by themselves be antigenic; however, these low molecular weight compounds penetrate the epidermis and become conjugated, either covalently or non-covalently, to normal body proteins. Knowledge of the chemical configuration of a compound will not predict whether it will become allergenic, although certain contact allergens have unsaturated carbon bonds and are easily oxidized. Some haptens, for example, dinitrochlorobenzene (DNCB), will sensitize nearly all individuals. About 85% of epicutaneously applied DNCB binds to the epidermal cell proteins, by their lysine–NH_2 residues, and the conjugates thus formed serve to sensitize the animal. T cell recognition of the conjugate is specific for the hapten/carrier conjugate and is not dependent on the separate recognition of hapten and carrier, which occurs in antibody formation.

Contact hypersensitivity is mainly an epidermal phenomenon, as distinct from tuberculin-type hypersensitivity, which is predominantly dermal in nature. The principal antigen-presenting cell for contact sensitization is the Langerhans' cell (Fig. 22.4).

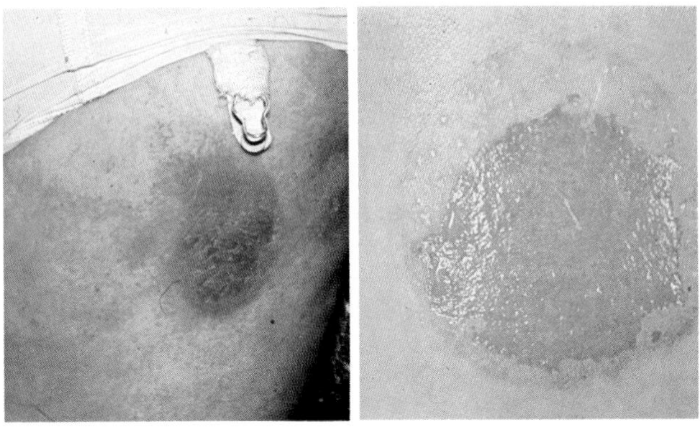

Fig. 22.3 Clinical and patch test appearances of contact hypersensitivity. The eczematous area is due to sensitivity to the rubber component of this individual's undergarment (left). The suspected allergen may be confirmed by applying it, in a weak, non-irritant concentration to a patch of skin (patch test). An eczematous reaction (right) induced between 48 and 72 hours, confirms the allergen.

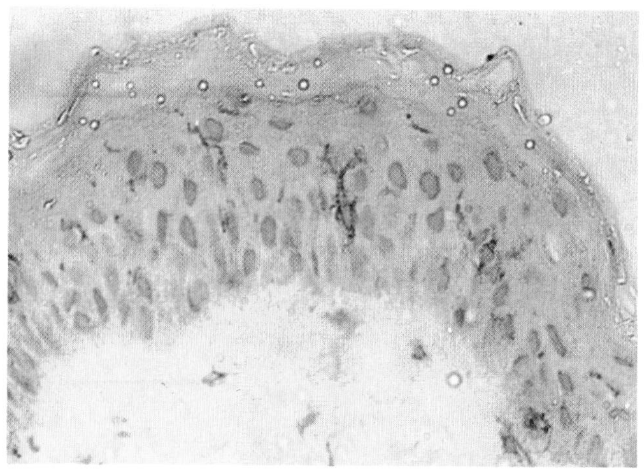

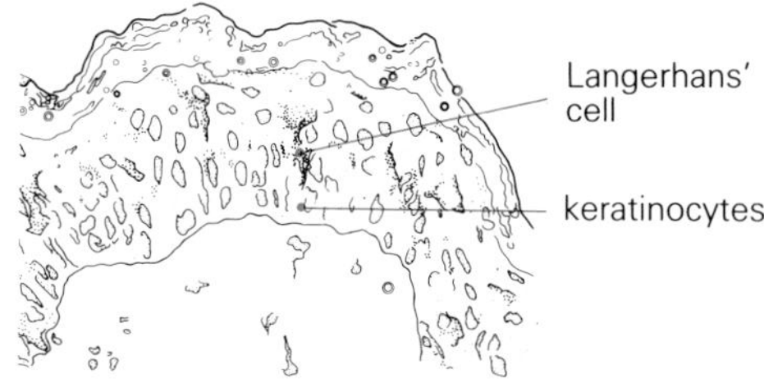

Fig. 22.4 Langerhans' cells seen in a skin section. These dendritic cells constitute 3% of all the cells in the epidermis. They express a variety of surface markers which allow them to be visualized. Here they have been revealed using a monoclonal antibody which reacts with the CD1 antigen (counterstained with Mayer's haemalum). ×312.

Langerhans' cells are dendritic and are located in the suprabasal epidermis. They are derived from the bone marrow and express the cortical thymocyte antigen CD1 and MHC class II antigens. These cells also have surface receptors for Fc and complement. Electron microscopy identifies an organelle, the Birbeck granule, which is specific for Langerhans' cells (Fig. 22.5). The Birbeck granule is endocytotic but its function is unknown.

Direct evidence for the participation of Langerhans' cells in contact hypersensitivity includes the finding of Langerhans'-like cells (veiled cells) in the efferent lymph after the epicutaneous application of dinitrofluorobenzene (DNFB) in pigs sensitive to DNFB and the *in vitro* observation that Langerhans' cells can act as antigen-presenting cells in lieu of macrophages. Langerhans' cells are found in the paracortical areas of lymph nodes as early as 4 hours after DNCB challenge in mice.

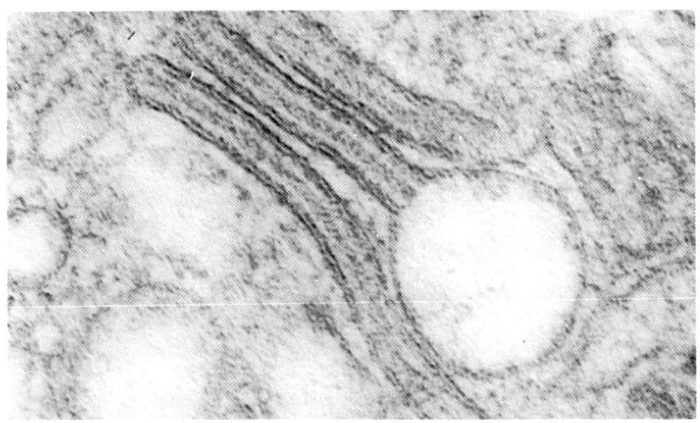

Fig. 22.5 Langerhans' cell under electron microscopy showing the characteristic 'Birbeck granule'. This organelle is a plate-like structure with a distinct central striation and often has a bleb-like extension at one end. ×132,000.

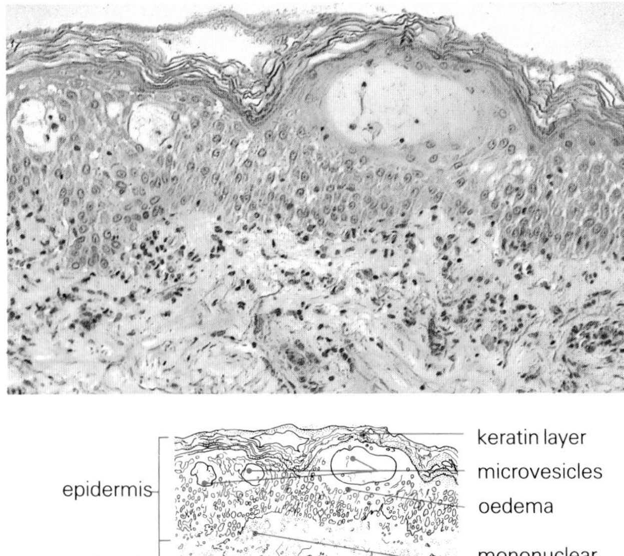

Fig. 22.6 Histological appearance of the lesion in contact hypersensitivity. There is infiltration of the epidermis (which is pushed outwards) by mononuclear cells, and microvesicle formation with oedema of the epidermis. The dermis is infiltrated by mononuclear cells. H&E stain, ×130.

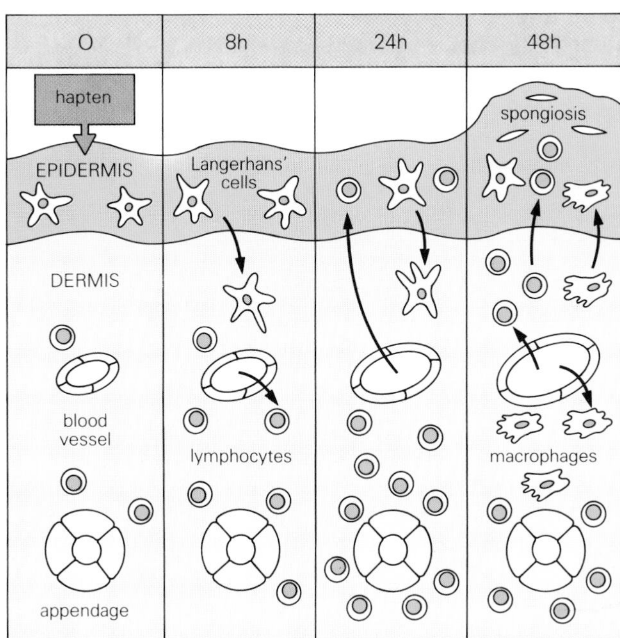

Fig. 22.7 Contact hypersensitivity. This diagram illustrates cellular movements in the elicitation phase of contact hypersensitivity, following epicutaneous application of a hapten. By 8 hours, Langerhans' cells have begun to migrate from the epidermis and there is lymphocyte emigration from blood vessels. At 24 hours, lymphocytes have entered the epidermis and started to accumulate around appendages. By 48 hours, macrophages are present in all areas, including the epidermis. Appendage cells and keratinocytes of the epidermis now express MHC class II molecules and disruption of the epidermis (spongiosis) occurs.

The earliest histological change in the challenge reaction of contact hypersensitivity is observed after 3–4 hours, when a mononuclear cell infiltrate is noted around the appendages or blood vessels. By 8 hours, mononuclear cells have begun to infiltrate the epidermis. The epidermal and dermal infiltrates increase, reaching a maximum at 48–72 hours, by which time the epidermis has become oedematous (Fig. 22.6).

Immunophenotyping shows that the majority of infiltrating mononuclear cells are $CD4^+$ and are presumed to be T_D cells. Lesser numbers of $CD8^+$ (T suppressor/cytotoxic) cells are seen in the infiltrate. The number of Langerhans' cells in the epidermis is increased at 24 and 48 hours in the contact hypersensitivity reaction, and Langerhans'-like cells are found in the dermal infiltrate. Macrophages invade the dermis and epidermis by 48 hours. Basophils have been observed, as early as 8 hours, in some reactions. Antigen-conjugated epidermal cells may be destroyed by hapten-specific T cytotoxic cells: epidermal Langerhans' cells show ultrastructural signs of damage early in the contact hypersensitivity reaction, but there is little corroborative evidence that they act as 'target' cells. Fig. 22.7 shows the time course of events after epicutaneous challenge.

Keratinocytes do not normally express surface MHC class II antigens but in the contact hypersensitivity reaction such expression may occur. At 48 hours after challenge, keratinocytes usually express HLA–DR but can give positive reactions for HLA–DP and HLA–DQ as well.

Infiltrating lymphocytes and macrophages are often DR-positive (and occasionally express HLA–DP or HLA–DQ). Their presence may induce class II antigen expression by keratinocytes. The functional significance of class II gene product synthesis by keratinocytes is unknown, though it may contribute to the induction and perpetuation of the immune response.

TUBERCULIN-TYPE HYPERSENSITIVITY

This form of hypersensitivity was originally described by Koch, who observed that patients with tuberculosis reacted with fever and generalized sickness following a subcutaneous injection of tuberculin, a lipoprotein antigen derived from the tubercle bacillus. This reaction was accompanied by an area of induration and swelling at the site of injection.

Soluble antigens from a number of organisms, including *Mycobacterium tuberculosis, M. leprae* and *Leishmania tropica,* induce similar reactions in sensitive people. The skin reaction is frequently used as the basis of a test for sensitivity to the organisms following previous exposure (Fig. 22.8). This form of hypersensitivity may also be induced by non-microbial antigens.

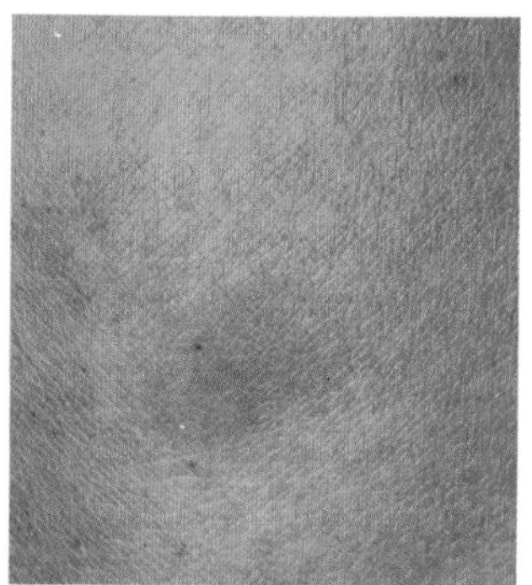

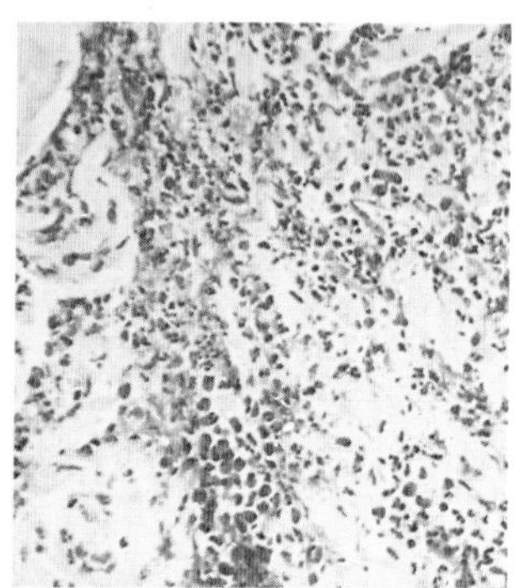

Fig. 22.8 Clinical and histological appearances of tuberculin-type sensitivity. Shown here is the dermal reaction to antigens of the leprosy bacillus in a sensitive individual (Fernandez reaction). The response is characterized clinically by red induration of the skin, maximal at 48–72 hours after challenge (left), and histologically (right) by a dense dermal infiltrate of lymphocytes and macrophages. H&E stain, ×80.

Twelve hours after intradermal tuberculin challenge in a sensitive individual, T lymphocytes are present at perivascular sites and this infiltrate, which extends outwards and disrupts the collagen bundles of the dermis, increases to a peak at 48 hours. $CD4^+$ cells outnumber $CD8^+$ cells by about 2:1; $CD1^+$ cells (Langerhans'-like cells) are also found in the dermal infiltrate at 24 and 48 hours, and a few $CD4^+$ cells infiltrate the epidermis between 24 and 48 hours. Polymorphs are uncommon in this reaction in man, but macrophages start to accumulate around dermal vessels at 12 hours, their numbers increasing up to 72 hours. Infiltrating lymphocytes and macrophages may express HLA–DR. Overlying keratinocytes express HLA–DR molecules 48–96 hours after the appearance of the lymphocytic infiltrate. These events are summarized in Fig. 22.9.

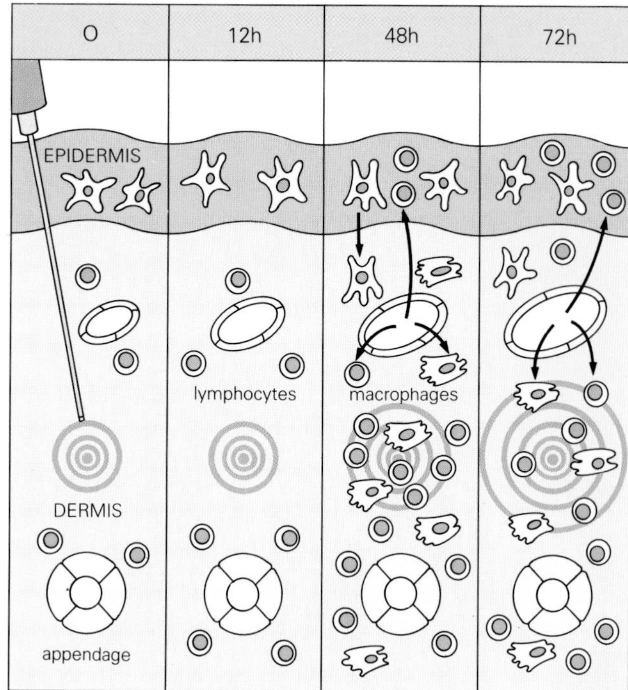

Fig. 22.9 Tuberculin-type hypersensitivity. This diagram illustrates cellular movements following intradermal injection of tuberculin. At 12 hours, lymphocytes begin to migrate from local blood vessels and accumulate around appendages. By 48 hours, macrophages are also present and Langerhans' cells start to migrate out of the epidermis. The cellular traffic continues over the next 24 hours, and class II molecules appear on keratinocytes; there is no spongiosis (compare contact hypersensitivity).

Cells of the macrophage lineage are probably the main antigen-presenting cells in the tuberculin hypersensitivity reaction, but the finding of $CD1^+$ cells in the dermal infiltrate suggests that Langerhans' cells or indeterminate dendritic cells may also be involved. Afferent and efferent circulation of immunocompetent cells to and from the regional lymph nodes is thought to be similar to that for contact hypersensitivity (see Chapter 3).

As the tuberculin lesion develops it may become a granulomatous reaction, possibly as a consequence of the persistence of the antigen in the tissues. Subepidermal infiltration with basophils is not a characteristic of this reaction.

GRANULOMATOUS HYPERSENSITIVITY

Granulomatous hypersensitivity is clinically the most important form of delayed hypersensitivity, causing many of the pathological effects in diseases which involve T cell-mediated immunity. It results from the presence within macrophages of a persistent agent, usually a microorganism, which the cell is unable to destroy. On occasion it may also be caused by the continued presence of immune complexes, for example in allergic alveolitis. The process results in epithelioid cell granuloma formation.

The histological appearance of the granuloma reaction is quite different from the tuberculin-type reaction,

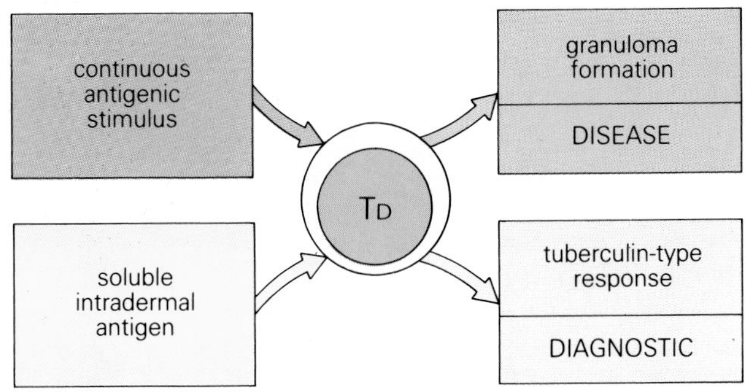

Fig. 22.10 Role of TD cells. Both tuberculin-type and granulomatous hypersensitivity reactions depend on a functionally defined group of T cells, TD cells, which consists primarily of T-helper cells. Where there is continuous antigenic stimulation due to persistent or recurrent infection, or when macrophages cannot destroy an antigen, granuloma formation occurs. The presence of antigen-sensitized TD cells can be detected by the tuberculin-type response to intradermal injection of antigen.

which is usually a self-limiting response to antigen rather than being due to the persistence of antigen. Nevertheless they often result from sensitization to similar microbial antigens, for example, *Mycobacterium tuberculosis* and *M. leprae* (Fig. 22.10).

Immunological granuloma formation also occurs in zirconium sensitivity and in sarcoidosis. Granulomas are also produced by certain non-antigenic stimuli, such as talc. In this case the macrophages are unable to digest the inorganic matter. These non-immunological granulomas may be distinguished by the absence of lymphocytes in the lesion. Examples of granulomatous hypersensitivity in various diseases will be discussed later.

The characteristic cell of granulomatous hypersensitivity is the epithelioid cell. On electron microscopic examination this appears as a large flattened cell with increased endoplasmic reticulum (Fig. 22.11). The nature of the cell is poorly understood; it has been suggested that epithelioid cells are derived from activated macrophages but examination reveals that whereas activated macrophages have many phagosomes this is not true of epithelioid cells. Also seen in this type of reaction are multinucleate giant cells, sometimes referred to as Langhans' giant cells (not to be confused with the Langerhans' cell discussed earlier). Giant cells have several peripherally distributed nuclei, leaving the central area of the cytoplasm free. The cytoplasm contains membrane-lined vesicles and intracellular particles. The giant cell has little endoplasmic reticulum, and its mitochondria and lysosomes appear to be undergoing degeneration. For this reason it is thought that the cell may be a terminal differentiation stage of the monocyte/macrophage line (Fig. 22.12).

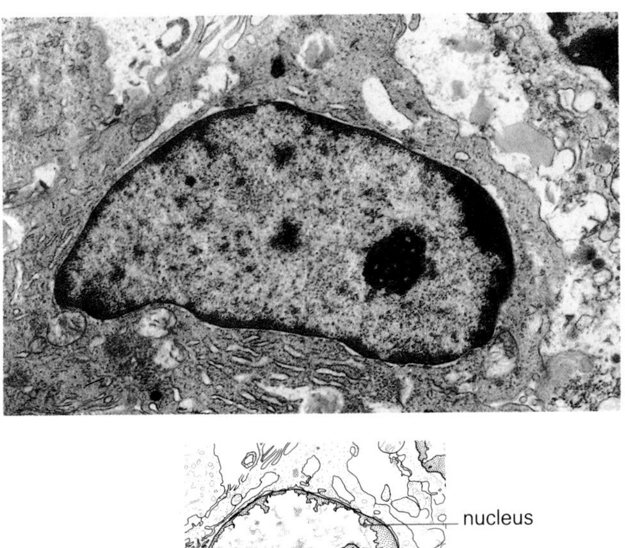

Fig. 22.11 Electronmicrograph of an epithelioid cell. This is the characteristic cell of granulomatous hypersensitivity. Note the increased endoplasmic reticulum compared with a monocyte/macrophage. ×4,800.

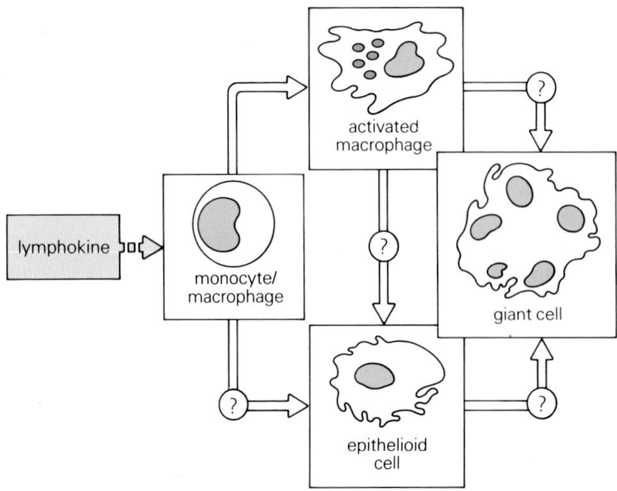

Fig. 22.12 A proposed scheme for the terminal differentiation of cells of the monocyte/macrophage system. The pathological changes result from the inability of the macrophage to deal effectively with the pathogen. Lymphokines from active T cells induce monocytes and macrophages to become activated macrophages. Where prolonged antigenic stimulation exists, activated macrophages may differentiate into epithelioid cells and then into giant cells *in vivo*, in granulomatous tissue. The multinucleate giant cell may be derived from fusion of several epithelioid cells.

The typical immunologically induced granulomatous lesion has a core of epithelioid cells and macrophages, sometimes with giant cells. In some diseases, such as tuberculosis, this central area may have a zone of necrosis (cell death), with complete destruction of all cellular architecture. The macrophage/epithelioid core is surrounded by a cuff of lymphocytes, and there may also be considerable fibrosis (deposition of collagen fibres) caused by proliferation of fibroblasts and increased collagen synthesis. An example of a granulomatous reaction can be seen in the Mitsuda reaction to leprosy antigens or in the Kveim test, where patients suffering from sarcoidosis (a disease of unknown aetiology) react to splenic antigens derived from other sarcoid patients. The Mitsuda reaction is illustrated in Fig. 22.13.

The four types of delayed hypersensitivity reaction are summarized in Fig. 22.14.

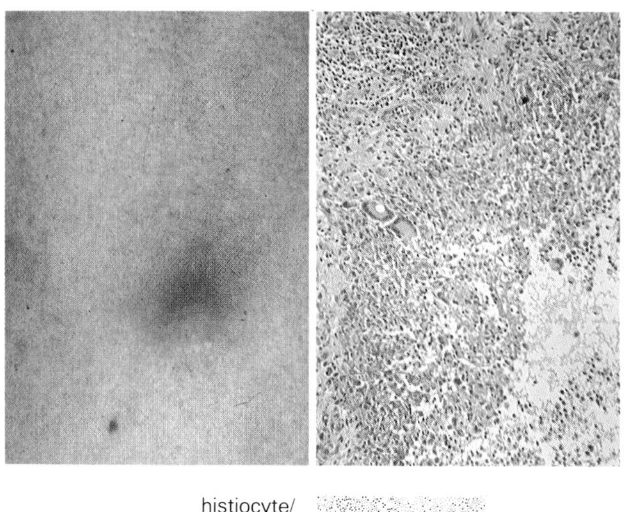

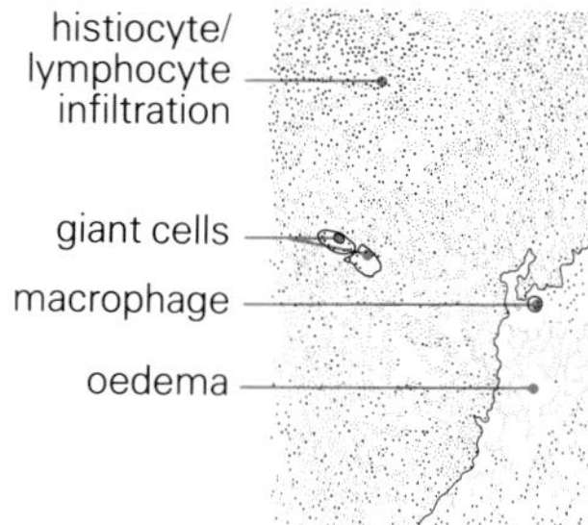

Fig. 22.13 Clinical and histological appearances of the Mitsuda reaction in leprosy seen at 28 days. The resultant skin swelling (which may be ulcerated) is much more indurated, and is better defined than at 48 hours. Histology demonstrates a typical epithelioid cell granuloma. Giant cells are visible in the centre of the lesion, which is surrounded by a cuff of lymphocytes (right, H & E stain, ×60). This response is more akin to the pathological processes in delayed hypersensitivity diseases than the self-resolving tuberculin-type reaction. The reaction is due to the continued presence of antigen.

type	Jones–Mote	contact	tuberculin	granulomatous
reaction time	24 hours	48 hours	48 hours	4 weeks
clinical appearance	skin swelling	eczema	local induration and swelling ± fever	skin induration
histological appearance	basophils, lymphocytes, mononuclear cells	infiltration of lymphocytes and, later, macrophages: oedema of epidermis	mononuclear cells (lymphocytes and monocytes), macrophages	epithelioid cell granuloma, giant cells, macrophages, fibrosis, ± necrosis
antigen	intradermal antigen, e.g. ovalbumin	epidermal: e.g. nickel, rubber, poison ivy	dermal: tuberculin, mycobacterial and leishmanial antigens	persistent Ag or Ag/Ab complexes in macrophages or 'non-immunological', e.g. talcum powder

Fig. 22.14 The four types of delayed hypersensitivity reaction; a summary of their most important characteristics. The four types of delayed hypersensitivity reaction can be distinguished not only by their time of onset, but also by the cell types seen histologically at the reaction site.

CELLULAR REACTIONS IN DELAYED HYPERSENSITIVITY

Delayed hypersensitivity reactions are initiated by cells rather than antibody. It was shown by Simon and Rackeman in 1934 that there was no association between the tuberculin-type reaction and the incidence of serum antibodies to the sensitizing antigen. Moreover, in 1942 Landsteiner and Chase showed that the reactivity may only be transferred to a non-sensitive individual by cell suspensions containing lymphocytes. By eliminating T lymphocytes in the transfer it is relatively easy to show that these cells are the effectors in tuberculin-type hypersensitivity (Fig. 22.15).

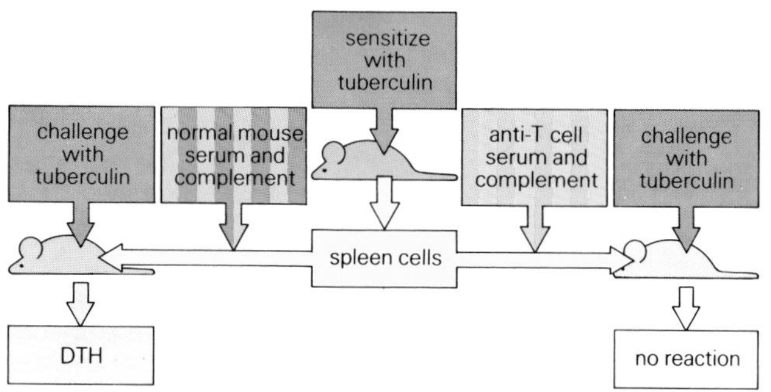

Fig. 22.15 Demonstration of the role of T lymphocytes in the tuberculin response. A mouse is sensitized to tuberculin by intradermal injection. Its spleen cells are later removed and treated with either normal serum and complement, or anti-T lymphocyte serum and complement. The treated cells are injected into recipient mice which are challenged with tuberculin. The mouse with spleen cells treated with normal serum develops a tuberculin-type reaction, whereas the mouse given anti-T cell-treated spleen cells fails to respond. It is concluded that sensitized T cells are responsible for producing the response to tuberculin.

Similarly, T cells are responsible for initiating the other delayed hypersensitivity reactions. Sensitized T cells which are stimulated with the appropriate antigen undergo lymphoblastoid transformation prior to cell division (Fig. 22.16). This forms the basis of the lymphocyte transformation test which is detailed in Chapter 25, and is useful in the diagnosis of delayed hypersensitivity. Lymphocyte transformation is accompanied by DNA synthesis and this can be measured by assaying the uptake of radiolabelled thymidine, a nucleotide which is required for DNA synthesis. Lymphocytes from a patient are cultured with the suspect antigen to determine whether it induces transformation. It is important to stress that this is a test for T cell memory and does not necessarily imply the presence of protective immunity in the host against microorganisms carrying the antigen.

Following activation, T cells produce a number of lymphokines which are important in causing the localization and activation of macrophages at the site of reaction. Of these lymphokines, macrophage activating factor (MAF) and macrophage migration inhibition factor (MIF) are particularly important in the development of delayed hypersensitivity reactions. MAF activity is primarily

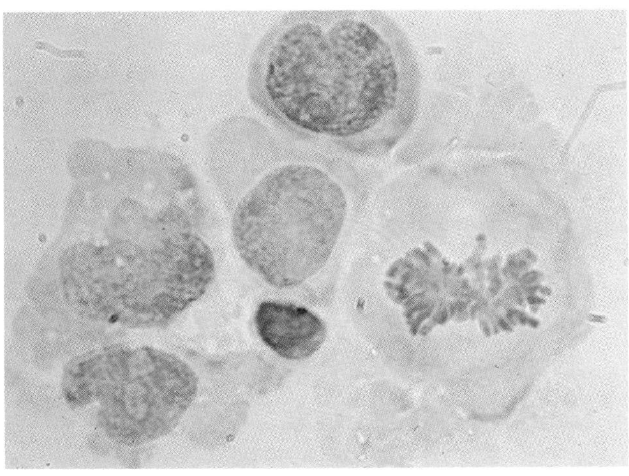

Fig. 22.16 Transformed lymphocytes. Following stimulation with appropriate antigen, T cells undergo lymphoblastoid transformation prior to cell division. Blast cells with expanded nuclei and cytoplasm (as well as one lymphocyte in the metaphase of cell division) are shown.

constituted by IFNY and is important in enhancing macrophage activity, promoting the killing of intracellular organisms (Fig. 22.17); it also induces class II molecules on many facultative antigen-presenting cells in the tissues. One of the tests for T cell reactivity measures MIF production by T cells in the presence of antigen. MIF inhibits the normal migration of macrophages (Fig. 22.18). The characteristics of lymphokines involved in these types of hypersensitivity reaction are detailed in Chapters 8 and 9.

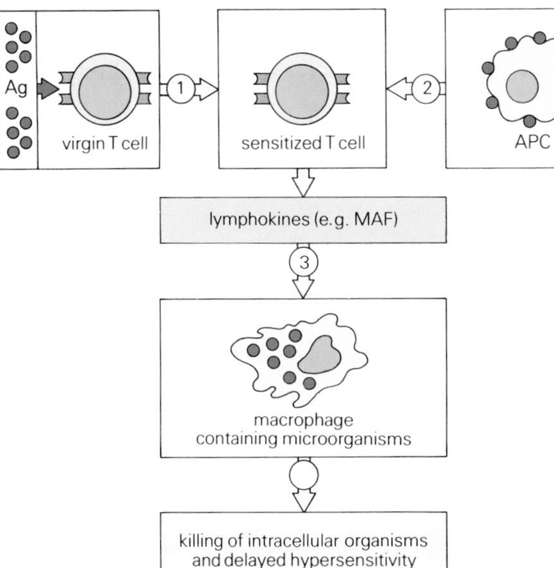

Fig. 22.17 The production and role of lymphokines in delayed hypersensitivity. During infection, T cells recognize the microorganism's antigens and proliferate, giving rise to a population of sensitized T cells (1). When these cells are presented with antigen by the antigen-presenting cell (2), they release lymphokines. The lymphokine macrophage activating factor (MAF) activates the macrophages (3), stimulating them to kill any microorganisms they may contain. These macrophages may participate in a delayed hypersensitivity response.

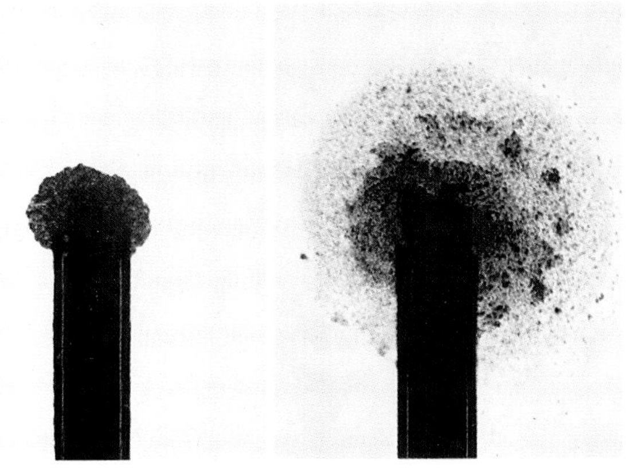

Fig. 22.18 Macrophage Migration Inhibition Test. Macrophages are packed into capillary tubes with either test lymphocytes (suspected as being sensitized to an antigen) together with antigen (left) or control lymphocytes and the antigen (right), and set up in short-term tissue culture. Where migration is inhibited (left), it is concluded that the lymphocytes are sensitized to the antigen and produce the lymphokine, migration inhibition factor, which inhibits the normal migration of macrophages.

DISEASES MANIFESTING DELAYED HYPERSENSITIVITY

There is a considerable number of chronic diseases in man which manifest delayed hypersensitivity, and most are due to infectious agents such as mycobacteria, protozoa and fungi. Important diseases in this respect include the following.

1. Tuberculosis.
2. Leprosy.
3. Leishmaniasis.
4. Listeriosis.
5. Deep fungal infections (e.g. blastomycosis).
6. Helminthic infections (e.g. schistosomiasis).

These diseases are caused by pathogens which present a persistent chronic antigenic stimulus. The threat they pose is met by lymphocytes and macrophages. Although these diseases are liable to induce protective immunity, as previously stated, protective immunity and delayed hypersensitivity are not always coincident.

LEPROSY

A dramatic example of delayed hypersensitivity occurs in the borderline leprosy reaction. Leprosy is a disease where protective immunity depends on cell-mediated immunity and where humoral immunity apparently plays no protective role.

There is a spectrum of disease dependent on the competence of the host's immune response; those with good responsiveness to the organism are 'tuberculoid', and those with no response, 'lepromatous'. In between these two extremes lies borderline leprosy, and these patients tend to develop characteristic reactions to the leprosy bacillus.

Borderline reactions occur either naturally or following drug treatment; the hypopigmented skin lesions become swollen and inflamed following sensitization to antigens of *Mycobacterium leprae* (Fig. 22.19, left)

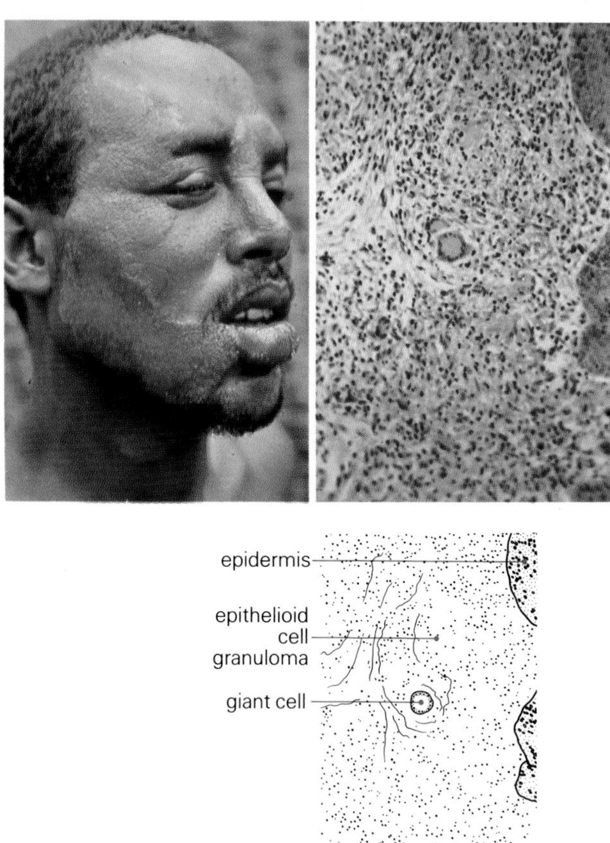

Fig. 22.19 A borderline leprosy reaction. The previously hypopigmented skin lesions have become swollen and inflamed following sensitization to antigens of *M. leprae* (left). The histological appearance of the borderline leprosy reaction (right) is typical of granulomatous hypersensitivity. Note the giant cell and infiltration by monocytes and lymphocytes. H&E stain, ×140.

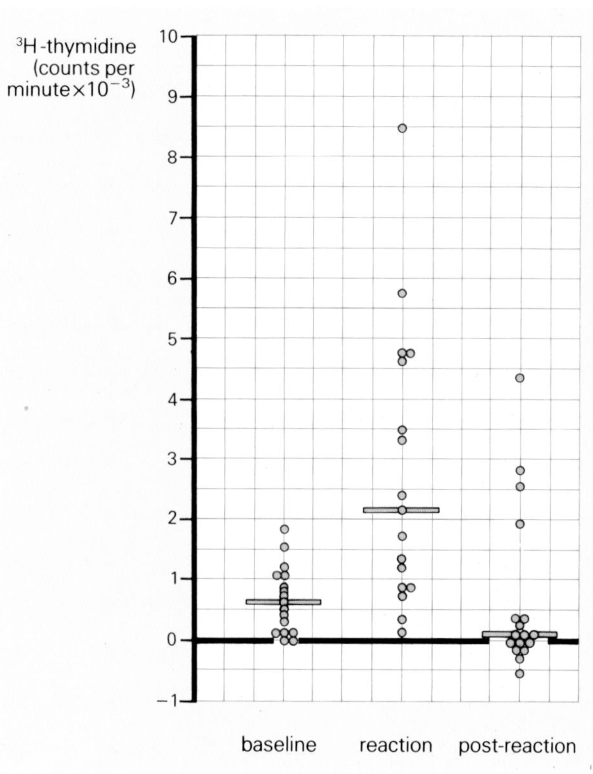

Fig. 22.20 Results of a lymphocyte transformation test in a borderline leprosy reaction. During a borderline leprosy reaction, the lymphocyte transformation response to *M. leprae* rises, and there is a fall in response when the reaction is treated successfully. The lymphocyte transformation responses (uptake of [^{3}H]-thymidine) to sonicated *M. leprae* are shown for 17 patients who developed such reactions: (a) before starting leprosy treatment (baseline); (b) during the reaction; and (c) on cessation of steroids. Medians are indicated by horizontal bars.

and the histological appearance becomes more tuberculoid. The same process may occur in peripheral nerves, and this is the most important cause of nerve destruction in this disease. The lesion in leprosy patients who have borderline reactivity is typical of granulomatous hypersensitivity (Fig. 22.19, right).

When a patient develops immunity associated with tuberculoid-type hypersensitivity, T cell sensitization may be assessed *in vitro* by the lymphocyte transformation test using either whole or sonicated *M. leprae* as the source of antigen (Fig. 22.20).

TUBERCULOSIS

In tuberculosis there is granuloma formation in the lung and other infected organs. Lung damage caused by the granulomatous reaction leads to cavitation and spread of bacteria.

The reactions are frequently accompanied by extensive fibrosis and the lesions may be seen in the chest radiographs of affected patients (Fig. 22.21).

The histological appearance of the lesion is typical of a granulomatous reaction, with central caseous (cheesy) necrosis (Fig. 22.22), which is surrounded by an area of epithelioid cells containing multinucleate giant cells. Monocyte infiltration occurs at the periphery of the lesion.

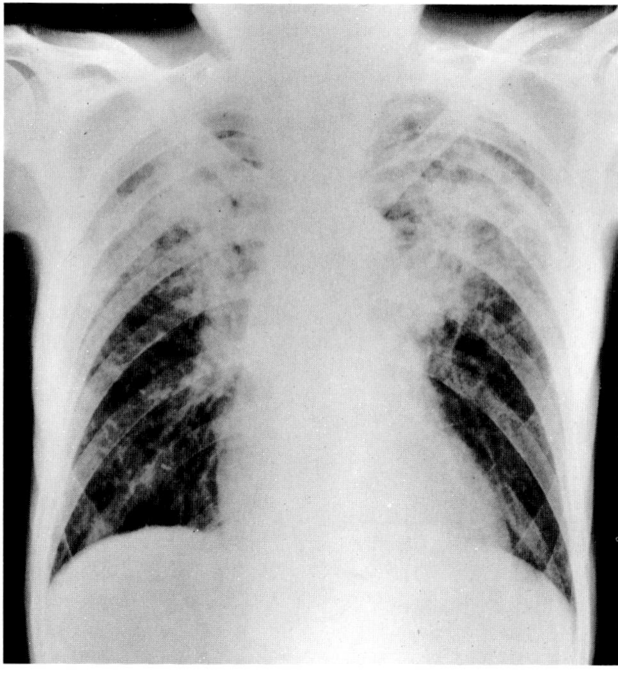

Fig. 22.21 Chest radiograph of a patient with pulmonary tuberculosis. This shows marked tuberculous infiltration of both lungs.

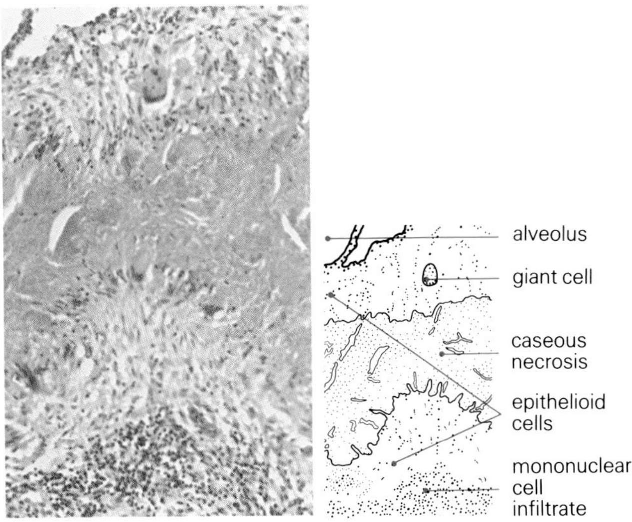

Fig. 22.22 Histological appearance of a tuberculous section of lung. This demonstrates an epithelioid cell granuloma and giant cells typical of a granulomatous reaction. There is also marked caseation and necrosis within the area of the granulomatous reaction. H&E stain, ×75.

SARCOIDOSIS

Sarcoidosis is a disease of unknown aetiology, although it has been postulated that it might be due to an infectious agent such as a mycobacterium, since the condition produces all the features of immunological granuloma formation frequently accompanied by fibrosis typical of mycobacterial infection (Fig. 22.23).

There may also be manifestations of Type III hypersensitivity, such as cutaneous vasculitis or uveitis. The disease particularly affects lymphoid tissue and lymphadenopathy may be detected in chest radiographs of affected patients (Fig. 22.24).

One of the paradoxes of clinical immunology is that this disease is usually associated with depression of delayed hypersensitivity both *in vivo* and *in vitro*. These patients are anergic on testing with tuberculin but when cortisone is injected with tuberculin antigen, skin tests become positive, suggesting that cortisone-sensitive suppressor T cells are responsible for the anergy. Cortisone would normally suppress these responses.

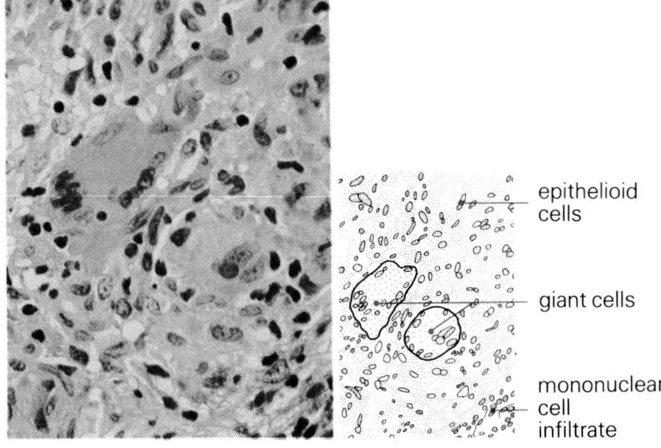

Fig. 22.23 Histological appearance of sarcoid lymph node tissue. This appearance is typical of an epithelioid cell granuloma without necrosis. H&E stain, ×240.

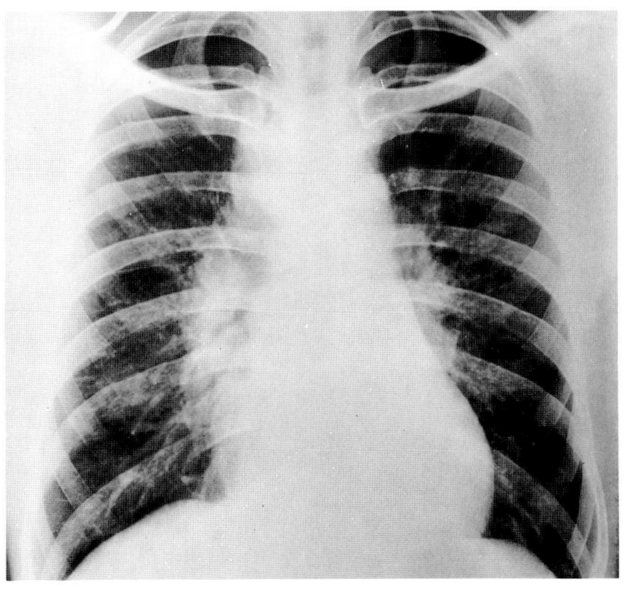

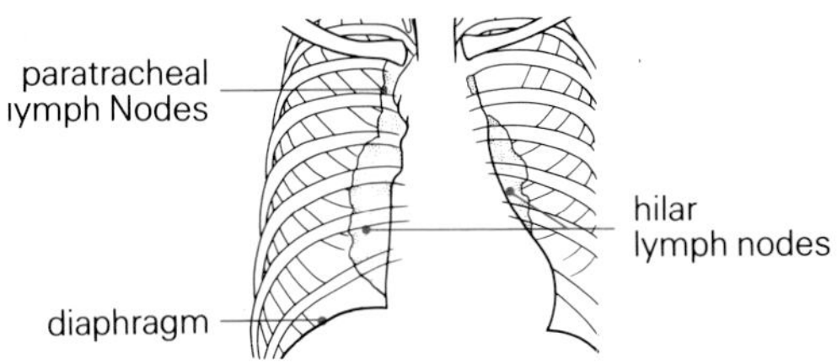

Fig. 22.24 The chest radiograph of a patient with sarcoidosis. There is bilateral hilar and paratracheal lymphadenopathy, with diffuse pulmonary infiltration characteristic of the disease.

SCHISTOSOMIASIS

Another disease exemplifying granulomatous hypersensitivity is schistosomiasis, caused by parasitic trematode worms (schistosomes). The host becomes sensitized to the ova of the worms, leading to a typical granulomatous reaction in the parasitized tissue (Fig. 22.25).

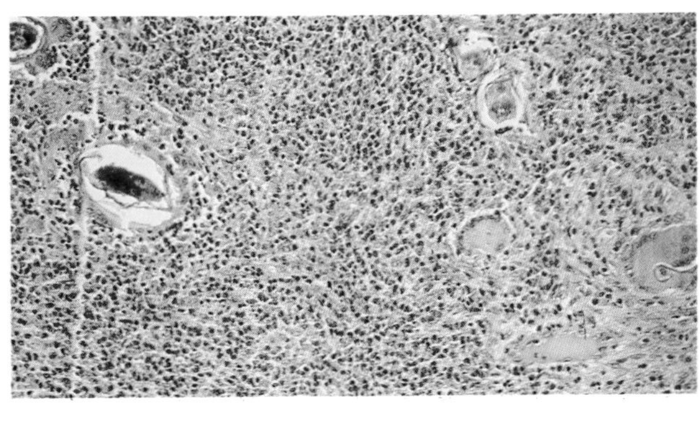

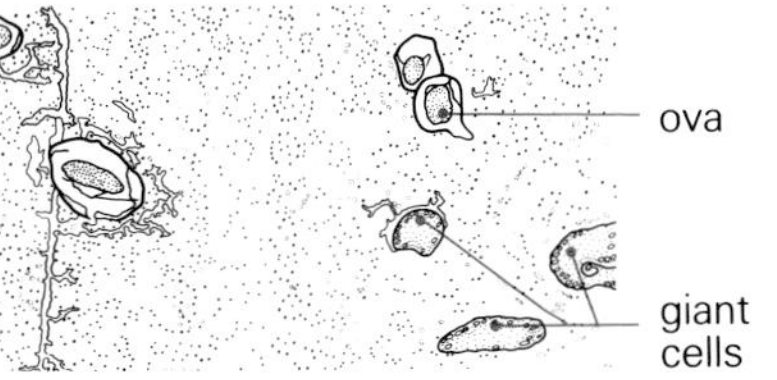

Fig. 22.25 Histological appearance of the liver in schistosomiasis. The epithelioid cell granuloma is surrounding ova of schistosomes. Note also the giant cells. H&E stain, ×100.

FURTHER READING

Bjune, G., Barnetson, R. StC., Ridley, D. S. & Kronvall, G. (1976) Lymphocyte transformation test in leprosy: correlation of the response with inflammation of lesions. *Clinical and Experimental Immunology*, **25**, 85–94.

Gawkrodger, D. J., McVittie, E., Carr, M. M., Ross, J. A. & Hunter, J. A. A. (1986) Phenotypic characterization of the early cellular responses in allergic and irritant contact dermatitis. *Clinical and Experimental Immunology*, **66**, 590–598.

Gawkrodger, D. J., Carr, M. M., McVittie, E., Guy, K. & Hunter, J. A. A. (1987) Keratinocyte expression of MHC class II antigens in allergic sensitization and challenge reactions and in irritant contact dermatitis. *Journal of Investigative Dermatology*, **88**, 11–16.

Lens, J. W., Drexhage, H. A., Benson, W. & Balfour, B. M. (1983) A study of cells present in lymph draining from a contact allergic reaction in pigs sensitized to DNFB. *Immunology*, **49**, 415–422.

Platt, J. L., Grant, B. W., Eddy, A. A., & Michael, A. F. (1983) Immune cell populations in cutaneous delayed hypersensitivity. *Journal of Experimental Medicine*, **158**, 1227–1242.

Poulter, L. W., Seymour, G. J., Duke, O., Janossy, G. & Panayi, G. (1982) Immunohistochemical analysis of delayed-type hypersensitivity in man. *Cellular Immunology*, **74**, 358–369.

Sauder, D. N. (1986) Allergic contact dermatitis. In *Pathogenesis of Skin Disease*. Edited by B. H. Thiers & R. L. Dobson. p. 3–12. New York: Churchill Livingstone.

Sonoda, Y., Asano, S., Miyazaki, T. & Sagami, S. (1985) Electron microscopic study on Langerhans cells and related cells in lymph nodes of DNCB-sensitive mice. *Archives of Dermatological Research*, **277**, 44–54.

Turk, J. L. (1980) *Delayed Hypersensitivity, 3rd edition*. Research Monographs in Immunology, **1**. Amsterdam: Elsevier.

Wolff, K. & Stingl, G. (1983) The Langerhans cell. *Journal of Investigative Dermatology*, **80**, supplement, 175–215.

23 Autoimmunity and Autoimmune Disease

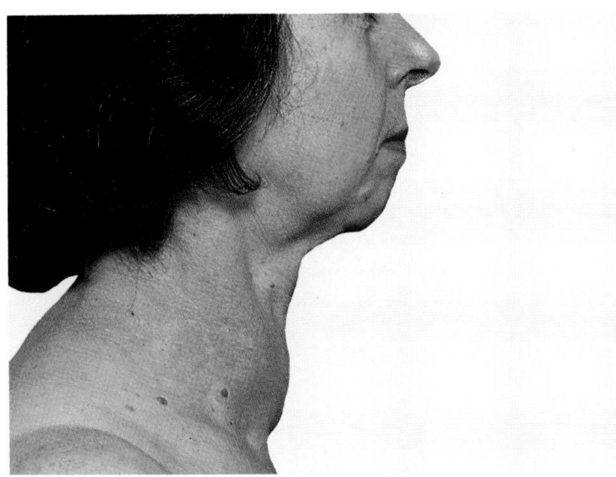

Fig. 23.1 Enlarged thyroid in Hashimoto's thyroiditis.

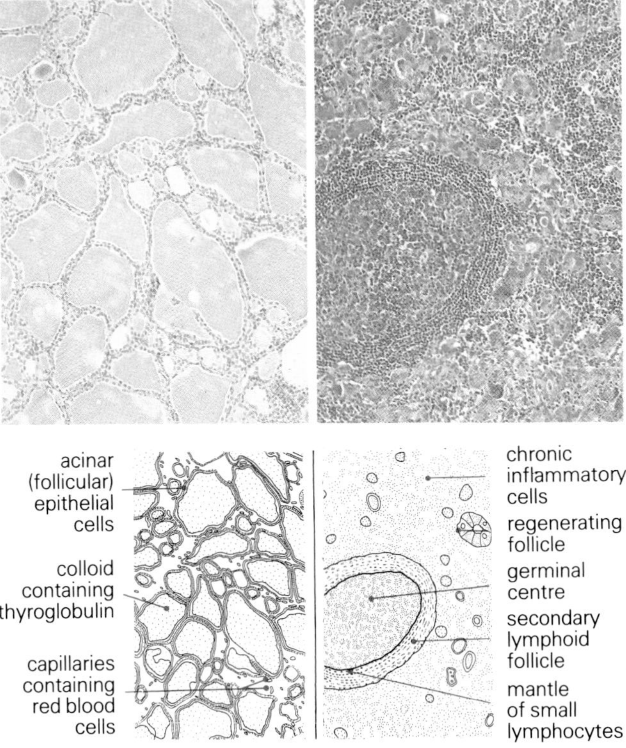

Fig. 23.2 Histological changes in Hashimoto's thyroiditis. A normal thyroid (left), showing the follicular cells lining the colloid space into which they secrete thyroglobulin, which is broken down on demand to provide thyroid hormones. A Hashimoto gland (right) in which the normal architecture is virtually destroyed and replaced by invading cells which consist essentially of lymphocytes, macrophages and plasma cells. A secondary lymphoid follicle with a germinal centre and a small regenerating thyroid follicle are present. H & E stain, ×80.

The immune system has tremendous diversity and the repertoire of specificities expressed by the B and T cell populations is bound to include many which are directed to self-components. In earlier chapters, we have discussed the complicated mechanisms which the body must establish to distinguish between self and non-self determinants so as to avoid the embarrassment of autoreactivity. However in the nature of things, all mechanisms have a risk of breakdown and the self-recognition mechanisms are no exception. So it is that a number of diseases have been identified in which there is copious production of autoantibodies and autoreactive T cells.

One of the earliest examples in which the production of autoantibodies was associated with disease in a given organ was Hashimoto's thyroiditis. This is a disease of the thyroid which is most common in middle-aged women and often leads to formation of a goitre (Fig. 23.1) and hypothyroidism. The gland is infiltrated, sometimes to an extraordinary extent, with inflammatory lymphoid cells. These are predominantly mononuclear cells of the lymphocytic and phagocytic series, and plasma cells: secondary lymphoid follicles are common (Fig. 23.2). The gland in Hashimoto's disease often shows regenerating follicles but this is not a feature of the thyroid in a related condition, primary myxoedema, in which comparable immunological features are seen but the gland undergoes almost complete destruction and shrinks (Fig. 23.3).

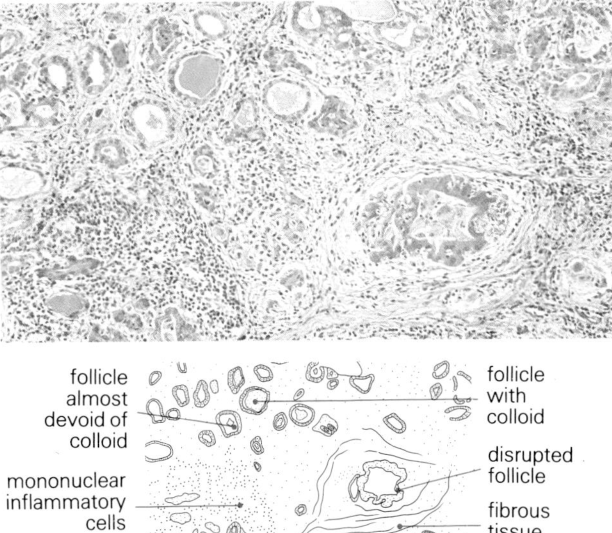

Fig. 23.3 Histological appearance of the thyroid in primary myxoedema. There is destruction of the gland by chronic inflammatory cells associated with fibrosis. Isolated thyroid follicles, some in the process of breakdown, are seen. Unlike the appearance in Hashimoto's disease, there is no tendency for follicular regeneration, and the thyroid shrinks instead of becoming a goitre. H & E stain, ×100.

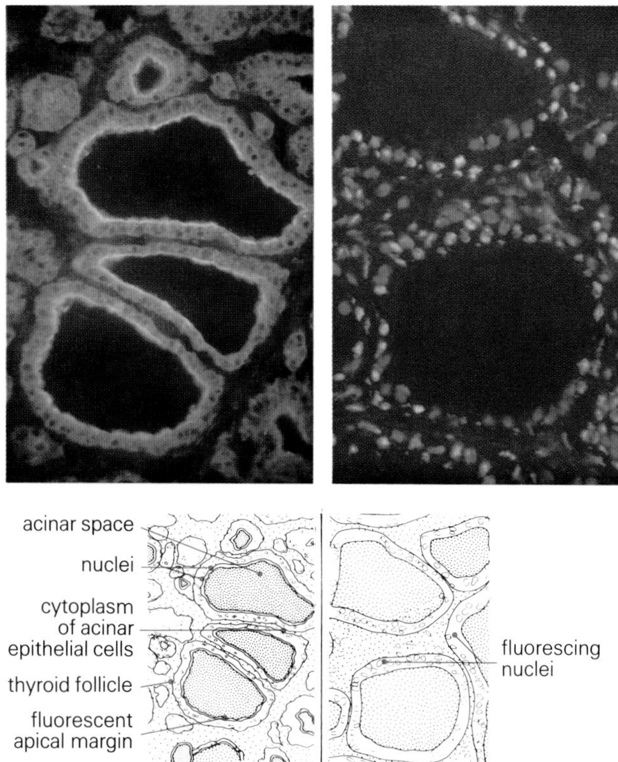

Fig. 23.4 Autoantibodies to thyroid demonstrated with double layer immunofluorescence. An unfixed human thyroid section was treated with a patient's serum and then a fluoresceinated rabbit anti-human immunoglobulin. The acinar epithelial cells are stained by antibody in serum from a patient with Hashimoto's disease, which reacts with cytoplasm (left). Note the unstained nuclei. The colloid is lost from the unfixed section so thyroglobulin staining is not seen. In contrast, serum from a patient with systemic lupus erythematosus contains antibodies which react with the nucleus but leave the cytoplasm unstained (right).

The serum of patients with Hashimoto's disease usually contains antibodies to thyroglobulin, which is the major iodine-containing protein in the follicular fluid of the thyroid acinae and acts as a depot for the thyroid hormone. These antibodies are demonstrable by immunofluorescence and also, when present in high titre, by precipitin reactions. The immunofluorescence method led to the finding of antibodies directed against a cytoplasmic or microsomal antigen which is also present on the apical surface of microvilli. This is now known to be thyroid peroxidase, which is responsible for the iodination of thyroglobulin (Fig. 23.4).

THE SPECTRUM OF AUTOIMMUNE DISEASES

The antibodies which have just been described in association with Hashimoto's disease and primary myxoedema react only with the thyroid: they do not react with any other tissues in the body. In contrast, the serum from patients with diseases such as systemic lupus erythematosus (SLE) reacts with many if not all tissues in the body. In SLE, one of the dominant antibodies is directed against the cell nucleus (Fig. 23.4).

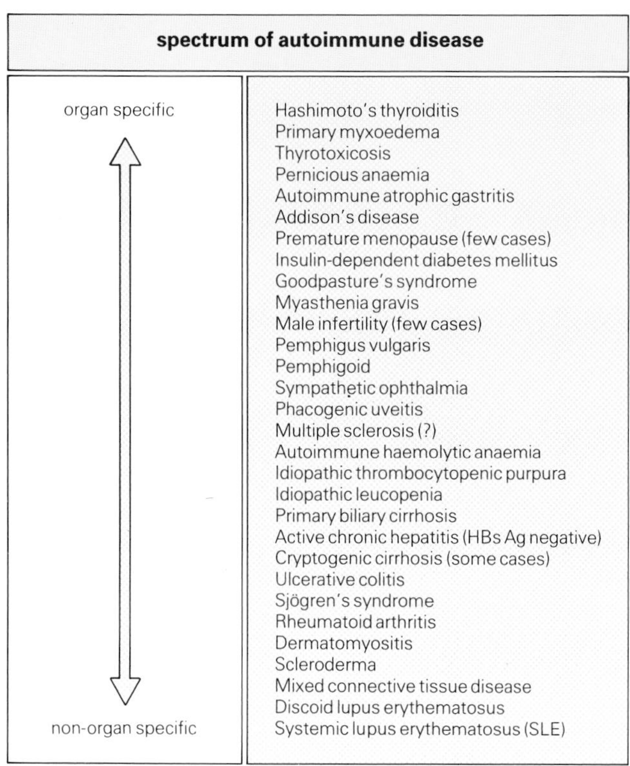

Fig. 23.5 The spectrum of autoimmune diseases. Autoimmune diseases may be classified as organ specific or non-organ specific depending on whether the response is primarily against either antigens localized to particular organs, or widespread antigens.

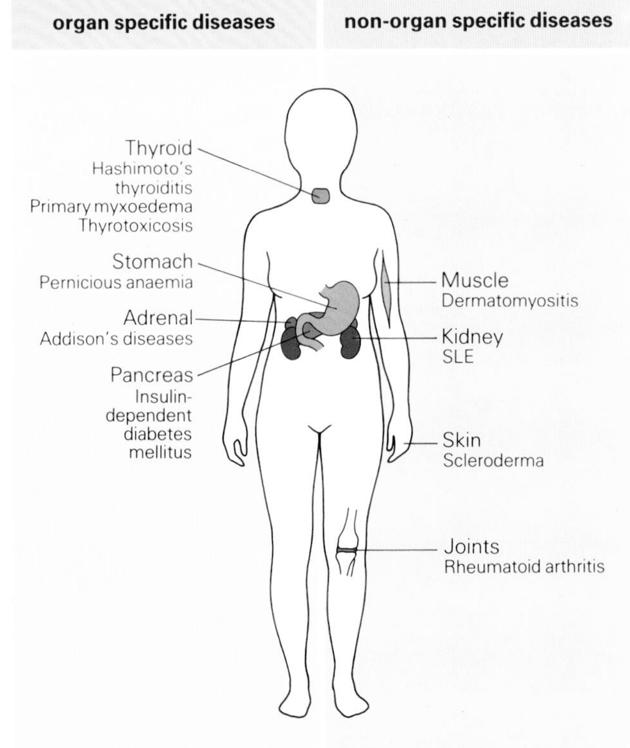

Fig. 23.6 Two types of autoimmune diseases – organ specific and non-organ specific. Although the non-organ specific diseases produce symptoms in different organs, particular organs are more markedly affected by particular diseases, for example the kidney in systemic lupus erythematosus (SLE) and the joint in rheumatoid arthritis.

Diseases associated with autoimmune phenomena tend to distribute themselves within a spectrum. At one pole, typified by Hashimoto's thyroiditis, the antibodies and the invasive destructive lesion are directed against just one organ in the body. At the other end of the spectrum, typified by SLE, the antibodies are directed to antigens which are widespread throughout the body and the characteristic lesions of the disease are also widely disseminated. Thus, we speak of organ specific and non-organ specific autoimmune diseases; in Fig. 23.5 the diseases are classified according to where they lie within this spectrum.

The common target organs in organ specific disease include the thyroid, adrenals, stomach and pancreas. On the other hand, the non-organ specific diseases, which include the so-called rheumatological disorders, involve skin, kidney, joints and muscle (Fig. 23.6).

Interestingly, there are remarkable overlaps at each end of the spectrum. For example, thyroid antibodies occur with a high frequency in patients with pernicious anaemia who have stomach autoimmunity, and these patients have a higher incidence of thyroid autoimmune disease than the normal population. Similarly, patients with thyroid autoimmunity have a high incidence of stomach autoantibodies and to a lesser extent, the clinical disease itself, pernicious anaemia.

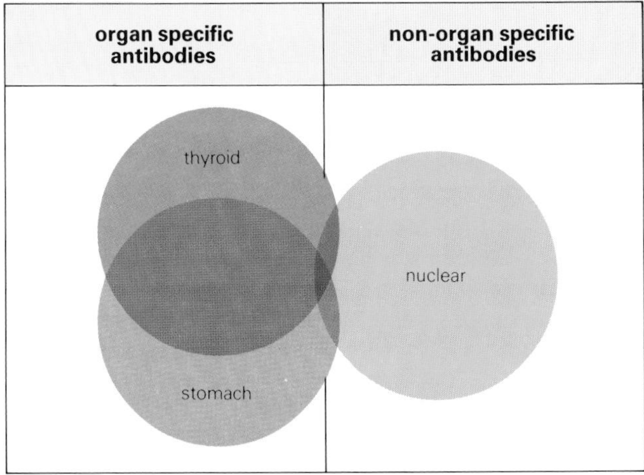

Fig. 23.7 Overlap of autoantibodies. The organ specific autoantibodies directed against thyroid and stomach often occur together in the same individual but there is little overlap with non-organ specific antibodies such as those with reactivity for nuclear components such as DNA and nucleoproteins.

	organ specific	non-organ specific
antigen	essentially localized to given organ	widespread throughout the body
lesions	antigen in organ is target for immunological attack	complexes deposit systemically particularly in kidneys, joints and skin
overlap	with other organ-specific antibodies and diseases	with other non-organ specific antibodies and diseases

Fig. 23.8 Comparison of organ specific and non-organ specific disorders.

The cluster of rheumatological disorders at the non-organ specific end of the spectrum also shows considerable overlap and features of rheumatoid arthritis, for example, are often associated with the clinical picture of SLE.

In non-organ specific disease, complexes formed with the antigens involved are deposited systemically, particularly in the kidney, joints and skin, so giving rise to the more disseminated features of the disease. In contrast, overlap between diseases at the two ends of the spectrum is relatively rare, and cases in which thyroiditis and SLE occur together are extremely unusual (Fig. 23.7).

In organ specific diseases, lesions are restricted because the antigen in the organ acts as a target for immunological attack.

The mechanisms by which immunopathological damage occur in autoimmunity vary depending on where the disease lies in the spectrum. Where the antigen is localized in a particular organ, type II hypersensitivity and cell-mediated reactions are most important (see Chapters 20 and 22). In non-organ specific autoimmunity, immune complex deposition at sites of filtration is also relevant (see Chapter 21). The features of organ specific and non-organ specific disorders are compared in Fig. 23.8.

GENETICS

There is an undoubted familial incidence of autoimmunity, a remarkable example of which is shown in Fig. 23.9. This familial incidence is almost certainly largely genetic rather than environmental, as may be seen from studies of identical and non-identical twins, and from the association of, for example, thyroid autoantibodies with abnormalities of the X-chromosome.

Just as there is an overlap between organ specific disorders in given individuals, so the tendency to develop

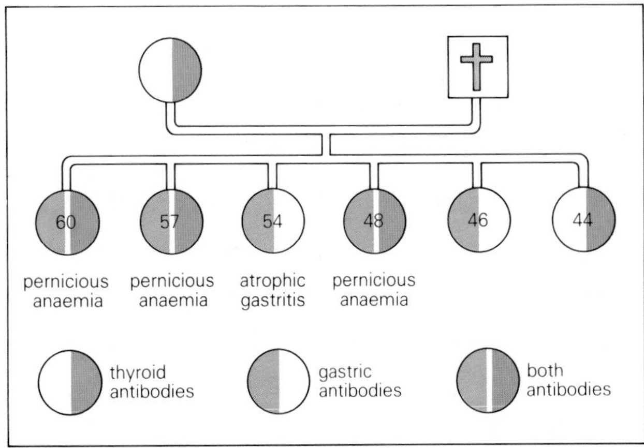

Fig. 23.9 Autoimmunity in a family. The family chart shows the incidence of organ specific abnormalities affecting the thyroid and stomach. Although the siblings presented with gastric autoimmune disease, unlike the mother, who has primary myxoedema, there is a striking overlap with thyroid autoimmunity at the serological level, although the subjects lack clinical symptoms of thyroid disease. Autoantibodies are more prevalent with increasing age (ages are given at which autoantibodies were detected).

autoimmunity within families shows a bias towards organ specific autoimmunity (Fig. 23.10). In addition to this predisposition to develop organ specific antibodies, it is clear that other genetically controlled factors tend to select the organ which will be mainly affected. It is interesting to note that although relatives of Hashimoto patients have a higher than expected incidence and titre of thyroid autoantibodies and that the same is seen in relatives of patients with pernicious anaemia, the latter are distinguished by having a far higher frequency of gastric autoantibodies indicating that the stomach is being differentially selected as the target organ within this group.

Further evidence for the operation of genetic factors in the development of autoimmune diseases comes from their tendency to be associated with particular HLA specificities (Fig. 23.11). The haplotype B8, DR3 is particularly common in the organ specific diseases, though Hashimoto's disease tends to be associated more with DR5. Rheumatoid arthritis showed no HLA associations when only the specificities at the A and B loci were studied, but has now been shown to be associated with HLA–DR4; individuals with this tissue type have a higher chance of developing the disease. Of note is the finding that in the organ specific disease, insulin-dependent or type 1 diabetes mellitus, heterozygotes for DR3 and DR4 have a greatly increased risk of developing the disease. This supports the concept of several genetic factors being involved in the development of autoimmune diseases. These must include factors predisposing individuals to develop autoimmunity, either organ specific or non-organ specific, and others which determine the particular antigen or antigens involved.

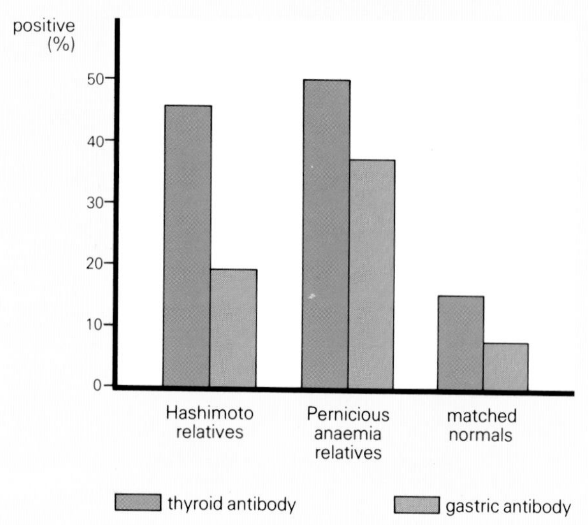

Fig. 23.10 Thyroid and stomach antibodies in first degree relatives of patients with Hashimoto's disease or pernicious anaemia. A remarkably high proportion of the first degree relatives of patients with Hashimoto's disease have thyroid autoantibodies and to a lesser degree, parietal cell (gastric) autoantibodies. The relatives of patients with pernicious anaemia also have a very high incidence of thyroid autoimmunity, indicative of a predisposition to develop organ specific autoantibodies; the percentage with gastric autoantibodies is also high even when compared with the Hashimoto relatives, suggesting an inherent bias of the immune system for reactivity against particular organs.

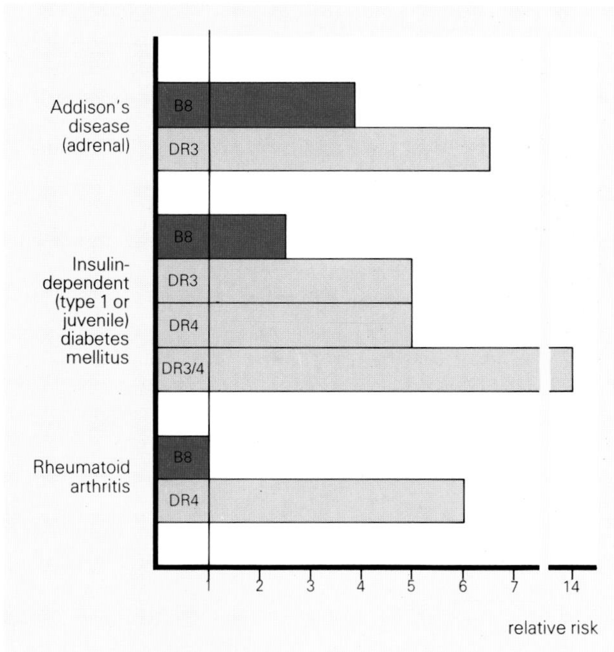

Fig. 23.11 HLA associations in autoimmune disease. The relative risk is a measure of the increased chance of contracting the disease for individuals bearing the antigen relative to those lacking it. Virtually all autoimmune diseases studied show an association with some HLA specificity. The greater relative risk for Addison's disease associated with DR3 as compared with B8 suggests that DR3 is closer to, if not identical with, the 'disease susceptibility gene'. In this case B8 has a relative risk greater than 1 because it is known to occur together with DR3 more often than expected by chance in the population, a phenomenon termed linkage disequilibrium. Both DR3 and DR4 are associated with type 1 diabetes mellitus but strikingly, the DR3/4 heterozygote shows a greatly increased relative risk supporting the concept of multiple genetic factors. Rheumatoid arthritis is linked to HLA–DR4 but not to any HLA–A or –B specificities.

PATHOGENESIS

If autoantibodies are found in association with a particular disease there are logically three possible implications.

1. The autoimmunity is responsible for producing the lesions of the disease.
2. There is a disease process which, through the production of tissue damage, leads secondarily to the development of autoantibodies.
3. There is a factor which produces both the lesions and the autoimmunity (Fig. 23.12).

Autoantibodies secondary to a lesion have been found in some circumstances. For example, cardiac autoantibodies may develop after myocardial infarction. However, autoantibodies are rarely induced following release of autoantigens by simple trauma. The first proposition, namely that a number of diseases are caused by the autoimmune process is an attractive hypothesis and evidence will be adduced that is consistent with this view.

The most direct test of the first proposition is to say that if autoimmunity is responsible for lesions of a given disease, then deliberate induction of autoimmunity in an experimental animal should lead to the production of the lesions. In fact, it is possible to provoke certain organ specific diseases in experimental animals by injecting the causative antigen with Complete Freund's Adjuvant. Thyroglobulin can induce an inflammatory disease of the thyroid while myelin basic protein can cause encephalomyelitis in animals that have been appropriately autoimmunized (Fig. 23.13). Strict organ specificity may be seen since the lesions are confined in both cases to the

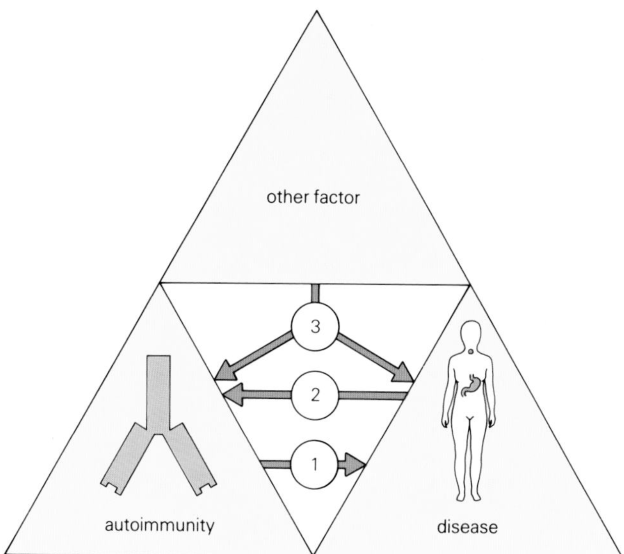

Fig. 23.12 Implications of an association of a disease with autoimmunity. There are three possible explanations for an association of a disease with autoimmunity.
1. Autoimmunity may produce the disease.
2. The disease is responsible for the generation of autoimmunity.
3. A third factor may lead to both.

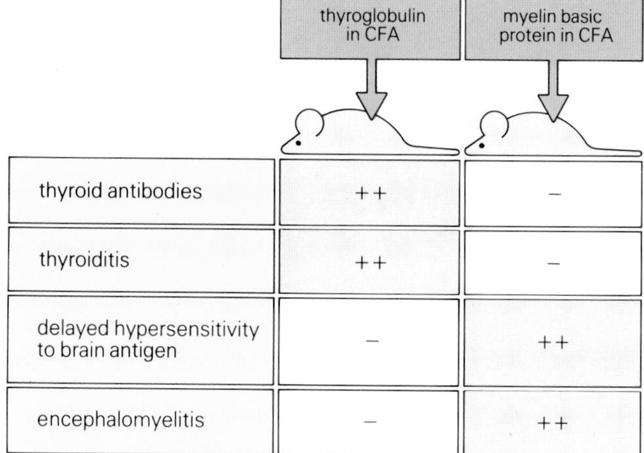

Fig. 23.13 Deliberate induction of autoimmunity to produce diseases in the organ containing the autoantigen. Injection of an aqueous solution of thyroglobulin in Complete Freund's Adjuvant (CFA) produces thyroid antibodies and a destructive inflammatory lesion in the thyroid reminiscent of that seen in Hashimoto's thyroiditis. Immunization with the basic protein from myelin in CFA induces T cell activity, demonstrable as delayed hypersensitivity, which leads to paralysis due to demyelination associated with lymphoid infiltration (encephalomyelitis).

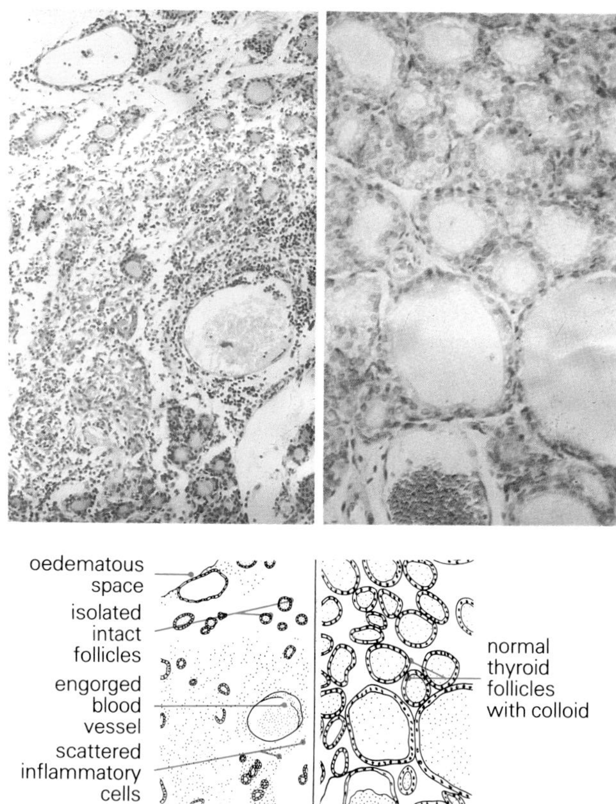

Fig. 23.14 The histological appearance of experimental autoallergic thyroiditis. In the section from a thyroglobulin-injected animal (left, H & E stain, ×200) there is gross destruction of the follicular architecture with extensive invasion by mononuclear inflammatory cells, associated with distended blood vessels, oedema and fibrosis. A control section is shown on the right (H & E stain, ×110).

organ or organ system in which the antigen used for immunization is located. In the case of the thyroglobulin-injected animals, not only are thyroid autoantibodies produced, but the gland becomes infiltrated with mononuclear cells and the acinar architecture crumbles under their influence (Fig. 23.14). Although not identical in every respect with Hashimoto's disease, the thyroiditis produced bears a remarkable overall similarity to the human condition.

The ability to induce these experimental autoimmune diseases depends on the strain of animal used. For example, it is found that the susceptibility of rats and mice to myelin basic protein-induced encephalomyelitis depends on a small number of gene loci, of which the most important are MHC class II genes. It is also possible to induce autoallergic encephalomyelitis in susceptible strains by injecting myelin basic protein-specific T cell lines. These lines are $CD4^+$ and it has been found that induction of the disease can be blocked by treating the recipients with antibody to CD4, just before the expected time of disease onset. The results indicate the importance of class II restricted autoreactive T cells in the development of these conditions, and emphasize the role of the MHC.

There is much to learn from spontaneous examples of autoimmune disease in animals. One well-established example is the Obese strain chicken in which thyroid autoantibodies occur spontaneously and the thyroid undergoes progressive destruction associated with a chronic inflammatory lesion (Fig. 23.15). The sera of these animals contain thyroglobulin autoantibodies. Furthermore, approximately 15% of the sera react with the proventriculus (stomach) of the normal chicken giving a pattern similar to that obtained when the test is carried out with sera from patients with pernicious anaemia who have parietal cell autoantibodies (Fig. 23.16). This example parallels spontaneous human autoimmune thyroid disease in terms of the lesion in the gland, the production of antibodies to different components in the thyroid, and the overlap with gastric autoimmunity. When the immunological status of these animals is altered, quite dramatic effects on the outcome of the disease are seen. For example, if the bursa of Fabricius is removed soon after hatching, the severity of the thyroiditis is greatly diminished, indicating a role for antibody in the pathogenesis of the disease. Paradoxically, removal of the thymus at birth appears to exacerbate the lesion, suggesting that the thymus exerts a controlling effect on the outcome of the disease (Fig. 23.17). Nonetheless, ablation of the T cell population in adult animals by draconian injections of anti-chick T cell serum completely inhibits both autoantibody production and the attack on the thyroid.

Clearly, the severity of the disease is significantly influenced by the state of the immune system and this is consistent with an important role for immunological processes in the causation of the disease.

In investigating human autoimmunity, it is of course more difficult to carry out direct experiments because of ethical limitations, but there is a great deal of evidence which favours the view that the autoantibodies are of importance in the pathogenesis. A number of diseases have been recognized in which there are autoantibodies to hormone receptors which may actually mimic the

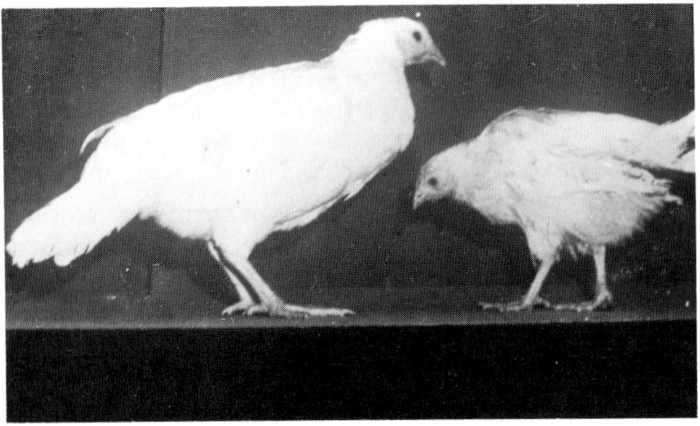

Fig. 23.15 The Obese strain (OS) chicken. This strain of chicken provides an example of spontaneously occurring autoimmune thyroid disease in animals (right). The birds grow poorly and look dishevelled because of the thyroxine deficiency which results from thyroid destruction.

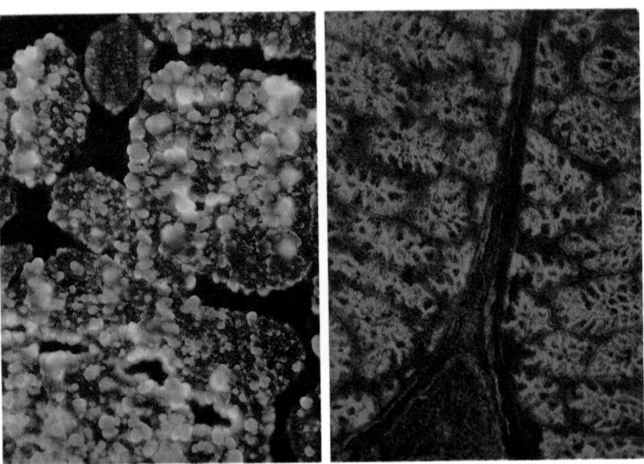

Fig. 23.16 Autoantibodies in OS chickens. Fluorescent staining of a fixed thyroid section showing reaction in the colloid (left). Approximately 15% of the birds have serum antibodies which stain the chicken stomach (proventriculus) giving the characteristic pattern shown (right); this pattern is also seen if human sera containing parietal cell antibodies are tested against this organ.

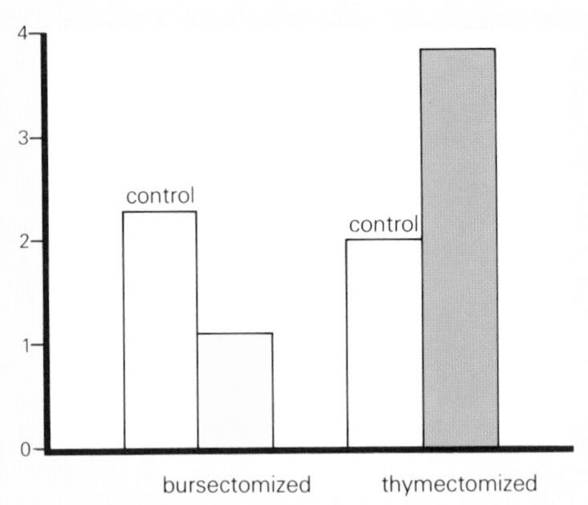

Fig. 23.17 Modification of thyroiditis in OS chickens by neonatal bursectomy and thymectomy. Neonatal bursectomy reduces the spontaneous development of thyroiditis suggesting an important role for antibody in the pathogenesis of the lesions. Paradoxically, removal of the thymus at birth exacerbates the disease indicating a controlling effect of T-suppressor cells. The severity of thyroiditis is assessed by lymphocyte infiltration.

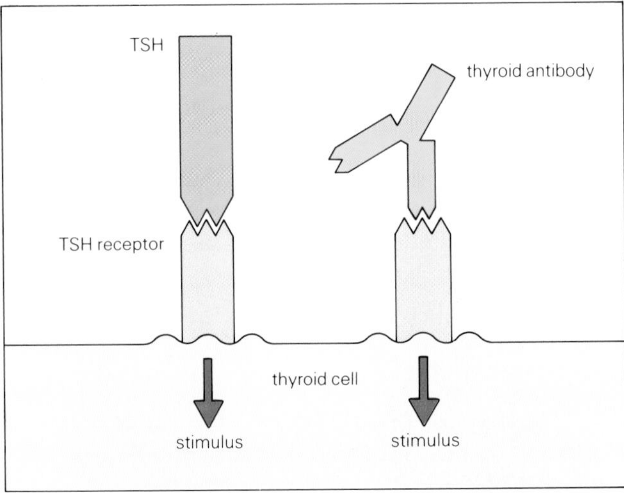

Fig. 23.18 Autoimmunity to cell surface receptors. The thyroid cell is stimulated when its receptors for thyroid stimulating hormone (TSH) from the pituitary, bind the hormone (left). Antibody to the TSH receptor present in the serum of a patient with thyrotoxicosis (Graves' or Basedow's disease) combines with the receptor in a similar fashion to pituitary TSH thereby delivering a comparable stimulus to the thyroid cell (right).

function of the normal hormone concerned (Fig. 23.18). Thyrotoxicosis was perhaps the first disorder in which anti-receptor antibodies were clearly recognized. The phenomenon of neonatal thyrotoxicosis provides us with a 'natural' passive transfer study in which the IgG antibodies from the mother can cross the placenta; if these antibodies are capable of acting *in vivo,* they should stimulate the thyroid of the baby. Indeed, many babies born to thyrotoxic mothers and showing thyroid hyperactivity have been reported (Fig. 23.19). As might be expected, the overactivity of the thyroid spontaneously resolves as the maternally derived thyroid stimulating IgG is catabolized in the baby over several weeks. A similar phenomenon has been observed in neonatal myasthenia gravis, where antibodies to acetylcholine receptors cross the placenta into the fetus and cause transient muscle weakness. Somewhat rarely, autoantibodies to insulin and to β-adrenergic receptors can be found, the latter occurring in a minority of patients with bronchial asthma.

Yet another example of autoimmune disease is seen in rare cases of male infertility where antibodies to spermatozoa lead to clumping of spermatozoa, either by their heads or by their tails, in the semen (Fig. 23.20). It is surely difficult to imagine that spermatozoa in this stage of aggregation are capable of the hard swim required to fertilize the ovum. A small proportion of cases of male infertility have been attributed to this cause.

In pernicious anaemia, an autoantibody interferes with the normal uptake of oral vitamin B_{12}. Vitamin B_{12} is not absorbed directly, but must first associate with a protein called intrinsic factor; the complex is then transported across the intestinal mucosa. Early studies of pernicious anaemia demonstrated that the intrinsic factor-mediated uptake of oral vitamin B_{12} could be inhibited if the intrinsic factor–B_{12} complex was fed together with serum from the patient. Evidently, there is a factor (antibody) in the serum of patients with pernicious anaemia which blocks the uptake of the vitamin B_{12}–intrinsic factor complex. It is known that plasma cells in the gastric mucosa of patients with pernicious anaemia secrete antibodies directed against intrinsic factor into the lumen of the stomach and it therefore seems probable, from the results of these experiments, that these antibodies mixed with intrinsic factor derived from parietal cells block the physiological action of intrinsic factor in transporting dietary vitamin B_{12} into the body (Fig. 23.21).

An excellent study bearing on the point in question, was carried out in Goodpasture's syndrome in which antibodies to the glomerular capillary basement membrane are bound to the kidney *in vivo* (see Fig. 21.3). These antibodies were eluted from the kidney of a patient who had died with this disease and transferred to a primate whose antigens were sufficiently similar to those of the human for the injected antibodies to localize on the glomerular basement membrane. The injected monkeys subsequently died with glomerulonephritis which was the cause of death in the original patient.

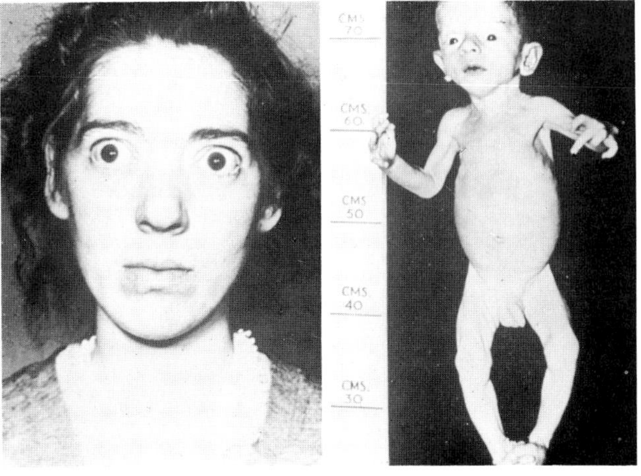

Fig. 23.19 Neonatal thyrotoxicosis. The TSH-receptor autoantibodies are IgG and therefore cross the placenta. If they act *in vivo* the baby should show evidence of thyroid stimulation. The appearances of both the mother and child shown above are characteristic of thyrotoxicosis.

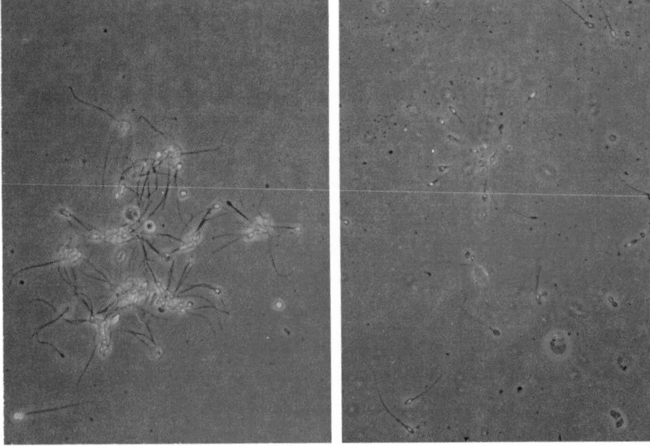

Fig. 23.20 Serum agglutination. The presence of sperm autoagglutinins produces either head-to-head (left) or tail-to-tail (right) agglutination.

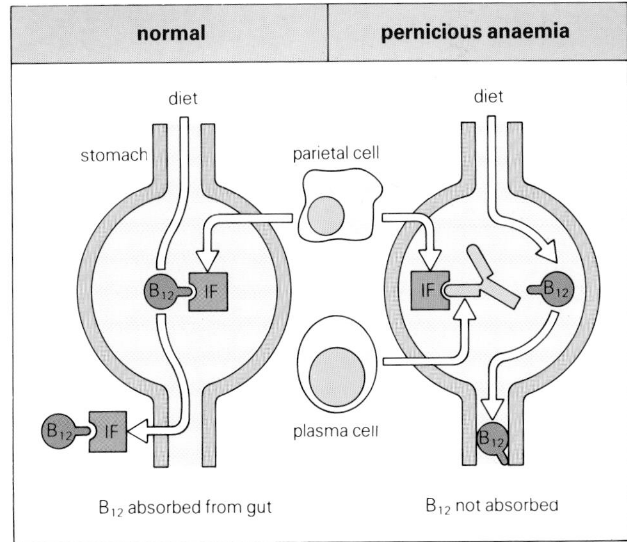

Fig. 23.21 Failure of vitamin B_{12} absorption in pernicious anaemia. Normally, dietary vitamin B_{12} is transported across the small intestine into the body as a complex with intrinsic factor, which is synthesized by the parietal cells in the gastric mucosa. In pernicious anaemia, locally synthesized autoantibodies which are specific for intrinsic factor occur in the gastric juice and combine with intrinsic factor to inhibit its role as a carrier for vitamin B_{12}; as a result vitamin B_{12} cannot be absorbed.

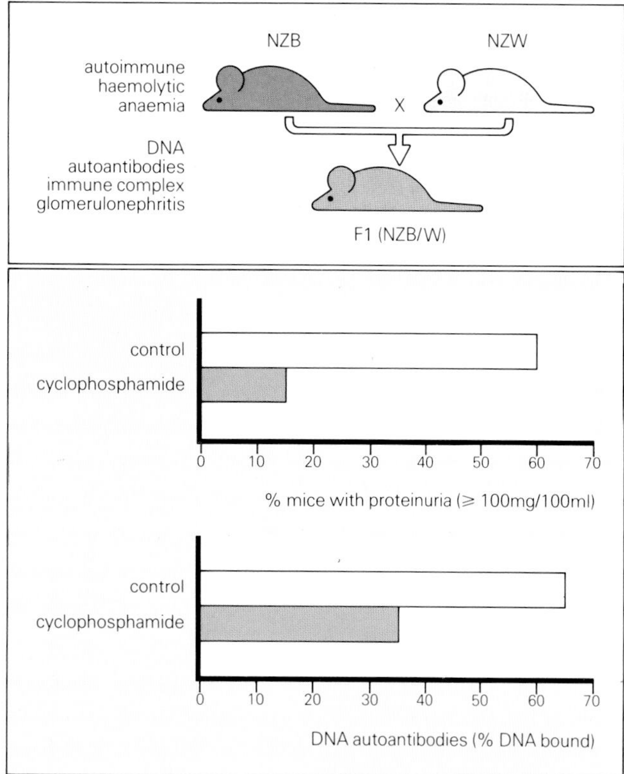

Fig. 23.22 Suppression of autoimmune disease in NZB/W hybrid mice. The New Zealand Black spontaneously develops autoimmune haemolytic anaemia and when crossed with the New Zealand White strain, the F1 develops DNA autoantibodies and immune complex glomerulonephritis like patients with SLE. Immunosuppression with cyclophosphamide (an anti-mitotic agent) considerably reduces the severity of the glomerulonephritis and the amount of DNA autoantibodies showing the relevance of the immune processes to the generation of the disease.

In contrast to the linear staining seen in Goodpasture's syndrome, kidney biopsies from patients with SLE show punctate staining of irregular deposits using fluorescent anti-human IgG (see Fig. 21.3).

Autoantigenic complexes deposited in the kidney of patients with SLE produce the hypersensitivity reactions outlined in Chapter 21. Glomerulonephritis and proteinuria can be induced by repeated injections of high doses of antigen which lead to chronic immune complex disease and deposition in the kidney. Even a single large dose of antigen can produce acute kidney damage, as occurs in serum sickness.

Turning to experimental animals, the hybrid of the New Zealand black and white strains of mice provides a spontaneous model of murine SLE in which immune complex glomerulonephritis and anti-DNA antibodies are major features (see Chapter 11). What is particularly relevant to our argument is that measures which suppress the immune response in these animals, for example the drug cyclophosphamide, likewise suppress the development of disease and prolong the survival of these mice (Fig. 23.22).

These studies provide powerful evidence that in many circumstances the autoimmune process appears to play a dominant role in the causation of disease.

AETIOLOGY

The aetiology of autoimmune disease can be considered only in relation to the mechanisms by which an individual maintains tolerance to self molecules. These mechanisms, which are detailed in Chapter 12, include:

1. isolation of the autoantigen from the immune system
2. deletion of the autoreactive T cell clones during development
3. absence of processing and presentation of self molecules
4. the action of T-suppressor cells in damping autoimmune responses.

evidence for self-reactive lymphocytes
thyroglobulin in Complete Freund's Adjuvant (CFA) and other adjuvants (e.g. lipopolysaccharide, poly A:U) induces autoimmunitv in normal animals
small percentage of normal B cells bind self-thyroglobulin to surface
brain specific T cell line from normal rat induces encephalomyelitis
lymphocytes cultured with syngeneic testes or thyroid become autosensitized

Fig. 23.23 Evidence for self-reactive lymphocytes.

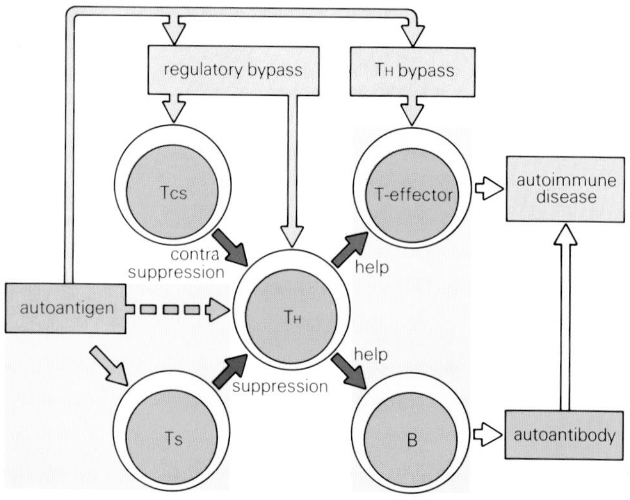

Fig. 23.24 Autoimmune disease resulting from evasion of the controls on autoreactivity. Self-reactive B cells, T- effector cells and autoantigens are all normally present (indicated in this and later figures by blue backshading), but T-helper (T_H) cells capable of inducing an autoimmune response are functionally absent, due either to clonal abortion or to the action of T-suppressor (T_S) cells (T_S antigen-, idiotype-, or non-specific). Thus the self-reactive T cells and B cells are not activated. (Idiotype-specific T_S cells may also act directly on B cells.) Autoimmunity may arise by a regulatory bypass which either causes direct activation of the T_H cell or, by activating another cell, the T-contrasuppressor (T_{CS}), renders the T_H cell resistant to suppression. The existence of contrasuppressors is still equivocal. Autoantigen could also bypass the T_H cell to directly stimulate T-effectors and B cells.

Some of these mechanisms are relevant for some autoantigens, and some for others. This section examines how these controls may be circumvented.

It is now generally accepted that self-reactive lymphocytes exist in the body for many potential autoantigens, and some of the evidence for this is listed in Fig. 23.23. In addition, many proteins previously thought to be isolated from the immune system, for example thyroglobulin, are now known to be available to the recirculating lymphocyte pool. This leads to a situation in which both self-reactive lymphocytes and autoantigen can make contact in the normal individual. For such antigens, autoreactivity must be controlled either by lack of antigen presentation or by T-suppressor cells. Fig. 23.24 outlines a possible scheme by which the normal controls on autoreactivity may be bypassed. These controls include different types of suppressor T cells, which go to make up a complex of T-suppressor activity. This subject is discussed more fully in Chapter 12. It has been postulated that defects in perhaps more than one type of T-suppressor cell may be important for the development of an autoimmune response. It is interesting to note that studies on the clinically unaffected relatives of patients with SLE have shown that these individuals share with the patients themselves a defect in the generation of non-specific T-suppressor cells, suggesting first that the defect is not a consequence of the disease, and secondly that it is unable by itself to cause SLE. This is consistent with the previous discussion suggesting that several factors may be implicated in the causation of autoimmune disease, and it may be necessary to postulate further abnormalities in either antigen-specific or idiotype-specific regulatory T cells.

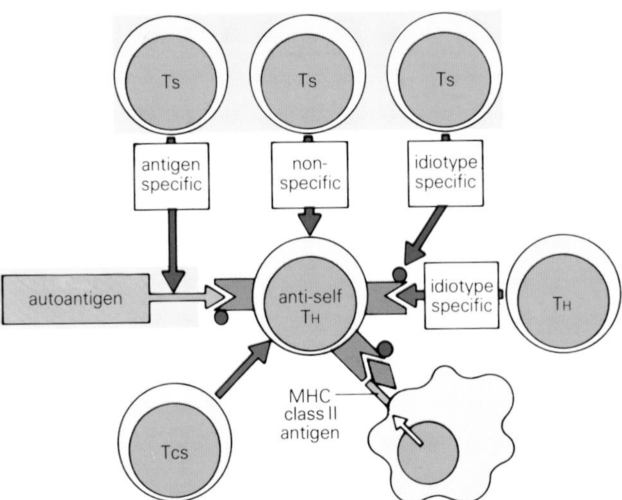

Fig. 23.25 Induction of autoimmunity through bypass of regulatory mechanisms. The anti-self T-helper (TH) cell may be triggered through defects in antigen-specific T-suppressor (Ts) cells, non-specific Ts cells, or idiotype-specific Ts cells, which would counteract the action of idiotype-specific TH cells. (There is evidence that the various types of Ts cell may induce the activity of the others via soluble factors.) Stimulation of contrasuppressors (Tcs) can render the anti-self TH cells insusceptible to suppression, while the inappropriate cellular expression of MHC class II antigens on a cell carrying an autoantigen could convert that cell into an antigen-presenting cell to the autoreactive TH cell. In this scheme an idiotype-specific TH cell is shown acting via the idiotype on the anti-self TH cell.

Another important factor in the maintenance of self-tolerance must be the inability of autoreactive T-helper cells to recognize potentially autoantigenic molecules on cells which do not normally express MHC class II genes. In these circumstances 'immunological silence' prevails because these T cells can only recognize antigen when it is presented in association with class II molecules. This 'immunological silence' could be broken by inappropriate expression of class II; it was therefore most exciting when cells in thyrotoxic thyroiditis were found to be actively synthesizing class II MHC molecules. In effect the tissue cells could now act as antigen presenters (Fig. 23.25).

Subsequently it has been shown that normal human thyroid cells could be induced to derepress their class II genes by treatment with interferon-γ. We are thus presented with an unresolved conundrum – is autoimmunity initiated by some non-T cell factor causing inappropriate class II expression, or is the class II expression induced by a pre-existing autoimmunity, in which case it could contribute to the continuation of the pathogenetic process.

These are not the only possibilities however, and other not necessarily exclusive factors could operate. Particular interest was aroused by the suggestions of Allison and Weigle that a T cell bypass mechanism might operate. They argued that since the unresponsiveness of the

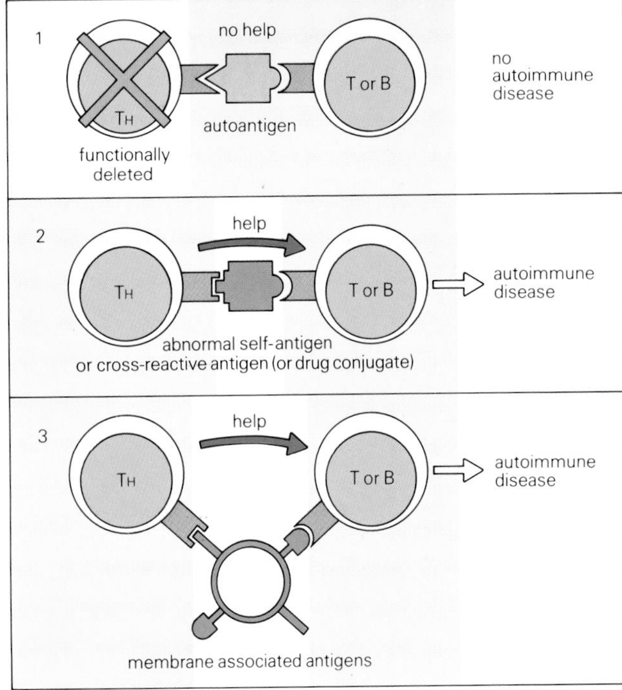

Fig. 23.26 Induction of autoimmunity by T cell bypass – I. Normally autoimmune disease does not occur since T cells reacting with autoantigen are functionally deleted or suppressed (1). In the presence of a cross-reacting antigen, a new population of T-helper (TH) cells reacting with a foreign carrier determinant can supply help (2). The binding of a drug to self-antigen may also act as the carrier determinant recognized by the TH cells. Another possibility is that the autoantigen can be structurally altered through abnormalities in synthesis or processing. The new carrier determinant can either be on a molecule which also bears the autoantigenic determinant (as in 2), or it can be on a different molecule associated with the autoantigen on a cell membrane (3).

final effector T and B cells could be a consequence of suppression or tolerization of the autoantigen-specific T-helper cells (inducer T cells), any circumstances leading to the circumvention of these tolerant T cells would lead directly to the triggering of effector lymphocytes. A number of different ways in which this could be achieved are outlined in Figs 23.26–23.28. For simplicity these diagrams show T cells and B cells interacting via antigen bridges, though in reality the T cell would probably recognize processed antigen on the B cell surface.

A disease in which this mechanism appears to operate is rheumatic fever, in which autoantibodies to heart can be detected. This condition occurs in a small proportion of individuals several weeks after a streptococcal infection of the throat. Carbohydrate antigens on the streptococci cross-react with an antigen on heart valves, so the infection may bypass T cell self-tolerance to heart valve antigens. Pertinent to Fig. 23.26 is the intriguing recent discovery that IgG in patients with rheumatoid arthritis shows defective addition of galactose to the Fc region oligosaccharides, probably as a result of lowered galactosyl transferase in the B cells. This gives added impetus to the view that abnormal sensitization to IgG in rheumatoid arthritis is a major factor contributing to the chronic synovial inflammatory process.

A novel idea presented in Fig. 23.28 suggests that the idiotype network could be involved through the triggering of a self-reactive T or B cell carrying a public idiotype cross-reacting with the idiotype on an antibody stimulated by a microbial agent, or with a structure on the microbe itself. Even in this case, it seems unlikely that the autoimmune response would be maintained unless there was some defect in the anti-idiotypic T-suppressor cell; this re-emphasizes the considerable importance of multiple factors in the establishment of prolonged autoimmunity.

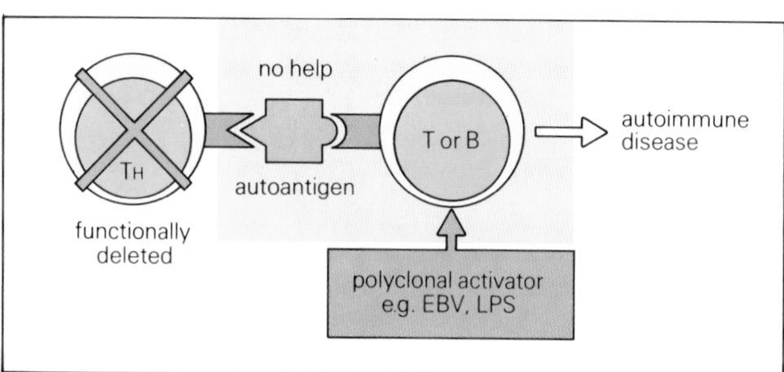

Fig. 23.27 Induction of autoimmunity by T cell bypass–2. Self-reactive cells can be stimulated directly by polyclonal activators, for example Epstein-Barr virus or bacterial lipopolysaccharides.

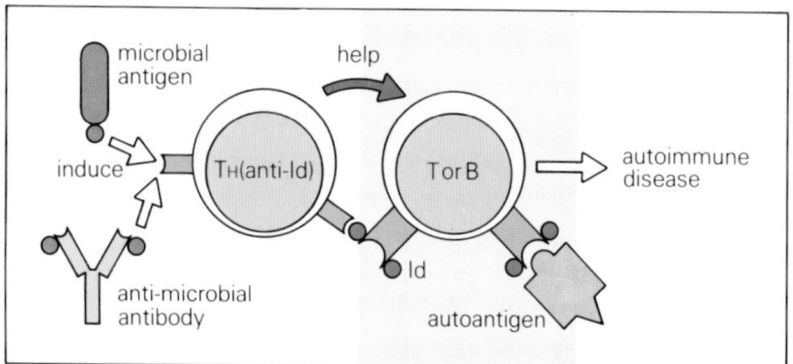

Fig. 23.28 Induction of autoimmunity by stimulation via idiotype. Autoimmunity could arise if self-reactive T or B cells carry a public idiotype (Id) which cross-reacts with the idiotype on antibody stimulated by a microbial agent or even with a structure on the microbe itself.

DIAGNOSTIC AND PROGNOSTIC ASPECTS

Whatever the relationship of autoantibodies to the disease process, they undeniably provide valuable markers which can be exploited for diagnostic purposes. In the clinical immunology laboratory of today, tests for a wide range of different autoantibodies are carried out with this end in view. A particularly good example is the test for mitochondrial antibodies for diagnosing primary biliary cirrhosis (Fig. 23.29); the need for exploratory laparotomy which was previously necessary to obtain this diagnosis, and was often hazardous because of the age and condition of the patients concerned, is consequently avoided.

Autoantibodies may also have a predictive value, as shown in Fig. 23.30. In this example, a child related to siblings with insulin-dependent diabetes mellitus shared an HLA haplotype with them, developed complement fixing antibodies to the islet cells of the pancreas,

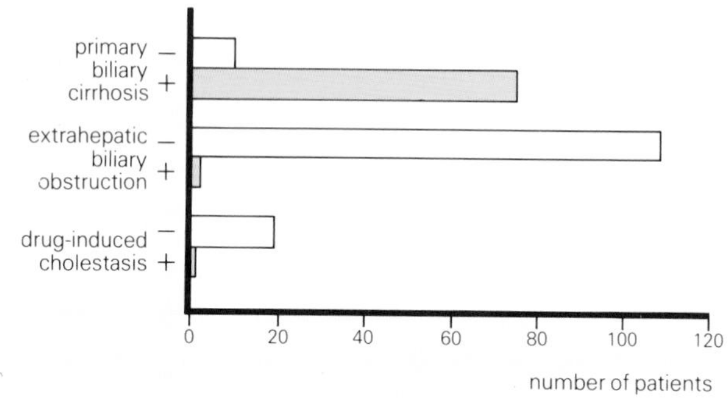

Fig. 23.29 Diagnostic value of anti-mitochondrial antibodies. Mitochondrial antibody tests using indirect immunofluorescence together with percutaneous liver biopsy can be used to assist in the differential diagnosis of the diseases listed above. A large proportion of patients with primary biliary cirrhosis have antimitochondrial antibodies but this is rare in the other diseases.

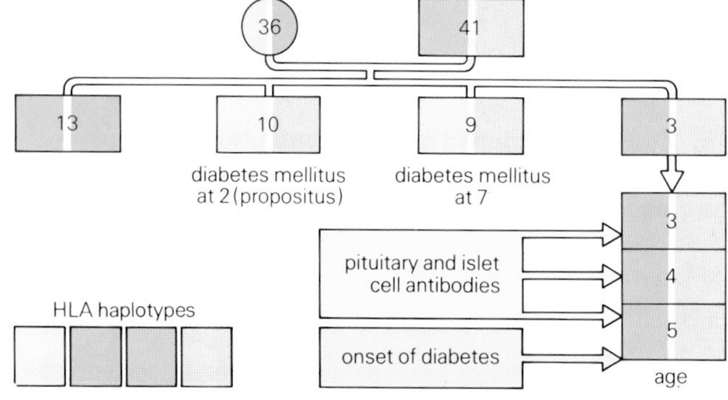

Fig. 23.30 Prospective study of a family with insulin-dependent diabetes mellitus. The sibling sharing a haplotype with the propositus and having complement fixing islet cell antibodies became diabetic 3 years after the study had begun.

and within 3 years after the study had begun, had become frankly diabetic. This illustrates the predictive value of these antibodies and the relatively long period of time before the disease becomes overt.

TREATMENT

Conventionally, in organ specific disorders, the lesion can often be corrected by metabolic control. For example, in hypothyroidism the lack of thyroid hormone can be controlled by administration of thyroxine, while in thyrotoxicosis, antithyroid drugs are normally prescribed. In pernicious anaemia, metabolic correction is achieved by injection of depot vitamin B_{12}, and in myasthenia gravis, by administration of cholinesterase inhibitors. Where function is lost and cannot be substituted by hormones, as may occur in lupus nephritis or chronic rheumatoid arthritis, mechanical or tissue grafts may be appropriate, though in the case of tissue grafts, protection from the immunological processes which originally necessitated the transplant may be required.

Conventional immunosuppressive therapy with anti-mitotic drugs may be employed to damp down the immune response, but because of the dangers involved, this tends to be used only in life-threatening disorders such as SLE and dermatomyositis. The potential of cyclosporin and possible derivatives in the therapy of autoimmune diseases has yet to be fully realized but quite dramatic results have been reported in the treatment of type I diabetes mellitus. Anti-inflammatory drugs are, of course, prescribed for rheumatoid disease.

As we understand more about the precise defects in different autoimmune diseases and learn how to manipulate the immunological status of the patient, a number of the less well established approaches may become practical (Fig. 23.31). In particular, the successful treatment of experimental autoimmune disease by 'vaccination' with antigen-specific T cell clones suggests that the exploitation of the idiotype network to inhibit the idiotypes on T-inducer and effector cells could prove to be a promising approach.

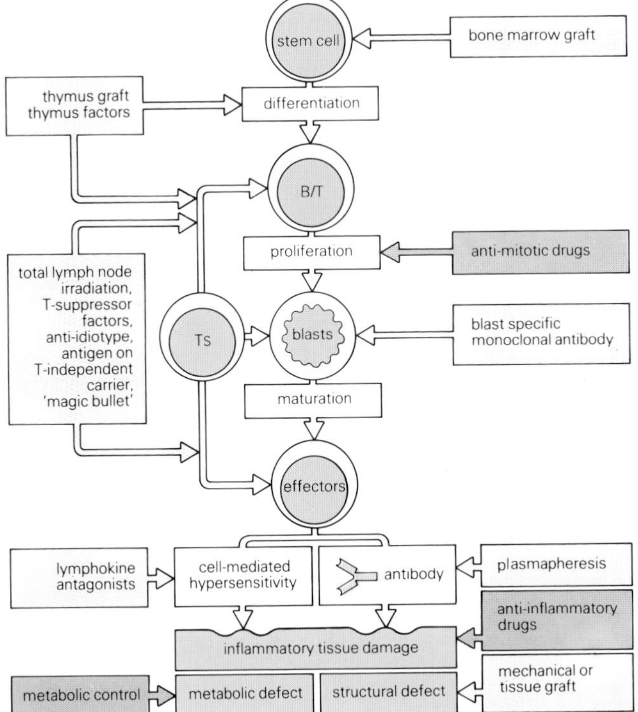

Fig. 23.31 The treatment of autoimmune disease. Current treatments for arresting the pathological developments in autoimmune disease are shown in dark grey, and those that may become feasible, in light grey. For example, anti-mitotic drugs are given in severe cases of systemic lupus erythematosus or chronic active hepatitis. Anti-inflammatory drugs are widely prescribed in rheumatoid arthritis. Organ specific disorders which lead to a metabolic defect, for example primary myxoedema or pernicious anaemia, can usually be treated by supplying the defective component; in these examples, thyroid hormone and depot vitamin B_{12}. Where a live graft becomes necessary, the immunosuppressive therapy used may protect the tissue from autoimmune damage.

POSITIVE INDUCTION OF AUTOIMMUNITY

There are areas in which the deliberate induction of an autoimmune response would be desirable (Fig. 23.32). Although these represent academically feasible enterprises, the major (but not the only) problems in man concern the identification of the correct autoreactive epitopes which do not cross-react with other autoantigens, the attachment to an effective carrier, and the identification of an acceptable adjuvant.

target	purpose
1. human chorionic gonadotrophin	control of fertility
2. LHRH	pseudocastration (cattle)
3. tumours	immunotherapy
4. idiotype	manipulation of the immune response

Fig. 23.32 Positive induction of autoimmunity.
1. Human chorionic gonadotrophin (HCG) is necessary for the maintenance of the implanted ovum at an early stage in pregnancy. Autoimmunization to the unique determinants on HCG (not shared with pituitary hormones such as LH) by coupling to a carrier such as tetanus toxoid provides a basis for a possible contraceptive vaccine.
2. Neutralization of the releasing hormone for LH by autoimmunization can produce pseudocastration in cattle.
3. The destruction of tumours through identification and exploration of tumour-specific antigens has long been a 'holy grail' for cancer immunologists.
4. Monoclonal anti-idiotypes may well have a potential for either boosting or damping down immune responses.

FURTHER READING

Brochier, J., Clot, J. & Sany, J (eds) (1986) Anti-Ia antibodies in treatment of autoimmune disease. *Immune Intervention, 2*. London: Academic Press.

Cinader, B. & Miller, R.G. (eds) (1987) *Progress in Immunology VI*. USA: Academic Press.

Lachmann, P.J. & Peters, D.K. (eds) (1982) *Clinical Aspects of Immunology,* 4th edition. Oxford: Blackwell Scientific Publications.

McGregor, A.M. (ed.) (1986) *Immunology of Endocrine Diseases*. Lancaster: MTP Press.

Morrow, J. & Isenberg, D.A. (eds) (1987) *Autoimmune Rheumatic Disease*. Oxford: Blackwell Scientific Publications.

Schwartz, R.S. & Rose, N.R. (eds) (1986) Autoimmunity: experimental and clinical aspects. *Annals of the New York Academy of Sciences,* **475**.

Sites, D.P., Stobo, J.D., Fudenberg, H.H. & Wells, J.V. (1987) *Basic and Clinical Immunology,* 6th edition. California: Lange Medical Publications.

24 Transplantation and Rejection

Tissue transplantation is the third area (after hypersensitivity and autoimmunity) in which the immune system acts detrimentally. The phenomenon of graft rejection between unrelated individuals has been recognized for a long time but it is only since the 1950s that this has been shown to be due to the adaptive immune system.

Graft rejection displays the two key features of adaptive immunity, namely memory and specificity. These characteristics can be demonstrated by grafting skin from one animal to another. Memory is demonstrated when a second allogeneic skin graft from one donor is rejected by the recipient more quickly than the first graft from that donor. This accelerated rejection is specific for the one donor – it is observed that grafts from other individuals applied at the same time do not suffer faster rejection (Fig. 24.1). These two types of rejection reaction are referred to as 'first set' and 'second set' reactions.

Only sites in the recipient which are accessible to the immune system are susceptible to the graft rejection phenomenon. There are certain 'privileged' sites in the body where allogeneic grafts can survive indefinitely. It is also found that the ability to reject grafts can be transferred with previously sensitized lymphocytes. These, and many other observations, confirm the responsibility of the immune system for graft rejection. In view of the unphysiological nature of tissue transplantation it may seem surprising that the immune system has thrown such a formidable barrier in the path of transplantation surgery, but it appears that this is an unfortunate side-effect of a system which has evolved to recognize and destroy virally altered cells.

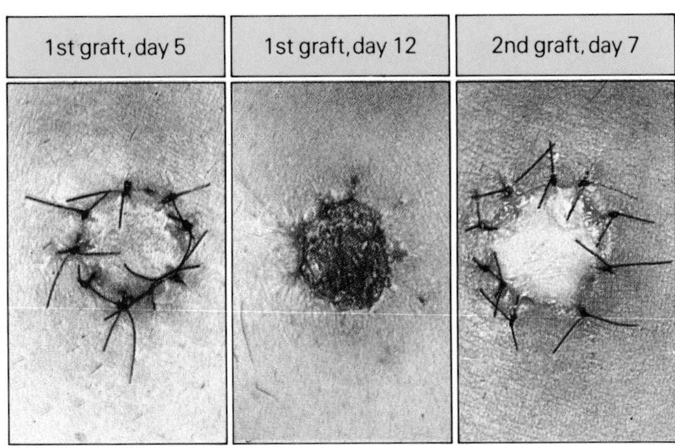

Fig. 24.1 Graft rejection displays immunological memory. A human skin allograft at day 5 (left) is fully vascularized and the cells are dividing, but by day 12 it is totally destroyed (middle). A second graft from the same donor (right) shown here on day 7 does not become vascularized and is destroyed rapidly. This indicates that sensitization to the first graft produces immunological memory.

GENETICS OF TRANSPLANTATION

In 1914 Little proposed that successful transplantation would depend on the donor and recipient sharing a number of independently segregating alleles, in effect histocompatibility genes. This hypothesis has been confirmed in all mammalian species studied, a process which was greatly facilitated by the development of haplotype identical inbred strains of mice (see Chapter 4). Grafting between such isogeneic mouse strains showed that animals could reject any graft carrying allogeneic histocompatibility determinants and would accept any graft that did not have allogeneic determinants (Fig. 24.2). These observations also confirm that histocompatibility genes are co-dominantly expressed in the F1 animals.

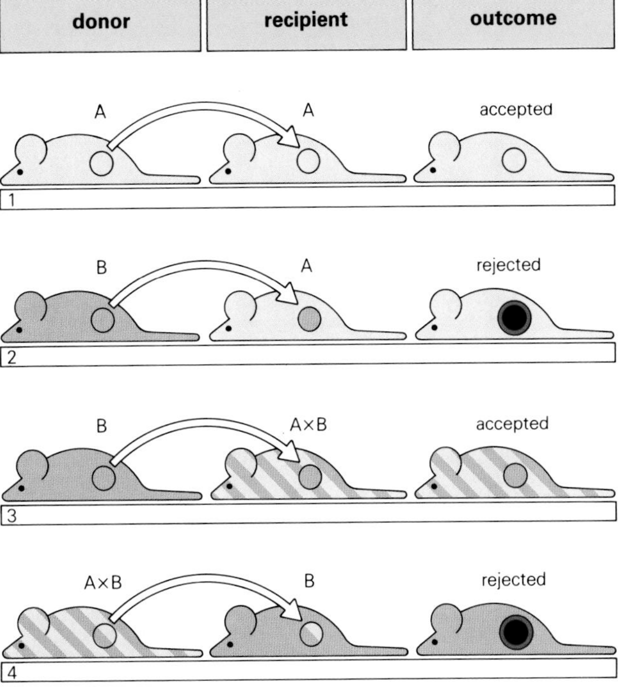

Fig. 24.2 The laws of transplantation. Grafts between genetically identical animals are accepted. Grafts between genetically non-identical animals are rejected with a speed which is dependent on where the genetic differences lie. For example, syngeneic animals which are identical at the MHC locus, accept grafts from each other (1). Animals which differ at the MHC locus reject grafts from each other (2). The ability to accept a graft is dependent on the recipient sharing all the donor's histocompatibility genes. This is illustrated by grafting between parental and F1 (A × B) animals (3 and 4). Animals which differ at loci other than the MHC reject grafts from each other, but much more slowly.

In special circumstances there are exceptions to these simple rules. The first is seen where animals have been tolerized to the donor tissue either by having encountered the donor tissue antigens during neonatal life, or through immunopharmacological manipulation as described in Chapter 12. Indeed, the ability to accept grafts between allogeneic individuals is viewed as the most stringent criterion of immunological tolerance to allogeneic tissue. The second exception can be seen when immunocompetent cells are transferred from a donor to an allogeneic recipient which is incapable of reacting against them. In this case the donor cells react to the recipient's tissues, particularly those of the skin, gut epithelia and the liver, and may destroy them. This is known as graft versus host (GVH) disease (Fig. 24.3). The precise mechanism by which the recipient's cells are damaged is uncertain since many of the cells seen at the sites of damage are of recipient origin. Nevertheless, the condition is frequently fatal and GVH disease is a problem particularly associated with bone marrow transplantation, where total obliteration of the host responsiveness is necessary to enable the graft to take. Less severe GVH disease has however also been reported after other types of transplantation especially heart and liver transplants. Removal of T cells from donor marrow can prevent GVH reactions. However this has two particularly interesting corollaries:

1. the percentage of successful transplants is lower
2. there is a higher recurrence rate for tumours in the host, presumably because GVH cytotoxicity is an effective mechanism for suppressing tumour cell expansion.

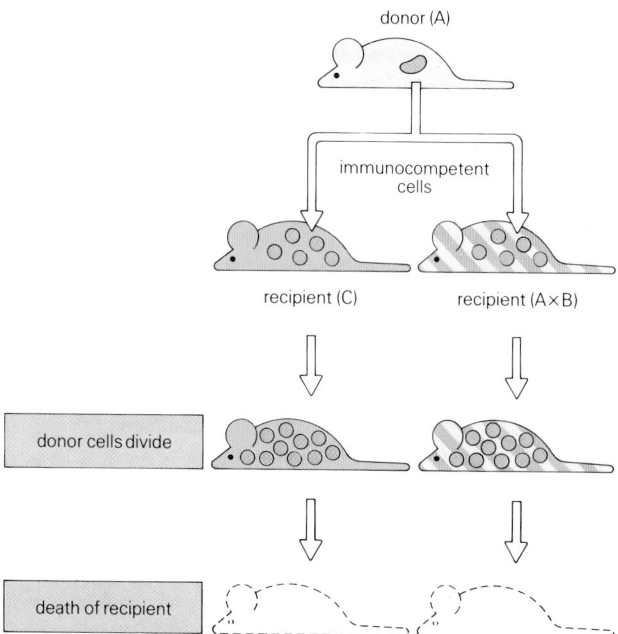

Fig. 24.3 Graft versus host disease. Immunocompetent cells from a donor of type 'A' are injected into an immunosuppressed (X-irradiated) host of type 'C' or a normal F1 (A × B) recipient. The immunosuppressed individual is unable to reject the cells and the F1 animal is fully tolerant to parental type 'A' cells. In both cases the donor cells recognize the foreign tissue types 'B' and 'C' of the recipient. They divide and react against the recipient tissue cells and recruit large numbers of host cells to inflammatory sites. Very often the process leads to the death of the recipient.

HISTOCOMPATIBILITY GENES

Genetic studies on the segregation of histocompatibility genes have demonstrated a large number of independently segregating loci in all species. As many as 30 different loci have been identified in mice designated H-1, H-2, etc. However, in all species there is one locus, the major histocompatibility complex (MHC), which elicits stronger allogeneic reactions than the others. With the discovery of the importance of the MHC in many other immune reactions, the minor histocompatibility loci have been less well studied. Nevertheless, second set allogeneic rejection reactions to minor locus antigens, or to minor locus differences may be as fast as to an MHC allogeneic graft (Fig. 24.4). In man, approximately 50% of kidney grafts between HLA-matched siblings are rejected after 5 years suggesting that in man also, minor loci differences are sufficient to cause rejection. In spite of this, the major obstacle to successful transplantation is the MHC, since rejection arising from allogeneic differences of minor loci can usually be overcome by immunosuppressive therapy provided the recipient has not been previously sensitized to the minor locus antigens.

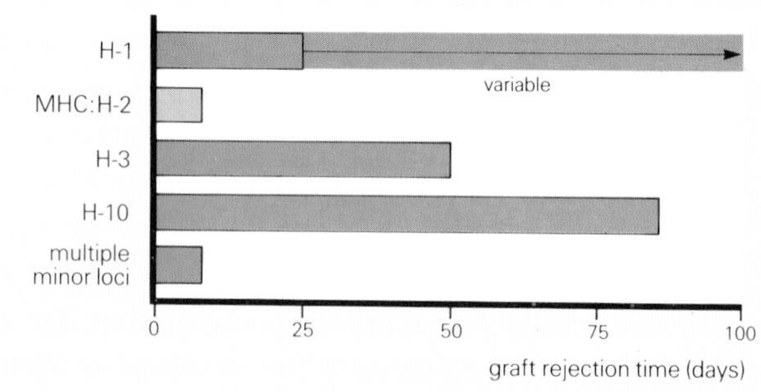

Fig. 24.4 Histocompatibility antigens and graft survival. This chart gives the rejection time for skin grafts between mice differing at the minor histocompatibility loci (red) or at the MHC locus (H-2) (blue) listed. Grafts which differ at multiple minor loci are rejected as quickly as those that differ at H-2. (Data from Graff & Bailey.)

ALLOGENEIC RECOGNITION

Allogeneic MHC molecules are highly immunogenic. They do not necessarily have to be recognized in association with self MHC molecules in order to stimulate T cells and they appear to be able to provide the dual signal of self MHC plus antigen. It is notable that some clones of T cells which can recognize antigen in association with self MHC molecules can also react against allogeneic MHC molecules. For example, one clone of mouse Tc cells recognizes myoglobin in association with $H\text{-}2^k$ and also responds to $H\text{-}2^b$ allogeneic cells. Such findings confirm the proposal that T cells can see allogeneic MHC in the same way as self MHC plus antigen, and also suggest that these cells are not exclusively alloreactive, but contribute to the T cell repertoire which recognizes foreign antigens. The number of T cells which can recognize a particular allogeneic MHC in unprimed animals is relatively high, perhaps as great as 0.1% of the total T cell pool.

The precise way in which allogeneic recognition occurs is still debated. One hypothesis proposes that fragments of allogeneic MHC molecules are processed in the same way as conventional antigens and are then presented in association with self molecules by antigen-presenting cells. A second hypothesis supported by the evidence above states that the T cells react directly with the foreign MHC molecules. One recent suggestion is that self MHC molecules normally carry a self peptide in the cleft of their binding sites and that this may become displaced by processed antigen, which is then recognized by T cells. A self peptide occupying the cleft could in the same way be recognized as an antigen by an allogeneic T cell.

In clinical transplantation, allogeneic recognition is considerably more complicated than recognition *in vitro*. As will be discussed below it seems clear that class I and II molecules present on dendritic cells in the graft provide the primary stimulus for the host immune response, with the class II molecules presenting class I. How this occurs in practice is less clear since one would expect the best presentation and the most vigorous graft rejection by matched class II and allogeneic class I, but this does not occur. Initial studies indicated the value of matching MHC molecules between donor and recipient and it appeared that matching class II molecules was particularly important for graft survival (Fig. 24.5). These findings have now been extended and analysed further to show that fully matched HLA–B and HLA–DR grafts do better than all other groups, and there are no significant differences between the other groups. In cases where a graft with several mismatches is rejected, antibody responses are not observed to all the mismatches. It is as if an HLA–B or HLA–DR mismatched graft causes the immune system to become activated to a particular level of aggression and that this is channelled to any class I differences which are present. The class I system is so polymorphic that there is less than a 1/40,000 chance of a full match between random individuals, and it has been shown in model systems that a single amino acid difference is sufficient to channel an allogeneic response.

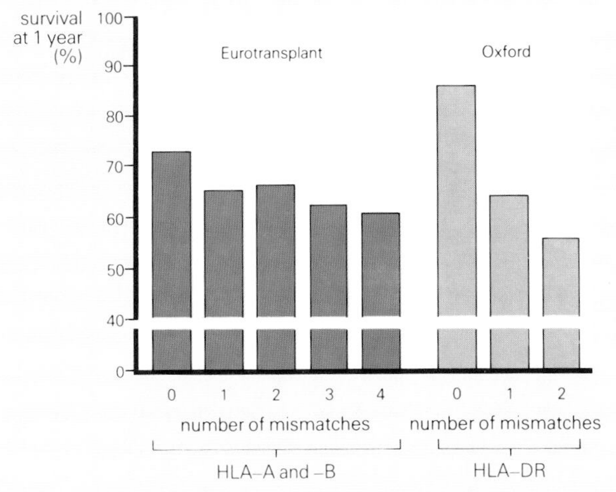

Fig. 24.5 Kidney graft survival and HLA matching. The bar chart shows the percentage survival of cadaver kidney grafts at 12 months in humans in two separate studies. In the first study (Eurotransplant), donors were matched as far as possible for the HLA–A and –B antigens (class I). In the second study (Oxford), the donors were matched for HLA–DR antigens (class II). Note that the fewer mismatches present, the greater the number of grafts surviving in both studies, but that DR matching has a greater effect on survival; the best results were obtained when the grafts were fully matched for HLA–DR and –B.

MECHANISMS OF GRAFT REJECTION

THE ROLE OF T CELLS

Evidence has accumulated which indicates that the T cell is mainly responsible for rejection of solid grafts. First, nude mice do not reject foreign skin grafts. It is even possible to give nude mice xenogeneic grafts (that is, from a different species) which are still accepted.

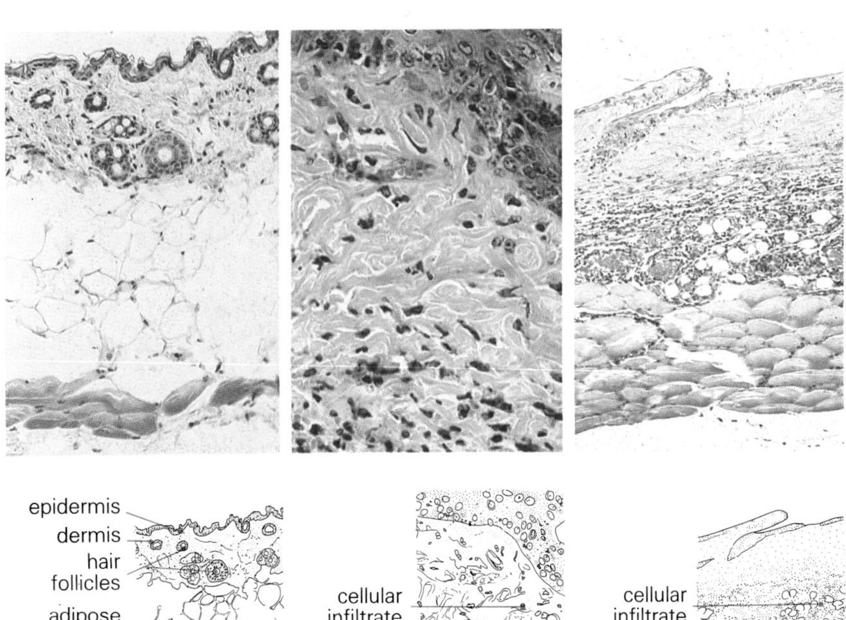

Fig. 24.6 Sections of strain A mouse skin showing the normal appearance (left) and the allograft 5 days (middle) and 12 days (right) after transplantation to a CBA host. At 5 days there is a substantial infiltration by host mononuclear cells. At 12 days the epithelium has been totally destroyed and is lifting off the dermis, which is now free of cells; the infiltrating host cells have been destroyed by anoxia but there is still a brisk cellular traffic in the graft bed between the dermis and the panniculus carnosus. (Courtesy of Professor L. Brent.)

Furthermore, it appears that the T cells alone are sufficient to cause graft rejection since neonatally bursectomized chickens, which totally lack B cells, are still able to reject allogeneic grafts. This does not mean that antibody has no role in graft rejection. As indicated below, antibody can cause rapid graft rejection but it usually plays a lesser role than cell-mediated immunity except in some cases where the recipient has been previously sensitized to particular donor antigens, or in reactions to haemopoietic cells.

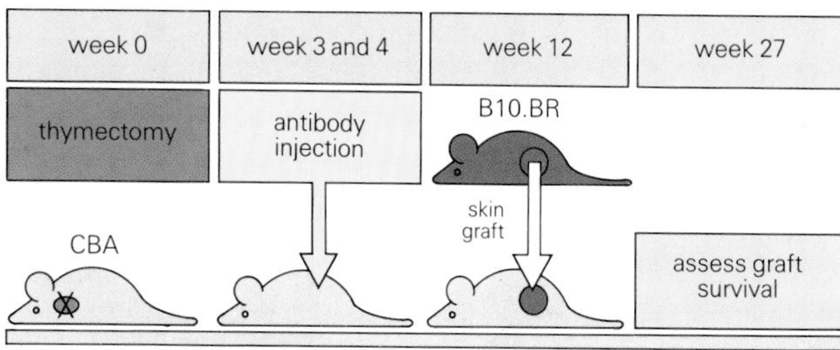

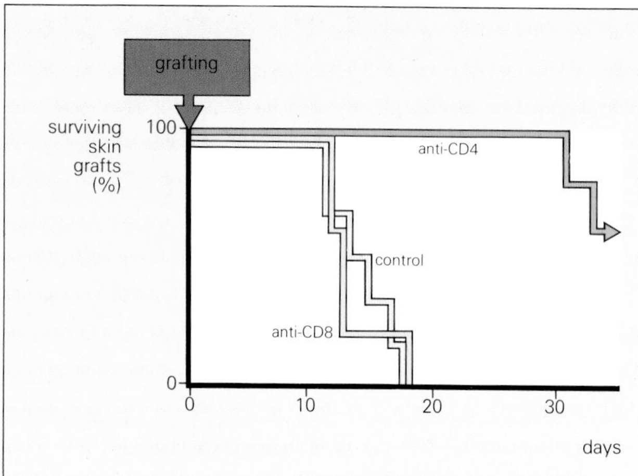

Fig. 24.7 Role of T cells in graft rejection. Thymectomized CBA mice aged 6 weeks were treated with cytotoxic monoclonal antibodies to CD4 or CD8 to selectively deplete those T cell populations. They were then grafted with skin from B10.BR mice which differ at minor histocompatibility loci. The survival of the grafts was assessed. Animals treated with anti-CD4 had greatly extended graft survival by comparison with untreated animals (control) or those treated with anti-CD8. This emphasizes the importance of the CD4 population in graft rejection. (Based on data of Cobbold & colleagues.)

Histological examination of an allogeneic skin graft during rejection shows the dermis becoming infiltrated by mononuclear cells, many of which are small lymphocytes (Fig. 24.6). The accumulation of these lymphocytes precedes destruction of the graft by several days. It is assumed that these cells are responsible for graft rejection and for some time it was thought that graft destruction was effected by cytotoxic T cells. However several pieces of evidence point to the importance of $CD4^+$ cells in graft rejection. For example, rats made T cell deficient by adult thymectomy and irradiation, and then reconstituted with bone marrow cells are able to accept allogeneic skin grafts, but inoculation of these animals with $CD4^+$, $CD8^-$ T-helper cells restores alloreactivity. In another series of experiments, mice treated with anti-CD4 antibody showed delayed rejection or tolerance of skin allografts, whereas mice treated with anti-CD8 rejected the grafts at the same rate as control animals (Fig. 24.7). Furthermore, in H-Y-mediated allograft rejection in syngeneic mice the ability of female mice to reject male skin grafts was not related to their ability to generate H-Y-specific cytotoxic T cells. (The H-Y antigen complex is expressed on cells of male animals only.)

These observations have led to the idea that graft rejection may be a specialized form of response related to delayed hypersensitivity reactions, in which case the ultimate effector of graft destruction would be monocytes and macrophages which may be recruited to the site. On the other hand, a number of observations confirm the importance of $CD8^+$ cytotoxic T cells, particularly where the major difference between donor and recipient is at class I loci. An example of this is the observation that sublethally irradiated rats will reject heart allografts only if they are reconstituted with a cell population containing $CD8^+$ T cells. Moreover several experiments imply that graft cell destruction is specific for the allogeneic cells and does not affect nearby cells, this being more typical of cytotoxic T cell-mediated damage than the promiscuous damage produced by macrophage activation. These two mechanisms are presented in Fig. 24.8. It is likely that different mechanisms operate in different circumstances.

ANTIGEN PRESENTATION

Since allogeneic MHC antigens are capable of stimulating recipient T cells without needing to associate with host MHC antigens the graft cells

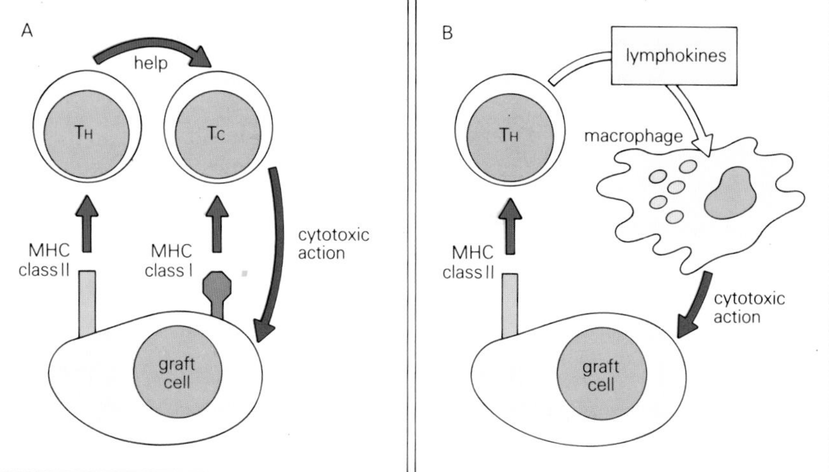

Fig. 24.8 Graft cell destruction. Two ways in which T cells may mediate graft cell destruction are illustrated. A. Foreign MHC class II antigens on the graft stimulate host T-helper (TH) cells to help cytotoxic T (Tc) cells destroy the target graft cell. Tc cells recognize the graft via the foreign MHC class I antigens. B. TH cells reacting to the graft release lymphokines, which stimulate macrophages to enter the graft and destroy it.

themselves are capable of eliciting rejection reactions. Allogeneic MHC molecules are most immunogenic when presented on viable cells; purified MHC antigens or membrane fragments containing the antigens are no more immunogenic than other non-MHC antigens. Thus, the presence of antigen-presenting cells in the graft tissues is particularly likely to elicit graft rejection. Originally it was thought that leucocytes in the graft would act as antigen presenters but it is now thought that dendritic cells are most important in inducing responses in the host. These cells express MHC class II molecules constitutively and are very potent stimulators of mixed lymphocyte reactivity. They are also present in all tissues with the single exception of the brain parenchyma. Such antigen-presenting cells are referred to as passenger cells (Fig. 24.9). In human transplantation a problem may arise from immunogenic passenger cells leaving the graft after transplantation and entering the draining lymphatic system where they are particularly effective in sensitizing the host. Various manoeuvres have been performed to circumvent this problem including infusion of donor kidney with cytotoxic drugs before transplantation and ultraviolet irradiation of donor skin grafts, which induces emigration of Langerhans' cells.

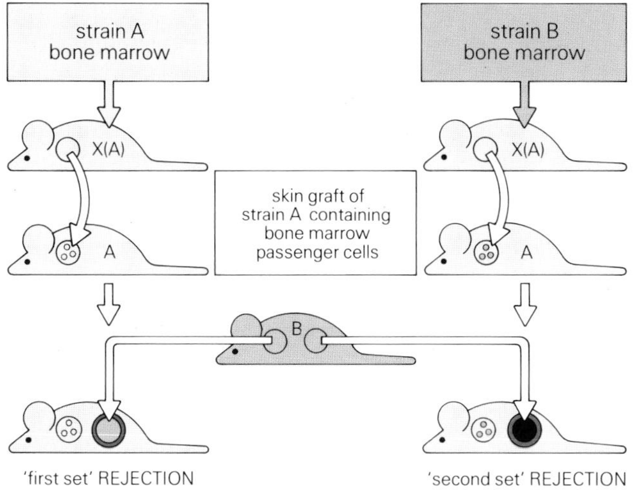

Fig. 24.9 The role of passenger cells in graft destruction. Strain A mice were X-irradiated and reconstituted with bone marrow cells of either strain A or strain B. Skin grafts from these mice were transplanted to strain A recipients and are accepted. The recipients subsequently received skin grafts from strain B animals. Animals whose first graft came from an animal reconstituted with strain A cells reject the strain B graft more slowly than animals whose first graft came from a mouse reconstituted with strain B bone marrow. This implies that strain B bone marrow cells which were carried as passengers in the first graft primed the recipient to the strain B alloantigen.

Depletion of dendritic cells in grafts leads to greatly enhanced graft survival but does not necessarily ensure success. This leads to the possibilities either that the host dendritic cells can process alloantigens emanating from the graft or that other cells from the graft can initiate the allogeneic reaction. As indicated in Chapter 8, a great number of cell types can be induced to express class II molecules in response to interferon-γ and can stimulate T cell responses.

Organs vary with respect to their susceptibility to rejection (Fig. 24.10). This is probably due to two factors.
1. The expression of class II MHC antigens by the graft varies for different tissues. For example, some strains of pig are able to accept liver grafts from other strains without immunosuppression but cannot accept kidney grafts from the same animals: swine liver parenchymal cells lack MHC class II antigens but tolerance in this system may also be due to a second factor.
2. There is a lack of suitable antigen-presenting cells in some tissues. It is noted that the most immunogenic tissues (bone marrow and skin), contain high numbers of dendritic cells or Langerhans' cells which develop into dendritic cells.

EFFECTS OF ANTIBODY

While cell-mediated immunity is the major effector in graft rejection, antibodies can also be involved (Fig. 24.11). This is particularly true if the individual is

immunogenicity of different tissues
bone marrow
skin
islets of Langerhans
heart
kidney
liver

Fig. 24.10 Immunogenicity of different tissues. In this table, different tissues are ordered according to their capacity to induce allogeneic reactions. Bone marrow is the most immunogenic.

type	time of damage	effector mechanism	cause
hyperacute rejection	within minutes	Ab	preformed cytotoxic antibodies to donor antigens
accelerated rejection	2–5 days	CMI ± Ab	previous sensitization to donor antigens
acute rejection	7–21 days	CMI (± Ab)	development of allogeneic reaction to donor antigens
chronic rejection	later than 3 months	CMI (± Ab)	disturbance of host/graft tolerance
immuno-pathological	later than 3 months	immunopathological events related to those which necessitated the transplant damage the new organ	

Fig. 24.11 Immune destruction of kidney grafts. This table lists the ways in which kidney grafts may be rejected. Acute rejection is equivalent to a first set allograft in experimental animals and accelerated rejection is equivalent to a second set allograft; both are primarily mediated by cells. Immunopathological changes include immune complex deposition and other hypersensitivity reactions already present in the recipient.

already sensitized to donor antigens, and antibodies are either present before grafting or develop concomitantly with the cell-mediated immunity. The effects of antibody are most frequently seen in grafts which are connected directly to the host's blood supply, for example, the kidney. Rejection of kidney grafts can be subdivided according to the time of occurrence and the effector mechanisms involved (see Fig. 24.11).

Hyperacute graft rejection (Fig. 24.12) is caused entirely by cytotoxic antibodies, usually those to A1 or B blood group substances or to class I MHC antigens (see Chapter 20). This type of rejection is now rare since red cell matching prevents problems due to A1 or B blood group substances and white cell cross-matching (donor cells + recipient serum + complement) is carried out prior to most forms of allografting. Liver transplantation is a notable exception since there is no evidence for hyperacute rejection occurring in transplanted livers. This may be because the liver is a great sink for antibody removal in general and is a very large organ containing many more antigenic sites than kidney; thus a much greater amount of antibody would be necessary to cause damage. It is also apparent that there is only a very narrow window, perhaps only 0–72 hours after a kidney transplant, when hyperacute rejection can occur. Thus retransplantation of an organ expressing a previously mismatched antigen can lead to a secondary response within 48 hours and cases of delayed hyperacute rejection have been reported. In contrast, however, many groups have reported circulating anti-donor antibody more than 1 week post transplantation without rejection occurring. In cases where antibody-mediated damage is recognized early, plasma exchange can be used to reduce the antibody titre until the window is closed. In kidneys, existing or rapidly produced anti-donor responses are generally damaging whereas subsequent ones are often not harmful. For livers, the situation is roughly the opposite with hyperacute rejection being absent and later anti-HLA antibody

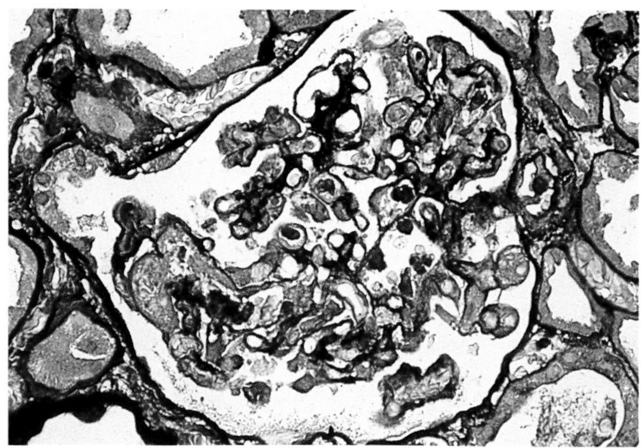

Fig. 24.12 Renal histology showing hyperacute graft rejection. There is extensive necrosis of the glomerular capillary associated with massive interstitial haemorrhage. This extensive necrosis is preceded by an intense polymorphonuclear infiltration which occurs within the first hour of the graft's revascularization. The changes shown here occur 24–48 hours after this. H&E stain, × 200.

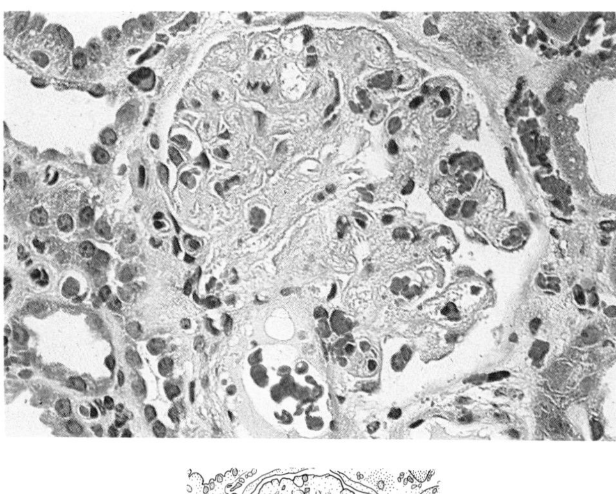

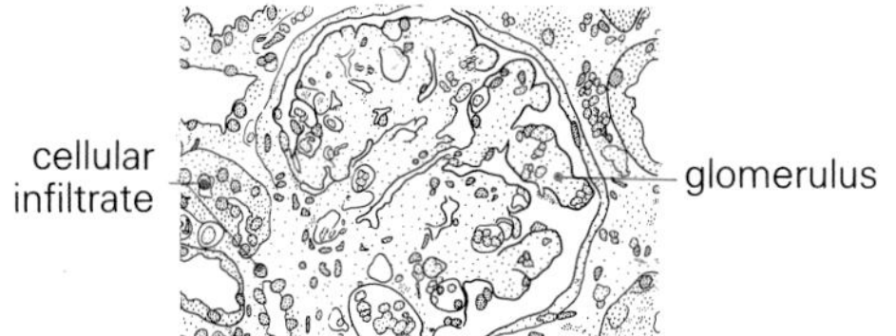

Fig. 24.13 Renal histology showing acute graft rejection – I. Small lymphocytes and other cells are accumulating in the interstitium of the graft. Such infiltration is characteristic of acute rejection and occurs before the appearance of any clinical signs. H&E stain, × 200.

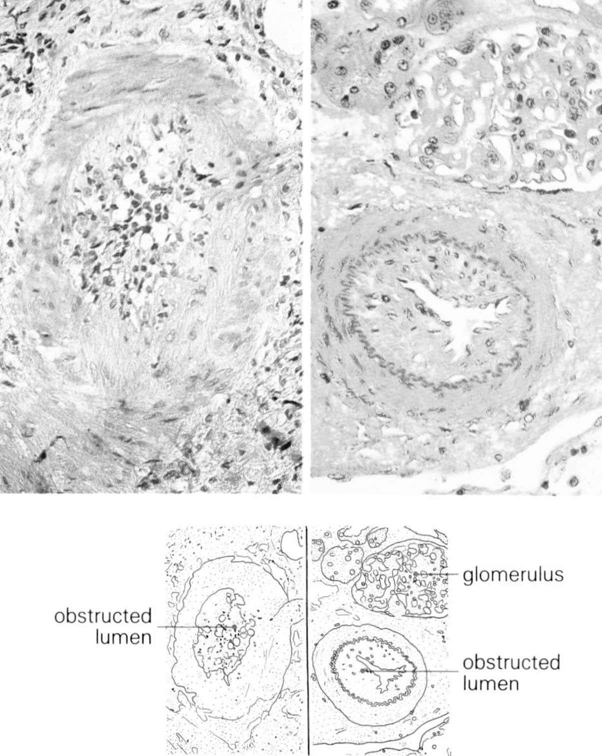

Fig. 24.14 Renal histology showing acute graft rejection – II. The section of acutely rejecting kidney shown on the left (H&E stain) shows vascular obstruction and that on the right (Van Giesen stain) shows the end-stage of this process. × 140.

production often being accompanied by graft loss. The graft loss occurs as a result of the vanishing bile duct syndrome and as yet there is no proof that the anti-HLA antibodies are directly involved in the process. In heart transplantation, the situation is roughly half way between that of kidney transplantation and liver transplantation, with hyperacute rejection being rare and HLA antibody production having a detrimental effect on long-term graft survival.

With accelerated and acute graft rejection the importance of antibodies depends on circumstances. Acute graft rejection is more usually mediated by T cells although antibodies may develop concomitantly. The second set accelerated rejection is more likely to involve antibody-mediated damage since secondary antibody responses develop early after implantation. The histological appearance of an acutely rejecting kidney is illustrated in Figs 24.13 and 24.14.

GRAFT FACTORS AFFECTING REJECTION

As mentioned above, different tissues vary considerably in their immunogenicity, but in addition, the site of implantation also affects the eventual outcome. Tissues of low immunogenicity are referred to as 'privileged tissues' and sites, such as the brain, cornea and specially prepared skin flaps, which lack normal lymphatic drainage, are referred to as 'privileged sites'. With corneal transplantation the rate of rejection is dependent upon whether the cornea becomes vascularized, and so accessible to the recipient's immune system (Fig. 24.15). It is only within vascularized corneal transplants that HLA incompatibility increases the likelihood of rejection.

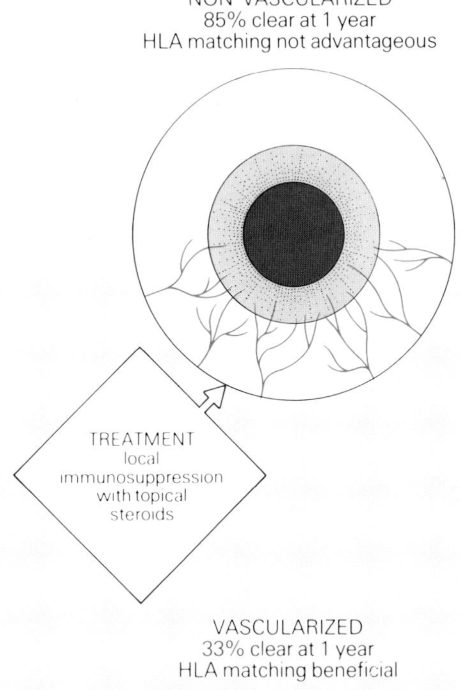

Fig. 24.15 Corneal transplantation. The success of corneal transplantation depends on whether the graft becomes vascularized. Grafts which do become vascularized are treatable with topical steroids to produce local immunosuppression.

CLINICAL TISSUE TRANSPLANTATION

The most frequent types of transplantation in humans are listed in Fig. 24.16. In practical terms the frequency with which transplants are performed depends upon the availability of suitable alternatives to transplantation and the availability of donor organs. The success rate of transplantation also depends on these factors as well as on the rejection reactions discussed earlier and the amount of tissue damage which the graft can tolerate and still function effectively. For example, a kidney graft can recover from a certain amount of damage following death of the donor before transplantation. It can also withstand some immunological damage caused by rejection reactions provided they are checked by immunosuppressive therapy. By contrast, the heart graft is liable to go into a fatal arrhythmia following only a moderate amount of damage.

Undoubtedly, the most successful transplantation programmes have been with kidneys and corneas. Success rates have improved with practice and statistical analysis of previous results in order to identify which factors are important in improving the level of

organ	comment
kidney	kidney transplantation is treatment of choice in most patients with end-stage renal failure; HLA–B and –DR identity advantageous
cornea	high success rate without matching for first grafts; HLA–B and –DR matching advantageous for second grafts (<5%)
liver	for hepatoma and biliary atresia, not HLA matched; graft loss usually due to factors other than rejection
pancreas/ islets of Langerhans	treatment for IDDM patients who have had, have or are likely to have end-stage renal failure
bone marrow	autologous bone marrow transplantation used where possible – HLA matched siblings or 'washed' autologous tissue is prefered, HLA matched unrelateds are the third choice; unmatched relateds are less successful.
heart	now as successful as kidneys at 1 year (>80%) but coronary artery disease is a significant problem within 3 years of transplantation; no HLA matching necessary, although preformed HLA antibodies indicate a lower survival chance
skin	treatment for burns; temporary cover provided by allograft, permanent replacement by autograft
lung	not HLA matched; poor success rate, but improving
fetal tissue (e.g. from brain or pancreas)	short term successes have been reported, but early experiments with fetal fibroblasts show a rapid functional deterioration

Fig. 24.16 Main areas of clinical tissue transplantation.

graft acceptance and function (Fig. 24.17). It appears that the acceptance of a graft depends on a balance of factors in the donor and the recipient (Figs 24.18 and 24.19).

XENOTRANSPLANTATION

There is a great world-wide shortage of most donor organs, especially kidneys, and this has led several groups to use organs from other primates (concordant species) and non-primates (discordant species). On the positive side, suitably treated pig skin and sections of blood vessels have been successfully used in humans. On the negative side, whole organs have nearly always been disastrous failures. The immunological reasons are unclear however, because even within a species, once we move away from perfect matching, increased mismatching appears to have little or no effect. It is probable that preformed antibodies, probably of the IgM anti-blood group type, are the most significant immunological problem to be faced in xenotransplantation. The relatively small sizes of primate kidneys, import restrictions, possible diseases, species rarity, and animal rights, are therefore a greater bar to xenotransplantation than immunological considerations.

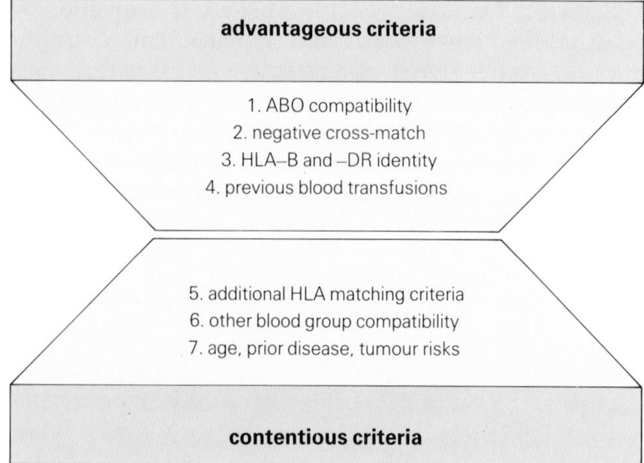

Fig. 24.17 Factors affecting kidney transplantation. There is no rigid consensus on the importance of all these criteria.

RECURRENCE OF ORIGINAL DISEASE

This subject provides endless hours of discussion for the immunologist. For example, Goodpasture's disease, associated with HLA–DR2 is mediated by an antibody to the non-collagenous sections of type 4 collagen molecules. After renal transplantation, the antibody decreases with time but often causes renal failure before it vanishes completely. If the DR on the kidney is responsible for disease induction then transplantation with a DR matched kidney might be expected to lead to disease recurrence whereas transplantation with a non-DR2 positive kidney might not. Unfortunately, although there are instances where the disease has recurred in DR2 transplants no control data are available.

There are many well documented cases of grafts being lost by a direct occurrence of the original disease. The time course is variable with certain forms of aggressive nephritis being capable of graft destruction within months. One recipient has lost 3 grafts by this mechanism. At the other extreme one graft in an identical twin survived for 15 years before a recurrence of diabetic nephropathy destroyed it. Pancreatic segment and whole organ grafts are particularly prone to being destroyed presumably by the immune-mediated processes which instigated the original diabetes mellitus. With liver and heart transplants, specific post-transplant diseases, not necessarily recurrent, are major causes for concern. With a liver transplant, the major problem is vanishing bile duct syndrome, a self explanatory disease, which can be difficult to distinguish from rejection. With hearts, some centres have reported that 60% of their recipients have coronary heart disease within 3 years of the transplant. The situation is also problematical for corneal grafts where loss of the first graft, or indeed the loss of the primary function,

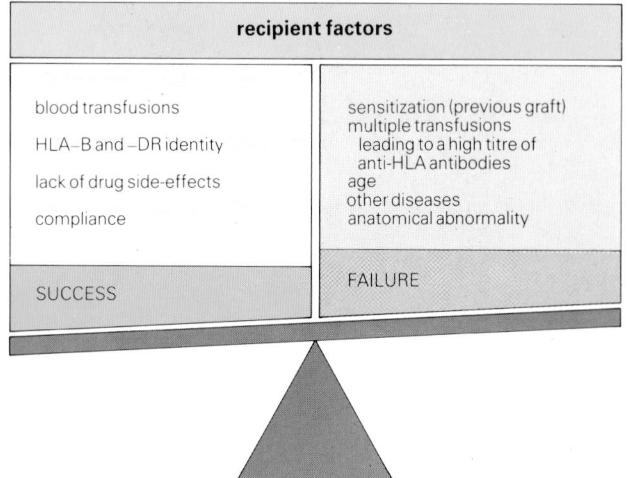

Fig. 24.18 Recipient factors affecting success in kidney transplantation. The success or failure of a kidney transplant depends on a balance of factors. Cross-matching the donor and recipient tends to produce success, especially if blood transfusions are performed prior to the operation – prior sensitization of the recipient to donor antigen is likely to end in rejection.

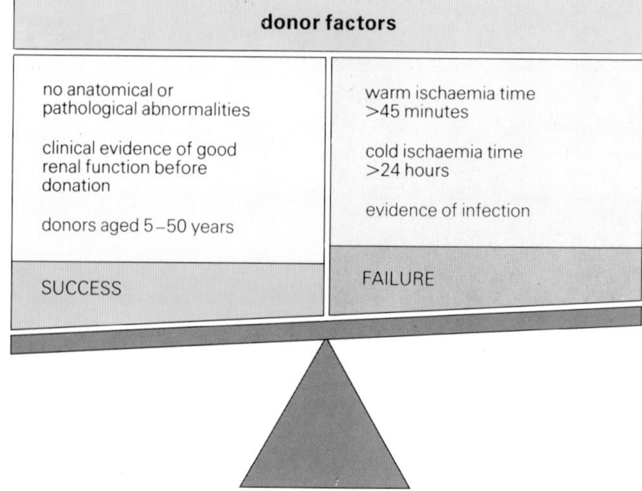

Fig. 24.19 Donor factors affecting success in kidney transplantation. Donor factors which affect graft success include the amount of time the donor organ is ischaemic, that is, lacking an effective blood supply. The length of time that a graft can tolerate ischaemia depends on its temperature before transplantation, that is, 37°C (warm) or 4°C (cold).

	kidney	heart	liver
first transplants into non-sensitized recipients	90%	85%	85%
first transplants into sensitized recipients	75%	70%	75%
second and subsequent transplants into sensitized recipients	70%	NA	NA

Fig. 24.20 Graft survival figures. The table shows the percentages of heart, liver and kidney transplants functioning at 1 year for good transplant centres using optimum donor and recipient pairs. (NA. Data not available.)

was caused by rejection or non-rejection induced vascularization.

We can see that transplanted tissue appears to be particularly prone to severe damage in certain circumstances and there is a definite art in defining and hence avoiding high-risk recipient and donor groups.

The percentages of heart, liver and kidney transplants, functioning at 1 year, from the best transplantation centres are summarized in Fig. 24.20. Success is highest with first transplants into unsensitized donors. Although these figures relate to optimum donor and recipient conditions, it is notable that graft survival is on average twice what it was 5 years ago.

IMMUNOSUPPRESSION

The success of any allogeneic transplantation is often due to the immunosuppressive measures adopted. These may be divided into two phases.

1. Immediately after the graft has been implanted it is necessary to prevent sensitization of pre-existing mature T cells capable of recognizing the graft.
2. After the graft has escaped the initial acute phase rejection reactions, a cumulative unresponsiveness to the graft develops as the recipient is continually exposed to donor MHC. This stable state sometimes depends on the development of antigen-specific T-suppressor cells. Unless the equilibrium is disturbed by other factors, such as infection, chronic rejection reactions may be avoided indefinitely.

Immunosuppressive measures may be antigen specific or antigen non-specific.

ANTIGEN NON-SPECIFIC IMMUNOSUPPRESSION

Antigen non-specific measures include the use of immunosuppressive drugs and other methods to specifically reduce T cell function. Many cytotoxic drugs are primarily active against dividing cells and therefore have some functional specificity for any cells activated to divide by donor antigens, but the use of these drugs is limited because they also damage other dividing tissues such as the gut epithelium. The drug cyclosporin A appears to have a greater specificity for lymphoid cells than others. It is an undecapeptide derived from the fungus *Trichoderma polysporum* and it is highly lipophilic.

The rapid expansion of allogeneic transplantation in recent years is undoubtedly due to the introduction of cyclosporin A. Its main contribution has been to greatly improve survival rates for first grafts, but it needs to be combined with the lymphocytotoxic reagents anti-thymocyte globulin (ATG) or anti-lymphocyte globulin (ALG) before results are improved in sensitized patients. This suggests that primed cells may be less easily controlled by cyclosporin alone. The primary action of cyclosporin A is in inhibiting the production of the lymphokine interleukin-2 (Fig. 24.21).

Theoretically the process defined in Fig. 24.21 could also be blocked by antibody to class I or class II molecules, or to the T cell receptor, or by the presence of solubilized forms of these molecules. A number of anti-CD3 monoclonal antibodies have been described and are available commercially.

A problem arising from all these measures is that the individual is more susceptible to infection and if infection occurs, immunosuppression has to be suspended and the graft is usually lost from rejection.

The major side-effect of cyclosporin A is nephrotoxicity, and the maintenance of an immunosuppressive non-nephrotoxic dose in transplant recipients is expensive and difficult. A common clinical scenario in renal transplantation is a rejection episode treated with high-dose steroid at the time of high cyclosporin A. The combination of rejection and nephrotoxicity often irreversibly damages the graft.

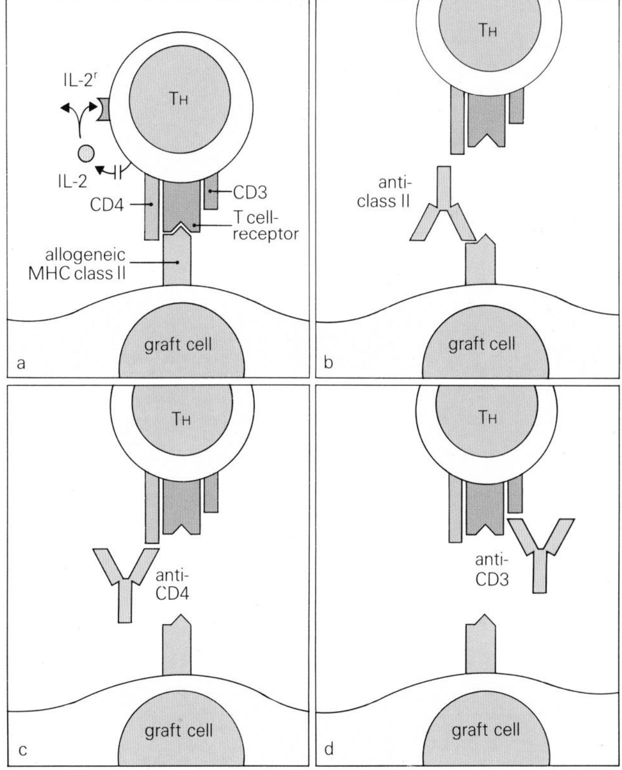

Fig. 24.21 Prevention of T cell activation. a) T-helper (TH) cells recognize allogeneic MHC, but production of interleukin-2 (IL-2) is blocked, hence this cell and other T cells fail to receive the signal to divide. Cyclosporin can act in this way. In b, c, and d, the antigen-specific recognition of the allogeneic MHC is blocked by antibodies. These can be against the MHC class II molecule itself (b), or against CD4 or CD3 (c, d) of the T cells which recognize the graft cell.

ANTIGEN-SPECIFIC IMMUNOSUPPRESSION

Antigen-specific immunosuppression is undoubtedly the most exciting area in transplantation with interest being focused on toxic lymphokines. After specific antigen activation, the responding T cells expand and express IL-2 receptors on their surface. Toxin coupled to IL-2 binds and specifically removes this population. The method has passed its probationary testing in species up to primates. A more specific technique based on observations that antigen-specific tolerance can be induced in the neonatal animal by infusion of donor cells has also been developed for rodent models. The process involves transfection of the recipient's cells with donor antigen and reinfusion under conditions to induce antigen-specific tolerance, but is not a practical proposition for human transplantation at present.

Potentially more useful is the phenomenon of immunological enhancement. This occurs when graft survival can be prolonged by the seemingly paradoxical treatment with antibodies directed towards the graft alloantigens. This is referred to as passive enhancement (in an analogous way to passive immunization). It is possible to produce the same effect by an active pre-immunization with allogeneic cells. Various suggestions have been put forward as to the mechanism by which the enhancement occurs, including the removal of donor passenger cells or recipient T-helper cells. Another suggestion is that the antibody shields the alloantigens on the graft from the responding host cells. In this sense the action of the antibody is similar to the action of anti-class II MHC antibodies in preventing T cell sensitization (see Fig. 24.21), and it is possible that transfusion does induce some anti-class II antibodies. None of these explanations seems wholly satisfactory because the enhancing antibodies appear to have a long-term action in reducing reactions to the graft which extend beyond the short-term allogeneic reactions and in some instances there is a development of graft-specific T-suppressor cells.

An interestingly similar phenomenon has been observed in human kidney grafting; those recipients immunosuppressed with corticosteroids and azathioprine and previously sensitized by donor blood, either by pregnancy or by transfusion before operation, have improved graft survival (Fig. 24.22). The mechanism for this observation is unknown but may be related to those discussed above. The improvement noticed with blood transfusions to recipients is less marked when donors and recipients are well matched for MHC antigens, which again suggests that the manoeuvre is in some way removing antigen-presenting cells or donor-specific T-helper cells. It is interesting to note that the preliminary indications are that if cyclosporin is used alone, or together with corticosteroids then the pre-transplant blood transfusion does not affect graft survival. The main problem with blood transfusion is that a number of patients develop cytotoxic antibodies and these are a major bar to transplantation.

Another immunosuppressive technique (described in Chapter 12) is the induction of anti-idiotypic antibodies to the T cells which recognize the graft. These antibodies block recognition of the MHC antigens on the graft. Although there has been considerable success in animals with this technique, the induction of suitable anti-idiotypic antibodies during an extended period before the grafting presents difficult immunological and procedural problems in man. The various forms of immunosuppression are summarized in Fig. 24.23.

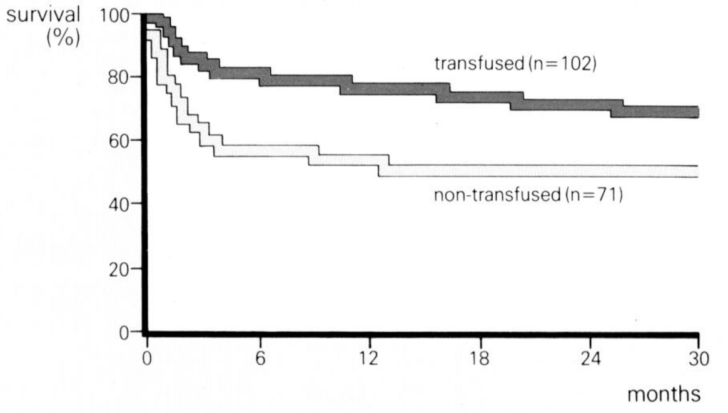

Fig. 24.22 The effect of blood transfusion on kidney transplantation. This graph plots the survival of kidney grafts in 102 transfused and 71 non-transfused patients.

antigen non-specific	antigen specific
1. cytotoxic drugs	7. neonatal tolerization
2. lymphoid irradiation	8. toxic lymphokines
3. anti-lymphocyte globulin	9. enhancing antibodies
4. cyclosporin A	10. anti-idiotypic antibodies
5. corticosteroids/ azathioprine	11. blood transfusions in human kidney transplants
6. monoclonal antibodies to T cells	

Fig. 24.23 Immunological suppression for transplantation. Various immunosuppressive treatments are listed. Items 7 and 10 are of theoretical interest and have not found practical application in human organ transplantation.

FURTHER READING

Billingham, R.E. & Silvers, E.S. (1971) *The Immunobiology of Transplantation*. New Jersey: Prentice-Hall.

Cerilli, C.J. (1988) *Organ Transplantation and Replacement*. Maryland: J.B. Lippincott.

Kahan, D. (ed.) (1984) *Cyclosporin A: Biological Activity and Clinical Applications*. New York: Grune & Stratton Inc.

Klein, J. (1987) *Natural History of the Major Histocompatibility Complex*. New York: John Wiley & Sons.

25 Immunological Techniques

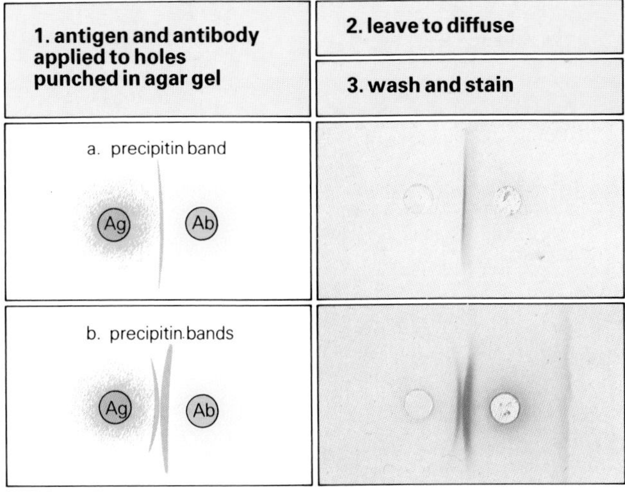

Fig. 25.1 Immuno-double diffusion—I. Agar gels are poured onto slides and allowed to set (1–2% agar in buffer at pH 7–8.5). Wells are then punched in the gel and the test solutions of antigen (Ag) and antibody (Ab) are added. The solutions diffuse out and where Ag and Ab meet they bind to each other, cross-link and precipitate leaving a line of precipitation (a). If two antigens are present in the solution and both can be recognized by the antibody two lines of precipitation form independently (b). The precipitin bands can be better visualized by washing the gel to remove soluble proteins and then staining the precipitin arcs with a protein stain such as Coomassie Blue (right).

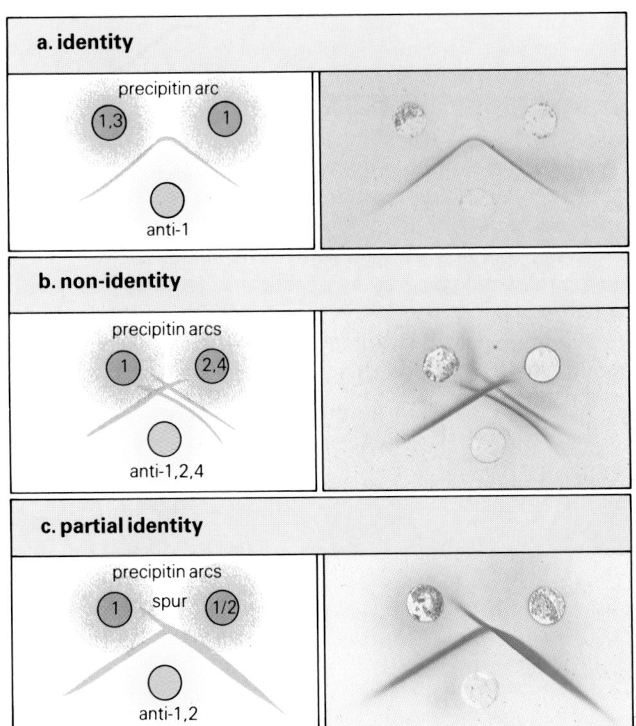

Immunologists employ a number of techniques which are common to other biological sciences. For example, the methods used to isolate antigens and antibodies are those of biochemistry and protein fractionation, while the gene structure of immunologically important molecules has been elucidated by molecular biological techniques. Immunology has however developed a number of its own techniques, particularly those based on the specificity of the antigen–antibody interaction. These are finding increasing use in many of the biological sciences. Examples are the quantification of low concentrations of antigenic molecules by radioimmunoassay (RIA) and enzyme-linked immunosorbent assay (ELISA), and the identification of particular antigens in tissues by immunocytochemical methods. There are hundreds of different immunological methods now in use and some of the most common are outlined in this chapter.

ANTIGEN – ANTIBODY INTERACTIONS

PRECIPITATION REACTION IN GELS

One of the first observations of antigen–antibody reactions was their ability to precipitate when combined in proportions at or near equivalence. By performing these reactions in agar gels it is possible to distinguish separate antigen–antibody reactions produced by different populations of antibody present in a serum – the immuno-double diffusion technique. This technique has been extended to the examination of the relationship between different antigens (Figs 25.1 and 25.2).

Some antigen mixtures however, are too complex to be resolved by simple diffusion and precipitation and so

Fig. 25.2 Immuno-double diffusion—II. The immuno-double diffusion technique may be used to determine the relationship between antigens (blue) and a particular test antibody (yellow). Three basic patterns appear. The numbers in the blue wells refer to the epitopes present on the test antigen. In reaction (a) the precipitin arcs formed between the antibody and the two test antigens fuse indicating that the antibody is precipitating identical epitopes in each preparation (epitope 1). This does not mean that the antigens are necessarily identical; they are only identical as far as the antibody can distinguish the difference. In reaction (b) the antibody preparation distinguishes the three different antigens which form independent precipitin arcs. In reaction (c) the antigens share epitope 1 but one antigen also has epitope 2. This is the same situation as in (a), but in this case the antibody can distinguish them, by virtue of being able to react against both epitopes. A line of identity forms with anti-epitope 1, with the addition of a 'spur' where the anti-epitope 2 has reacted with the second epitope, thus indicating partial identity between the antigen preparations.

the technique of immunoelectrophoresis was developed – antigens are separated on the basis of their charge before being visualized by precipitation (Fig. 25.3).

These gel techniques only identify antigens and antibodies qualitatively, but by further modification, using the technique of single radial immunodiffusion, they can be made quantitative (Fig. 25.4).

By applying a voltage across the gels to move the antigens and antibodies together, immuno-double diffusion becomes countercurrent electrophoresis, and single radial immunodiffusion becomes rocket electrophoresis (Fig. 25.5). These techniques operate in the range of 20 μg/ml to 2 mg/ml of antigen or antibody.

Another development of these techniques is crossed electrophoresis as described by Laurell. In this system an antigen mixture is first separated electrophoretically as in Fig. 25.3. The agar strip containing the separated proteins is then cut out of the gel and applied across the

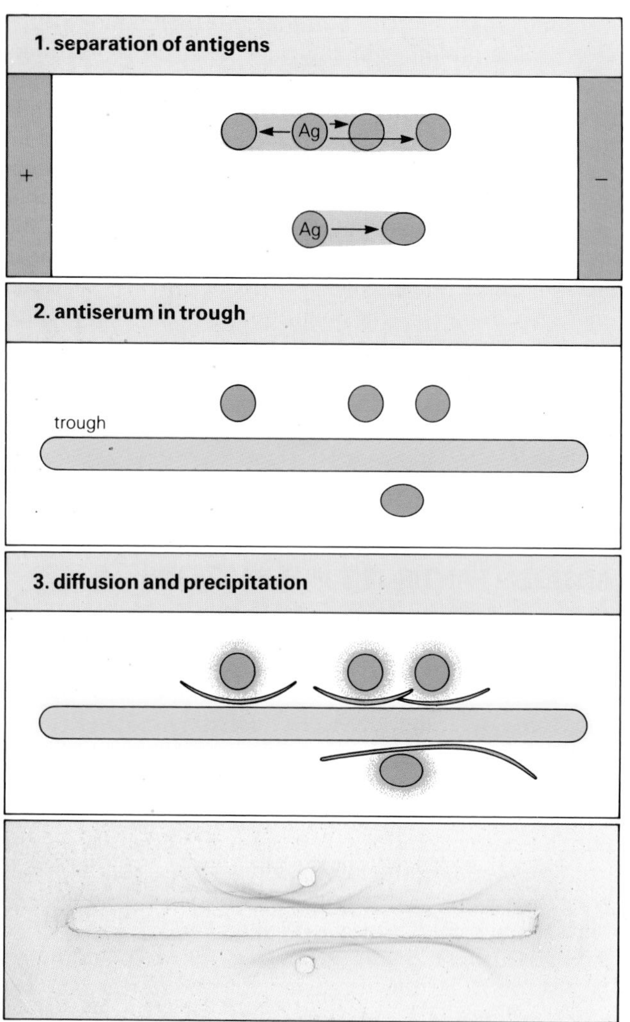

Fig. 25.3 Immunoelectrophoresis. 1. Antigens are separated in an agar gel by placing an electric charge across it. The pH is chosen so that positively charged proteins move to the negative electrode and negatively charged proteins to the positive. 2. A trough is then cut between the wells, filled with the antibody and the plate is left to diffuse. 3. The antigens and antibody form precipitin arcs. This method allows the comparison of complicated mixtures of antigens as found in serum.

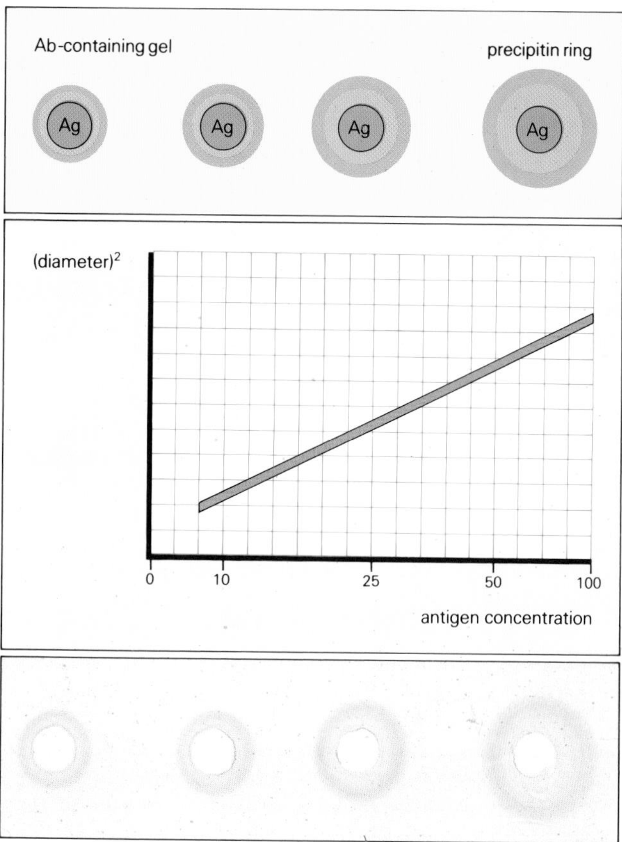

Fig. 25.4 Single radial immunodiffusion. Antibody is added to the agar gel which is then poured onto slides and allowed to set. Wells are punched in the agar and standard volumes of test antigen of different concentration are put in the wells. The plates are left for at least 24 hours, during which time the antigen diffuses out of the wells to form soluble complexes (in antigen excess) with the antibody. These continue to diffuse outwards, binding more antibody until an equivalence point is reached and the complexes precipitate in a ring. The area within the precipitin ring, measured as ring diameter squared, is proportional to the antigen concentration. Unknowns are derived by interpolation from the standard curve (graph). The whole process may be reversed to determine unknown concentrations of antibody.

bottom of an antibody-containing gel, as in Fig.25.5. The separated proteins are electrophoresed into the antibody-containing gel where they immunoprecipitate, in a similar way to that occurring in rocket electrophoresis. The area under the precipitin curve is proportional to the antigen concentration. This technique permits the quantification of electrophoretically different forms of an antigen in a complex mixture.

HAEMAGGLUTINATION AND COMPLEMENT FIXATION

Antibody may be detected at lower concentrations than those detectable by countercurrent electrophoresis and rocket electrophoresis by haemagglutination which relies on the ability of antibody to cross-link red blood cells by interacting with the antigen on their surface (Fig.25.6). The haemagglutination test is a direct development of the Coombs' test described in Chapter 20.

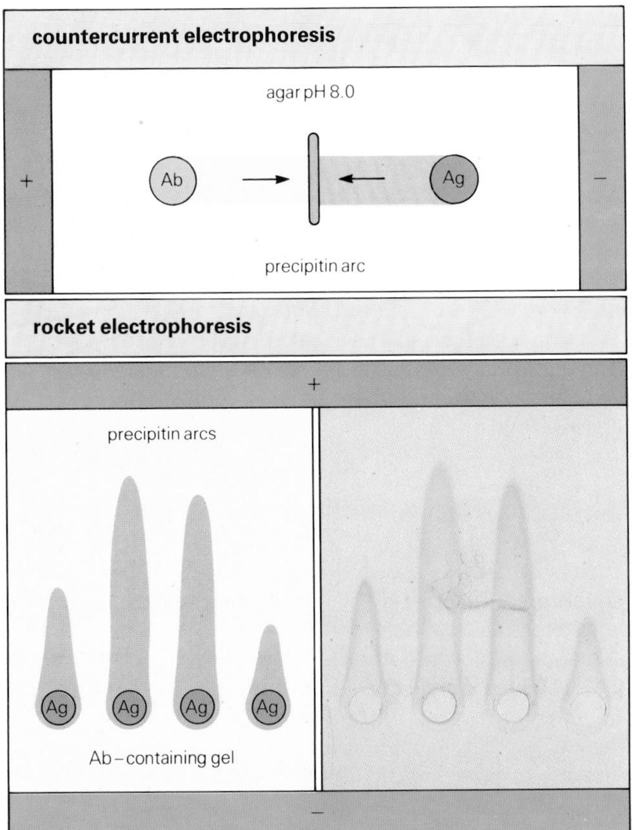

Fig. 25.5 Countercurrent electrophoresis and rocket electrophoresis. Countercurrent electrophoresis is performed in agar gels where the pH is chosen so that the antibody is positively charged and the antigen is negatively charged. By applying a voltage across the gel the antigen and antibody move towards each other and precipitate. The principle is the same as immuno-double diffusion but the sensitivity is increased 10–20-fold. Antigens may be quantitated by electrophoresing them into an antibody-containing gel in the technique termed rocket electrophoresis. The pH of the gel is chosen so that the antibodies are immobile and the antigen is negatively charged. Precipitin rockets form; the height of the rocket is proportional to antigen concentration, and unknowns are determined by interpolation from standards. The appearance of stained rockets is shown on the right. Both techniques rely on the antigen and antibody having different charges at the selected pH; this is true for most antigens since antibodies have a relatively high isoelectric point (i.e. they are neutrally charged at a more alkaline pH than most antigens). If the charges on the antigen and antibody do not differ sufficiently, the antibody or antigen can be chemically modified to alter its isoelectric point. Rocket electrophoresis can be reversed to estimate antibody concentration if a suitable pH gel to immobilize the antigen, without damaging it or preventing the antigen–antibody reaction, can be found.

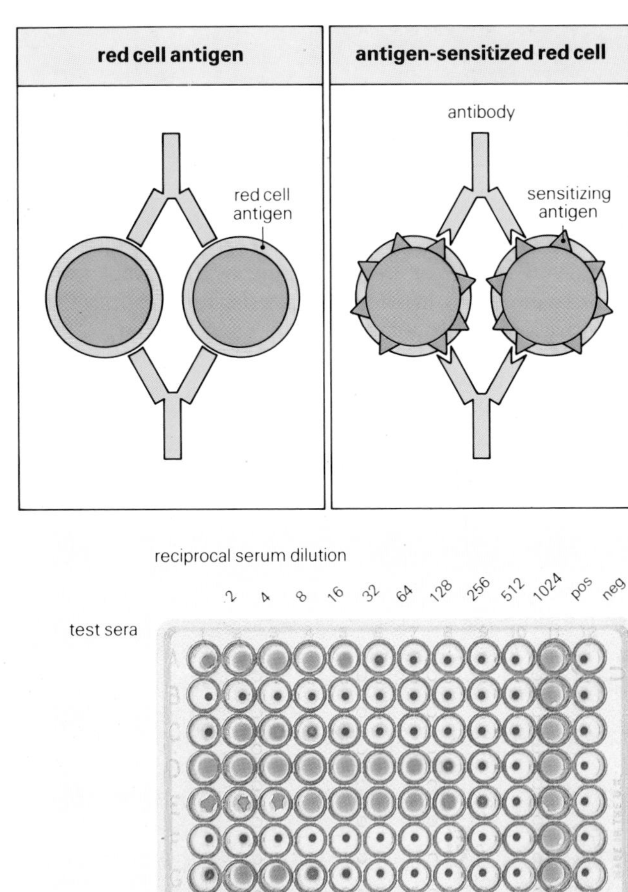

Fig. 25.6 Haemagglutination. The active haemagglutination test (left) detects antibodies to red blood cell antigens. The antibody is serially diluted (usually in doubling dilutions) in physiological saline and placed in the wells (rows 1–10) of the haemagglutination plate. Positive controls (row 11) and negative controls (row 12) are included. A suspension of red cells (containing a protein to prevent the red cells agglutinating non-specifically) is added to each well to give a final concentration of about 1% cells. If sufficient antibody is present to agglutinate (cross-link) the cells they sink as a mat to the bottom of the well (direct Coombs' test). If insufficient antibody is present, the cells roll down the sloping sides of the plate to form a red pellet at the bottom. Some antibodies do not agglutinate red cells very effectively and may be detected in the indirect agglutination test (indirect Coombs' test) by the addition of a second antibody which binds to the antibody on the red cell. By binding different antigens onto the red cell surface, covalently or non-covalently, the test can be extended to detect antibodies to antigens other than those on red cells (right). Chromic chloride, tannic acid, glutaraldehyde and a number of other chemicals are used to cross-link the antigen to the cells.

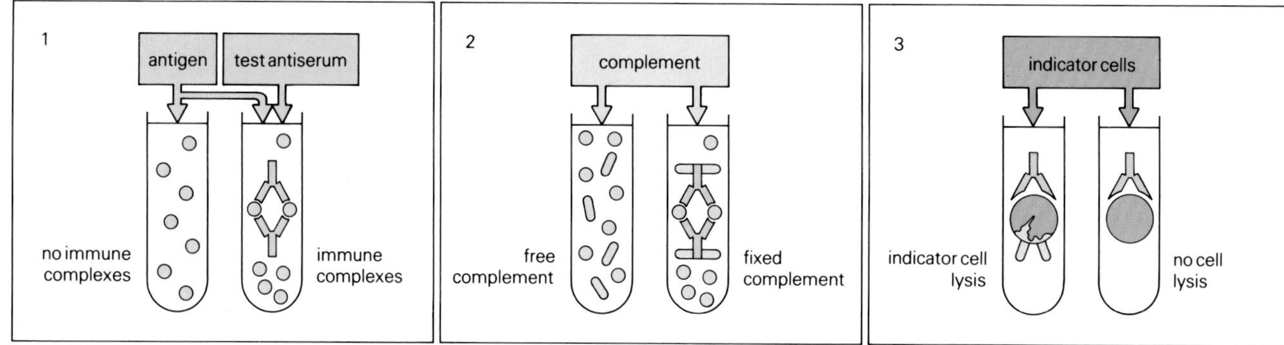

Fig. 25.7 Complement fixation. The complement fixation test detects antibody. 1. A test antiserum is titred in doubling dilutions and a fixed amount of antigen is added to each well or tube. If antibody is present in the test serum, immune complexes will form. 2. Complement is then added to the mixture. If complexes are present, they will fix complement and consume it. 3. In the final step, indicator cells (red cells) together with a subagglutinating amount of antibody (erythrocyte antibody) are added to the mixture. If there is any complement remaining these cells will be lysed; if it was consumed by immune complexes there will be insufficient to lyse the red cells. A quantity of complement is used which is just enough to lyse the indicator cells if none is consumed by the complexes. The assay is often performed on plastic plates. By using constant amounts of antibody and titrations of antigen, the assay can be applied to testing for antigens. Appropriate controls are most important in this assay because some antibody preparations consume complement without the addition of antigen, for example, if the antibody preparation is serum already containing immune complexes. Some antigens can also have anti-complement activity. The controls should therefore include antibody alone and antigen alone to check that neither fix complement by themselves.

Antigen–antibody reactions lead to immune complex formation which produces complement fixation via the classical pathway and this may be exploited to determine the amount of antigen or antibody present (Fig. 25.7). Haemagglutination and complement fixation can detect antibody at levels less than 1 μg/ml.

DIRECT AND INDIRECT IMMUNOFLUORESCENCE

Immunofluorescence is used extensively to detect autoantibodies and antibodies to tissue and cellular antigens (Fig. 25.8). Although the techniques are more cumbersome than those described above if a quantitative measure of antibody concentration is required, they do have advantages. By using tissue sections (which contain a large number of antigens), antibodies to several different antigens can be identified in a single test. The antigens are differentiated by their different staining patterns. Furthermore, the immunofluorescence tests can be used to identify particular cells in suspension, that is, to identify antigens on live cells. When a live stained cell

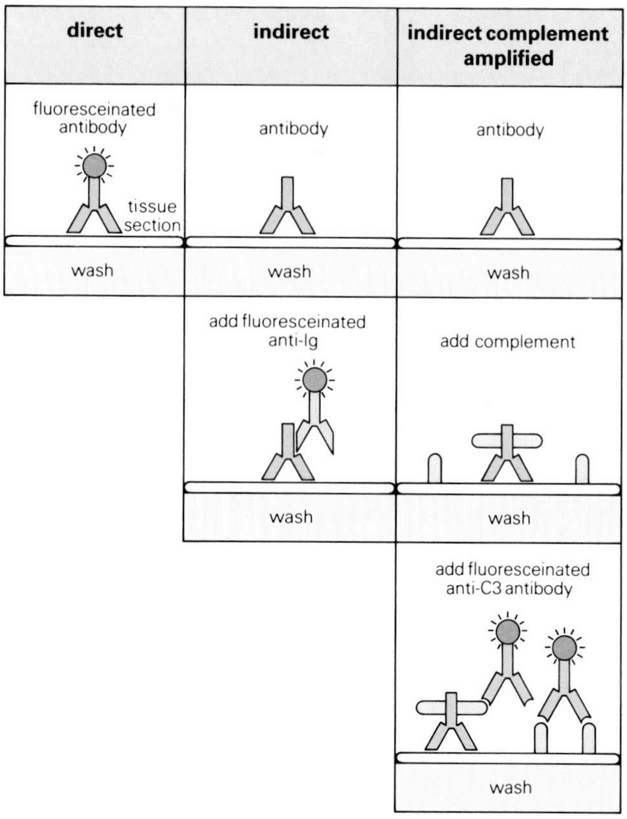

direct	indirect	indirect complement amplified
fluoresceinated antibody; tissue section	antibody	antibody
wash	wash	wash
	add fluoresceinated anti-Ig	add complement
	wash	wash
		add fluoresceinated anti-C3 antibody
		wash

Fig. 25.8 Direct and indirect immunofluorescence. A section is cut on a cryostat from a deep frozen tissue block. This ensures that labile antigens are not damaged by fixatives.
Direct. The test solution of fluoresceinated antibody is applied to the section in a drop, incubated and washed off. Any bound antibody is then revealed under the microscope; UV light is directed onto the section through the objective, thus the field is dark and areas with bound fluorescent antibody fluoresce green. The pattern of fluorescence is characteristic for each tissue antigen.
Indirect. Antibody applied to the section as a solution is visualized using fluoresceinated anti-immunoglobulin.
Indirect complement amplified. This is an elaboration of the indirect method for the detection of complement fixing antibody. In the second step fresh complement is added which becomes fixed around the site of antibody binding. Due to the amplification steps in the classical complement pathway one antibody molecule can cause many C3b molecules to bind to the section; these are then visualized with fluoresceinated anti-C3.

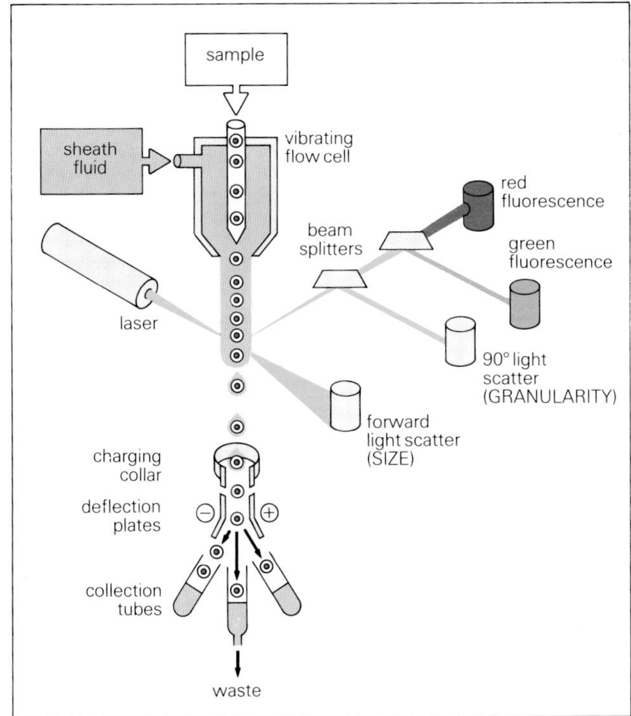

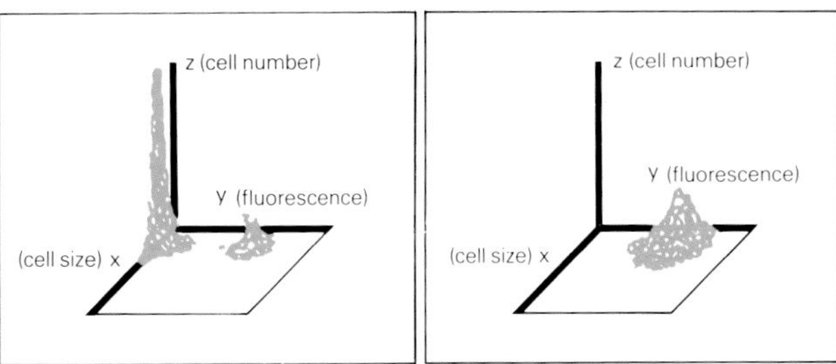

Fig. 25.9 Fluorescence Activated Cell Sorter (FACS). Cells in the sample are stained with specific fluorescent reagents to detect surface molecules and are then introduced into a vibrating flow chamber. The cell stream passing out of the chamber is encased in a sheath of buffer fluid. The stream is illuminated by laser and each cell is measured for size (forward light scatter) and granularity (90° light scatter), as well as for red and green fluorescence, to detect two different surface markers. The vibration in the cell stream causes it to break into droplets which are charged and may then be steered by deflection plates under computer control to collect different cell populations according to the parameters measured. The 3-dimensional plots above show a whole lymphocyte population (left) and a $CD8^+$ population obtained by cell sorting (right), stained with anti-CD8.

suspension is put through a fluorescence activated cell sorter (FACS) the machine measures the fluorescence intensity of each cell and then the cells are separated according to their particular fluorescent brightness. This technique permits the isolation of different cell populations with different surface antigens (stained with different fluorescent antibodies) (Fig. 25.9).

RADIOIMMUNOASSAY AND ENZYME-LINKED IMMUNOSORBENT ASSAY

The techniques of radioimmunoassay (RIA) and enzyme-linked immunosorbent assay (ELISA) are exquisitely sensitive for detecting antigens and antibodies, and are extremely economical in the use of reagents (Figs 25.10 and 25.11).

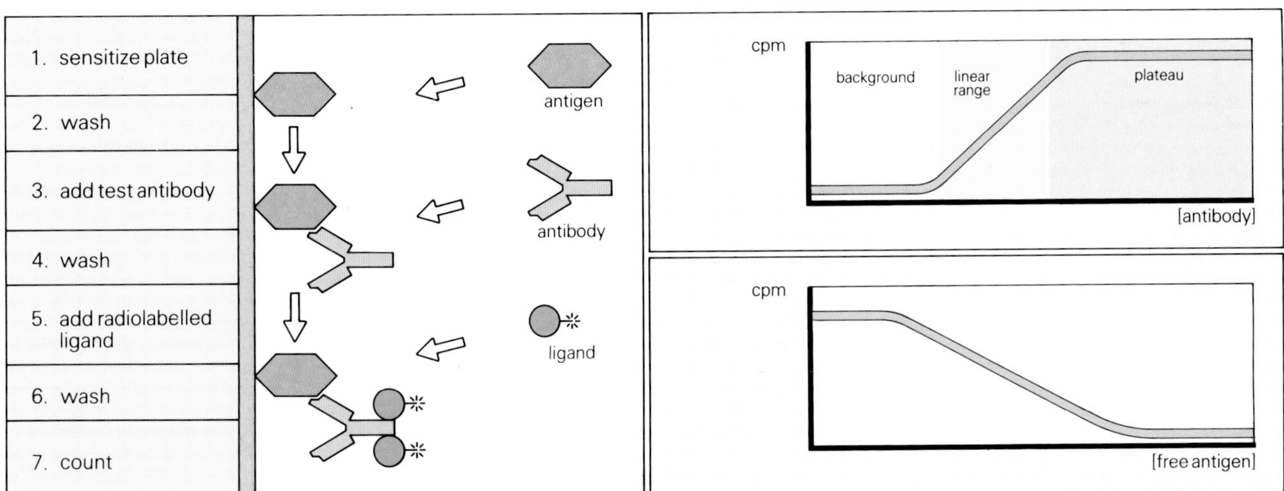

Fig. 25.10 Radioimmunoassay (RIA). 1. Antigen in saline is incubated on a plastic plate or tube, and small quantities become absorbed onto the plastic surface. 2. Free antigen is washed away. (The plate may then be blocked with excess of an irrelevant protein to prevent any subsequent non-specific binding of proteins.) 3. Test antibody is added, which binds to the antigen. 4. Unbound proteins are washed away and 5. the antibody is detected by a radiolabelled ligand. The ligand may be a molecule such as staphylococcal protein A which binds to the Fc region of IgG or more often it is another antibody specific for the test antibody. By using a ligand which binds to particular classes or subclasses of test antibody it is possible to distinguish isotypes. 6. Unbound ligand is washed away and 7. the radioactivity of the plate is counted on a gamma counter. A typical titration curve is shown in the upper graph. With increasing amounts of test antibody the counts per minute (cpm) rise from a background level through a linear range to a plateau. Antibody titres can only be detected correctly within the linear range. Typically the plateau binding is 20–100 times the background. The sensitivity of the technique is usually about 1–50 ng/ml of specific antibody. Specificity of the assay may be checked by adding increasing concentrations of free test antigen to the test antibody at step 3; this binds to the antibody and blocks it from binding to the antigen on the plate. Addition of increasing amounts of free antigen reduces the cpm (lower graph).

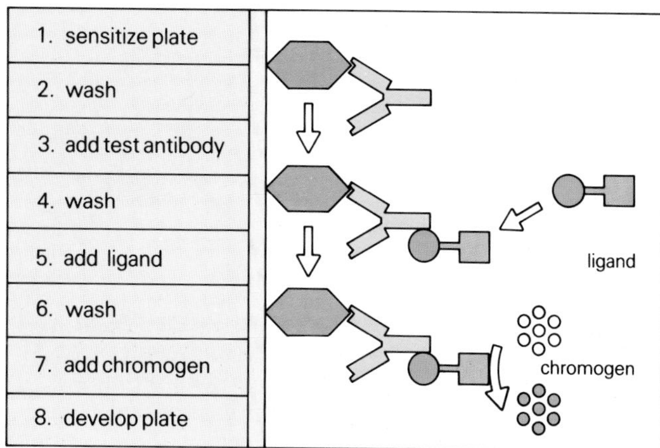

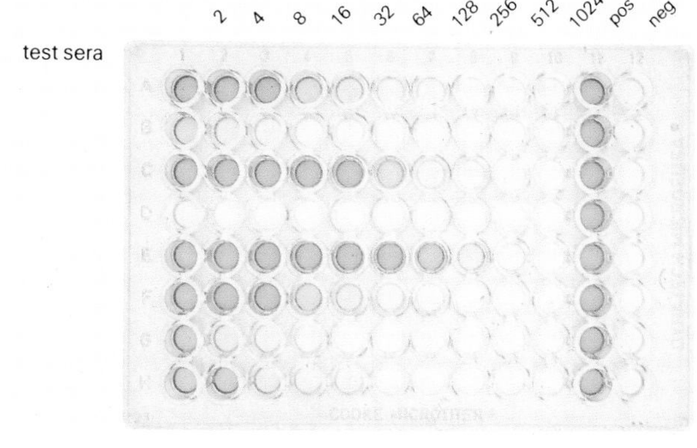

Fig. 25.11 Enzyme linked immunosorbent assay (ELISA). The ELISA plate is prepared in the same way as an RIA plate up to step 4. At this point a different kind of ligand is used. The ligand is a molecule which can detect the antibody and is covalently coupled to an enzyme such as peroxidase. This binds the test antibody and after free ligand is washed away (6) the bound ligand is visualized by the addition of chromogen (7) – a colourless substrate which is acted on by the enzyme portion of the ligand to produce a coloured end-product. A developed plate is shown on the right. The amount of test antibody is measured by assessing the amount of coloured end-product by optical density scanning of the plate.

RIA and ELISA are probably the most widely used of all immunological assays for antibodies since large numbers of tests can be performed in a relatively short time. Modification of the basic system as illustrated by the radioallergosorbent test (RAST) allows identification of antibodies of a particular isotype (Fig. 25.12). RIA can also be turned into a competition type of assay as illustrated by the radioimmunosorbent test (RIST) which may be used as a very sensitive assay for antigens (Fig. 25.13). Indeed, this form of competition was the first type of RIA. The serum concentration of a number of drugs and hormones are also measured by competition RIA. (Note that in the RIST the IgE being measured is acting as an antigen).

IMMUNOBLOTTING

The methods described above are particularly useful for quantitating levels of certain known antigens or antibodies, but in many cases it is necessary to identify and biochemically characterize antigens from a complex mixture, in which case immunoblotting is very useful.

In immunoblotting, complex mixtures are resolved in analytical separation gels and then the molecules are transferred to membranes (blots) for the identification of individual antigens by specific antisera. By using SDS gels, isoelectric focusing gels or peptide mapping gels in the initial separation, it is possible to obtain data on the size, isoelectric point and molecular relationships of the antigens under investigation (Fig. 25.14).

Fig. 25.12 The radioallergosorbent test (RAST). This test measures antigen-specific IgE in a radioimmunoassay where the ligand is a labelled anti-IgE antibody. The steps are identical to the standard radioimmunoassay except that the antigen (allergen) is covalently bound to a cellulose disc rather than non-covalently to a radioimmunoassay plate. The availability of much more antigen on the disc permits the high sensitivity necessary to bind the small quantities of IgE present in the test serum.

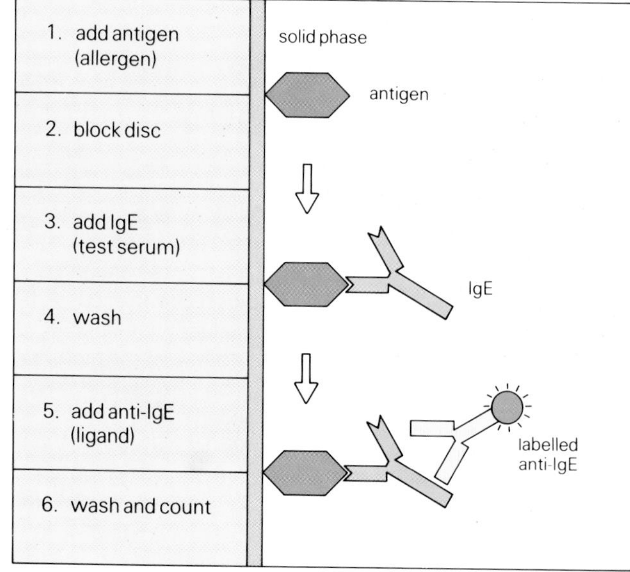

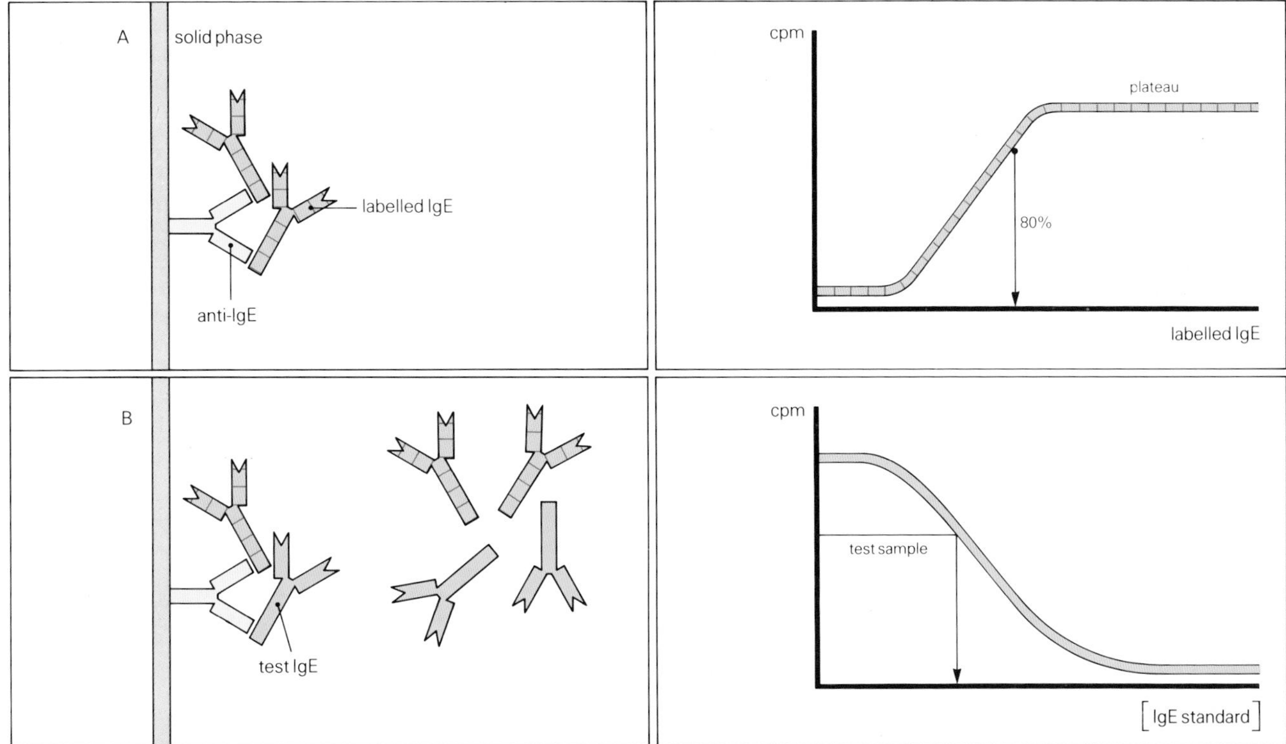

Fig. 25.13 The radioimmunosorbent test (RIST). This is a competition radioimmunoassay for total serum IgE. The plate is sensitized with anti-IgE and increasing amounts of labelled IgE are added to the plate to determine the maximum amount of IgE that the plate can bind (A). A quantity of labelled IgE equivalent to approximately 80% of the plateau binding is chosen. In the test experiments (B) this amount of labelled IgE is mixed with the serum containing the IgE to be tested The test IgE competes with the labelled IgE. Thus the more IgE present in the test serum the less the amount of labelled IgE that binds. This produces a standard curve of the type shown where dilutions of a serum containing a known IgE concentration are used. This type of test is widely used to measure hormone concentrations in serum.

Fig. 25.14 Immunoblotting. Antigen samples are separated in an analytical gel, for example an SDS polyacrylamide gel or an isoelectric focusing gel. The resolved molecules are transferred electrophoretically to a nitrocellulose membrane in a blotting tank. The blot is then treated sequentially with antibody to the specific antigen, and washed, and then a radiolabelled conjugate to detect antibodies is bound to the blot. The principle is similar to that of a radioimmunoassay or ELISA. After washing again, the blot is placed in contact with X-ray film in a cassette; the autoradiograph is developed and the antigen bands which have bound the antibody are visible. The technique can be modified for use with an enzyme coupled conjugate, and the bound material can be detected by treatment with a chromogen which deposits an insoluble reagent directly onto the blot.

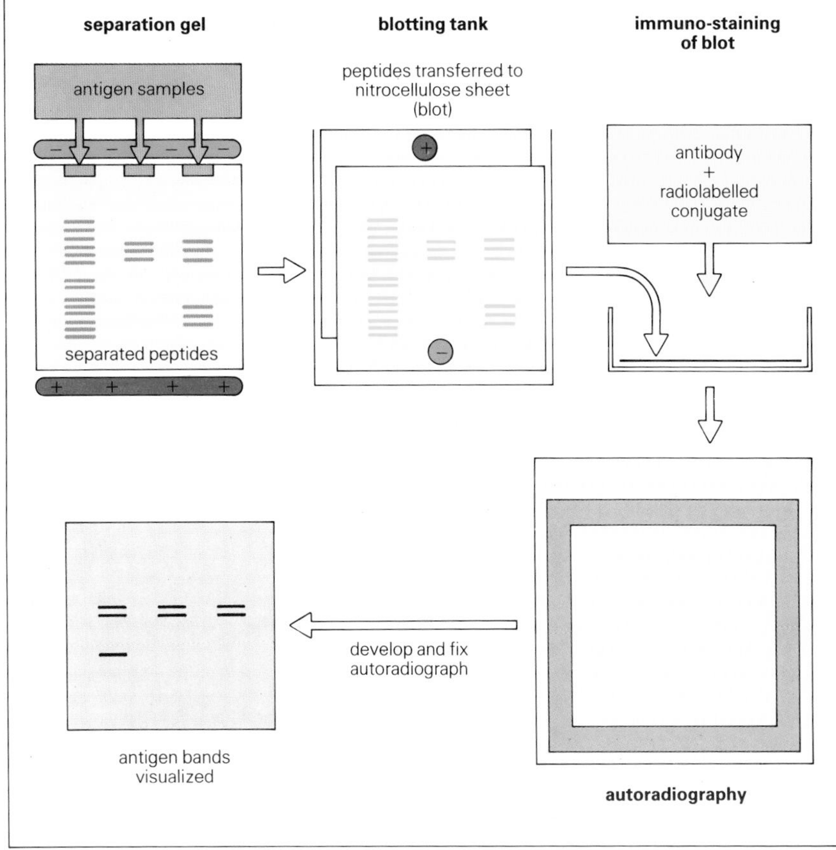

ISOLATION OF PURE ANTIBODIES

Immunologists often need to isolate pure antibodies, which may be either antigen-specific or non-specific immunoglobulin. Isolation of non-specific immunoglobulin from serum is usually carried out by sequential protein fractionation steps which may include:

1. precipitation of the gammaglobulins in 30 – 50% ammonium sulphate
2. gel filtration to obtain molecules of the correct size
3. ion exchange chromatography to isolate molecules which are positively charged at neutral pH
4. affinity chromatography on natural ligands for immunoglobulin, such as protein A (protein A is a component of staphylococcal cell walls which binds to a region in Cγ2 and Cγ3 of most IgG subclasses)

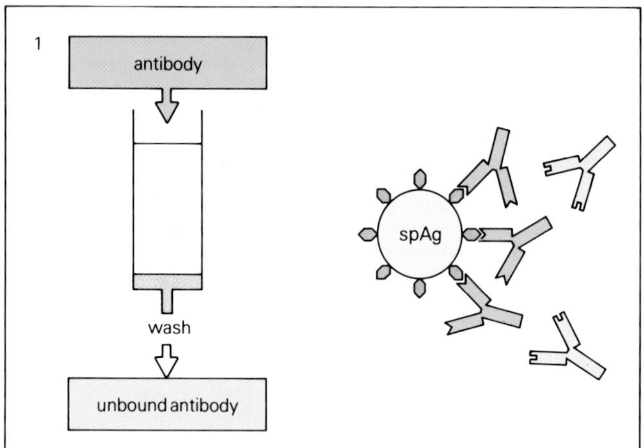

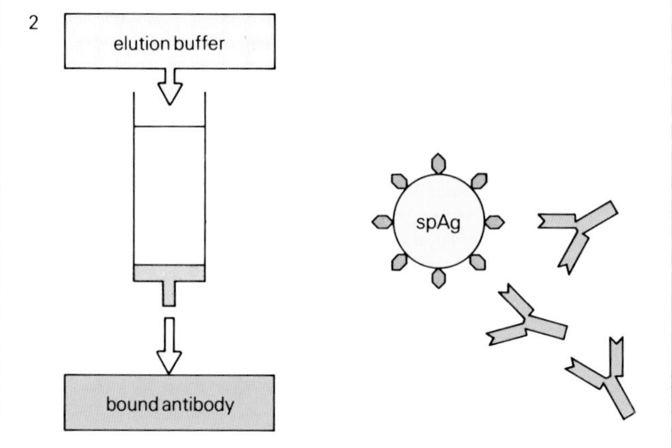

Fig. 25.15 Affinity chromatography. By using affinity chromatography a pure population of antibodies may be isolated. A solid phase immunoabsorbent is prepared (spAg); this is an antigen covalently coupled to an inert support (e.g. cross-linked dextran beads). The immunoabsorbent is placed in a column and the antibody mixture is run in under physiological conditions. Antibody to the antigen is bound to the column while unbound antibody washes through (1). In the second step the column is eluted to obtain the bound antibody using elution buffer (e.g. acetate pH 3.0, diethylamine pH 11.5, 3M guanidine, HCl), which dissociates the antigen–antibody bond (2). By placing antibody on the column the process can be reversed to obtain pure antigen. The technique can also be used to obtain other types of molecule. For example, a lectin column will absorb all molecules with particular sugar residues and these can be eluted in buffer containing the free sugar, which competes with the bound protein for the attachment site on the lectin.

Fig. 25.16 Monoclonal antibody production. Animals (usually mice or rats) are immunized with antigen. Once the animals are making a good antibody response the spleens are removed and a cell suspension prepared (lymph node cells may also be used). These cells are fused with a myeloma cell line by the addition of polyethylene glycol (PEG) which promotes membrane fusion. Only a small proportion of the cells fuse successfully. The fusion mixture is then set up in culture with medium containing 'HAT'. HAT is a mixture of Hypoxanthine, Aminopterin and Thymidine. Aminopterin is a powerful toxin which blocks a metabolic pathway. This pathway can be bypassed if the cell is provided with the intermediate metabolites hypoxanthine and thymidine. Thus spleen cells can grow in HAT medium, but the myeloma cells die in HAT medium because they have a metabolic defect and cannot use the bypass pathway. When the culture is set up in HAT medium it contains spleen cells, myeloma cells and fused cells. The spleen cells die in culture naturally after 1–2 weeks and the myeloma cells are killed by the HAT. Fused cells survive however as they have the immortality of the myeloma and the metabolic bypass of the spleen cells. Some of them will also have the antibody producing capacity of the spleen cells. Any wells containing growing cells are tested for the production of the desired antibody (often by RIA or ELISA) and if positive the cultures are cloned, that is, plated out so that only one cell is in each well. This produces a clone of cells derived from a single progenitor, which is both immortal and produces monoclonal antibody.

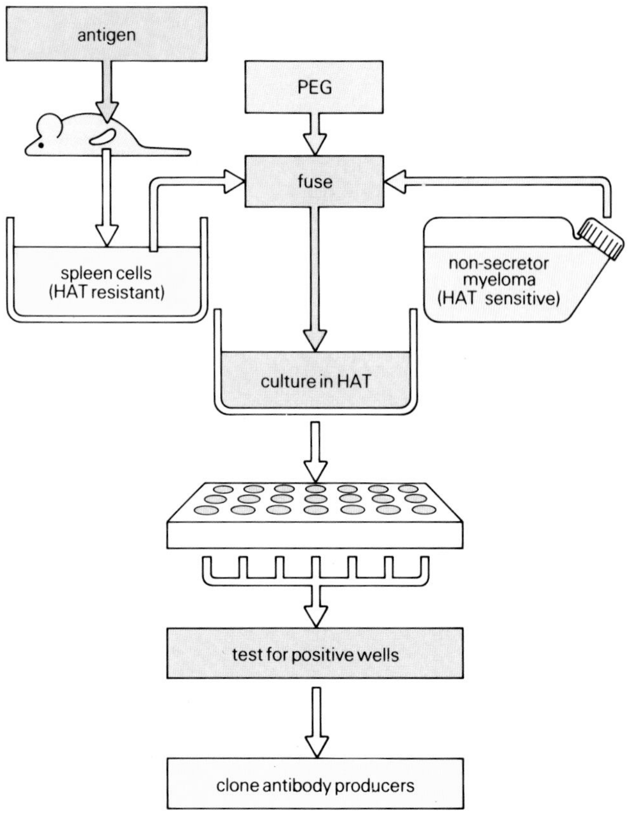

5. affinity chromatography using antigen coupled to Sepharose; pure antibody specific for the antigen is obtained by elution from the immunoadsorbent with chaotropic agents such as sodium thiocyanate, or glycine–HCL buffer, or diethylamine buffer.

Affinity chromatography is the technique used where the isolation of pure antibody or pure antigen is the objective (Fig. 25.15).

Another more recent way of obtaining pure antibody of a defined specificity is in the production of monoclonal antibodies. This technique involves the production of a cell which can manufacture a single antibody of defined specificity indefinitely, therefore obviating the vagaries of antiserum production (Fig. 25.16). The production of monoclonal antibodies has found widespread use in many biological sciences, where the antibody is used as a specific probe.

Since any particular B cell is effectively producing a monoclonal antibody, the requirement is to immortalize and propogate individual B cells. Most monoclonal antibodies are generated by the fusion of mouse splenocytes with a B cell tumour from the same strain which does not secrete its own antibody. It is possible to produce interstrain or even interspecies hybrids, however these are often unstable. An alternative method is to transform cells, and human B cells may be immortalized for monoclonal antibody production by infecting them with Epstein-Barr virus.

Although a monoclonal antibody is a well-defined reagent it does not have a greater specificity than a polyclonal antiserum which recognizes the antigen via a number of different epitopes.

ASSAYS FOR COMPLEMENT

The simplest measurement of complement activity is to determine the concentration of serum which will cause lysis of 50% of a standardized preparation of antibody-sensitized erythrocytes (EA). This is carried out in tubes or microwells. A simpler system, which provides a crude measure of complement activity is single radial haemolysis. The technique is similar to that of single radial immunodiffusion (Fig. 25.4) except that the wells contain the test serum and the gel contains EA. A zone of haemolysis develops around wells containing active complement, and the size of the zone is proportional to the amount of complement in the well. This technique measures the total activity of the classical and lytic pathways, but if a serum is deficient in complement activity it cannot identify which component is responsible.

Individual components may be measured separately to determine either their total level or their functional level. This is an important distinction, since a component may be present in normal quantities, but be functionally inactive. Total levels of individual components are usually measured by RIA or by ELISA using antibody specific for the component under investigation. Functional levels are measured in assays tailored to detect each individual component by providing a cocktail of sensitized red cells plus all the components required for lysis, except the one under investigation (Fig. 25.17). Again this can be performed in solution or by single radial haemolysis.

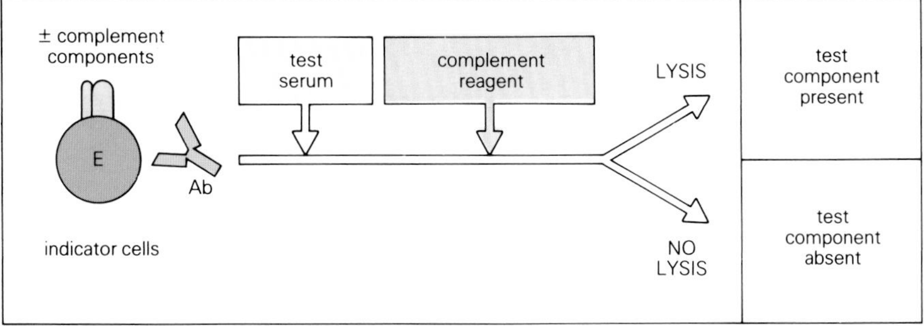

test	indicator cells	complement reagent
C1	EAC 4 (guinea-pig)	Cl reagent
C4	EA	C4 - deficient guinea-pig serum
C2	EAC4 (human) (antrypol)	C2 reagent
C3	EAC142 (guinea-pig)	C5-9 (NH_3 treated guinea-pig serum
C5	EAC14 oxy 23	C5 - deficient mouse serum
C6	EAC143 (human) (antrypol)	C6 - deficient rabbit serum
FB	EA + EGTA + Mg^{++}	B - deficient serum (50°C treated)
FD	EA + EGTA + Mg^{++}	D - deficient serum (Sephadex G75 exclusion peak)

Fig. 25.17 Assays for complement components. These assays detect specific complement components in a test serum. The principle of the assay is to mix sensitized red cells, with a 'complement reagent' so that the sensitized cells plus the reagent contain all the complement components needed to lyse the red cells except for the component being tested. For example to test for C4, erythrocytes sensitized with antibody (EA) are placed th C4-deficient guinea-pig serum. The cells will be lysed if there is C4 in the test serum, otherwise they will not. The table lists the combinations of reagents used for each test component. The red cells are prepared by blocking the reactions of EA with complement at a specific point. The complement reagents may be sera deficient in one component or sera treated physicochemically to remove or inactivate one component. In practice the assay would be performed quantitatively, for example, by single radial haemolysis, or in tubes to determine the point at which 50% of the red cells are lysed.

ISOLATION OF LYMPHOCYTE POPULATIONS

Many of the experiments performed by immunologists use populations of lymphocytes for either *in vivo* or *in vitro* work. The main sources of lymphocytes from experimental animals are the thymus, the spleen or the peripheral lymph nodes. Specialized studies may require isolation of cells from other areas such as Peyer's patches. Recirculating cells may be obtained by cannulating the thoracic duct and collecting the draining lymphocytes over a number of hours. In studies on humans, peripheral blood lymphocytes are the most readily available source of cells, but spleen tonsil or lymph nodes may become available following surgical resection. Problems can however arise with surgical material due to the presence of infectious agents or tumour cells, depending on the circumstances. It should be emphasized that the cell populations derived from each of these tissues is quite distinct, with respect to the maturational state of the lymphocytes and the proportions of different cell populations. The thymus is a source of fairly pure T cells but these are at varying stages of maturity. When working on lymphocytes from other sources, it is often desirable to separate the different cell populations so as to distinguish their effects.

Reference has already been made to the use of the fluorescence activated cell sorter (FACS) for the isolation of lymphocyte populations, based on their surface markers. The number of cells isolated is however limited by the flow-through rate of the sorter, since each cell is individually sorted. A number of bulk methods are also available for separating lymphocytes and the specific

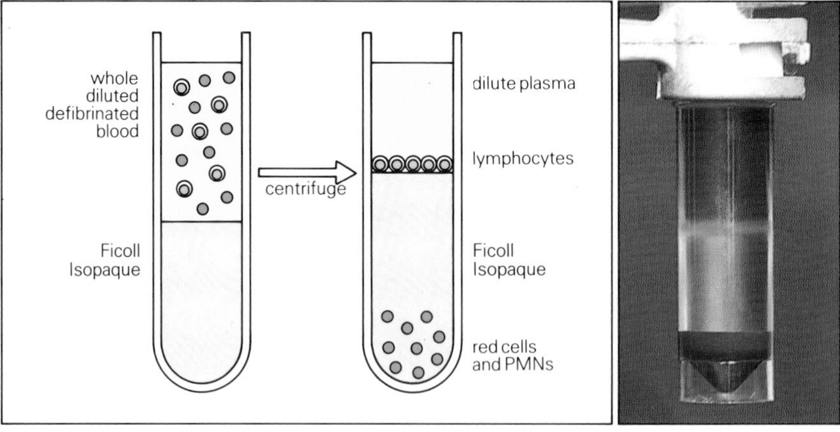

Fig. 25.18 Lymphocyte separation on Ficoll Isopaque. Whole blood is defibrinated by shaking with glass beads and the resulting clot removed. The blood is then diluted in tissue culture medium and layered on top of a tube half full of Ficoll. Ficoll has a density greater than that of lymphocytes but less than that of red cells and granulocytes (e.g. macrophages). After centrifugation the red cells and PMNs pass down through the Ficoll to form a pellet at the bottom of the tube while lymphocytes settle at the interface of the medium and Ficoll. The lymphocyte preparation can be further depleted of phagocytes by the addition of iron filings; these are taken up by the phagocytes which can then be drawn away with a strong magnet. Alternatively, macrophages can be removed by leaving the cell suspension to settle on a plastic dish. Macrophages adhere to plastic, whereas the lymphocytes can be washed off.

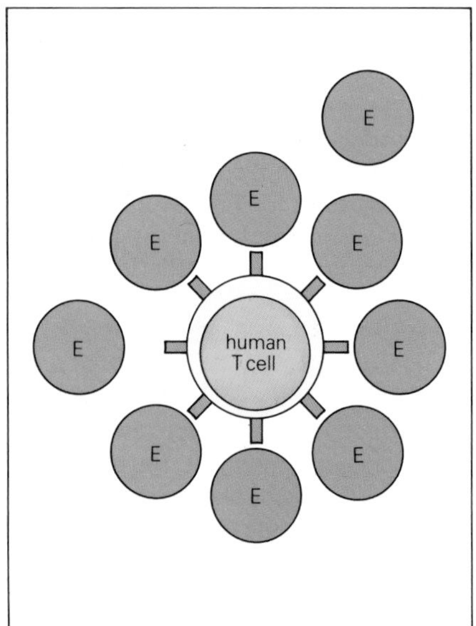

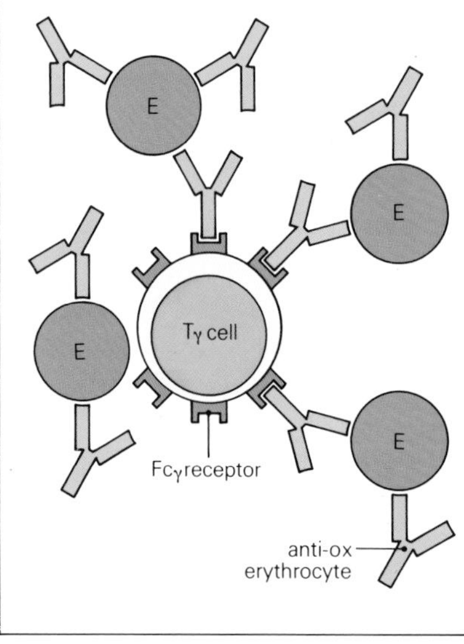

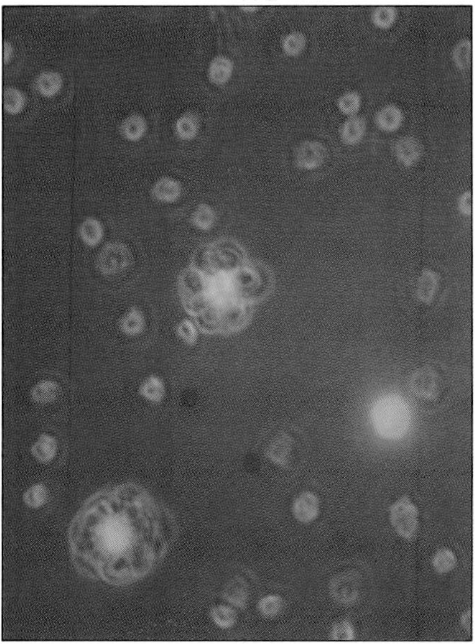

Fig. 25.19 Isolation of lymphocyte sub-populations – rosetting. Some lymphocytes have receptors for erythrocytes. Human T cells have receptors for sheep erythrocytes (E); these are CD2 molecules (left). They are not present on mouse T cells. When mixed together the T cells form rosettes with the erythrocytes and may be separated from non-rosetting B cells on Ficoll gradients. A modification of this technique to isolate cells with other receptors is also shown (middle). For example, some T cells have a receptor for the Fc of IgG (Fcγ). These cells may be identified and isolated by rosetting with ox erythrocytes sensitized with a subagglutinating amount of anti-ox erythrocyte. A rosetted lymphocyte is shown on the right. (Courtesy of Dr P. M. Lydyard.)

sub-populations. These include density gradient separation, rosetting and panning.

Density gradient separation relies on the differences in the density of lymphocytes compared with other cell populations (Fig. 25.18), and is used to isolate the majority of blood lymphocytes. Rosetting and panning (or plating) are used to isolate sub-populations (Figs 25.19 and 25.20). Lymphocyte panning is a type of affinity chromatography applied to lymphocytes. Another approach to the preparation of lymphocytes is the generation of antigen-specific lines of T cells, which may be propogated for an extended period (Fig. 25.21). This obviates the need for frequent isolation of primary cultures from animals.

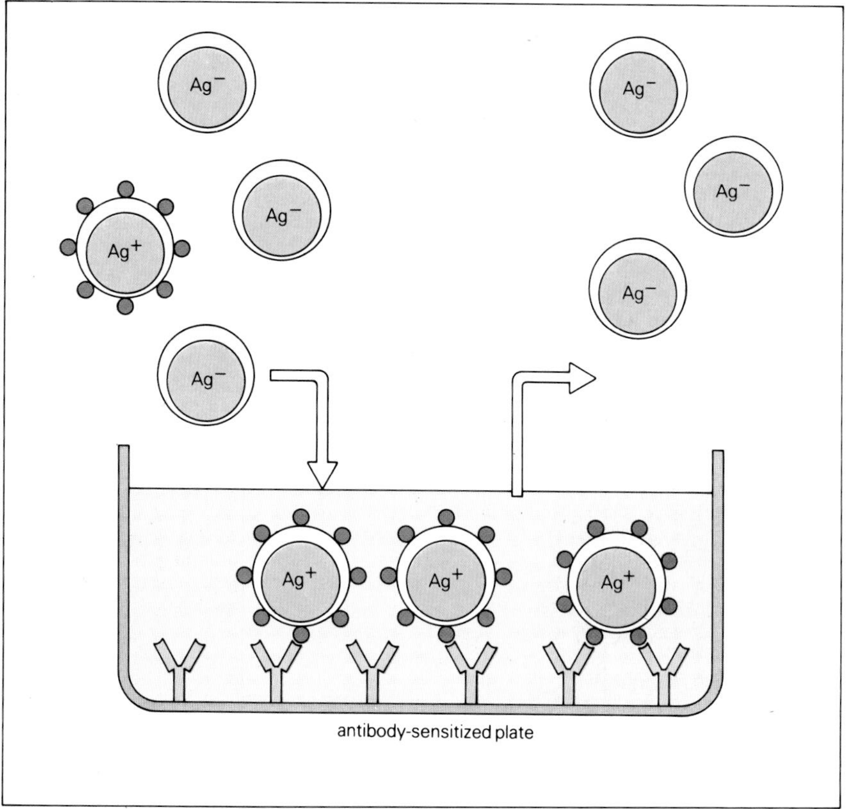

Fig. 25.20 Isolation of lymphocyte sub-populations – panning. Cell populations can be separated on antibody-sensitized plates. Antibody binds non-covalently to the plastic plate (as for RIA) and the cell mixture is applied to the plate. Antigen-positive cells (Ag^+) bind to the antibody and the antigen-negative cells (Ag^-) can be carefully washed off. By changing the culture conditions or by enzyme-digestion of the cells on the plate it is sometimes possible to recover the cells bound to the plate. Often the cells that have bound to the plate are altered by their binding, for example, binding to the plate cross-links the antigen which can cause cell activation. Thus, the method is most satisfactory for removing a cell population. Examples of the application of this method include separating T_H and T_S cell populations using antibodies to CD4 or CD8, and separating T cells from B cells using anti-Ig (which binds to the surface antibody of the B cell). By sensitizing the plate with antigen, antigen-binding cells can be separated from non-binding cells.

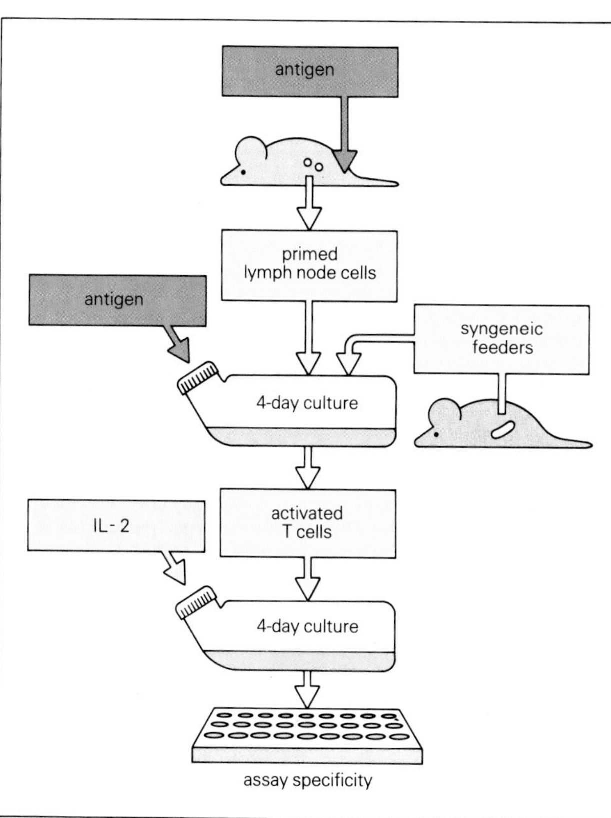

Fig. 25.21 T cell lines. The figure illustrates one protocol for the preparation of T cell lines, although many other protocols are used. Mice are primed with antigen (usually subcutaneously in the rear foot pad), and the draining lymph nodes (in this case the popliteal and inguinal) are removed 1 week later and set up in co-culture with syngeneic feeder cells (e.g. normal thymocytes or splenocytes) and antigen. After 4 days the lymphoblasts are isolated and induced to proliferate with interleukin-2 (IL-2). When the population of cells has expanded sufficiently they are checked for antigen and MHC specificity in a lymphocyte transformation test, and are maintained by alternate cycles of culture on antigen treated feeder cells and culture in IL-2 containing medium.

EFFECTOR CELL ASSAYS

The major lymphocyte effector functions include antibody production, cytotoxicity, and T cell-mediated help and suppression. Antibody-producing cells are measured by plaque forming cell assay (Fig. 25.22).

By modifying the plaque forming cell assay, it is possible to separately identify IgG and IgM producing cells specific for an antigen, as well as to identify the total number of antibody-producing cells (Fig. 25.23). It is also possible to identify antibody-producing cells by plating them onto an antigen-coated plate, which is then developed as for an ELISA but with the chromagen applied in an agar gel. The antibody-producing cells deposit antibody into their immediate vicinity onto the plates which is then visualized as a small dot of colour when the plate is developed (microdot assay).

Antigen-specific T cells are often detected by the lymphocyte stimulation test which detects their ability to respond to antigen by entering the cell cycle and incorporating precursors of DNA synthesis (Fig. 25.24). Cytotoxic T cells are usually detected by their ability to lyse target cells. Target cell lysis is determined in the chromium release assay (Fig. 25.25). Suppressor cell activity is often assessed by using the assays described above. For example, the action of suppressors may be

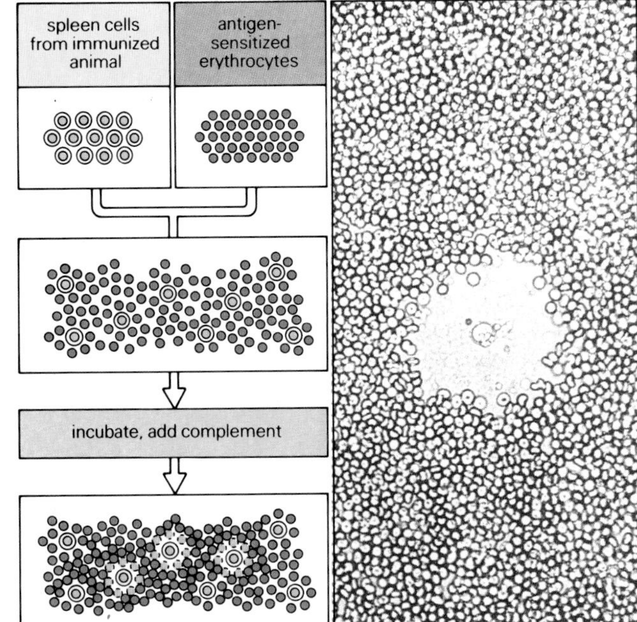

Fig. 25.22 Plaque forming cell assay – I. Antibody-forming cells are measured by mixing the test population with antigen sensitized red cells. Following incubation, the red cells surrounding the cells secreting specific antibody become coated with the antibody and may be lysed by complement.

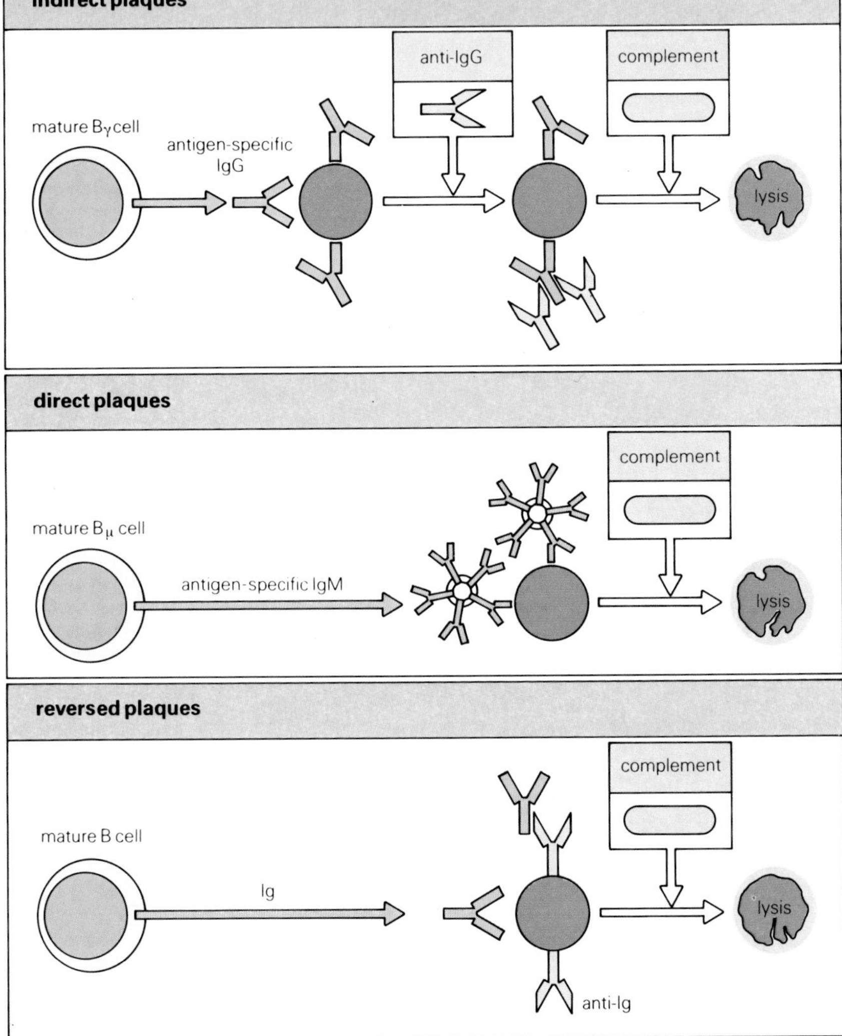

Fig. 25.23 Plaque forming cell assay – II. Plaque forming cell assays are used to detect antibody-forming cells. The assay may be performed in three different ways.

Indirect plaques. Cells producing antibody to a particular antigen release it, whence it diffuses and binds onto antigen on red cells. This may be red cell surface antigen, or the red cells may be sensitized with another antigen as in the haemagglutination assay. To detect the IgG antibodies bound to the red cells it is necessary to add anti-IgG antibody and then complement. Complexes formed on the cell fix complement and produce a zone of erythrocyte lysis around the B cell.

Direct plaques. Antigen-specific IgM antibodies are capable of causing complement-mediated lysis without the addition of an extra layer of anti-immunoglobulin. Thus the numbers of antigen-specific IgM and IgG plaque forming cells can be estimated separately.

Reversed plaques. The reversed plaque method measures total immunoglobulin-producing cells (not just antigen-specific cells). Released Ig binds onto red cells sensitized with anti-Ig. This complex can now fix complement and cause cell lysis. (Protein A, which binds IgG Fc regions, can be substituted for the anti-Ig on the red cells in this assay).

seen through their ability to reduce the number of plaque forming cells in a particular culture system.

Although this account is by no means exhaustive, the techniques described do form the basis of a great many experiments when used in combination, either together or sequentially. Furthermore, even complicated techniques found in research papers are frequently simple modifications of these basic systems.

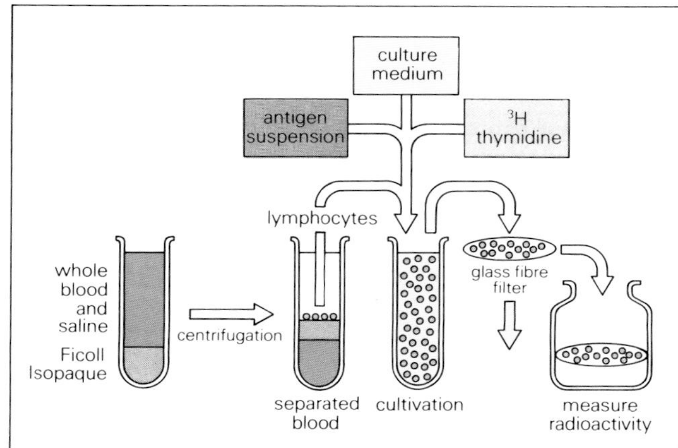

Fig. 25.24 The lymphocyte stimulation test. Whole blood in saline solution is layered on Ficoll Isopaque (which has a density between, and therefore separates, white cells and red cells) and centrifuged (400 × G). This separates the lymphocytes from the other cell and serum constituents. The cells are washed (to remove contaminants such as antigen) and then put into test tubes with a suspension of antigen and culture medium (cells from lymphoid tissues may also be used). Tritiated thymidine (^{3}H-thymidine) is added 16 hours before the cells are harvested. The cells are harvested on a glass fibre filter disc and their radioactivity is measured by placing the disc in a liquid scintillation counter. A high count indicates that the lymphocytes have undergone transformation and confirms their sensitivity to the antigen.

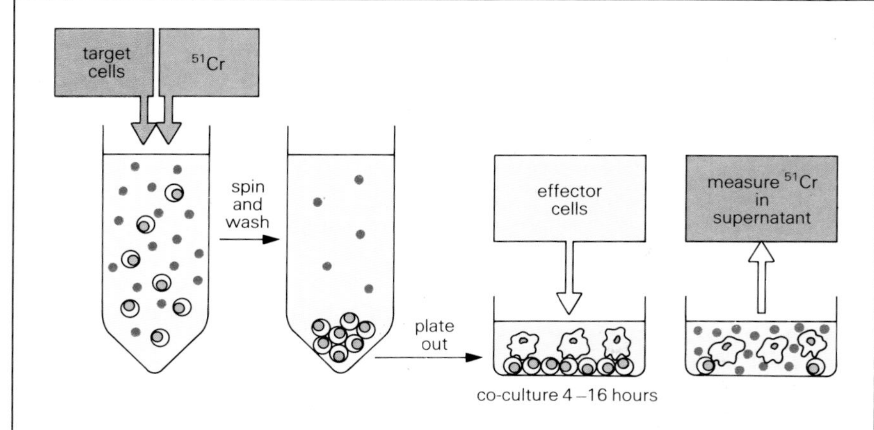

Fig. 25.25 Cytotoxicity assay by chromium release. Target cells are incubated with ^{51}Cr, which is taken up into the cells and binds to protein. After incubation the free ^{51}Cr is washed away and the target cells plated out. They are then co-cultured with the effector cells for 4–16 hours and the supernatant is removed and counted to detect chromium released from lysed target cells.

FURTHER READING

Hudson, L. & Hay, F.C. (1980) *Practical Immunology*. 2nd edition. Oxford: Blackwell Scientific Publications.

Johnstone, A. & Thorpe, R. (1987) *Immunochemistry in Practice*. 2nd edition. Oxford: Blackwell Scientific Publications.

Nairn, R.C. (ed.) (1980–1984) *Practical Methods in Clinical Immunology* Series. Edinburgh: Churchill Livingstone.

Weir, D.M. (1986) *Handbook of Experimental Immunology*. Vols I & II. 4th edition. Oxford: Blackwell Scientific Publications.

Glossary

Acute phase proteins. Serum proteins whose levels increase during infection or inflammatory reactions.

ADCC (antibody-dependent cell-mediated cytotoxicity). A cytotoxic reaction in which Fc receptor-bearing killer cells recognize target cells via specific antibodies.

Adjuvant. A substance that non-specifically enhances the immune response to an antigen.

AFCs (antibody-forming cells). Functionally equivalent to plasma cells.

Affinity. A measure of the binding strength between an antigenic determinant (epitope) and an antibody-combining site (paratope).

Affinity maturation. The increase in average antibody affinity frequently seen during a secondary immune response.

Agretope. The portion of an antigen or antigen fragment which interacts with an MHC molecule.

Allele. Intraspecies variance at a particular gene locus.

Allergy. Originally defined as altered reactivity on second contact with antigen; now usually refers to a Type I hypersensitivity reaction.

Allogeneic. Refers to intraspecies genetic variations.

Allotype. The protein product of an allele which may be detectable as an antigen by another member of the same species.

Altered self. The concept that the combination of antigen and a self MHC molecule interacts with the immune system in the same way as an allogeneic MHC molecule.

Alternative pathway. The activation pathways of the complement system involving C3 and factors B, D, P, H and I, which interact in the vicinity of an activator surface to form an alternative pathway C3 convertase.

Amplification loop. The alternative complement activation pathway, which acts as a positive feedback loop when C3 is split in the presence of an activator surface.

Anaphylatoxins. Complement peptides (C3a and C5a) which cause mast cell degranulation and smooth muscle contraction.

Anaphylaxis. An antigen-specific immune reaction mediated primarily by IgE which results in vasodilation and constriction of smooth muscles, including those of the bronchus, and which may result in death of the animal.

Antibody. A molecule produced by animals in response to antigen which has the particular property of combining specifically with the antigen which induced its formation.

Antigen. A molecule which induces the formation of antibody.

Antigen presentation. The process by which certain cells in the body (antigen-presenting cells) express antigen on their cell surface in a form recognizable by lymphocytes.

Antigen processing. The conversion of an antigen into a form in which it can be recognized by lymphocytes.

APCs (antigen-presenting cells). A variety of cell types which carry antigen in a form that can stimulate lymphocytes.

Atopy. The clinical manifestation of Type I hypersensitivity reactions including eczema, asthma and rhinitis.

Autologous. Part of the same individual.

Autosomes. Chromosomes other than the X or Y sex chromosomes.

Avidity. The functional combining strength of an antibody with its antigen which is related to both the affinity of the reaction between the epitopes and paratopes, and the valencies of the antibody and antigen.

β_2-microglobulin. A polypeptide which constitutes part of some membrane proteins including the Class I MHC molecules.

BCG (Bacille Calmette Guérin). An attenuated strain of *Mycobacterium tuberculosis* used as a vaccine, an adjuvant or a biological response modifier in different circumstances.

Biozzi mice. Lines of mice selectively bred to produce low or high antibody responses to a variety of antigens (originally sheep erythrocytes).

Bradykinin. A vasoactive nonapeptide which is the most important mediator generated by the kinin system.

BSFs (B cell stimulating factors). A group of compounds required for B cell maturation and proliferation. Several of these factors have been given interleukin designations.

Bursa of Fabricius. A lymphoepithelial organ found at the junction of the hind gut and cloaca in birds which is the site of B cell maturation.

Bystander lysis. Complement-mediated lysis of cells in the immediate vicinity of a complement activation site, which are not themselves responsible for the activation.

C domains. The constant domains of antibody and the T cell receptor. These domains do not contribute to the antigen-binding site and show relatively little variability between receptor molecules.

C genes. The gene segments which encode the constant portion of the immunoglobulin heavy and light chains and the α, β, γ and δ chains of the T cell antigen receptor.

C1–C9. The components of the complement classical and lytic pathways which are responsible for mediating inflammaory reactions, opsonization of particles and lysis of cell membranes.

Capping. A process by which cell surface molecules are caused to aggregate (usually using antibody) on the cell membrane.

Carrier. An immunogenic molecule, or part of a molecule, that is recognized by T cells in an antibody response.

CD markers. Cell surface molecules of leucocytes and platelets that are distinguishable with monoclonal antibodies and may be used to differentiate different cell populations.

CDRs (complementarity determining regions). The sections of an antibody or T cell receptor V region responsible for antigen or antigen–MHC binding.

Cell cycle. The process of cell division which is divisible into four phases: G1, S, G2 and M. DNA replicates during the S phase and the cell divides in the M (mitotic) phase.

Chemokinesis. Increased random migratory activity of cells.

Chemotaxis. Increased directional migration of cells particularly in response to concentration gradients of certain chemotactic factors.

Chimaerism. The situation in which cells from genetically different individuals coexist in one body.

Class I/II/III MHC molecules. Three major classes of molecule coded within the MHC. Class I molecules have one MHC encoded peptide associated with β_2-microglobulin. Class II molecules have two MHC encoded peptides which are non-covalently associated, and Class III molecules are other molecules including complement components.

Class I/II restriction. The observation that immunologically active cells will only cooperate effectively when they share MHC haplotypes at either the class I or class II loci.

Classical pathway. The pathway by which antigen–antibody complexes can activate the complement system, involving components C1, C2 and C4, and generating a classical pathway C3 convertase.

Class switching. The process by which an individual B cell can link new immunoglobulin heavy chain C genes to its recombined V gene to produce a different class of antibody with the same specificity. This process is also reflected in the overall class switch seen during the maturation of an immune response.

Clonal selection. The fundamental basis of lymphocyte activation in which antigen selectively stimulates only those cells which express receptors for it to divide and differentiate.

Clone. A family of cells or organisms having a genetically identical constitution.

CMI (cell-mediated immunity). A term used to refer to immune reactions that are mediated by cells rather than by antibody or other humoral factors.

Cobra venom factor. A cobra complement component equivalent to mammalian C3b.

Complement. A group of serum proteins involved in the control of inflammation, the activation of phagocytes and the lytic attack on cell membranes. The system can be activated by interaction with the immune system.

ConA (concanavalin A). A mitogen for T cells.

Congenic. Animals which are genetically constructed to differ at one particular locus.

Conjugate. A reagent which is formed by covalently coupling two molecules together such as fluorescein coupled to an immunogloblin molecule.

Contrasuppression. The action of a group of T cells which renders T-helper cells resistant to action of T- suppressors.

Constant regions. The relatively invariant parts of immunoglobulin heavy and light chains, and the α, β, γ and δ chains of the T cell receptor.

CR1, CR2, CR3. Receptors for activated C3 fragments.

CSFs (colony stimulating factors). A group of cytokines which control the differentiation of haemopoietic stem cells.

Cyclophosphamide. A cytotoxic drug frequently used as an immunosuppressive.

Cyclosporin. An immunosuppresive drug that is particularly useful in suppression of graft rejection.

Cytokines. A generic term for soluble molecules which mediate interactions between cells.

Cytophilic. Having a propensity to bind to cells.

Cytostatic. Having the ability to stop cell growth.

Cytotoxic. Having the ability to kill cells.

D genes. Sets of gene segments lying between the V and J genes in the immunoglobulin heavy chain genes, and in the T cell receptor β and δ chain genes which are recombined with V and J genes during ontogeny.

Degranulation. Exocytosis of granules from cells such as mast cells and basophils.

Dendritic cells. A set of antigen-presenting cells present in lymph nodes, spleen and at low levels in blood, which are particularly active in stimulating T cells.

Desetope. The part of an MHC molecule which links to antigen or processed antigen.

DTH (delayed type hypersensitivity). This term includes the delayed skin reactions associated with Type IV hypersensitivity.

DNP (dinitrophenol). A commonly used hapten.

Domain. A region of a peptide having a coherent tertiary structure. Both immunoglobulins and MHC Class I and Class II molecules have domains.

Dominant idiotypes. Individual idiotypes which are present on a large proportion of the antibodies generated to a particular antigen.

dsDNA. Double-stranded DNA.

Epstein–Barr virus (EBV). Causal agent of Burkitt's lymphoma and infectious mononucleosis, which has the ability to transform human B cells into stable cell lines.

Effector cells. A functional concept which in context means those lymphocytes or phagocytes which produce the end effect.

Endogenous. Originating within the organism.

Endothelium. Cells lining blood vessels and lymphatics.

Enhancement. Prolongation of graft survival by treatment with antibodies directed towards the graft alloantigens.

Epitope. A single antigenic determinant. Functionally it is the portion of an antigen which combines with the antibody paratope.

Exon. Gene segment encoding protein.

Fab. The part of an antibody molecule which contains the antigen combining site, consisting of a light chain and part of the heavy chain; it is produced by enzymatic digestion.

Factors B, P, D, H and I. Components of the alternative complement pathway.

Fc. The portion of an antibody that is responsible for binding to antibody receptors on cells and the C1q component of complement.

Framework segments. Sections of antibody V regions which lie between the hypervariable regions.

Freund's adjuvant. An emulsion of aqueous antigen in oil. Complete Freund's adjuvant also contains killed *Mycobacterium tuberculosis*, while incomplete Freund's adjuvant does not.

GALT (gut-associated lymphoid tissue). Refers to the accumulations of lymphoid tissue associated with the gastrointestinal tract.

Genetic association. A term used to describe the condition where particular genotypes are associated with other phenomena, such as particular diseases.

Genetic restriction. The term used to be describe the observation that lymphocytes and antigen-presenting cells cooperate most effectively when they share particular haplotypes.

Genome. The total genetic material contained within the cell.

Genotype. The genetic material inherited from parents; not all of it is necessarily expressed in the individual.

Germ line. The genetic material which is passed down through the gametes before it is modified by somatic recombination or mutation.

Giant cells. Large multinucleated cells sometimes seen in granulomatous reactions and thought to result from the fusion of macrophages.

GVH (graft versus host) disease. A condition cuased by allogeneic donor lymphocytes reacting against host tissue in an immunologically compromised recipient.

H-2. The mouse major histocompatibility complex.

Haplotype. A set of genetic determinants located on a single chromosome.

Hapten. A small molecule which can act as an epitope but is incapable by itself of eliciting an antibody response.

Helper (T_H) cells. A functional subclass of T cells which can help to generate cytotoxic T cells and cooperate with B cells in production of antibody response. Helper cells recognize antigen in association with class II MHC molecules.

Heterologous. Refers to interspecies antigenic differences.

HEV (high endothelial venule). An area of venule from which lymphocytes migrate into lymph nodes.

Hinge. The portion of an immunoglobulin heavy chain between the Fc and Fab regions, which permits flexibility within the molecule and allows the two combining sites to operate independently. The hinge region is usually encoded by a separate exon.

Histamine. A major vasoactive amine released from mast cell and basophil granules.

Histocompatibility. The ability to accept grafts between individuals.

HLA. The human major histocompatibility complex.

Homologous. The same species.

hnRNA (heteronuclear RNA). The fraction of nuclear RNA which contains primary transcripts of the DNA prior to processing to form messenger RNA.

Humoral. Pertaining to the extracellular fluids, including the serum and lymph.

Hybridoma. Cell lines created *in vitro* by fusing two different cell types, usually lymphocytes, one of which is a tumour cell.

5-hydroxytryptamine (5-HT). A vasoactive amine present in platelets and a major mediator of inflammation in rodents.

Hypervariable region. The most variable areas (3) of the V domains of immunoglobulin and T cell receptor chains. These regions are clustered at the distal portion of the V domain and contribute to the antigen-binding site.

ICAM-1 (intercellular adhesion molecule-1). Cell surface molecule found on a variety of leucocytes and non-haematogenous cells which interacts with LFA-1 and is involved in cell traffic.

Idiotope. A single antigenic determinant on an antibody V region.

Idiotype. The antigenic characteristic of the V region of an antibody.

Immune complex. The product of an antigen–antibody reaction which may also contain components of the complement system.

Immunofluorescence. A technique used to identify particular antigens microscopically in tissues or on cells by the binding of a fluorescent antibody conjugate.

Interferons (IFNs). A group of mediators which increase the resistance of cells to viral infection, and act as cytokines. IFNγ is also an important immunological mediator.

Interleukins (IL-1–IL-7). A group of molecules involved in signalling between cells of the immune system.

Intron. Gene segment between exons not encoding protein.

Ir gene. A group of immune response (Ir) genes determine the level of an immune response to a particular antigen or foreign stimulus. A number of them are found in the major histocompatibility complex.

Isoelectric focusing. Separation of molecules on the basis of charge. Each molecule will migrate to the point in a pH gradient where it has no net charge.

Isologous. Of identical genetic constitution.

Isotype. Refers to genetic variation within a family of proteins or peptides such that every member of the species will have each isotype of the family represented in its genome (e.g. immunoglobulin classes).

J chain. A monomorphic polypeptide present in, and required for the polymerization of polymeric IgA and IgM.

J genes. Sets of gene segments in the immunoglobulin heavy and light chain genes and in the genes for the chains of the T cell receptor, which are recombined during lymphocyte ontogeny and contribute towards the genes for variable domains.

K cell. A group of lymphocytes which are able to destroy their targets by antibody-dependent cell-mediated cytotoxicity. They have Fc receptors.

κ chains. One of the immunoglobulin light chain isotypes.

Karyotype. The chromosomal constitution of a cell which may vary between individuals of a single species, depending on the presence or absence of particular sex chromosomes or on the incidence of translocations between sections of different chromosomes.

Kinins. A group of vasoactive mediators produced following tissue injury.

Kupffer cells. Phagocytic cells which line the liver sinusoids.

λ chains. One of the immunoglobulin light chain isotypes.

Langerhans' cells. Antigen-presenting cells of the skin which emigrate to local lymph nodes to become dendritic cells; they are very active in presenting antigen to T cells.

Large granular lymphocytes (LGLs). A group of morphologically defined lymphocytes containing the majority of K cell and NK cell activity. They have both lymphocyte and monocyte/macrophage markers.

Leukotrienes. A collection of metabolites of arachidonic acid which have powerful pharmacological effects.

LFAs (leucocyte functional antigens). A group of three molecules which mediate intercellular adhesion between leucocytes and other cells in an antigen non-specific fashion.

Ligand. A linking (or binding) molecule.

Line. A collection of cells produced by continuously growing a particular cell culture *in vitro*. Such cell lines will usually contain a number of individual clones.

Linkage. The condition where two genes are both present in close proximity on a single chromosome and are usually inherited together.

Linkage disequilibrium. A condition where two genes are found together in a population at a greater frequency than that predicted simply by the product of their individual gene frequencies.

Locus. The position on a chromosome at which a particular gene is found.

LPR (lymphoproliferation gene). A gene found in MRL mice which is involved in the generation of autoimmune phenomena.

LPS (lipopolysaccharide). A product of some Gram-negative bacterial cell walls which can act as a B cell mitogen.

Lymphokines. A generic term for molecules other than antibodies which are involved in signalling between cells of the immune system and are produced by lymphocytes (cf. interleukins).

Ly antigens. A group of cell surface markers found on murine T cells which permit the differentiation of T cell subpopulations.

Lytic pathway. The complement pathway effected by components C5–C9 that is responsible for lysis of sensitized cell plasma membranes.

MALT (mucosa-associated lymphoid tissue). Generic term for lymphoid tissue associated with the gastrointestinal tract, bronchial tree and other mucosa.

Membrane attack complex (MAC). The assembled terminal complement components C5b–C9 of the lytic pathway which becomes inserted into cell membranes.

MHC (major histocompatibility complex). A genetic region found in all mammals whose products are primarily responsible for the rapid rejection of grafts between individuals, and function in signalling between lymphocytes and cells expressing antigen.

MHC restriction. A characteristic of many immune reactions in which cells cooperate most effectively with other cells sharing an MHC haplotype.

β_2-microglobulin. A monomorphic polypeptide encoded outside the MHC that is non-covalently associated with the MHC-encoded polypeptides of class I molecules.

MIF (migration inhibition factor). A group of peptides produced by lymphocytes which are capable of inhibiting macrophage migration.

MLR/MLC (mixed lymphocyte reaction/mixed lymphocyte culture). Assay system for T cell recognition of allogeneic cells in which response is measured by proliferation in the presence of the stimulating cells.

Mitogens. Substances which cause cells, particularly lymphocytes, to undergo cell division.

Monoclonal. Derived from a single clone, for example, monoclonal antibodies, which are produced by a single clone and are homogenous.

Myeloma. A lymphoma produced from cells of the B cell lineage.

Neoplasm. A synonym for cancerous tissue.

Network theory. A proposal first put forward by Jerne and since developed which states that T cells and B cells mutually inter-regulate by recognizing idiotopes on their antigen receptors.

NIP (4-hydroxy, 5–iodo, 3-nitrophenylacetyl). A commonly used hapten.

NK (natural killer) cells. A group of lymphocytes which have the intrinsic ability to recognize and destroy some virally infected cells and some tumour cells.

NP (4-hydroxy, 3-nitrophenylacetyl). A hapten which partially cross-reacts with NIP.

Nude mouse. A genetically athymic mouse which also carries a closely linked gene producing a defect in hair production.

NZB/W. A strain of mouse which is a model for systemic lupus erythematosus. The parental NZB strain also suffers from autoimmunity.

OKT. A group of monoconal antibodies used to identify T cell surface markers in humans.

Opsonization. A process by which phagocytosis is facilitated by the deposition of opsonins (e.g. antibody and C3b) on the antigen.

PAF (platelet activating factor). A factor released by basophils which causes platelets to aggregate.

PALS (periarteriolar lymphatic sheath). The accumulations of lymphoid tissue constituting the white pulp of the spleen.

Paratope. The part of an antibody molecule which makes contact with the antigenic determinant (epitope).

Pathogen. An organism which causes disease.

PC (phosphorylcholine). A commonly used hapten which is also found on the surface of a number of microorganisms.

PCA (passive cutaneous anaphylaxis). The technique used to detect antigen-specific IgE, in which the test animal is injected intravenously with the antigen and dye, the skin having previously been sensitized with antibody.

PFC (plaque forming cell). An antibody producing cell detected *in vitro* by its ability to lyse antigen-sensitized erythrocytes in the presence of complement.

PHA (phytohaemagglutinin). A mitogen for T cells.

Phagocytosis. The process by which cells engulf material and enclose it within a vacuole (phagosome) in the cytoplasm.

Phenotype. The expressed characteristics of an individual (cf. genotype).

Pinocytosis. The process by which liquids or very small particles are taken into the cell.

Plasma cell. An antibody producing B cell which has reached the end of its differentiation pathway.

Pokeweed mitogen. A mitogen for B cells.

Polyclonal. A term which describes the products of a number of different cell types (cf. monoclonal).

Primary lymphoid tissues. Lymphoid organs in which lymphocytes complete their initial maturation steps; they include the fetal liver, adult bone marrow and thymus, and the bursa of Fabricius in birds.

Primary response. The immune response (cellular or humoral) following an initial encounter with a particular antigen.

Prime. To give an initial sensitization to antigen.

Prostaglandins. Pharmacologically active derivatives of arachidonic acid. Different prostaglandins are capable of modulating cell mobility and immune responses.

Pseudoalleles. Tandem variants of a gene: they do not occupy a homologous position on the chromosome (e.g. C4).

Pseudogenes. Genes which have homologous structures to other genes but which are incapable of being expressed (e.g. $J_\kappa 3$ in the mouse).

Radioimmunoassay (RIA). A number of different, sensitive techniques for measuring antigen or antibody titres, using radiolabelled reagents.

Receptor. A cell surface molecule which binds specifically to particular proteins or peptides in the fluid phase.

Recombination. A process by which genetic information is rearranged during meiosis. This process also occurs during the somatic rearrangements of DNA which occur in the formation of genes encoding antibody molecules and T cell antigen receptors.

Recurrent idiotype. An idiotype present in the immune response of different animals or strains to a particular antigen.

Respiratory burst. Increase in oxidative metabolism of phagocytes following uptake of opsonized particles.

Reticuloendothelial system. A diffuse system of phagocytic cells derived from the bone marrow stem cell which are associated with the connective tissue framework of the liver, spleen, lymph nodes and other serous cavities.

Rosetting. A technique for identifying or isolating cells by mixing them with particles or cells to which they bind (e.g. sheep erythrocytes to human T cells). The rosettes consist of a central cell surrounded by bound cells.

Secondary response. The immune response which follows a second or subsequent encounter with a particular antigen.

Secretory component. A polypeptide produced by cells of some secretory epithelia which is involved in transporting secreted polymeric IgA across the cell and protecting it from digestion in the gastrointestinal tract.

SLE (systemic lupus erythematosus). An autoimmune disease of humans usually involving anti-nuclear antibodies.

Somatic mutation. A process occurring during B cell maturation and affecting the antibody gene region, which permits refinement of antibody specificity.

Suppressor (Ts) cell. A subpopulation of T cells which act to reduce the immune responses of other T cells or B cells. Suppression may be antigen-specific, idiotype-specific, or non-specific in different circumstances.

Synergism. Cooperative interaction.

Syngeneic. Strains of animals produced by repeated inbreeding so that each pair of autosomes within an individual is identical.

T15. An idiotype associated with anti-phosphorylcholine antibodies, named after the TEPC15 myeloma prototype sequence.

Tandem duplicates. Adjacent copies of related genes linked together on a chromosome.

TCR T cell receptor. The T cell antigen receptor consisting of either an α/β dimer (TCR2) or a γ/δ dimer (TCR1) associated with the CD3 molecular complex.

T-dependent/T-independent antigens. T-dependent antigens require immune recognition by both T and B cells to produce an immune response. T-independent antigens can directly stimulate B cells to produce specific antibody.

Thy. A cell surface antigen of mouse T cells which has allotypic variants.

TNF (tumour necrosis factor). A cytokine released by activated macrophages that is structurally related to lymphotoxin released by activated T cells.

Tolerance. A state of specific immunological unresponsiveness.

Transformation. Morphological changes in a lymphocyte associated with the onset of division. Also used to denote the change to the autonomously dividing state of a cancer cell.

V domains. The *N*-terminal domains of antibody heavy and light chains and the α, β, γ and δ chains of the T cell receptor which vary between different clones and form the antigen-binding site.

V genes. Sets of genes which encode the major part of the V domains of antibody heavy and light chains and the α, β, γ and δ chains of the T cell receptor, and become recombined with appropriate sets of D and J genes during lymphocyte ontogeny.

Vasoactive amines. Products such as histamine and 5–hydroxytryptamine released by basophils, mast cells and platelets which act on the endothelium and smooth muscle of the local vasculature.

White pulp. The lymphoid component of spleen, consisting of periarteriolar sheaths of lymphocytes and antigen-presenting cells.

Xenogeneic. Referring to interspecies antigenic differences (cf. heterologous).

Index

B

C

D

E

I

J

K

L

M

N

U

V

W

X

Z